ESSENTIALS OF BODY MRI

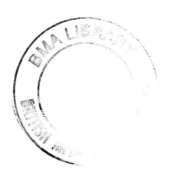

ESSENTIALS OF BODY MRI

William E. Brant, MD, FACR

PROFESSOR OF RADIOLOGY

DIRECTOR, THORACOABDOMINAL IMAGING DIVISION

DEPARTMENT OF RADIOLOGY AND MEDICAL IMAGING

UNIVERSITY OF VIRGINIA

CHARLOTTESVILLE, VIRGINIA

Eduard E. de Lange, MD

PROFESSOR OF RADIOLOGY

DIRECTOR, BODY MRI

DEPARTMENT OF RADIOLOGY AND MEDICAL IMAGING

UNIVERSITY OF VIRGINIA

CHARLOTTESVILLE, VIRGINIA

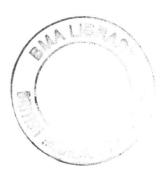

OXFORD
UNIVERSITY PRESS

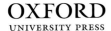

Oxford University Press, Inc., publishes works that further
Oxford University's objective of excellence
in research, scholarship, and education.

Oxford New York
Auckland   Cape Town   Dar es Salaam   Hong Kong   Karachi
Kuala Lumpur   Madrid   Melbourne   Mexico City   Nairobi
New Delhi   Shanghai   Taipei   Toronto

With offices in
Argentina   Austria   Brazil   Chile   Czech Republic   France   Greece
Guatemala   Hungary   Italy   Japan   Poland   Portugal   Singapore
South Korea   Switzerland   Thailand   Turkey   Ukraine   Vietnam

Published by Oxford University Press, Inc.
198 Madison Avenue, New York, New York 10016
www.oup.com

Library of Congress Cataloging-in-Publication Data

Essentials of body MRI / [edited by] William E. Brant, Eduard E. de Lange.
p. ; cm.
Includes bibliographical references and index.
ISBN 978-0-19-973849-6
I. Brant, William E. II. De Lange, Eduard E.
[DNLM: 1. Magnetic Resonance Imaging. WN 185]

616.07548—dc23
2011039714

987654321

Printed in China
on acid-free paper

We dedicate this book in memory of our friend, mentor and colleague, Dr. Theodore E. Keats, who served as Professor of Radiology for 47 years at the University of Virginia Health Sciences Center, and was the department's chairman for 29 years. He was a visionary and pioneer in promoting new imaging technologies, including MRI, and a great inspiration to all who worked with him and observed his exemplary dedication to teaching. This text can be viewed, in part, as a reflection of Dr. Keats's inspiration for the mission of teaching radiology.

William E. Brant, MD
Eduard E. de Lange, MD

To my daughter, Rachel, who brings tremendous joy, graciousness, strength, and humor to our lives, and to my wife, Barbara, whose patience and support grants me many hours working at my desk.
W.E.B.

To Cesca, Mabet, and Sacha
E.E.d.L.

PREFACE

Magnetic resonance imaging (MRI) has finally found its place as an invaluable diagnostic tool for the primary diagnosis and problem solving of diseases of the body, including the abdomen, pelvis, heart, and great vessels. Reasons for the slow implementation of the modality for routine use in body imaging was that the acquisition of data was relatively slow making it difficult for the patients to undergo the examination, and images were often nondiagnostic because of artifacts from breathing, the moving bowel, and the beating heart. The continuing improvement of the MR scanner hardware and the development of fast pulse sequences that allow acquisition of high-quality, motion-artifact-free images within a breath hold have made the modality as important a tool for imaging the body as it has been for imaging the brain and musculoskeletal system. Many radiology residency training programs now have dedicated rotations devoted entirely to body MRI. This creates the need for a text that introduces the resident, fellow, or medical student to the intricacies of the modality and allows for a quick understanding of the essential points in this difficult field.

To fully understand body MRI and comprehend the workings of specific pulse sequences that allow for rapid acquisition of high-quality, motion-artifact-free images within a breath hold, an understanding of MR physics is essential. Although there are many available texts and reviews describing MR physics, these are often written at a level of complexity that escapes the beginning student radiologist. Further, most texts provide broad coverage of the field but do not primarily focus on the specific issues related to body MRI. We felt, therefore, that a description of the physics, pulse sequences, and other practical considerations specifically related to body MRI is necessary to help the reader fully understand the imaging appearance of clinical disease. This text is provided in the first two chapters. When writing these, we strove to simplify the topics to a level that is easily understandable to the neophyte as well as to the practicing radiologist who has limited experience in this area. In the nine other chapters the clinical applications of body MRI are discussed with respect to the appearance of normal anatomic structures; the diagnosis of diseases of the abdomen, pelvis, heart, and great vessels; and the role of the modality in solving diagnostic problems. We tried to keep the discussions short and concise while allowing for a maximum number of figures to illustrate each subject.

To facilitate the learning process, the key points of each topic are emphasized as "Essentials to Remember," highlighted in separate, boxed sections throughout the text. We feel that these "Essentials" will greatly aid the reader in comprehending the material and understanding the important points. This text reflects the practice of body MRI at the University of Virginia. All authors are, or have been, associated with our institution. The format of the chapters and the discussed topics are based on years of teaching our residents, fellows, and medical students in body MRI.

We express our thanks to our associate authors for contributing to this venture, to the residents and fellows for their suggestions and criticisms, and to the MR technologists who performed the many clinical studies that provided the figures for this book. We further want to thank James R. Brookeman, Ph.D., for his critical review of the text on MR physics; Brian T. Burkholder, R.T.R. (MR), for obtaining the images on the normal volunteers; Sherry S. Deane and Shirley M. Naylor for their administrative work; and Andrea Seils, Senior Editor, and Staci Hou, Assistant Editor, of Oxford University Press USA for their encouragement, support, and, most importantly, tolerance as we worked on this book.

William E. Brant, MD, FACR
Eduard E. de Lange, MD

TABLE OF CONTENTS

CONTRIBUTORS

Matthew J. Bassignani, MD
Associate Professor of Radiology
Department of Radiology and Medical Imaging
University of Virginia School of Medicine
Charlottesville, VA
currently
Radiologist
Virginia Urology
Richmond, VA

Gia A. DeAngelis, MD
Associate Professor of Radiology
Department of Radiology and Medical Imaging
University of Virginia School of Medicine
Charlottesville, VA

Klaus D. Hagspiel, MD
Professor of Radiology, Medicine (Cardiology) and
  Pediatrics
Division Head, Noninvasive Cardiovascular Imaging
Department of Radiology and Medical Imaging
University of Virginia School of Medicine
Charlottesville, VA

Thomas D. Henry, MD
Assistant Professor of Radiology
Department of Radiology and Medical Imaging
University of Virginia School of Medicine
Charlottesville, VA
currently
Radiologist, Virtual Radiologic
Charlottesville, VA

Drew L. Lambert, MD
Assistant Professor of Radiology
Department of Radiology and Medical Imaging
University of Virginia School of Medicine
Charlottesville, VA

John P. Mugler, III, PhD
Professor of Radiology and Medical Imaging
Professor of Biomedical Engineering
Department of Radiology and Medical Imaging
University of Virginia School of Medicine
Charlottesville, VA

Patrick T. Norton, MD
Assistant Professor of Radiology
Department of Radiology and Medical Imaging
University of Virginia School of Medicine
Charlottesville, VA

Juan Olazagasti, MD
Associate Professor of Radiology
Department of Radiology and Medical Imaging
University of Virginia School of Medicine
Charlottesville, VA

Tereza Poghosyan, MD
Assistant Professor of Radiology
Department of Radiology and Medical Imaging
University of Virginia School of Medicine
Charlottesville, VA
currently
Radiologist
Carolina Regional Radiology
Fayetteville, NC

Marc Sarti, MD
Assistant Professor of Radiology
Department of Radiology and Medical Imaging
University of Virginia School of Medicine
Charlottesville, VA
currently
Radiologist
Diversified Radiology of Colorado
Denver, CO

UNIVERSAL ABBREVIATIONS

CT – computed tomography
DWI – diffusion-weighted imaging
GRE – gradient echo
MIP – maximum intensity projection
MR – magnetic resonance
MRI – magnetic resonance imaging
MRCP – magnetic resonance cholangiopancreatography

MRA – magnetic resonance angiography
MRV – magnetic resonance venography
TE – echo time
TR – repetition time
FSE/TSE – fast/turbo spin echo
US – ultrasound

1.

BASIC MR PHYSICS

Eduard E. de Lange, MD and John P. Mugler, III, PhD

INTRODUCTION

Magnetic resonance (MR) imaging has become an important modality for evaluating the abdomen and pelvis. However, acceptance of the modality as a routine clinical test in these areas has been relatively slow compared to, for example, MR imaging of the brain or musculoskeletal system. Important reasons for its slow development are that acquisition of the data for MR images is, for many routinely used methods, relatively slow, and that the technique is inherently sensitive to motion, leading to image artifacts. Sampling of the data for diagnostic, high-quality images is best performed when tissues are stationary.

The most important cause of motion-related image artifacts in the abdomen is breathing, followed by the moving bowel and vascular flow. Over the years, many improvements in MRI-scanner hardware and software have been made that were particularly focused on suppressing these artifacts from motion so that high-quality abdominal images could be routinely obtained in clinical patients. In particular, the development of a variety of fast imaging techniques, which allow acquisition of the data within a breath hold, have had a major impact on the ability to routinely obtain diagnostically useful, high-quality MR images of the abdomen.

To lay the foundation for the remainder of the book, we will discuss a variety of fast MR pulse-sequence techniques, focusing particularly on the methods that, in our experience, have proven to be most useful clinically, including those that permit acquisition of images relatively free of motion artifacts even in patients unable to hold their breath. However, before discussing the specifics of these pulse sequences in Chapter 2, it is important to first obtain an understanding of the basics of MR physics and the general design of T1- and T2-weighted pulse sequences.[1] Having this knowledge is essential to better understand the various schemes that are used to design pulse sequences that allow imaging to be completed within a short period of time, and thus within a breath hold, to minimize the effect of motion on the images. Our discussion is certainly not comprehensive, and the techniques discussed form only a subset of the many pulse sequences that are currently available on most clinical scanners.

MAGNETIZATION, RELAXATION AND CONTRAST

In the first half of this chapter, we will describe the origin and basic characteristics of the MR signal, and introduce the most commonly used types of image contrast.

NUCLEAR MAGNETIC MOMENTS AND THE NET MAGNETIZATION

The nuclei of atoms are composed of protons and neutrons, each of which intrinsically possesses angular momentum and can be regarded qualitatively as a collection of electrical charges spinning about an axis. In classical physics, angular momentum, symbolized by a vector directed along the axis of rotation, represents the intensity of the spinning motion. Thus, the intrinsic angular momentum of a proton or neutron is called its *spin*; these particles are often depicted in MRI textbooks as a circle (or sphere) with an arrow (vector) through it, and are commonly referred to simply as "spins." Protons and neutrons also possess a magnetic dipole moment proportional to their intrinsic spin. The *gyromagnetic ratio* is defined as the ratio of the magnetic moment to the spin. As we will discuss below, the magnetic properties of spins are at the heart of MRI.

The nucleus of the hydrogen atom is composed of one proton. Because hydrogen nuclei are present in large quantities in the water and fat molecules of the body, and have a relatively high gyromagnetic ratio (i.e., have a high magnetic moment relative to their spin), these are used as the source of signal for most clinical MR studies.

The magnet of an MRI scanner generates a strong static (constant) magnetic field, which is typically denoted by the symbol $\mathbf{B}_o$. In clinical MRI, the magnitude of $\mathbf{B}_o$ is usually expressed using the unit Tesla (abbreviated T, 1 Tesla = 20,000 times the Earth's magnetic-field strength) and ranges from a few tenths of Tesla to several Tesla. The most common field strengths are 1.5T and 3T. By convention, $\mathbf{B}_o$ is considered to point along the z axis of a Cartesian x-y-z coordinate system. The z axis is also called the *longitudinal* axis, and the plane defined by the x and y axes, and perpendicular to the z axis, is called the *transverse* plane.

In the absence of an externally applied magnetic field, the magnetic moments associated with hydrogen nuclei in a volume of tissue within a subject are oriented in random directions, and the *net magnetization*, which is the vector sum of the magnetic moments of all of the nuclei, is zero. However, when the subject is placed in the scanner, and thus within the magnetic field $\mathbf{B}_o$, the hydrogen nuclei in water and fat in the tissues experience an aligning force that, in essence, positions them either aligned with $\mathbf{B}_o$ (low energy state) or aligned in the opposite direction to $\mathbf{B}_o$ (high energy state). The number of nuclei, or spins, in the low energy state, aligned with $\mathbf{B}_o$, is slightly larger than the number aligned opposite to $\mathbf{B}_o$, leading to a non-zero net magnetization aligned with the longitudinal (z) axis and called the *thermal equilibrium* magnetization, denoted by the vector $\mathbf{M}_o$ (Fig. 1.1). The strength of the MR signal is directly related to the size of $\mathbf{M}_o$, which in turn is directly proportional to the applied field $\mathbf{B}_o$. This is why higher magnetic-field strengths are desirable—they result in a stronger MR signal, which in general leads to higher image quality.

The net magnetization vector is often discussed in terms of its component parallel to the z axis, called the longitudinal component of the net magnetization, or simply the longitudinal magnetization, and its component lying in the x-y plane, called the transverse component of the net magnetization, or simply the transverse magnetization. For example, the thermal equilibrium magnetization just described has a longitudinal component of length $\mathbf{M}_o$ but no transverse component. If the net magnetization vector were moved away from alignment with the z axis (in a moment we will discuss how this can happen), we would then have both longitudinal magnetization and transverse magnetization. Although it is often useful to discuss the behavior of the longitudinal magnetization separately from that for the transverse magnetization, as we will do in this chapter, it is nonetheless important to remember that these are the two components of a <u>single</u> net magnetization vector.

MANIPULATING THE MAGNETIZATION USING RF PULSES

A *radiofrequency pulse* (RF pulse) is used to manipulate the net magnetization vector corresponding to a volume of tissue, for example to tip it away from alignment with the z axis. Before we discuss how an RF pulse affects the magnetization, we first need to understand the concept of what such a pulse is. Consider a subject who is placed within the magnet of an MRI scanner and surrounded by an *RF coil*, which, in simplest terms, is one or more loops of wire either mounted within the bore of the scanner magnet or within a plastic case surrounding a portion of the subject. An RF pulse occurs when a voltage, alternating in amplitude at a frequency in the radiofrequency range (e.g., 63 MHz), is applied across the coil for a short period (e.g., 1 ms), causing an alternating electric current to flow through the coil. This current produces a magnetic field within the tissue that oscillates at the frequency of the applied voltage; this time-varying magnetic field, which is much weaker than $\mathbf{B}_o$, lies in the transverse plane.

The *resonant*, or Larmor, frequency is the product of the gyromagnetic ratio and the strength of the applied field $\mathbf{B}_o$. (For example, the resonant frequency is about 42.6 MHz at a magnetic-field strength of 1.0T and approximately 63.9 MHz at 1.5T.) This is the "natural" frequency of the spin system, and when an RF pulse is applied at the resonant frequency, the net magnetization vector will rotate, or *precess*, about the time-varying magnetic field induced by the RF pulse. In addition, once the RF pulse moves the net magnetization vector away from alignment with the z axis, the magnetization will also precess about the static magnetic field $\mathbf{B}_o$ generated by the scanner magnet (i.e., about the z axis) at the resonant frequency. Thus, while the RF pulse is turned on, the net magnetization simultaneously precesses about <u>both</u> the time-varying magnetic field induced by the RF pulse and $\mathbf{B}_o$. As a result, the magnetization spirals toward the transverse plane, as illustrated in Figure 1.2, which shows an RF pulse applied to magnetization that was initially at thermal equilibrium.

Before discussing key characteristics of RF pulses, we will briefly describe an important consequence of applying an RF pulse—generation of the MR signal. Since an RF pulse applied to thermal equilibrium magnetization rotates it away from alignment with the longitudinal axis, the resulting magnetization has both longitudinal and transverse components (Fig. 1.2). Once the RF pulse is switched off, the net magnetization

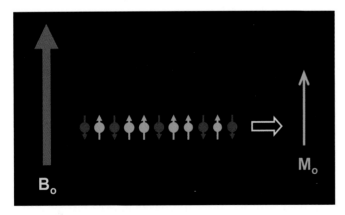

Figure 1.1 *Thermal equilibrium magnetization.* When the subject is placed in the strong static magnetic field of the scanner (indicated by the *large brown arrow*, labeled $\mathbf{B}_o$), hydrogen nuclei in water and fat in the tissues experience an aligning force that, in essence, positions them either aligned with $\mathbf{B}_o$ (shown in green, low energy state), or opposite to $\mathbf{B}_o$ (shown in red, high energy state). The number of nuclei (spins) in the low energy state is slightly larger than the number in the high energy state, leading to a net magnetization aligned with the z, or longitudinal, axis and called the thermal equilibrium magnetization (indicated by the *light green arrow*, labeled $\mathbf{M}_o$).

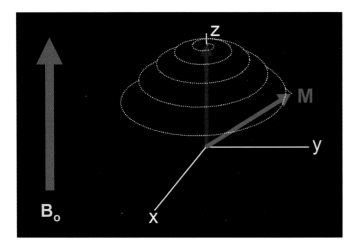

Figure 1.2 *How an RF pulse affects the magnetization.* The net magnetization vector **M** precesses about the time-varying magnetic field (not shown) induced by the RF pulse, as well as about the static magnetic field **B**₀ (*brown arrow*) generated by the scanner magnet. As a result, the RF pulse causes the magnetization to spiral toward the transverse (*x-y*) plane. The *white dotted line* shows the path traced out by the tip of the net magnetization vector as it "nutates" toward the *x-y* plane. The dark-purple vector on the *z* axis represents the position of the magnetization just before the RF pulse is applied. (Adapted from Mugler JP III. Basic principles. In: Edelman RR, Hesselink JR, Zlatkin MB, Crues JV III, eds. *Clinical Magnetic Resonance Imaging*, 3rd ed. Philadelphia: Saunders Elsevier, 2006.)

induce a voltage across the coil by Faraday's law of electromagnetic induction (Fig. 1.3). This is how the MR signal, which we sample to produce the data required for MR images, is generated. The generation of the MR signal is analogous to the generation of electricity by a dynamo.

The MR signal generated by precessing transverse magnetization, immediately after an RF pulse, is called a *free induction decay* (FID). The term "free" denotes that once the time-varying magnetic field induced by the RF pulse is switched off, the net magnetization vector precesses "freely" in the scanner's magnetic field **B**₀. The term "induction" is used because the precessing magnetization induces a voltage across the RF coil by Faraday's law. The term "decay" denotes that the magnitude of the transverse magnetization, and thus the associated signal, decreases (decays) over time, as discussed below in the section "Transverse magnetization and T2 relaxation." The FID signal oscillates at the resonant frequency, so it appears as a sinusoidal waveform that decays gradually (Fig. 1.4A). Before the signal is processed to calculate an MR image, the component of the signal oscillating at the resonant frequency is removed using a process called *demodulation*. This yields the envelope of the FID, which exhibits decay over time, as illustrated in Figure 1.4B.

Now, returning to the characteristics of RF pulses themselves, we see in Figure 1.2 that the motion of the net magnetization during an RF pulse, as it simultaneously precesses about both the time-varying magnetic field induced by the RF pulse and **B**₀, is somewhat complicated. Therefore, when illustrating the effects of RF pulses on the magnetization, it is customary to show only the effect of the time-varying magnetic field induced by the RF pulse, resulting in a simpler and easier-to-understand depiction (e.g., as shown in Fig. 1.5).

The effect of an RF pulse on the net magnetization is directly related to the magnitude of the time-varying magnetic field induced by the RF pulse. The larger its magnitude, the faster the magnetization precesses about this time-varying field. The angle through which the magnetization precesses during the RF pulse is called the *flip angle*. We can obtain a desired flip

vector continues to precess about the *z* axis under the influence of the static magnetic field **B**₀. Viewed in terms of the longitudinal and transverse components, the longitudinal magnetization appears stationary, while the transverse magnetization rotates in the *x-y* plane, about the *z* axis, at the resonant frequency. Conceptually, the precessing transverse magnetization vector can be considered to be a small rotating bar magnet. When placed in a coil of wire (analogous to the RF coil of the MRI scanner), such a rotating magnet will

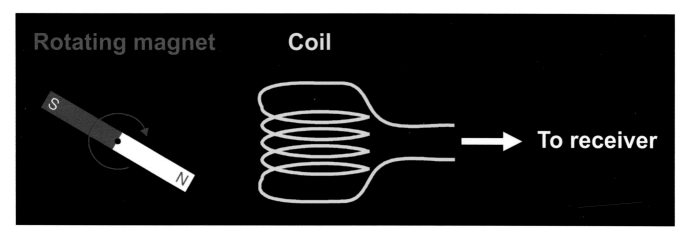

Figure 1.3 *Generation of the MR signal.* Conceptually, the precessing transverse magnetization vector is like a small rotating bar magnet. When placed in or near a coil of wire (corresponding to the RF coil of the MRI scanner), such a rotating magnet induces a voltage across the coil by Faraday's law of electromagnetic induction. This voltage, which represents the MR signal, is then amplified and sent to the receiver electronics to produce the data for the MR images. (Adapted from Mugler JP III. Basic principles. In: Edelman RR, Hesselink JR, Zlatkin MB, Crues JV III, eds. *Clinical Magnetic Resonance Imaging*, 3rd ed. Philadelphia: Saunders Elsevier, 2006.)

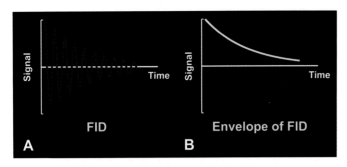

Figure 1.4 *The free induction decay (FID) signal produced following an RF pulse.* (**A**) Measured and (**B**) demodulated FID signals generated by precessing transverse magnetization, just after an RF pulse. The demodulated signal shows the envelope of the FID, which exhibits its characteristic decay over time (see Fig. 1.13). (Adapted from Mugler JP III. Basic principles. In: Edelman RR, Hesselink JR, Zlatkin MB, Crues JV III, eds. *Clinical Magnetic Resonance Imaging*, 3rd ed. Philadelphia: Saunders Elsevier, 2006.)

angle by varying the strength or duration of the RF pulse (i.e., by making the time-varying magnetic field induced by the RF pulse larger or leaving it on for a longer period of time).

The most common RF pulses used in MRI have flip angles of 90° or 180°. A 90° RF pulse is typically used to move, or "flip," the net magnetization from being aligned with the *z* axis onto the transverse (*x-y*) plane. In this case, the 90° RF pulse converts longitudinal magnetization into transverse magnetization, as illustrated in Figure 1.5. In terms of the low and high energy states discussed above, the application of a 90° RF pulse to thermal equilibrium magnetization equalizes the numbers of spins in the two energy states, corresponding to a longitudinal component of zero.

In general, an RF pulse that is used to move some or all of the net magnetization onto the transverse plane for the purpose of subsequently producing an MR signal is called an *excitation* RF pulse. In techniques designed for fast imaging, the flip angle of the excitation RF pulse is often less than 90°.

As its name implies, a 180° RF pulse is used to rotate the net magnetization through 180°. The common applications of a 180° RF pulse are (1) rotating magnetization that is aligned with the positive *z* axis to be aligned with the negative *z* axis, and (2) rotating magnetization that is in the transverse plane to the opposite side of the transverse plane. For the first case, the pulse is called an *inversion* RF pulse and is used in certain pulse sequences for suppressing the signal from a selected tissue or for improving image contrast, as discussed further below. In terms of the low and high energy states discussed above, the application of a 180° inversion RF pulse to thermal

---

***Box 1.1* ESSENTIALS TO REMEMBER**

- The signal for clinical MRI is derived from the hydrogen nuclei in the water and fat molecules of the body.

- In the absence of an externally applied magnetic field, the magnetic moments associated with hydrogen nuclei in tissue are oriented in random directions, and the net magnetization, which is the vector sum of the magnetic moments of all of the nuclei, is zero.

- When tissue is placed in a magnetic field, the number of hydrogen nuclei, or spins, in the low energy state (aligned with the field) is slightly larger than the number in the high energy state (aligned opposite to the field), leading to a net positive magnetization aligned parallel to the field, called the thermal equilibrium magnetization.

- The coordinate axis parallel to the direction of the scanner's static magnetic field is labeled the *z* axis, and is also known as the longitudinal axis; the plane perpendicular to the longitudinal axis, defined by the *x* and *y* axes, is called the transverse plane. The component of a magnetization vector parallel to the *z* axis is called the longitudinal magnetization, and that perpendicular to the z axis is called the transverse magnetization.

- The thermal equilibrium magnetization has only a longitudinal component.

- The longitudinal and transverse magnetizations are the two components of a single net magnetization vector and are not two separate, independent entities.

- The resonant, or Larmor, frequency is the "natural" frequency of the spin system and is the product of the gyromagnetic ratio and the strength of the applied magnetic field.

- When an RF pulse is applied to thermal equilibrium magnetization, the magnetization is moved away from alignment with the static magnetic field and, following the RF pulse, it rotates, or precesses, "freely" at the resonant frequency about the longitudinal axis, which is parallel to the static magnetic field.

- The precessing transverse magnetization vector is analogous to a small rotating bar magnet. When placed in or near a coil of wire, such a rotating magnet will induce a voltage across the coil, which is how the MR signal is generated.

- The magnitude of the transverse magnetization immediately after the application of a 90° RF pulse is equal to that of the longitudinal magnetization just before the RF pulse. Thus, by sampling the transverse magnetization immediately after a 90° RF pulse, information (signal) is obtained that essentially reflects the magnitude of the longitudinal magnetization that existed just before the RF pulse.

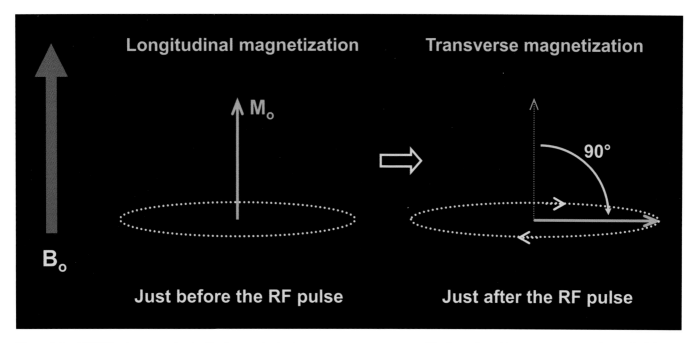

Figure 1.5 *A 90° RF pulse converts longitudinal magnetization into transverse magnetization.* The thermal equilibrium magnetization (*vertical solid green arrow*, labeled **M**$_o$) is parallel to the static magnetic field **B**$_o$ (*solid brown arrow*), and has only a longitudinal component just before the RF pulse is applied. The 90° RF pulse rotates the thermal equilibrium magnetization through 90° to become transverse magnetization (*horizontal solid green arrow*). Hence, just after the 90° RF pulse, the longitudinal component of the magnetization is zero (for reference, the original longitudinal component is indicated on the right by a *thin dotted arrow*), and the transverse magnetization generated by the RF pulse precesses (rotates) about the *z* axis at the resonant frequency. The magnitude of the transverse magnetization immediately after the RF pulse is equal to that of the longitudinal magnetization just before the RF pulse.

equilibrium magnetization inverts the numbers of spins in the two energy states, resulting in a larger number in the high energy state. For the second case, the pulse is called a *refocusing* RF pulse and is used in so-called *spin-echo* pulse sequences to compensate for spatial variations in magnetic-field strength, as described below in the section "Spin echoes."

LONGITUDINAL MAGNETIZATION AND T1 RELAXATION

As noted above, the thermal equilibrium magnetization **M**$_o$ is, by definition, aligned with the longitudinal (positive *z*) axis. If **M**$_o$ is perturbed by an RF pulse (e.g., Figs. 1.2 and 1.5), the resulting longitudinal magnetization will then grow back, or *relax*, toward its equilibrium state. This process is called *longitudinal relaxation*. For example, immediately following a 90° RF pulse, the component of the net magnetization vector parallel to the *z* axis, and thus the longitudinal magnetization, is zero (Fig 1.5). Subsequently, the longitudinal magnetization grows back toward the thermal equilibrium value **M**$_o$, as illustrated in Figure 1.6. Mathematically, this regrowth of the longitudinal magnetization is described by a monoexponential term with a time constant typically labeled either T1 or T$_1$ (here we will use T1). Thus, longitudinal relaxation is also called *T1 relaxation*. At time T1 after a 90° RF pulse, the longitudinal magnetization has recovered to 63% of the thermal-equilibrium value.

As described in the previous section, a 90° RF pulse equalizes the numbers of spins in the high and low energy states.

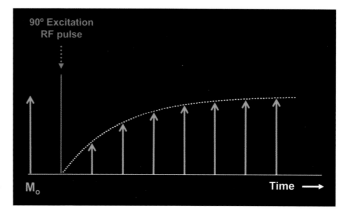

Figure 1.6 *Longitudinal (T1) relaxation.* At thermal equilibrium, the net magnetization **M**$_o$ (*green arrow* on left) is aligned with the longitudinal axis, parallel to the direction of the static magnetic field **B**$_o$. The longitudinal magnetization is positive at thermal equilibrium because the number of spins in the low energy state, aligned with the static field **B**$_o$, is slightly larger than the number in the high energy state, aligned opposite to the static field **B**$_o$ (Fig. 1.1). When an RF pulse is applied, the number of spins in the high energy state increases, leading to a decrease of the longitudinal magnetization. Specifically, when a 90° RF pulse is applied, the numbers of spins in the high and low energy states become equal and, as a result, the longitudinal magnetization is zero just after the pulse. Subsequently, through the process called longitudinal (T1) relaxation, the number of spins in the low energy state increases as the number in the high energy state decreases, and the longitudinal magnetization therefore grows back toward its equilibrium state, as illustrated by the series of green arrows with progressively increasing lengths.

Then, stimulated by the effect of molecular motion in the tissue surroundings, termed the "lattice," energy is transferred from the spin system to the lattice reservoir as the longitudinal magnetization regrows toward thermal equilibrium. Because of this interaction between the spins and the lattice, longitudinal relaxation is also termed spin-lattice relaxation.

The T1 relaxation time is an intrinsic property of a given tissue, and depends on the structure of the tissue at a molecular level. Thus, different types of tissue typically have different T1 values. For example, fat has a relatively short T1 of a few hundred milliseconds, while fluid, such as in a liver cyst, has a relatively long T1 of several seconds (Fig. 1.7). Large macromolecules, such as proteins, restrict the molecular motion of nearby water molecules and, consequently, shorten the associated T1 relaxation time. As a result, fluids with high protein content, such as mucus, have shorter T1 values than less viscous, more watery fluids. The T1 relaxation time also depends on the strength of the static magnetic field $\mathbf{B}_o$. Over the range of field strengths used for clinical imaging, T1 values for most tissues increase as the field strength is increased.

As a second example of longitudinal relaxation, consider that which occurs following a 180° inversion RF pulse. Just as discussed for the case of a 90° RF pulse, the longitudinal magnetization will relax toward $\mathbf{M}_o$ with an exponential time constant T1. However, since following the inversion RF pulse the longitudinal magnetization begins aligned along the negative z axis, the magnitude of the net magnetization vector must first decrease to zero before growing back to its equilibrium value, with the net magnetization vector aligned along the positive z axis (Fig. 1.8).

The time at which the magnitude of the longitudinal magnetization is zero following an inversion RF pulse (called the "null" point) depends on the T1 relaxation time, and hence depends on the tissue type since T1 values are tissue dependent. Longitudinal relaxation following an inversion RF pulse is also termed *inversion recovery*. Several MRI acquisition methods take advantage of the inversion-recovery process to generate high T1-dependent contrast, or to suppress the signal from a selected tissue by applying the excitation RF pulse when the relaxing longitudinal magnetization for the tissue passes through zero (which thus generates no signal from the selected tissue).

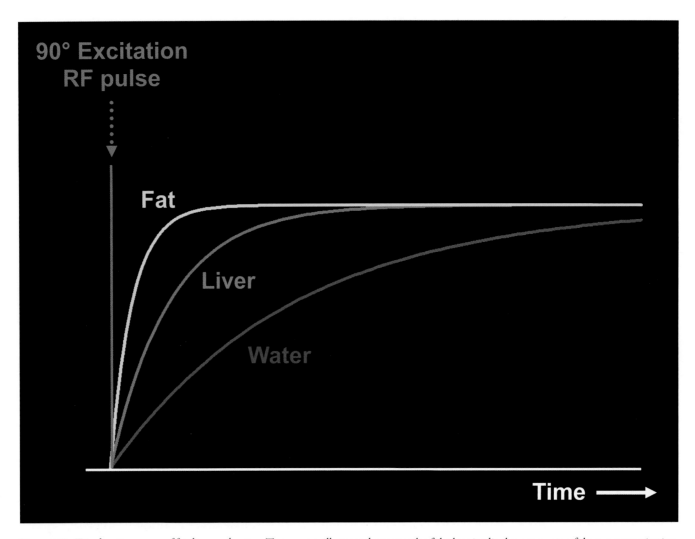

Figure 1.7 *T1 relaxation curves of fat, liver, and water.* These curves illustrate the regrowth of the longitudinal components of the net magnetization for fat (yellow), liver (orange), and water (blue) following a 90° excitation RF pulse. The T1 relaxation time is relatively short for fat (i.e., it grows back quickly), intermediate for liver, and relatively long for water (i.e., it grows back slowly). As described in a subsequent section, T1-weighted images emphasize the differences among the T1 relaxation times of the tissues.

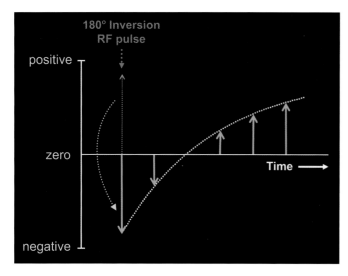

Figure 1.8 *T1 relaxation following a 180° inversion RF pulse.* When a 180° RF pulse is applied to thermal equilibrium magnetization, the numbers of spins in the low and high energy states are inverted, resulting in a larger number in the high energy state. Thus, the longitudinal magnetization after the RF pulse has the same magnitude as before the pulse, but is aligned along the negative *z* axis. Immediately following the inversion RF pulse, the longitudinal magnetization begins to grow back, from its negative value, toward thermal equilibrium with an exponential time constant T1. The longitudinal magnetization thus passes from negative, through zero, to positive values during its recovery. (For reference, the longitudinal magnetization just before the 180° RF pulse is indicated by the *thin, dotted green arrow.*)

This concept will be discussed further when we review magnetization-prepared gradient-echo imaging in Chapter 2.

TRANSVERSE MAGNETIZATION AND T2 RELAXATION

As discussed in the section "Manipulating the magnetization using RF pulses," an RF pulse that tips the thermal equilibrium magnetization away from alignment with the *z* axis generates transverse magnetization, which will then precess about the *z* axis at the resonant frequency. (Recall that this precessing transverse magnetization generates the MR signal, which we sample to produce the data required for MR images.) For example, a 90° excitation RF pulse creates transverse magnetization that is equal in magnitude to the longitudinal magnetization that existed just before the pulse (Fig. 1.5). To describe the magnetization's behavior following an RF pulse, it is useful to consider two different representations for the transverse magnetization corresponding to a tissue volume of interest, which, for convenience, we will call the "spin-level" representation and the "tissue-subvolume" representation. The spin-level representation is based on the fact that the net magnetization is the vector sum of the magnetic moments for the spins (as described above in the section "Nuclear magnetic moments and the net magnetization"). Thus, for this representation, we view the transverse magnetization as a collection of vectors, each associated with the magnetic moment of an individual spin. For the tissue-subvolume representation, we instead consider the transverse magnetization to be subdivided into a group of transverse magnetization vectors, each of which corresponds to a small portion ("subvolume") of the tissue volume of interest. Each tissue subvolume includes a large number of

---

Box 1.2 **ESSENTIALS TO REMEMBER**

- When a 90° RF pulse is applied to thermal equilibrium magnetization, the numbers of spins in the high and low energy states become equal and, as a result, the longitudinal magnetization is zero just after the pulse.

- When a 180° inversion RF pulse is applied to thermal equilibrium magnetization, the number of spins in the low energy state decreases and the number in the high energy state increases until the numbers of spins in the two energy states are inverted, resulting in a larger number in the high energy state. Consequently, the longitudinal magnetization is aligned along the negative *z* axis following the RF pulse, in the opposite direction as the static magnetic field, but has the same magnitude as before the pulse, when the magnetization was aligned along the positive *z* axis.

- Immediately following either a 90° or 180° RF pulse, the longitudinal magnetization grows back toward its thermal equilibrium value via the process of longitudinal, or T1, relaxation. Through this process, the number of spins in the high energy state decreases as the number in the low energy state increases, until the spin system has returned to its thermal equilibrium configuration.

- The T1 relaxation time is an intrinsic property of a given tissue, and depends on the structure of the tissue at a molecular level. Large macromolecules, such as proteins, can restrict the rapid molecular motion of nearby water molecules and, consequently, shorten the associated T1 relaxation time.

- The T1 relaxation time also depends on the strength of the main magnetic field. For the range of field strengths used for clinical imaging, T1 values for most tissues increase as the field strength is increased.

- At time T1 after a 90° RF pulse, the longitudinal magnetization has recovered to 63% of its thermal-equilibrium value.

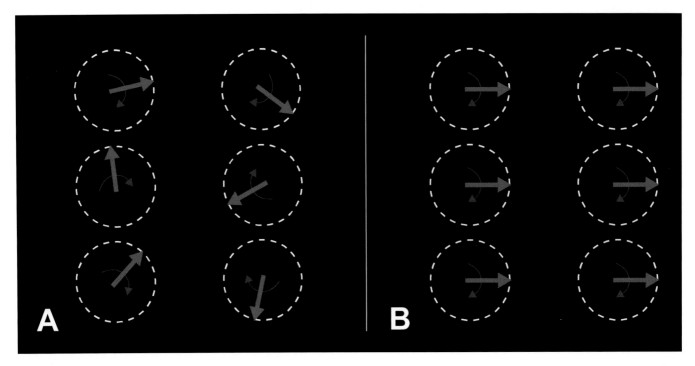

Figure 1.9 *Phase coherence.* (**A**) The vectors (*magenta arrows*) are precessing with random phases relative to one another. These vectors are out of phase with one another and thus do not exhibit phase coherence. (**B**) The vectors are precessing in synchrony and are in phase with one another. These vectors exhibit phase coherence. The *dashed, white circles* illustrate the paths traced out by the tips of the magnetization vectors as they precess. (Adapted from Mugler JP III. Basic principles. In: Edelman RR, Hesselink JR, Zlatkin MB, Crues JV III, eds. *Clinical Magnetic Resonance Imaging,* 3rd ed. Philadlephia: Saunders Elsevier, 2006.)

spins that experience a uniform magnetic-field strength (i.e., the resonant frequency is the same for all spins within the subvolume). As described below, the spin-level representation pertains to the process called transverse relaxation, and the tissue-subvolume representation pertains to the additional transverse-magnetization decay that occurs due to magnetic-field inhomogeneity, leading to so-called T2* relaxation, which includes the effects of both transverse relaxation and field-inhomogeneity-induced decay. Nonetheless, the common aspect of both representations is that the transverse magnetization corresponds to a collection of small vectors.

With regard to either the spin-level or tissue-subvolume representation, the concept of *phase coherence* is key to understanding the behavior of the associated transverse magnetization following an RF pulse. This concept is illustrated in Figure 1.9, which shows six precessing vectors on each side of the diagram; each vector could correspond to a magnetic moment, or to the transverse magnetization associated with a subvolume of tissue. Recall that, in our context, "phase" refers to the angular orientation of a vector with respect to a reference axis. The precessing vectors on the left of the diagram have random orientations with respect to one another, or, in other words, are out of phase with one another, whereas the vectors on the right are precessing in synchrony and are aligned with one another; the vectors on the right are said to possess phase coherence.

Immediately following an RF pulse, the collection of small vectors (either for the spin-level or the tissue-subvolume representation) that correspond to the transverse magnetization exhibit a high degree of phase coherence. If some physical influence (as described below) causes a loss of alignment among the vectors (i.e., a loss of phase coherence), then the magnitude of the transverse magnetization will decrease as a result.

At the level of the spins, random, atomic-level, magnetic interactions cause a gradual loss of phase coherence among the associated magnetic moments, which results in a corresponding decrease over time in the magnitude of the transverse magnetization. Since the equilibrium value of the transverse magnetization is zero, the magnitude of the transverse magnetization decreases, or *decays*, toward zero following an RF pulse (Fig. 1.10). This process of "spin-spin" interactions, whereby the transverse magnetization relaxes toward zero through a loss of phase coherence at the spin level, is called *transverse relaxation*. In view of the fundamental role of spin-spin interactions in transverse relaxation, this process is also called spin-spin relaxation. It is important to note that the loss of phase coherence due to random spin-spin interactions (transverse relaxation) is irreversible, in contrast to loss of phase coherence on the tissue-subvolume scale (field-inhomogeneity contribution to T2* relaxation), discussed below.

Analogous to longitudinal relaxation, transverse relaxation is typically described mathematically by a monoexponential decay with a time constant labeled either T2 or T_2 (here we will use T2). Thus, transverse relaxation is also called *T2 relaxation*. At time T2 after a 90° RF pulse, the transverse magnetization has decayed to 37% of its initial value. The T2 relaxation time, like the T1 relaxation time, is an intrinsic property of the tissue. Thus, as is the case for T1, different types of tissue typically have different T2 values. For example, fat has a relatively short T2 of less than

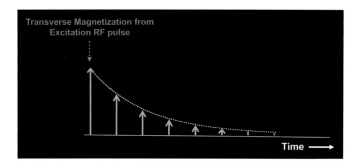

Figure 1.10 *Transverse (T2) relaxation.* Application of an RF pulse generates transverse magnetization (Fig. 1.5). Immediately following the RF pulse, random, atomic-level, magnetic interactions among the spins cause a gradual loss of phase coherence, which results in a corresponding decrease over time in the magnitude of the transverse magnetization. The transverse magnetization thus irreversibly *decays* toward zero, as illustrated by the series of green arrows with progressively decreasing lengths. This process is called transverse, or T2, relaxation.

100 milliseconds, while fluid has a relatively long T2 of more than 1 second (Fig. 1.11). In contrast to T1, the T2 relaxation times remain approximately constant for most tissues with increasing field strength up to approximately 1.5T. However, with higher field strengths, the T2 values for many tissues decrease.

At the level of tissue-subvolumes that were introduced above, inhomogeneity of the static magnetic field, for example due to imperfections in the scanner magnet or due to local field gradients generated secondary to differences in the magnetic properties (see the section "Magnetic susceptibility" in Chapter 2) of adjacent substances (e.g., at interfaces between tissue and air, or tissue and metal objects), also plays an important role in the decay of the transverse magnetization. Recall, as noted above, that the frequency of precession (resonant frequency) is directly proportional to the applied magnetic-field strength. Thus, for subvolumes of tissue for which the magnetic-field strength is higher than its average value, the associated transverse magnetization will precess faster than

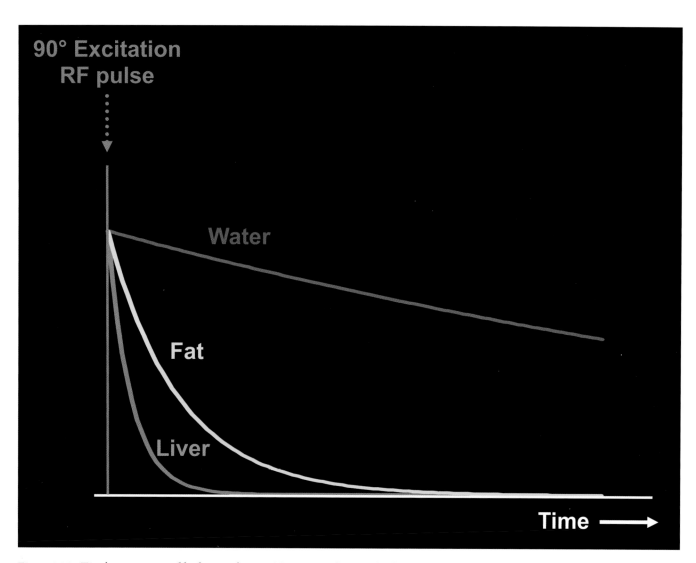

Figure 1.11 *T2 relaxation curves of fat, liver, and water.* These curves illustrate the decay of the transverse components of the net magnetization for fat (yellow), liver (orange), and water (blue) following an RF pulse. The T2 relaxation time is relatively short for liver (i.e., it decays quickly), intermediate for fat, and relatively long for water (i.e., it decays slowly). As described in a subsequent section, T2-weighted images emphasize the differences among the T2 relaxation times of the tissues.

the average frequency, and for subvolumes for which the average field strength is lower, the associated transverse magnetization will precess slower. As a result, due to the presence of magnetic-field inhomogeneity, phase coherence is lost among the transverse magnetization vectors corresponding to the subvolumes of tissue, and the magnitude of the total transverse magnetization decreases as time passes (Fig. 1.12); this decay of the magnetization is the field-inhomogeneity contribution to T2* relaxation. In general, loss of phase coherence caused by spatial variations in the strength of the magnetic field at the tissue-subvolume scale is called *dephasing*. In contrast to loss of phase coherence due to spin-spin interactions (i.e., at the level of the spins—T2 relaxation), dephasing caused by spatial variations in magnetic-field strength can often be reversed, as discussed in the section below, "Spin echoes."

The time constant T2* ("T2 star") is used to express the decay of the transverse magnetization associated with T2* relaxation, which, as noted above, includes the effects of both transverse relaxation and field-inhomogeneity-induced decay. Thus, T2* is based on <u>both</u> the intrinsic T2 value of the tissue (decay from spin-level interactions) *and* the effects of dephasing due to inhomogeneity of the static magnetic field (decay due to different frequencies of precession among tissue subvolumes, Fig. 1.12). In the absence of field inhomogeneity, T2 and T2* are equal; in the presence of field inhomogeneity, T2* must be shorter than T2 since field inhomogeneity accelerates the decay of the transverse magnetization. The general relationship between T2 and T2* is illustrated in Figure 1.13.

For all tissues, the T2 relaxation time is equal to or shorter than the T1 relaxation time, and for most tissues T2 is substantially less than T1 (Fig. 1.14). Interactions between large macromolecules, such as proteins, and water molecules accelerate the decay of the transverse magnetization. Thus, the T2 values for soft tissues (e.g., brain matter, liver, muscle) are much shorter than those for fluids. It is important to note that multiple time constants (i.e., multiple T2 values) are required to accurately describe the transverse-magnetization decay of some tissues.

In the previous section we described T1 relaxation, and in this section we described T2 relaxation. Although for the most part these phenomena were discussed as distinct processes, it is important to remember that both occur simultaneously as soon as the magnetization is disturbed from thermal equilibrium. For example, immediately following a 90° excitation RF pulse, the longitudinal component of the magnetization begins to regrow from zero, and, at the same time, the transverse component begins to decay toward zero. Figure 1.15 illustrates the coexistence of these two relaxation processes.

SPIN ECHOES

Two RF pulses applied in succession, and closely spaced compared to the T2 relaxation time(s) for the tissue(s) of interest, generate an MR signal called a *spin echo*. We can understand the generation of a spin echo by combining the concepts of

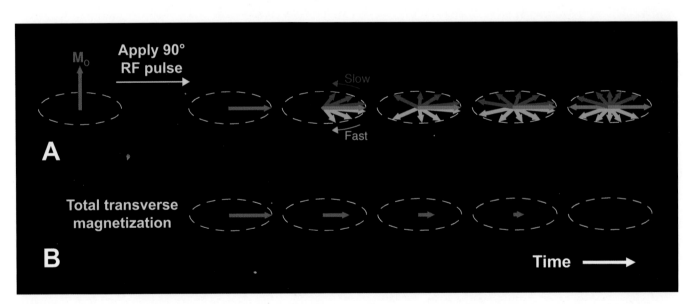

Figure 1.12 *Dephasing of the transverse magnetization in a volume of tissue in the presence of magnetic-field inhomogeneity.* (**A**) A 90° excitation RF pulse applied to longitudinal magnetization at thermal equilibrium (*vertical magenta arrow* labeled **M₀**) generates a total transverse magnetization (*horizontal magenta arrow*) for which the transverse magnetization vectors that correspond to subvolumes of tissue volume are in phase. (For the initial transverse magnetization [*leftmost horizontal magenta arrow*], the magnetization vectors corresponding to the subvolumes are superimposed, so that only one vector is visible.) As time progresses, transverse magnetization that experiences a higher-than-average magnetic-field strength within its subvolume, due to the presence of magnetic-field inhomogeneity, precesses faster (*green arrows*) than the average frequency, while transverse magnetization that experiences a lower-than-average field strength precesses slower (*red arrows*). Thus, phase coherence among the transverse magnetization vectors corresponding to the subvolumes of tissue is gradually lost over time. (**B**) The total transverse magnetization, which is the sum of the transverse magnetization vectors corresponding to the subvolumes, decays as dephasing progresses; this decay is the field-inhomogeneity contribution to T2* relaxation. For simplicity, the effects of T1 and T2 relaxation are neglected in the figure. (Adapted from Mugler JP III. Basic principles. In: Edelman RR, Hesselink JR, Zlatkin MB, Crues JV III, eds. *Clinical Magnetic Resonance Imaging*, 3rd ed. Philadelphia: Saunders Elsevier, 2006.)

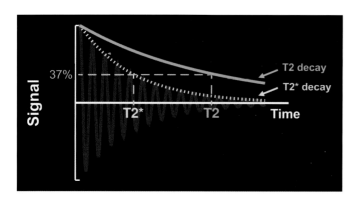

Figure 1.13 *Relationship between T2 and T2*.* As illustrated in Figure 1.4, an FID (*oscillating dark-purple curve*), which is the MR signal from precessing transverse magnetization, is generated following an excitation RF pulse. In the presence of field inhomogeneity, the FID decays with the time constant T2* (*dashed yellow curve*), which combines the intrinsic T2 decay associated which the tissue (*solid green curve*) and the dephasing effects of field inhomogeneity (Fig. 1.12). Note that the T2* curve decreases more quickly than the T2 curve, because decay of the transverse magnetization is accelerated by magnetic-field inhomogeneity. For both T2 and T2* decay, the respective curves decrease to 37% of their initial values when time is equal to the corresponding time constant. (Adapted from Mugler JP III. Basic principles. In: Edelman RR, Hesselink JR, Zlatkin MB, Crues JV III, eds. *Clinical Magnetic Resonance Imaging*, 3rd ed. Philadelphia: Saunders Elsevier, 2006.)

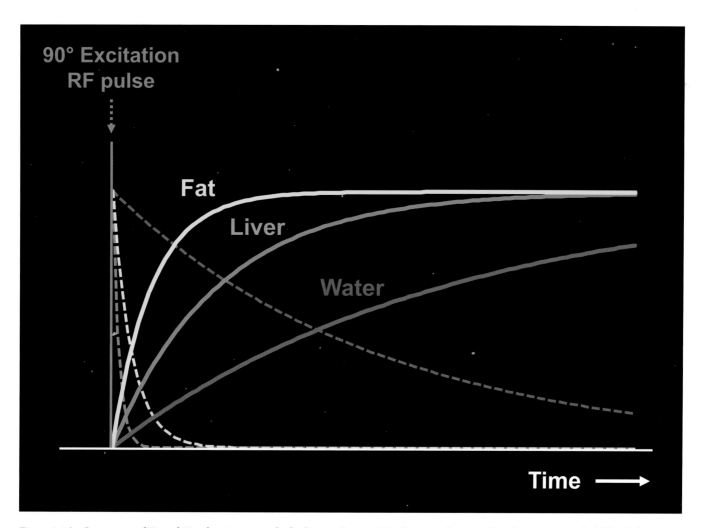

Figure 1.14 *Comparison of T1 and T2 relaxation curves for fat, liver, and water.* This figure combines the T1 relaxation curves (*solid lines*) shown in Figure 1.7, and the T2 relaxation curves (*dashed lines*) shown in Figure 1.11, plotted on the same time scale of 0 to 4 s. We see that the T2 relaxation times for the three tissues are shorter than the corresponding T1 relaxation times. This is particularly evident for liver; its transverse component of the magnetization (*dashed orange line*) is close to zero long before its longitudinal component (*solid orange line*) approaches thermal equilibrium. Any differences in proton (spin) densities among the tissues are neglected in the figure.

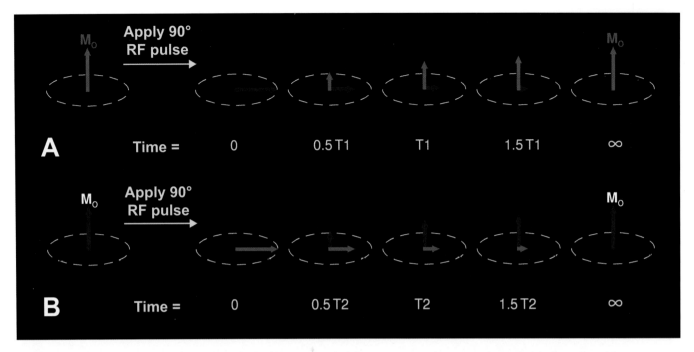

Figure 1.15 *T1 and T2 relaxation occur simultaneously.* (**A**) Immediately following a 90° excitation RF pulse applied to thermal equilibrium magnetization (*vertical magenta arrow* labeled M_o), the longitudinal component of the magnetization is zero (time = 0). Subsequently, the longitudinal magnetization grows back toward thermal equilibrium (*vertical magenta arrows* with increasing heights). (**B**) By rotating the thermal equilibrium magnetization through 90°, the excitation RF pulse also creates transverse magnetization having a magnitude that equals that of M_o (*horizontal magenta arrow* at time = 0). At the same time that the longitudinal magnetization is growing back to thermal equilibrium, the transverse magnetization is decaying toward zero (*horizontal magenta arrows* with decreasing lengths). The *dark-purple arrows* in A and B emphasize that the T1 and T2 relaxation processes occur at the same time. For this illustration, the T1 and T2 values were assumed to be similar. (Adapted from Mugler JP III. Basic principles. In: Edelman RR, Hesselink JR, Zlatkin MB, Crues JV III, eds. *Clinical Magnetic Resonance Imaging*, 3rd ed. Philadelphia: Saunders Elsevier, 2006.)

Box 1.3 ESSENTIALS TO REMEMBER

- The transverse magnetization corresponding to a volume of tissue can be considered to be composed of a collection of small vectors. Immediately following an RF pulse, these vectors exhibit a high degree of alignment with one another, or, in other words, they possess phase coherence.

- The transverse magnetization generated by an RF pulse decays toward zero via the process of transverse, or T2, relaxation. This process occurs through random, atomic-level, magnetic interactions among the spins, leading to loss of phase coherence, and thus decay of the transverse magnetization. This decay is irreversible.

- The T2 relaxation time is an intrinsic property of the tissue, and depends on the structure of the tissue at a molecular level. Large macromolecules, such as proteins, can restrict the rapid molecular motion of nearby water molecules and, consequently, shorten the associated T2 relaxation time.

- At time T2 after a 90° RF pulse, the transverse magnetization has decayed to 37% of its initial value.

- T2* expresses the decay of the transverse magnetization including both the intrinsic T2 value of the tissue *and* any effects of dephasing due to inhomogeneity of the static magnetic field. T2* is always shorter than T2 in the presence of field inhomogeneity.

- For all tissues, T1 > T2 > T2*.

- Longitudinal and transverse relaxation occur at the same time; as the longitudinal magnetization regrows, the transverse magnetization decays.

phase coherence and dephasing, discussed in the preceding section, and the properties of excitation and refocusing RF pulses, discussed in the section "Manipulating the magnetization using RF pulses." Consider the behavior of the transverse magnetization for a volume of tissue in an inhomogeneous magnetic field following a 90° excitation RF pulse. Figure 1.16A illustrates the evolution of transverse magnetization vectors corresponding to various subvolumes of a tissue volume located in the inhomogeneous magnetic field, with reference to the transverse magnetization for a subvolume that experiences the average field strength. Note that this situation is the same as that discussed above with reference to Figure 1.12, where we saw that for subvolumes of tissue experiencing a field strength higher than the average value, the transverse magnetization

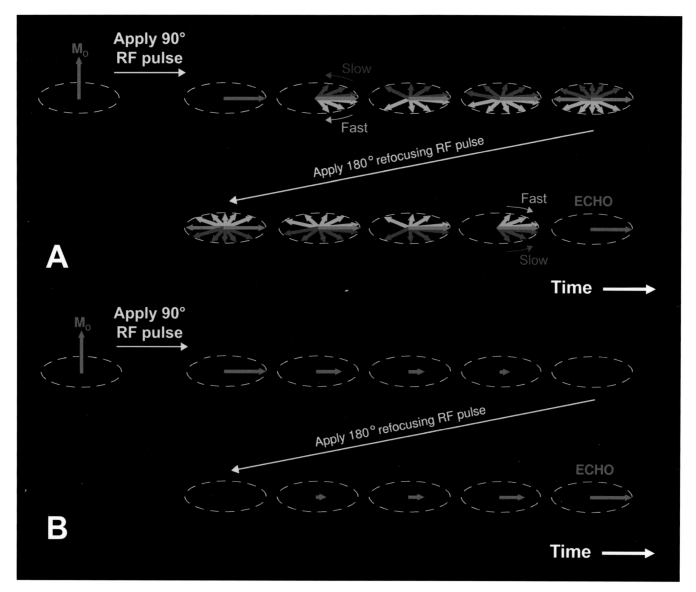

Figure 1.16 *Formation of a spin echo.* (**A**) Directly analogous to Figure 1.12, the transverse magnetization vectors that correspond to subvolumes of tissue volume are in phase (and superimposed on one another, such that only one vector is visible) immediately after a 90° excitation RF pulse. As time progresses, transverse magnetization that experiences a higher-than-average magnetic-field strength within its subvolume precesses faster (*green arrows*) than the average frequency, while transverse magnetization that experiences a lower-than-average field strength precesses slower (*red arrows*). As a result, the transverse magnetization vectors corresponding to the subvolumes of tissue dephase as shown in the upper row. A 180° refocusing RF pulse is applied to the transverse magnetization, which "flips" the vectors such that those precessing slower swap positions with those precessing faster. As time progresses further (lower row of A), the transverse magnetization vectors rephase (refocus) and form an echo (i.e., the transverse magnetization vectors return to their original orientations as existed immediately after the excitation RF pulse) when the time period following the 180° RF pulse matches that between the 90° and 180° RF pulses. (**B**) Also analogous to Figure 1.12, the total transverse magnetization, which is the sum of the transverse magnetization vectors corresponding to the subvolumes, gradually decays as dephasing progresses (upper row of B); recall, as indicated in Figure 1.12, that this decay is the field-inhomogeneity contribution to T2* relaxation. Following the 180° refocusing RF pulse, the total transverse magnetization then grows back to its original magnitude as the echo is formed at the echo time. In this illustration, the magnitude of the total transverse magnetization immediately after the 90° excitation RF pulse is equal to that at the echo time because, for simplicity, T2 decay was not included. (Adapted from Mugler JP III. Basic principles. In: Edelman RR, Hesselink JR, Zlatkin MB, Crues JV III, eds. *Clinical Magnetic Resonance Imaging*, 3rd ed. Philadelphia: Saunders Elsevier, 2006.)

vectors precess faster (green in Fig. 1.16A) than the average frequency, and for subvolumes experiencing a field strength lower than the average value, the transverse magnetization vectors precess slower (red in Fig. 1.16A). As time progresses following the excitation RF pulse, the transverse magnetization vectors dephase (lose phase coherence) due to the inhomogeneity of the field, and hence the total transverse magnetization decays as shown in the figure. As noted in the preceding section, the decay of the transverse magnetization in an inhomogeneous magnetic field is described by the T2* relaxation time.

If now, following the 90° excitation RF pulse, we apply a 180° refocusing RF pulse such that the time between the two RF pulses is short relative to the T2 relaxation time(s) of interest, a spin echo will be generated. This 180° RF pulse rotates the transverse magnetization to the opposite side of the transverse plane. Thus, the "fast" and "slow" transverse magnetization vectors exchange positions (Fig. 1.16A). As additional time passes and precession continues, the transverse magnetization vectors return to their original orientations that existed immediately after the excitation RF pulse. As a result, the total transverse magnetization grows, as phase coherence is reestablished (Fig. 1.16B), until a spin echo forms at the *echo time* (abbreviated TE, for time to echo). The echo time is that at which the time elapsed after the refocusing RF pulse matches the time period between the excitation and refocusing RF pulses. Although formation of the spin echo compensates for the magnetic-field inhomogeneity contribution to T2* relaxation, T2 relaxation nonetheless reduces the magnitude of the transverse magnetization vectors as time passes following the excitation RF pulse (not shown in Fig. 1.16). Therefore, the transverse magnetization at the time of the spin echo is reduced by T2 decay compared to the transverse magnetization that existed immediately following the excitation RF pulse (Fig. 1.17).

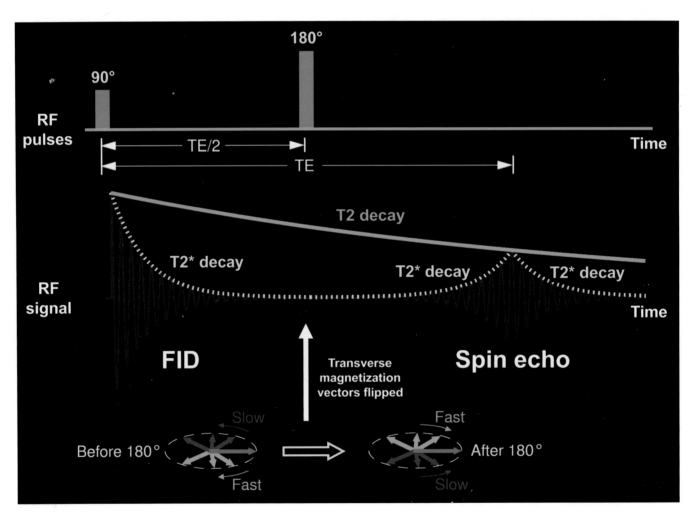

Figure 1.17 *Signal evolution during formation of a spin echo.* Just after a 90° excitation RF pulse, precessing transverse magnetization creates an MR signal that decays with a time constant T2* due to dephasing in the presence of magnetic-field inhomogeneity (Figs. 1.4 and 1.13). The 180° refocusing RF pulse, applied at time TE/2, swaps the positions of transverse magnetization vectors that precess slower than the average frequency with those that precess faster (Fig. 1.16), leading to a regrowth of the signal and formation of a spin echo at time TE. Although formation of the spin echo compensates for inhomogeneity of the magnetic field, T2 relaxation reduces the magnitude of the transverse magnetization, and hence the associated signal, as time passes following the excitation RF pulse. The signal at the time of the spin echo is thus reduced by T2 decay compared to that immediately following the excitation RF pulse. (Adapted from Mugler JP III. Basic principles. In: Edelman RR, Hesselink JR, Zlatkin MB, Crues JV III, eds. *Clinical Magnetic Resonance Imaging*, 3rd ed. Philadelphia: Saunders Elsevier, 2006.)

Following the first spin echo, one or more additional spin echoes can be created by simply applying one or more additional 180° refocusing RF pulses. Analogous to the case for the first spin echo, the second spin echo will form when the time elapsed after the second refocusing RF pulse matches the time period between the first spin echo and the second refocusing RF pulse. Additional spin echoes can be formed by using additional refocusing RF pulses up to the point when relaxation depletes the available magnetization.

Although the prototypical spin echo is generated by using a 90° excitation RF pulse followed by a 180° refocusing RF pulse, it is important to note that any RF pulse that "excites" (i.e., converts some portion of the longitudinal magnetization into transverse magnetization) followed by any RF pulse that "refocuses" (i.e., effectively rotates some portion of the transverse magnetization generated by the excitation RF pulse to the opposite side of the transverse plane) will generate a spin echo. For example, a 30° RF pulse followed by a 45° RF pulse generates a spin echo, although the amplitude of such a spin echo will be much less than that generated by a 90°-180° pair of RF pulses. (For this example, the spin-echo amplitude would be 7% of that generated by a 90°-180° pair.) The fact that two consecutive RF pulses having almost any flip-angle values generate a spin echo is relevant to the design of certain fast imaging methods used in the abdomen, as discussed further in the section "Short-TR gradient-echo imaging" in Chapter 2.

T1-WEIGHTED AND T2-WEIGHTED CONTRAST

The term *contrast* in MR imaging refers to differences in the signal intensities from the various tissues in the imaging volume. The most basic form of contrast in MRI is based on differences in the tissue relaxation times T1 and T2. It is important to realize that a single MR acquisition cannot generate contrast based solely on either T1 or T2. Instead, images are generated for which the contrast is determined primarily by one of the two parameters. That is, we may generate an image for which the contrast primarily reflects differences in T1 among the tissues, with only a minor contribution due to differences in T2. Nonetheless, both T1 and T2 always contribute to some extent.

A *T1-weighted* image primarily reflects differences in the T1 relaxation times among tissues while minimizing signal-intensity variations due to T2 differences. In such an image, tissues with short T1 values appear relatively bright and those with long T1 values appear relatively dark. For a standard spin-echo pulse sequence using a 90° excitation RF pulse, a T1-weighted image is obtained by choosing a relatively short period (the *repetition time*, abbreviated TR) for the longitudinal magnetization to recover following each application of the excitation RF pulse. This choice of TR emphasizes differences in T1 relaxation times among the tissues because it allows tissues with relatively short T1 values to recover substantially, and thus yield a relatively high signal, while those with relatively long T1 values recover only a small amount, and thus yield a relatively low signal. Signal-intensity variations due to T2 differences are minimized by acquiring the signal as soon as possible following the application of the excitation RF pulse, so there is little time for the transverse magnetization to decay. Thus, the echo time, TE (which corresponds to the formation of a spin echo, as discussed above, or a gradient echo, as discussed below, and which typically occurs at the middle of the data sampling period), is chosen to be as short as possible given the other constraints of the pulse sequence.

A *T2-weighted* image primarily reflects differences in the T2 relaxation times among tissues while minimizing signal-intensity variations due to T1 differences. In a T2-weighted image, tissues with long T2 values appear relatively bright and those with short T2 values appear relatively dark. In principle, as explained in more detail in Chapter 2, a T2-weighted image is obtained by choosing a relatively long TR, which allows the longitudinal magnetization of all tissues to essentially return to thermal equilibrium between successive excitation RF pulses regardless of the associated T1 values. This therefore minimizes signal-intensity differences due to differences in T1 values. Further, by choosing a relatively long TE, substantial transverse relaxation occurs following each excitation RF pulse before acquiring the signal, so that the transverse magnetization for tissues with long T2 values will remain relatively large, and hence yield a relatively high signal, while that for tissues with short T2 values will decay significantly, and hence yield a relatively low signal. As a result, choosing a relatively long TE emphasizes differences in T2 relaxation times among the tissues.

Finally, it is important to note that the signal intensity for every tissue is modulated by its associated *proton density*. This term refers to the number per volume (density) of signal-producing protons, typically normalized with respect to pure water. For example, cerebral spinal fluid has a (normalized) proton density of approximately 1, whereas that for brain white matter is less, in the range of 0.7 to 0.8.

In summary, the repetition time, TR, controls the degree of T1 weighting, wherein decreasing TR from a relatively long value increases T1 weighting, and the echo time, TE, controls the degree of T2 weighting, wherein increasing TE from a relatively short value increases T2 weighting. A T1-weighted image uses a short TR and short TE, whereas a T2-weighted image uses a long TR and long TE. If both T1 weighting and T2 weighting are suppressed, proton-density weighting is obtained. The details of creating T1-weighted and T2-weighted contrast are discussed in the section "Conventional two-dimensional spin-echo imaging" in Chapter 2.

SPATIAL LOCALIZATION AND *k* SPACE

The next step, before discussing details of specific MR pulse sequences in the following chapter, is to briefly review the basic concepts of spatial localization and *k* space.

Box 1.4 ESSENTIALS TO REMEMBER

- Following a 90° excitation RF pulse and a subsequent time period during which the transverse magnetization vectors dephase, the application of a 180° refocusing RF pulse rotates the vectors to the opposite side of the transverse plane. Transverse magnetization vectors that dephased faster than others due to field inhomogeneity will also rephase faster, and likewise for those that dephased slower. As a result, the transverse magnetization vectors return to their original orientations and phase coherence is reestablished, forming a spin echo when the time after the 180° RF pulse matches that between the 90° and 180° RF pulses.

- The echo time (TE) is the time between the excitation RF pulse and the formation of the spin echo. The 180° refocusing RF pulse is applied halfway between the excitation RF pulse and the formation of the spin echo (i.e., at ½ of TE).

- Even though formation of the spin echo compensates for inhomogeneity of the magnetic field, the magnitude of the transverse magnetization is reduced at the time of the spin echo (compared to the magnitude immediately after the excitation RF pulse) due to T2 relaxation.

- A single MR acquisition cannot generate contrast based solely on either T1 or T2; instead, images are generated for which the contrast is determined primarily by one of the two parameters. Thus, in general, both T1 and T2 contribute to some extent to the image contrast.

- For a T1-weighted image, contrast from differences among T1 relaxation times of the tissues is emphasized by using a relatively short TR, while that from differences among T2 relaxation times is suppressed by using a short TE. For a T2-weighted image, contrast from differences among T1 relaxation times is suppressed by using a relatively long TR, while that from differences among T2 relaxation times is emphasized by using a relatively long TE.

MAGNETIC-FIELD GRADIENTS

As described above, placing a subject within the static magnetic field of an MRI scanner results in a magnetization vector, associated with the hydrogen nuclei of the water and fat molecules of the body, which, once perturbed from alignment with the field, precesses about the axis of the field with a frequency that is directly proportional to the field strength. For the ideal condition of a perfectly homogeneous static magnetic field, the resonant frequency will be identical for all spatial locations within the subject. However, by purposely superimposing a second, supplementary magnetic field having a strength that varies with spatial location, we can cause the resonant frequency to also vary with spatial location. This spatial variation in the resonant frequency is analogous to that discussed in the context of T2* relaxation, except now we <u>want</u> to achieve different field strengths at different locations, whereas in the case of T2* relaxation there are <u>unwanted</u> variations in field strength with position that result in signal loss. Thus, for the case of the supplementary magnetic field, the resultant dephasing (loss of phase coherence) of the transverse magnetization is both intentional and useful, as described in more detail below.

The supplementary magnetic field is called a *magnetic-field gradient*, and in clinical MRI three orthogonal (along the *x, y,* and *z* axes), linear magnetic-field gradients are used. The term *linear* gradient means that the variation in magnetic-field strength is linearly related to position along the gradient, and the *gradient strength* is the change in field strength per unit of length along the direction of the gradient (Fig. 1.18). Gradient strengths can be positive or negative (Fig. 1.18B), and are typically expressed in either milliTesla per meter (abbreviated mT/m) or Gauss per centimeter (abbreviated G/cm; 1 G/cm = 10 mT/m). For example, an *x* gradient with a strength of +5 mT/m means that the magnetic-field strength varies along the *x* direction and, moving in the positive *x* direction from any given position to a second position, the change in field strength, expressed in milliTesla (one thousandth of a Tesla), divided by the change in position, expressed in meters, equals 5. The maximum gradient strength is an important performance parameter for MRI scanners. State-of-the-art whole-body clinical MRI scanners typically have maximum gradient strengths of at least 40 mT/m.

The magnetic-field gradients used in MRI can be switched on and off as needed. Physically, switching on a gradient corresponds to sending an electric current through a coil of wire mounted in the bore of the MRI scanner magnet. A given application of a magnetic-field gradient, wherein the gradient is switched on, maintained at a selected strength for some period of time (typically a few hundred microseconds to several milliseconds), and then switched off, is called a *gradient pulse* (Fig. 1.18C). With this concept in mind, we can now formally define an MRI *pulse sequence* as the collection of RF pulses, gradient pulses, and data sampling that together generate a particular type of image. The speed of switching of the magnetic-field gradient, commonly called the slew rate, is also an important performance parameter for the MRI scanner. Slew rates are typically expressed in units of mT/m/ms or T/m/s; state-of-the-art whole-body scanners have maximum slew rates of at least 150 mT/m/ms.

Magnetic-field gradients are used to perform spatial localization (i.e., to determine the locations from which the MR signals originate and are measured). Next, we will describe how RF excitation can be localized to a desired *slice* (or *section*) of tissue by using a magnetic-field gradient. Subsequently, we will discuss how the locations of the magnetization vectors within a given slice are determined.

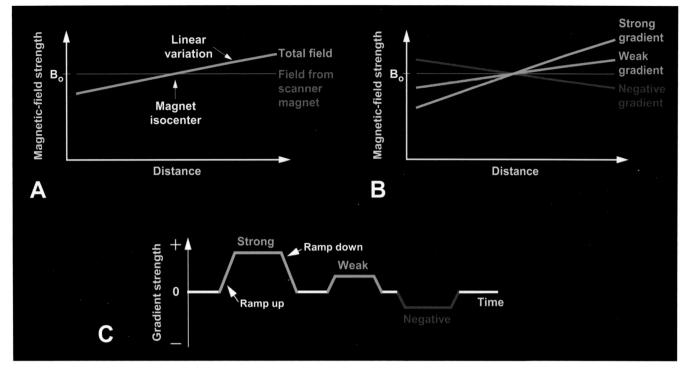

Figure 1.18 *Linear magnetic-field gradients.* (**A**) Plot of magnetic-field strength versus distance during application of a linear magnetic-field gradient. Note that the field strength varies linearly with distance (*bright green line*). At the "isocenter" of the magnet, the applied gradient has no effect on the magnetic-field strength (i.e., the magnetic-field strength at the isocenter equals B_o). (**B**) The slope of the line showing the relationship between magnetic-field strength and distance provides the strength of the magnetic-field gradient; a steeper slope corresponds to a stronger gradient. A positive slope (increasing to the right) corresponds to a positive gradient (*bright-green* and *medium-green lines*), and a negative slope (decreasing to the right) corresponds to a negative gradient (red line). (**C**) A gradient timing diagram is used to illustrate how the strength (slope) and polarity of a magnetic-field gradient change over time. The portions of the gradient waveform labeled "strong," "weak," and "negative" correspond to the three lines shown in **B**. Each of the three colored sections of **C** corresponds to a gradient pulse. In **A** and **B**, the amount of field-strength variation with distance, relative to B_o, is exaggerated for clarity. (Adapted from Mugler JP III. Basic principles. In: Edelman RR, Hesselink JR, Zlatkin MB, Crues JV III, eds. *Clinical Magnetic Resonance Imaging*, 3rd ed. Philadelphia: Saunders Elsevier, 2006.)

SLICE SELECTION

The duration and waveform of an RF pulse determine the range of frequencies (the *transmit bandwidth*) affected by the pulse. As described above, applying a magnetic-field gradient causes the resonant frequency to vary linearly with position along the gradient. Therefore, if an RF pulse is applied simultaneously with a gradient pulse (called the *slice-select* gradient pulse, typically abbreviated G_S or G_{SS}), the RF pulse will affect only those magnetization vectors whose resonant frequencies fall within the transmit bandwidth of the pulse. This means that only a certain slice (section) of the tissue, oriented perpendicular to the direction of the slice-select gradient, is "selected" by the RF pulse (Fig. 1.19). The *slice thickness* is determined by the relationship between the slice-select gradient strength and the transmit bandwidth (Fig. 1.19); the slice thickness can be decreased either by increasing the gradient strength (thus mapping the transmit bandwidth into a smaller range of spatial locations) or by decreasing the transmit bandwidth (requiring a longer RF pulse since bandwidth is inversely proportional to duration). The center frequency of the RF pulse is that which lies at the middle of the transmit bandwidth. Selection of the center frequency determines the *slice position*—the position of the center of the slice along the gradient (Fig. 1.19).

Since MRI scanners include magnetic-field gradients along the x, y, and z directions, a slice can be selected perpendicular to any of these directions by applying the RF pulse in conjunction with the associated gradient. Specifically, applying the RF pulse with the x gradient yields a sagittal slice, with the y gradient yields a coronal slice, or with the z gradient yields a transverse (axial) slice (assuming the subject is either prone or supine on the scanner table). Further, two or three gradients can be switched on simultaneously, permitting a linear magnetic-field gradient to be generated along any selected direction. In this manner, an oblique (angled with respect to the x, y, or z axis) or double-oblique (angled with respect to two coordinate axes) slice can be selected.

The waveform of the RF pulse also determines the spatial uniformity of the effect of the pulse (i.e., the *slice profile*). An RF pulse with an ideal slice profile would provide a uniform flip angle across the thickness of the desired slice, and would have no effect on magnetization outside of this slice (Fig. 1.20A). In contrast, for a realistic slice profile, the flip angle varies to some degree across the thickness of the desired slice, and the RF pulse has some effect (i.e., non-zero flip angle) outside of the slice (Fig. 1.20B). Depending on their severity, these non-ideal features may affect image contrast or create image artifacts. In particular, if the RF pulse affects the magnetization associated

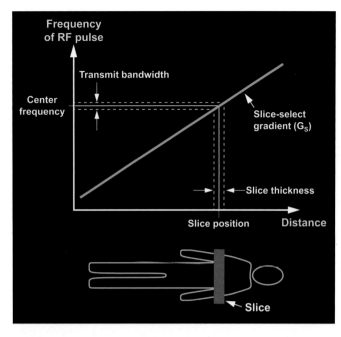

Figure 1.19 *Slice selection.* The image slice is "selected" by applying an RF pulse simultaneously with the slice-select gradient (*green line*, G_s); this gradient establishes a linear relationship between frequency and distance as illustrated in the plot. As a result, the RF pulse affects magnetization only within the slice of interest (*magenta rectangle*). The center frequency of the RF pulse is chosen to yield the desired slice position (*solid yellow line*), and the transmit bandwidth of the RF pulse and the gradient strength (slope) determine the slice thickness (pair of *dashed yellow lines*). (Adapted from Mugler JP III. Basic principles. In: Edelman RR, Hesselink JR, Zlatkin MB, Crues JV III, eds. *Clinical Magnetic Resonance Imaging*, 3rd ed. Philadelphia: Saunders Elsevier, 2006.)

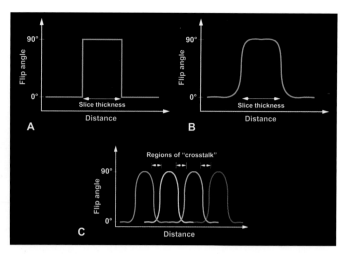

Figure 1.20 *Slice profile and crosstalk.* (**A**) Plot of the flip angle generated by a 90°, slice-selective, excitation RF pulse versus distance perpendicular to the slice for an ideal rectangular slice profile. The flip angle is 90° across the thickness of the slice and zero outside of the slice. (**B**) A realistic slice profile for a slice-selective excitation RF pulse shows that the flip angle varies from the intended value of 90° to zero over a finite distance. In addition, the flip angle is greater than zero beyond the slice thickness, meaning that the RF pulse has an effect on tissue outside of the desired slice. (**C**) When slices are positioned close to one another, the profiles of the slice-selective RF pulses may overlap, as illustrated, which can result in slice-to-slice interference, also known as slice "crosstalk." This interference can cause decreased signal intensities, modified contrast, and other image artifacts. This source of image degradation is one of the reasons that, in clinical practice, gaps between the slices are often used. (Adapted from Mugler JP III. Basic principles. In: Edelman RR, Hesselink JR, Zlatkin MB, Crues JV III, eds. *Clinical Magnetic Resonance Imaging*, 3rd ed. Philadelphia: Saunders Elsevier, 2006.)

with tissues outside of the desired slice, changes in tissue contrast or other artifacts may be generated when slices are acquired relatively close to one another (so-called "crosstalk" between slices, Fig. 1.20C). For this reason, a *slice gap* is often used between adjacent slices. A common method is also to acquire the slices in interleaved order such that odd-numbered slices (1, 3, 5, ...) are obtained first, followed by even-numbered slices (2, 4, 6, ...), effectively creating gaps between consecutively acquired slices that are at least as large as the thickness of the slice. In practice, an improved slice profile comes at the expense of a longer duration of the RF pulse and/or increased power deposited in the subject. As a result, the quality of the slice profile is often sacrificed for a faster acquisition or decreased power deposition.

SPATIAL ENCODING

Once we have selected a slice, it is necessary to determine the locations of the magnetization vectors within this slice by appropriate application of magnetic-field gradients along the two directions orthogonal to that used to define the slice. For purposes of illustration, let us assume that a transverse slice was selected by applying an RF pulse in the presence of a gradient pulse along the z axis. In this case, we will use the x and y gradients to perform *spatial encoding*—that is, to manipulate the magnetization vectors within the slice in a manner that allows us to determine their locations from the MR signals

acquired from the slice. A number of strategies exist for spatial encoding, but we will concentrate on the most common method, which uses *frequency encoding* along one direction (e.g., the x direction) and *phase encoding* along the other (e.g., the y direction).

Frequency encoding

To perform frequency encoding, the MR signal generated by precessing transverse magnetization is recorded, or *sampled*, during the application of a gradient pulse along a selected direction (the x direction for our example), which is termed the frequency-encoding direction. The data-sampling process converts ("digitizes") the MR signal from the subject into a set of numbers (which can be then processed by a computer) using a common electronic device called an analog-to-digital converter (ADC). Since a magnetic-field gradient causes the resonant frequency to vary linearly with position along the gradient, the frequency of the MR signal for any given spatial location is distinct from that for any other spatial location (Fig. 1.21). Thus, the sampled data from the subject contains the sum of all of the different frequencies generated by the associated precessing magnetization vectors. If we can somehow separate the various frequency components of the signal (how to do this is discussed in a subsequent section), the frequency corresponding to a specific component gives the spatial location of that component along the gradient, and the magnitude of the

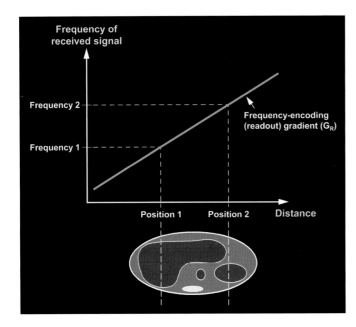

Figure 1.21 *Frequency encoding*. When MR signals are sampled during the application of a linear magnetic-field gradient (frequency-encoding gradient, G_R), the signal from tissues at any given position along the gradient corresponds to a unique frequency. For example, tissues at the location labeled "Position 1" yield a signal at the frequency value labeled "Frequency 1." Thus, the frequency of the signal corresponding to specific tissues gives the spatial location of those tissues along the gradient. (Adapted from Mugler JP III. Basic principles. In: Edelman RR, Hesselink JR, Zlatkin MB, Crues JV III, eds. *Clinical Magnetic Resonance Imaging*, 3rd ed. Philadelphia: Saunders Elsevier, 2006.)

component gives the signal strength, which is proportional to the signal intensity in the image. Therefore, in our example, the frequency-encoding process allows us to determine the signal intensity at each position along the *x* axis (Fig. 1.21).

Ideally, frequency encoding can be performed by simply switching on the frequency-encoding gradient while simultaneously sampling the MR signal. However, due to non-ideal factors that are beyond the scope of our discussion, it is usually necessary to apply a preparatory (sometimes called prephasing) gradient pulse along the same direction prior to application of the frequency-encoding gradient. This preparatory gradient pulse has a polarity that is the opposite of that for the frequency-encoding gradient pulse, and is configured such that the area is approximately half of that for the frequency-encoding gradient pulse (see Fig. 2.9 in Chapter 2, line labeled G_R). At the point during the frequency-encoding gradient pulse when the area under the pulse matches that for the preparatory gradient pulse, the dephasing (loss of phase coherence) caused by the preparatory gradient pulse is *balanced* by the *rephasing* (regaining of phase coherence) caused by the frequency-encoding gradient pulse, leading to the formation of a *gradient echo*. Analogous to the spin-echo case (wherein an echo is generated by an excitation RF pulse followed by a refocusing RF pulse), the point in time at which the echo forms is called the echo time. However, because static field inhomogeneity is not compensated in the case of a gradient echo (i.e., there is no refocusing RF pulse), the amplitude of the gradient echo is determined by T2* decay, not T2 decay.

Since the data are sampled, or *read out*, during the frequency-encoding gradient, this gradient and the corresponding direction are also called the readout gradient and the readout direction, respectively. The frequency-encoding gradient is typically abbreviated G_{FE}, G_R, or G_{RO}.

Phase encoding

To obtain sufficient data to permit calculation of a two-dimensional (2D) MR image, as widely used in clinical MRI, the process of applying an excitation RF pulse and then sampling data during application of the frequency-encoding gradient must be repeated numerous times, wherein, as described below, each repetition corresponds to a distinct value of the phase-encoding gradient. For example, if it is desired to obtain an image that contains 256 points, or *pixels*, along the *x* direction, and 128 pixels along the *y* direction, excitation followed by frequency encoding is repeated 128 times, and for each repetition 256 data points are sampled during the application of the frequency-encoding gradient. Thus the complete set of MR data acquired from the subject (commonly called the raw data or the *k*-space data) is composed of 128 "lines" of samples, each of which includes 256 samples, and likewise the MR image is composed of 256 pixels along the spatial direction that corresponds to the frequency-encoding gradient and 128 pixels along the direction that corresponds to the phase-encoding gradient. For this example, the image is said to have a 256 × 128 *matrix*. Each line of raw (*k*-space) data is often is referred to as a *phase-encoding line* or a *phase-encoding view*.

The phase-encoding process is performed by applying, for each repetition, a gradient pulse that occurs after the excitation RF pulse, with its accompanying slice-select gradient pulse, but before the frequency-encoding gradient pulse (see Fig. 2.9 in Chapter 2, line labeled G_P). The phase-encoding gradient pulse (typically abbreviated G_P or G_{PE}) is configured such that its net effect (the phase accumulated at a given position; see below) on the transverse magnetization changes by a fixed increment between successive repetitions. Since the net effect of a gradient pulse is determined by the area under the gradient waveform (e.g., for a rectangular waveform, this area is the strength of the gradient times the duration of the gradient pulse), the area of the phase-encoding gradient pulse increases by a fixed amount between successive repetitions. This variation of the phase-encoding gradient pulse from repetition to repetition manipulates the transverse magnetization vectors along the phase-encoding direction in exactly the same manner as the frequency-encoding gradient manipulates the transverse magnetization vectors along the frequency-encoding direction. The key difference is that the frequency-encoding gradient performs the desired manipulation of the magnetization vectors in a continuous fashion during the relatively short time it takes to sample each line of raw data (typically 1 to 10 ms), whereas the phase-encoding gradient performs the desired manipulation in an incremental, step-by-step, fashion during the acquisition time for the complete image, which may be up to several minutes. This time difference is why motion artifacts appear along the phase-encoding, but not frequency-encoding, direction: no structure in the human body moves an appreciable amount in a few milliseconds. An example may help to illustrate the equivalence between the fundamental effects of frequency encoding and phase encoding.

Consider a transverse magnetization vector at a specific location along the frequency-encoding gradient whose resonant frequency is increased by 2,500 Hz during the application of the gradient. If data samples are read out every 50 microseconds, this 2,500-Hz frequency increase causes the phase of the transverse magnetization vector to increase by a fixed amount, which happens to be 45° (given by the product of the frequency and the time period), between successive samples. Thus, for this magnetization vector, the effect of the frequency-encoding process is: increase phase by 45°, sample, increase phase by 45°, sample, etc. With reference to any given data sample, the phase change for the magnetization vector at the time of the next data sample is 45°, and at the time of the next data sample after that is 2 × 45°, etc.

Since the phase-encoding gradient is turned on and then off before the data are sampled, the gradient does not affect the resonant frequency <u>during</u> sampling. In contrast, along the direction of the phase-encoding gradient, a given transverse magnetization vector accumulates a change in phase that is proportional to the gradient-pulse area and the position of the vector relative to the magnet isocenter. (The phase-encoding gradient is named as such because its role in the spatial-encoding process is to generate specific changes in the phase of the magnetization vectors.) Since, as described above, the area for the phase-encoding gradient pulse is incremented by a fixed amount between successive lines, the change in phase is also incremented by a fixed amount. For example, consider a transverse magnetization vector located at a specific position along the phase-encoding gradient, analogous to the magnetization vector considered above that was located at a specific location along the frequency-encoding gradient. If, for this second magnetization vector, the change in phase between successive phase-encoding lines is also 45°, then, with reference to any given phase-encoding line, the phase change for the next phase-encoding line is 45°, and for next phase-encoding line after that is 2 × 45°, etc. This is exactly the same pattern described for the frequency-encoding gradient, and therefore the frequency-encoding and phase-encoding gradients manipulate transverse magnetization vectors at corresponding positions along the respective gradients in exactly the same manner. Therefore, for our example, the phase-encoding process allows us to determine the signal intensity at each position along the y axis.

We described above how a preparatory (or prephasing) gradient is generally required before the frequency-encoding gradient pulse is applied. There is an analogous requirement for phase encoding. In the ideal case, the amplitude of the phase-encoding gradient pulse would step from zero to the appropriate maximum value in equally spaced increments. In practice, however, the amplitude of the phase-encoding gradient pulse steps from a negative maximum value, through zero, to a positive maximum value (or vice versa). This stepping of the phase-encoding gradient-pulse amplitude as the pulse sequence repeats is generally illustrated in pulse-sequence diagrams by a series of equally spaced horizontal lines within the overall envelope depicting the gradient pulse. This representation

is often called a *phase-encoding gradient table* (see Fig. 2.9 in Chapter 2, line labeled G_p).

Just as two or more of the x, y, and z gradients can be switched on simultaneously to select a slice with an arbitrary orientation, a combination of these gradients can be used to perform frequency or phase encoding along an arbitrary direction.

Spatial resolution

A critical aspect of the frequency- and phase-encoding processes is the spatial resolution they achieve in the resulting image. Each pixel in an image represents the signal intensity from a volume, or *voxel*, of tissue within the subject. For most purposes, the voxel can be considered to be a rectangular solid (i.e., shaped like a shoebox). The dimensions of this voxel along the frequency-encoding, phase-encoding, and slice-select directions correspond to the spatial resolution, typically stated in millimeters or centimeters, along these directions. For example, a representative spatial resolution for a clinical MR image is 0.8 mm (frequency encoding) by 1.0 mm (phase encoding) by 5.0 mm (slice select). The *field of view*, or size, of the image in either the frequency-encoding or phase-encoding direction is given by the spatial resolution in that direction multiplied by the corresponding number of pixels. The field of view is typically abbreviated as FOV.

The voxel dimension along the frequency-encoding direction is inversely proportional to the area under the frequency-encoding gradient pulse. Therefore, to decrease the voxel dimension (i.e., to achieve "higher" resolution), either the strength of the frequency-encoding gradient pulse or the duration of sampling during the gradient pulse is increased. The relationship for the phase-encoding direction is analogous. The voxel dimension along the slice-select direction (i.e., the slice thickness) is decreased by increasing the slice-select gradient strength or by decreasing the transmit bandwidth of the RF pulse(s), as described above.

EFFECTS OF CHEMICAL SHIFT

In our discussion of spatial localization, we saw that the fundamental effect of applying a magnetic-field gradient (i.e., causing the resonant frequency to vary linearly with position along the gradient) was used to perform slice selection and frequency encoding. It is important to note that any factor other than the applied gradient that causes a variation in resonant frequency with position will interfere with the slice-selection or frequency-encoding process. Such a factor of particular relevance in clinical MRI is the *chemical shift* difference between the hydrogen nuclei in water-containing tissues and those in fat tissues.

The resonant frequency of a hydrogen nucleus is determined by the static magnetic field that it experiences. The electrons in the molecule containing the hydrogen nucleus partially "shield" it from the applied static magnetic field and, as a result, the field strength experienced by the nucleus is slightly modified, or "shifted," compared to the field that is applied. Since this effect depends on the chemical structure of the molecule, the associated change in the resonant frequency is called the chemical shift. Chemical shifts are typically expressed in parts per million (abbreviated ppm); a chemical shift expressed in ppm is independent of the applied field strength. Since the hydrogen nuclei in water and fat molecules are shielded by different amounts, they have different chemical shifts and thus different resonant frequencies. (The hydrogen nuclei in fat are more shielded than those in water, and thus the resonant frequency for fat is lower.) The chemical shift difference between water and fat is approximately 3.5 ppm, which corresponds to about 224 Hz at 1.5T.

For slice selection, the difference in resonant frequency between hydrogen nuclei in water-containing tissues and those in fat causes a shift in the slice position for water-containing tissues relative to that for fat. For example, if an RF pulse is chosen to select a 10-mm-thick slice at a position of 20 mm, the RF pulse may excite hydrogen nuclei in water-containing tissues between positions 15 mm and 25 mm, in contrast to exciting hydrogen nuclei in fat between positions 14 mm and 24 mm. The relative shift between the water and fat slices depends on the characteristics of the RF pulse. In practice the shift is often negligible, but can nonetheless become significant for certain pulse-sequence techniques. For frequency encoding, the difference in resonant frequency causes an artifactual (i.e., not real) displacement in the image between structures containing water and those containing fat. That is, fat tissue appears slightly shifted relative to water-containing tissue along the frequency-encoding direction. As a result, at interfaces between water-containing tissues and fat, a band of increased signal intensity is seen where the tissues appear to overlap and a band of no signal is seen on the opposite side (see Fig. 2.31 in Chapter 2). The bright or dark bands run generally perpendicular to the frequency-encoding direction, since the apparent shift is parallel to this direction. This *chemical-shift artifact* (sometimes called a Type 1 chemical-shift artifact) increases with static magnetic-field strength (because the frequency difference expressed in Hz scales with field strength) and with the sampling time for the echo. The artifact can be essentially eliminated by using one of the standard approaches for selectively suppressing the signal from fat, as discussed next.

Fat-signal suppression

Fat often displays one of the highest signal intensities in an MR image, and, due to this high signal, may detract from the evaluation of lower-intensity tissues of interest. In addition, the resonant-frequency (chemical shift) difference between fat and water-containing tissues may lead to undesirable artifacts as discussed in the preceding section. Thus, it is often desirable to suppress the signal from fat. There are two common approaches for achieving this goal; the first is based on the chemical-shift difference between fat and water, and the second is based on the relatively short T1 relaxation time of fat.

At moderate to high magnetic-field strengths (i.e., at approximately 1T and above), the resonant-frequency difference between fat and water-containing tissues is sufficiently large that appropriately designed RF pulses can be used to manipulate the fat magnetization while leaving the water magnetization unaffected. Such RF pulses are often referred to as CHESS (chemical-shift selective) pulses. A common approach for suppressing the

signal from fat is to apply a 90° CHESS RF pulse, followed by gradient pulse to "spoil" the resulting transverse magnetization, just before each excitation RF pulse for the pulse sequence of interest. The strength and duration for the spoiling gradient pulse are chosen such that the transverse magnetization from fat is dephased substantially and thus does not contribute significantly to signals acquired during the pulse sequence. Since the 90° CHESS RF pulse is applied immediately before the excitation RF pulse, there is little time for T1 relaxation between the two RF pulses, and thus the longitudinal magnetization associated with fat is close to zero when the excitation RF pulse is applied. As a result, the signal from fat will be close to zero in the resulting image (see Fig. 2.26 in Chapter 2 for a comparison of images with and without fat suppression). This method of suppressing the signal from fat is called chemical-shift selective fat saturation, or fat saturation, or simply *ChemSat* or *FatSat*.

A refinement of the FatSat method is to use a flip angle higher than 90° for the CHESS RF pulse, chosen based on the time period between the CHESS and excitation RF pulses, such that the longitudinal magnetization for fat is relaxing through zero (as discussed in the section "Longitudinal magnetization and T1 relaxation") when the excitation RF pulse is applied. A particular implementation of this concept uses an *adiabatic* 180° CHESS RF pulse. An adiabatic RF pulse is one specially designed to produce the desired flip angle in the presence of non-ideal variations in the strength of the time-varying magnetic field induced by the RF pulse. Another common variation of the general chemical-shift selective approach is to use a *water-excitation* RF pulse instead of a fat-saturation RF pulse. In this case, the excitation RF pulse for the pulse sequence is designed to excite the water magnetization while leaving the fat magnetization unaffected. Likewise, although not as commonly used, one can take advantage of the chemical-shift difference between water and fat to selectively suppress the signal from water-containing tissues, resulting in images that show only fat.

The second common approach for suppressing the signal from fat is based on the fact that, for many applications, the T1 relaxation time for fat is substantially shorter than that for all other tissues of interest. We can take advantage of this fact to suppress fat by simply applying an inversion RF pulse before each excitation RF pulse for the pulse sequence of interest, and choosing the time between the inversion and excitation RF pulses (often called the <u>t</u>ime to <u>i</u>nversion, abbreviated TI) such that the longitudinal magnetization for fat is relaxing through zero when the excitation RF pulse is applied. As a result, fat produces no signal in the resulting image. (This approach is similar to that discussed above with regard to the adiabatic 180° CHESS RF pulse, except here the inversion RF pulse affects the magnetization associated with all tissues, not just that associated with fat.) Since fat has a relatively short T1 relaxation time, the TI value required for this approach is also relatively short. This led to the common name for the approach, STIR, which stands for <u>s</u>hort <u>TI</u> <u>i</u>nversion <u>r</u>ecovery. Since STIR is based on the T1 relaxation time for fat and not its resonant frequency, it can also be used at relatively low magnetic-field strengths where the resonant-frequency difference between fat and water-containing tissues is too small to permit chemical-shift selective suppression of fat.

A general disadvantage of using either CHESS RF pulses or STIR RF pulses to suppress the signal from fat is that additional time is required for these events within the pulse sequence. Depending on the specific application and the nature of the underlying pulse sequence, this may translate to anywhere from a minor to a substantial increase in acquisition time. Further, these additional RF pulses increase the power deposition (i.e., specific absorption rate or SAR, which quantifies potential tissue heating caused by RF pulses) for the pulse sequence, which may be particularly problematic at relatively high magnetic-field strengths (3T or higher).

Fat suppression is often used in abdominal imaging. In T1-weighted images, fat suppression is particularly useful with contrast-agent (gadolinium) enhancement as it greatly increases the contrast between fat and gadolinium-enhanced tissues, which, because of their short T1, can sometimes look remarkably similar to fat on images without fat suppression. In T2-weighted images, fat suppression can be helpful for detecting edema or fluid within fat, such as in the mesenteric fat. This is particularly true when fast T2-weighted techniques such as FSE/TSE methods are used in which the fat signal can be relatively strong (see section "Fast T2-weighted imaging" in Chapter 2 and Fig. 2.22). The downside of using fat suppression in T2-weighted imaging is that the contours of organs, such as the liver and pancreas, may become less clear as these structures can also appear relatively dark in the image, and this can sometimes lead to difficulty in interpretation.

Another advantage of using of fat suppression is that it diminishes "ghost" artifacts (i.e., replicas of a moving structure or portion of the structure, displaced from the actual structure along the phase-encoding direction) from breathing (see Fig. 2.26 in Chapter 2). These ghosts are particularly prominent when the signal intensity associated with the moving structures is high, such as with subcutaneous fat. Thus, suppression of the fat signal greatly reduces these breathing artifacts. For additional details, see the section "Artifacts" in Chapter 2.

THE FOURIER TRANSFORM AND k SPACE

In our discussion of the frequency-encoding process, we noted that each line of raw data acquired from the subject contains the sum of all of the different frequencies generated by the associated precessing magnetization vectors, and that we need to separate the various frequency components of the signal to determine the signal intensity at each position along the frequency-encoding direction. This separation of the frequency components is performed using a mathematical tool called the *Fourier transform*. To help understand what the Fourier transform does, we can use the example of sunlight refracted by a glass prism, or by raindrops in the atmosphere, to form a rainbow. The prism or raindrop in essence physically performs a Fourier transform, letting us see the various frequencies of electromagnetic radiation, and thus the various colors, of which white light is composed (Fig. 1.22A).

Given the raw data from the subject as a function of time as input to the Fourier transform, the corresponding frequency components at a number of equally spaced frequencies are obtained. For example, if a line of raw data from the subject contains 256 samples recorded over a period of 10 ms, the Fourier transform yields 256 frequency components spaced 100 Hz apart; the frequency separation is simply the reciprocal of the data-sampling time (10 ms; 1/10 ms = 100 Hz). Recall, as noted in the description of frequency encoding, that the frequency corresponding to a specific component gives the spatial location of that component along the gradient, and the magnitude of the component gives the signal strength, which is proportional to the signal intensity in the image. The correspondence between frequency and position is determined by the strength of the frequency-encoding gradient applied during sampling. For our example, if the gradient strength is 5 mT/m, which corresponds to a frequency change of approximately 200 Hz/mm (given by the product of the gradient strength and the gyromagnetic ratio), then 100 Hz corresponds to 0.5 mm (i.e., the spatial resolution in the frequency-encoding direction). In practical terms, the Fourier transform is implemented as an optimized computer program on the image-calculation computer of the MRI scanner. This optimized implementation is called a fast Fourier transform, often abbreviated FFT.

We just described how the raw data acquired from the subject (a series of signals at different points in time) are related to the MR image data (a series of signals at different frequencies) through the mathematical process called a Fourier transform. In this context, the raw data acquired from the subject are said to exist in the "time domain," while the MR image data are said to exist in the "frequency domain." Thus, the Fourier transform provides the correspondence between the data in the time

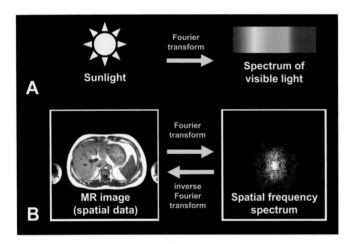

Figure 1.22 *The Fourier transform provides the frequency components contained in a signal.* (**A**) When sunlight is refracted by raindrops in the atmosphere to form a rainbow, the raindrops in essence physically perform a Fourier transform, letting us see the various frequencies of electromagnetic radiation, and thus various colors, of which sunlight is composed. (**B**) An MR image is composed of a collection of spatial intensity variations. The image's spatial-frequency (k-space) spectrum specifies the amplitudes, orientations, and spatial frequencies of these intensity variations. Because the signals acquired from a subject during MR imaging are the k-space components of the image, the image itself is obtained by applying an inverse Fourier transform. (Adapted from Mugler JP III. Basic principles. In: Edelman RR, Hesselink JR, Zlatkin MB, Crues JV III, eds. *Clinical Magnetic Resonance Imaging*, 3rd ed. Philadelphia: Saunders Elsevier, 2006.)

domain and those in the frequency domain, and time and frequency are said to be a Fourier transform "pair."

There is an alternative, and very useful, way to view the relationship between the raw and image data. Since the MR image is a collection of signal intensities at various positions in space, the MR image can be considered to be data in the "spatial domain." The corresponding Fourier transform partner for the spatial domain is the spatial-frequency domain; spatial frequency is commonly abbreviated by the letter *k*, and thus the spatial-frequency domain is called *k space*. In this context, the raw data acquired from the subject are the spatial frequency (*k* space) spectrum corresponding to the MR image; the MR image is thus obtained from the raw data by applying an inverse Fourier transform (Fig. 1.22B).

Viewing the raw data acquired from the subject as *k*-space data is very important in MRI because the established properties of the Fourier transform can be used to understand essential relationships between the timing and order of data sampling, and the resulting signal and contrast properties of the image. In this context, it is important to remember that each data point in *k* space corresponds to information for the complete image, as illustrated in Figure 1.23. As an example of the utility of the *k*-space framework for describing MR images, consider the behavior of a rapid MRI method (e.g., fast or turbo spin echo imaging, as discussed in Chapter 2) for which the

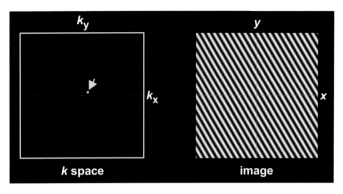

Figure 1.23 *Each data point in k space corresponds to information for the entire image.* The *k* space shown on the left contains a single spatial-frequency component (*yellow dot*, indicated by *arrow*). The image on the right, obtained using an inverse Fourier transform, corresponds to this single spatial-frequency component. We see a signal-intensity oscillation that spans the entire image. The frequency and orientation of the signal-intensity oscillation corresponding to a spatial-frequency component are determined by the distance of the component from the center of *k* space (the frequency increases with distance from the center of *k* space) and the position of the component relative to the *k*-space axes (a component lying off the axes, as shown on the left in this example, corresponds to a signal-intensity oscillation that propagates at an angle relative to the *x* and *y* axes), respectively. (Adapted from Mugler JP III. Basic principles. In: Edelman RR, Hesselink JR, Zlatkin MB, Crues JV III, eds. *Clinical Magnetic Resonance Imaging*, 3rd ed. Philadelphia: Saunders Elsevier, 2006.)

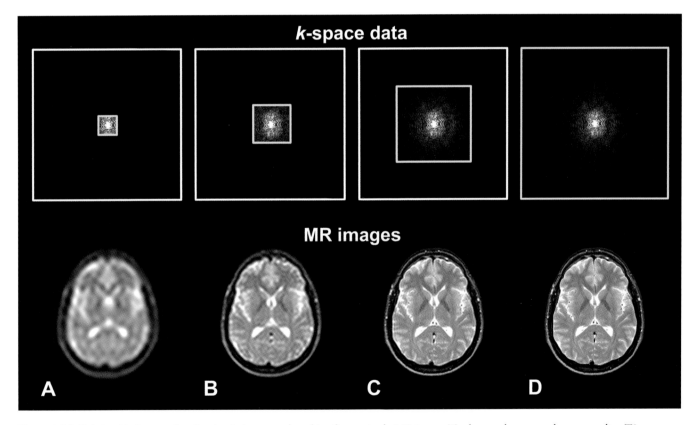

Figure 1.24 *Relationship between data location in k space and resulting features in the MR image.* The *k*-space data sets and corresponding T2-weighted MR images of the brain are shown for (**A**) the central 32 × 32 data values in *k* space, (**B**) the central 64 × 64 data values in *k* space, (**C**) the central 128 × 128 data values in *k* space, and (**D**) the complete 256 × 256 data set. In **A**–**C**, the *white squares* mark the extent of *k* space for the 256 × 256 data set, and the *yellow squares* enclose the *k*-space data used to calculate the corresponding images. As demonstrated in **A**, the data in the central portion of *k* space (low spatial-frequency components) primarily determine the contrast and gross structure in the image. As higher spatial-frequency components are added, proceeding from **B** to **D**, the sharpness (spatial resolution) of the images improves, because the high spatial-frequency components primarily describe the detailed structure of the image.

Box 1.5 ESSENTIALS TO REMEMBER

- Magnetic-field gradients are used to (1) select an image slice by localizing the effects of the RF pulses to the desired section of tissue, and (2) perform spatial encoding (i.e., determine the locations from which the MR signals from the slice originate).

- The *slice thickness* is determined by the relationship between the slice-select gradient strength and the RF-pulse transmit bandwidth; the slice thickness can be decreased either by increasing the gradient strength or by decreasing the transmit bandwidth.

- The effect of an RF pulse used for slice selection is not perfectly confined to the thickness of the selected slice; the RF pulse also affects tissues immediately adjacent to the slice, resulting in some signal from those tissues. This may lead to image artifacts if slices are acquired close to one another. A gap between slices is therefore often included to avoid these artifacts.

- Determination of the location of the signals within a slice (spatial encoding) is done most commonly by using differences in frequency among the transverse magnetization vectors in one direction (*frequency encoding*), and differences in phase in the perpendicular direction (*phase encoding*).

- Frequency encoding typically occurs in a much shorter time (usually 1 to 10 ms, during the brief period that each line of raw data is sampled) than phase encoding (which may span several minutes as it occurs in a step-by-step fashion during the full acquisition time of the image). This is why motion artifacts are much more likely to occur in the phase-encoding direction than in the frequency-encoding direction.

- The chemical shift expressed in parts per million (ppm) is independent of the applied field strength and depends on the chemical structure of the molecule. The chemical shift difference between hydrogen nuclei in water and fat is approximately 3.5 ppm, which corresponds to about 224 Hz at 1.5T. Since chemical shift is determined by differences in resonant frequency, signal misregistration artifacts related to chemical shift appear in the frequency-encoding direction.

- There are two common approaches for fat suppression. One is based on the chemical-shift, and hence frequency, difference between hydrogen nuclei in fat and those in water, and uses a frequency-selective RF pulse followed by a spoiler gradient to excite and then dephase the transverse magnetization from fat so that it does not contribute signal. The other makes use of the relatively short T1 relaxation time of fat by applying an inversion RF pulse before each excitation RF pulse, and choosing an inversion time such that the longitudinal magnetization for fat is relaxing through zero and, hence, generates no signal when the excitation RF pulse is applied.

- The Fourier transform is used to separate the various frequency components of the raw data acquired from a subject.

- The data in the central portion of *k* space (low spatial-frequency components) primarily determines the contrast and gross structure in the image; the data in the outer regions of *k* space (high spatial-frequency components) primarily describe the detailed structure (sharpness) of the image.

signal strength for a given tissue relative to that for another tissue changes as the acquisition proceeds. Since the image contrast is determined by the differences in signal intensities among tissues, what is the contrast in the corresponding image? From the Fourier transform relationship between the *k*-space domain (i.e., the raw data acquired from the subject) and the spatial domain (i.e., the MR image), we know that the data in the central portion of *k* space (the so-called low spatial-frequency components) primarily determines the contrast and gross structure in the image (Fig. 1.24A). Therefore, the relative signal strengths for the tissues that exist when the lines of data are sampled corresponding to the central region of *k* space primarily determine the contrast for the image. Another important relationship is that the data in the outer regions of *k* space (the so-called high spatial-frequency components) primarily describe the detailed structure (sharpness) of the image (Fig. 1.24B–D), although these data also contribute to the image contrast for detailed features in the image. Thus, if the high spatial-frequency components are attenuated relative to those in the central region of *k* space, the details will be suppressed, or, stated another way, the image will be blurred. There are a number of other Fourier-transform relationships that permit us to understand various image properties and artifacts. While these are beyond the scope

of our current discussion, additional information can be found in the MRI literature.

The order in which the raw data are sampled, as viewed in the *k*-space domain, determines the *k-space trajectory* for the pulse sequence. Many clinical MRI techniques use a simple *k*-space trajectory whereby the data are sampled sequentially, line by line, moving from one extreme of *k* space to the opposite extreme. When nothing changes during data sampling (i.e., if the anatomy is stationary and the signal strengths are the same for every line of raw data), the resulting image is unaffected by the choice of *k*-space trajectory. However, if something does change, such as the relative signal strengths as described for the example in the preceding paragraph, then the *k*-space trajectory is critical in determining the properties of the resulting image. We will see this latter case for the fast T2-weighted techniques used for body imaging, discussed in Chapter 2.

REFERENCE

1. Mugler JP III. Chapter 2: Basic principles. In: Edelman RR, Hesselink JR, Zlatkin MB, Crues JV III, eds. *Clinical Magnetic Resonance Imaging,* 3rd ed. Philadelphia: Saunders Elsevier, 2006:23–57.

2.

MR ACQUISITION TECHNIQUES & PRACTICAL CONSIDERATIONS FOR ABDOMINAL IMAGING

Eduard E. de Lange, MD and John P. Mugler, III, PhD

In this chapter we will discuss commonly used pulse sequences for clinical abdominal imaging, focusing on those techniques that can be completed within the duration of a breath hold. However, to understand why certain pulse-sequence techniques are preferable over others with respect to acquiring images with relatively few breathing artifacts, we begin our review with conventional 2D, multislice spin-echo imaging to lay the foundation for subsequent discussion of techniques that are of particular relevance to abdominal MRI because of their short acquisition times. We will then review some of the major factors that contribute to the appearance of blood flow in vessels, and conclude the chapter with a review of several practical issues that are important to consider when performing abdominal MR imaging. The first practical issue we discuss is common image artifacts, including those related to motion and flow, aliasing or wraparound, and magnetic susceptibility, and those associated with gadolinium-containing contrast agents. We then describe briefly the appearances of hemorrhage and hematoma in MR images. At the end of the chapter we provide an overview of the effects of changing common imaging parameters, and finish with a listing of the pulse sequences used in most of the abdominal MR imaging protocols performed at our institution.

ACQUISITION TECHNIQUES

CONVENTIONAL 2D SPIN-ECHO IMAGING

Before discussing how images with T1-weighted and T2-weighted contrast are acquired, we need to first review the principles of standard single-echo, spin-echo imaging, referring to the *pulse-sequence timing diagram* shown in Figure 2.1A. Such timing diagrams show the temporal order of events used in a given pulse sequence.[1]

The diagram in Figure 2.1A for a T1-weighted spin-echo pulse sequence combines the following concepts discussed in Chapter 1: formation of a spin echo by using a 90° excitation RF pulse followed by a 180° refocusing RF pulse (RF pulses on the first line of Fig. 2.1A, spin-echo signal on the fifth line), slice selection (RF pulses on the first line applied together with slice-select gradients on the second line), spatial encoding based on phase encoding (gradient-pulse table on the third line) and frequency encoding (gradient pulses on the fourth line), and data sampling (sixth line). However, there are two aspects of the pulse-sequence timing diagram that we did not discuss in Chapter 1. First, on the line depicting the slice-select gradient pulses, there is a negative gradient pulse applied just after the slice-select gradient pulse for the 90° excitation RF pulse. As the excitation RF pulse tips longitudinal magnetization toward the transverse plane, the magnetization dephases across the thickness of the slice because the slice-select gradient causes the frequency of precession to vary along the direction of the gradient. If no action were taken to compensate for this effect, the resulting signal after the excitation RF pulse would be very small due to this dephasing. The negative gradient pulse, often called the *slice-select rephasing* gradient, corrects for this dephasing so that the full signal strength is obtained. Second, for the frequency-encoding gradients, the prephasing gradient (which occurs between the 90° and 180° RF pulses) is positive, instead of being negative as was the case

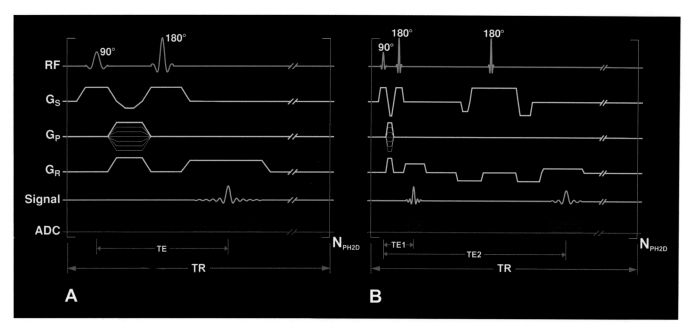

Figure 2.1 *Timing diagrams for (A) single-echo and (B) dual-echo spin-echo pulse sequences.* The first line of each diagram (in green) shows the radiofrequency (RF) pulses applied in each repetition of the respective pulse sequences. A 90° excitation RF pulse is followed by a single 180° refocusing RF pulse for the single-echo pulse sequence, generating a single spin-echo as illustrated on the fifth line (in cyan) of the diagram, whereas two 180° refocusing RF pulses follow the excitation RF pulse for the dual-echo pulse sequence, resulting in two spin echoes. The second, third, and fourth lines (in yellow) illustrate application of the slice-select (G_S), phase-encoding (G_P), and frequency-encoding (G_R) gradients, respectively, as discussed in the section "Spatial localization and *k* space" in Chapter 1. The slice-select and frequency-encoding gradients for the dual-echo pulse sequence look somewhat different than those for the single-echo pulse sequence because the dual-echo pulse sequence incorporates the *flow compensation* method to help suppress motion artifacts and signal loss from motion and flow. The last line of the diagrams (in magenta) shows when the analog-to-digital converter, or ADC, is turned on to sample the echo signals. The dual-echo pulse sequence uses a relatively short sampling time for the first echo (TE1) to achieve a short echo time for the first image, and a relatively long sampling time for the second echo (TE2) to provide increased signal-to-noise ratio for the second image. TR, the repetition time, is the time interval between equivalent points in successive repetitions of the basic timing events for the pulse sequence (for example, the time between 90° RF pulses in successive repetitions). The label N_{PH2D} denotes the number of times that the basic timing events for the pulse sequence are repeated and equals the number of phase-encoding steps for these conventional spin-echo pulse sequences. (Adapted from Mugler JP III. Basic principles. In: Edelman RR, Hesselink JR, Zlatkin MB, Crues JV III, eds. *Clinical Magnetic Resonance Imaging*, 3rd ed. Philadelphia: Saunders Elsevier, 2006.)

when the concept of the prephasing gradient was introduced in the section "Frequency encoding" in Chapter 1. The effect of a gradient pulse is reversed by a refocusing RF pulse. Thus, a positive gradient pulse occurring before the 180° refocusing RF pulse is equivalent to a negative gradient pulse occurring after the RF pulse.

Next, let us review how T1-weighted and T2-weighted contrast can be generated using this spin-echo pulse sequence. As described in Chapter 1, T1-weighted contrast is generated by using a short TR and a short TE. To understand how these parameter values yield the desired tissue contrast for a given spin echo, we must consider first what happens in the pulse-sequence repetition that immediately precedes the repetition in which the spin echo of interest is acquired. Just after the 90° excitation RF pulse for this preceding repetition, the longitudinal components of the magnetization for all tissues are zero, after which they begin to relax (recover) toward thermal equilibrium at different rates as determined by the T1 relaxation times of the tissues, as illustrated in Figure 2.2. For T1 weighting, a TR is chosen so that tissues with relatively short T1 values are allowed to recover substantially toward their respective thermal equilibrium values, whereas tissues with relatively long T1 values recover much less. (This condition essentially

defines the TR as being "short.") When the next 90° excitation RF pulse is applied to convert longitudinal magnetization to transverse magnetization, relatively large transverse magnetization values, and hence signals, are generated for tissues with short T1 values, while the opposite occurs for tissues with long T1 values. (Remember that the magnitude of the transverse magnetization immediately following a 90° excitation RF pulse is equal to that of the longitudinal magnetization immediately before the pulse.) Thus, when the signals are sampled, as soon as possible after the 90° excitation RF pulse (i.e., when the TE is chosen to be as short as possible), a relatively small amount of decay of transverse magnetization occurs between the excitation RF pulse and sampling of the signals. Thus, the image contrast is determined primarily by differences in T1 values, with short T1 values yielding high signal and long T1 values yielding low signal, and the contributions from T2 decay are minimal (Fig. 2.2). In practice, a T1-weighted spin-echo acquisition at 1.5T is typically performed using a TR of 500 to 1,000 ms and a TE of 10 to 15 ms.

As discussed in Chapter 1 and illustrated in Figure 2.1A, each 90° excitation RF pulse in a spin-echo pulse sequence is followed by a 180° refocusing RF pulse, applied midway between the excitation RF pulse and the echo time. This 180°

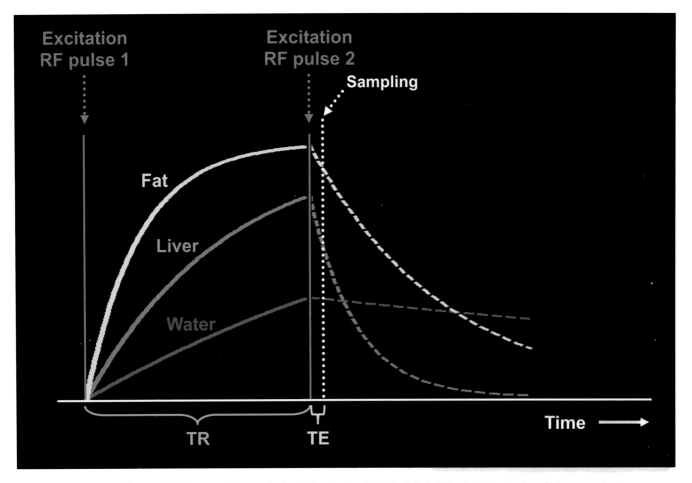

Figure 2.2 *Generation of T1-weighted contrast.* Prior to the first 90° excitation RF pulse (labeled "Excitation RF pulse 1") the magnetization vectors of all tissues are at thermal equilibrium, aligned with the longitudinal axis of the main field. When the pulse is applied, the magnetization vectors are rotated to the transverse plane and thus the longitudinal components become zero. Just after Excitation RF pulse 1, the longitudinal components of the magnetization vectors (fat, liver, and water depicted by *solid yellow, orange, and blue lines*, respectively) begin to recover toward thermal equilibrium at different rates as determined by the T1 relaxation times of the tissues. When the longitudinal components have recovered to the degree that reflects the desired contrast for the image, a second 90° excitation RF pulse (labeled "Excitation RF pulse 2") is applied at time TR (repetition time); this pulse converts the partially recovered longitudinal magnetization of the tissues to transverse magnetization, and brings the longitudinal components of the magnetization vectors back again to zero. Since the magnitude of transverse magnetization immediately following a 90° excitation RF pulse is equal to that of the associated longitudinal magnetization immediately before the pulse, tissues whose longitudinal magnetization had recovered most toward thermal equilibrium due to a short T1 value (such as fat) have relatively large transverse magnetization values, whereas tissues having a long T1 value (such as water) have relatively small transverse magnetization values. The transverse components of the magnetization vectors (depicted for fat, liver, and water by *dashed yellow, orange, and blue lines*, respectively) begin to decay due to T2 relaxation immediately following Excitation RF pulse 2; at the time of the spin echo this decay will reflect the respective T2 values. If the MR signals generated by the transverse components of the magnetization are sampled (shown as the *dotted white line*) as soon as possible after this RF pulse is applied, at time TE (echo time) after the pulse, relatively little decay of the transverse magnetization will have occurred and the MR signal from each tissue corresponds primarily to the magnitude of the longitudinal magnetization vectors immediately before Excitation RF pulse 2. Thus, in the image, the signal intensities of the tissues mostly reflect the differences in the longitudinal components of the magnetization vectors, which occur due to differences among T1 values, with little contribution from differences among T2 values. Hence, a T1-weighted image is obtained.

Notes: 1. Transverse magnetization is also generated by Excitation RF pulse 1; however, since the longitudinal magnetization vectors of all tissues were at thermal equilibrium prior to this pulse, the transverse magnetization vectors after this first RF pulse do not reflect the desired T1-weighted contrast, and are therefore omitted from the diagram for simplicity. For the same reason, data are not sampled following Excitation RF pulse 1.

2. Following Excitation RF pulse 2, the longitudinal components of the magnetization vectors also begin to recover, just as after Excitation RF pulse 1. However, for simplicity, these longitudinal components are omitted from the diagram since they do not contribute to the MR signals generated by the transverse magnetization vectors resulting from Excitation RF pulse 1.

3. In a spin-echo pulse sequence, a 180° refocusing RF pulse is applied after each 90° excitation RF pulse to create the echo, which occurs at twice the time between the 90° and 180° RF pulses. Sampling of the MR signals is performed at the time of the echo. The 180° refocusing RF pulse is applied to compensate for dephasing of transverse magnetization due to unwanted spatial variations in the magnetic-field strength, and hence the signal decay is governed by T2 as opposed to T2*. However, the 180° pulse is not essential for sampling of the MR signals, and therefore, for simplicity, the pulse and its effects on the evolution of the magnetization vectors are not depicted in the figure. The effect of the 180° pulse on longitudinal magnetization is negligible when TR is much larger than TE.

4. For clarity, the curves for the longitudinal and transverse magnetization are displayed at different time scales; in reality, the transverse magnetization curves decay more quickly than shown as the T2 values are much shorter than the T1 values as shown in Figure 1.14.

5. Any differences in proton (spin) densities among tissues are neglected.

RF pulse, which rotates transverse magnetization to the opposite side of the transverse plane, is applied to compensate for unwanted spatial variations in magnetic field strength; however, this pulse is not essential for sampling of the signals. Although the purpose of the 180° refocusing RF pulse is to rotate the transverse magnetization to the opposite side of the transverse plane, it also affects any longitudinal magnetization that exists when the pulse is applied, inverting it to point along the negative *z* axis, after which the longitudinal magnetization again begins to relax toward thermal equilibrium. The effect of the 180° refocusing RF pulse on the overall evolution of longitudinal magnetization is negligible because TE is typically many times shorter than TR in a T1-weighted spin-echo pulse sequence. As a result, at the end of the repetition time, the net recovery of longitudinal magnetization is nearly equal to that which would have occurred without the refocusing RF pulse.

The framework just described for T1 weighting also applies to the generation of T2 weighting, except that a long TR and a long TE are required, as described in the section "T1-weighted and T2-weighted contrast" in Chapter 1. For TR, "long" means that the time period is sufficient to allow all tissues to recover substantially toward their respective thermal equilibrium values, regardless of the corresponding T1 values, thereby suppressing contributions to contrast associated with differences among T1 values. For TE, "long" means that the transverse magnetization decays substantially for tissues with relatively short T2 values, whereas little to moderate decay occurs for tissues with relatively long T2 values. The final result is that the image contrast is determined primarily by differences in T2 values, with long T2 values yielding high signal and short T2 values yielding low signal (Fig. 2.3). In practice, a T2-weighted spin-echo acquisition at 1.5T

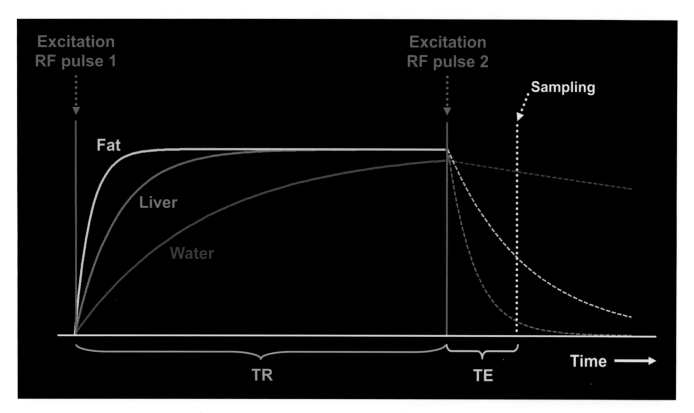

Figure 2.3 *Generation of T2-weighted contrast.* The longitudinal magnetization vectors of all tissues are rotated to the transverse plane by the first 90° excitation RF pulse (Excitation RF pulse 1) and the longitudinal components become zero, as described for a T1-weighted image. However, to suppress T1 contributions to contrast in the image, the longitudinal components of the magnetization vectors (fat, liver, and water depicted by *solid yellow, orange, and blue lines,* respectively) are allowed to recover substantially more than for a T1-weighted image. Thus, the longitudinal magnetization of most tissues approaches thermal equilibrium and, consequently, differences among the longitudinal magnetization vectors for the tissues become small. When the second 90° excitation RF pulse (Excitation RF pulse 2) is then applied at time TR, longitudinal magnetization of the tissues is converted to transverse magnetization, and the longitudinal components of the magnetization vectors are brought back again to zero. However, because the magnitude of the longitudinal magnetization immediately before Excitation RF pulse 2 is approximately the same for all tissues, the magnitudes of the transverse magnetization vectors immediately after this pulse will also be approximately the same. Just after the RF pulse, the transverse components of the magnetization vectors (depicted for fat, liver, and water by *dashed yellow, orange, and blue lines,* respectively) decay as determined by the T2 relaxation times of the tissues. Subsequently, the MR signals generated by the transverse components of the magnetization vectors are sampled (shown as the *dotted white line*) at time TE when the transverse magnetization vectors have decayed to the degree that reflects the desired image contrast. Differences among the magnitudes of the MR signals from the tissues correspond primarily to differences in the amount of decay that has occurred for the corresponding transverse magnetization, since the magnitudes of the longitudinal magnetization vectors just before Excitation RF pulse 2 were similar. Consequently, in the image, the signal intensities primarily reflect differences among T2 values, with relatively little contribution from differences among T1 values. Hence, a T2-weighted image is obtained. (The notes provided for Fig. 2.2 also apply to this figure.)

typically uses a TR value of 2,500 ms or greater and a TE value of about 100 ms.

In the section "Spin echoes" in Chapter 1, we noted that multiple echoes can be generated following an excitation RF pulse by simply applying multiple refocusing RF pulses. This creates a series of spin echoes, each with a different TE. For example, Figure 2.1B shows the timing diagram for a dual-echo spin-echo pulse sequence. From a pulse-sequence perspective, the number of echoes following each excitation RF pulse is limited only by the number of refocusing RF pulses and associated spatial-encoding gradient pulses that fit within TR. From a practical perspective, however, the number of echoes is limited by the relaxation times of the tissues; it is not useful to continue sampling data once the signal has decayed to essentially zero. Nonetheless, since the TR, and not the TE,

determines the acquisition time (as discussed in more detail below), sampling multiple spin echoes does not increase the acquisition time. (Strategies for using multiple spin echoes to speed up imaging are discussed later in the chapter.) For spin-echo imaging using a long TR, multiple spin echoes permit images with varying degrees of T2 weighting to be obtained from the same acquisition, as illustrated in Figure 2.4. For instance, if our pulse sequence includes three refocusing RF pulses after each excitation RF pulse to generate spin echoes at 20 ms, 100 ms, and 200 ms, we will obtain three images. The first image (TE = 20 ms) has relatively weak T2 weighting, the second image (TE = 100 ms) moderate T2 weighting, and the last image (TE = 200 ms) relatively strong T2 weighting. For this implementation of multiple spin-echo imaging, the phase-encoding gradient pulse is applied once during each

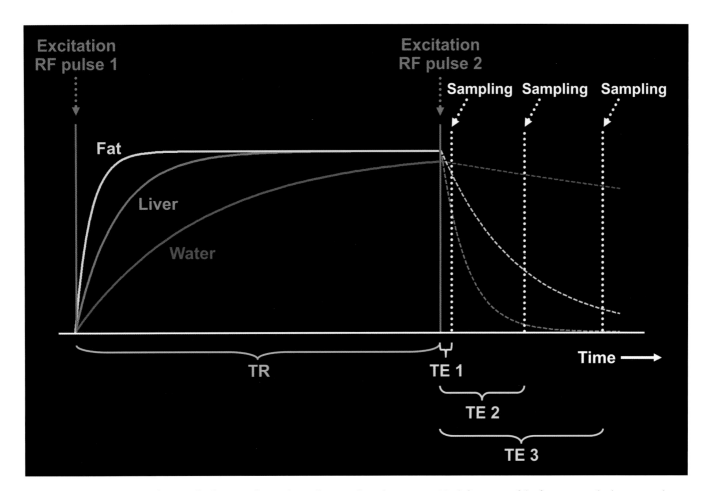

Figure 2.4 *Varying degrees of T2-weighted contrast from a three-echo spin-echo pulse sequence.* The left portion of the figure is exactly the same as the corresponding portion of Figure 2.3, which described a single-echo T2-weighted pulse sequence. Likewise, when the second 90° excitation RF pulse (Excitation RF pulse 2) is applied, the longitudinal magnetization vectors are rotated to the transverse plane, after which the transverse magnetization begins to decay. When the transverse magnetization is sampled shortly after Excitation RF pulse 2 (using a short echo time, labeled "TE 1"), there will be relatively small differences in signal intensities among tissues since relatively little decay has occurred. Consequently, there will be relatively weak T2-weighted contrast in the image and, as explained for Figure 2.3, there will be relatively little contribution from differences among T1 values. Thus, in the image with a long TR and short TE, differences in T1 and T2 values among tissues contribute little to the image contrast, which is primarily determined by any differences in the density of signal-producing protons among tissues. Hence, the image is called *proton-density* weighted. When, after Excitation RF pulse 2, the signals are sampled at a longer echo time (labeled "TE 2") for which more decay of the transverse magnetization has occurred, an image is obtained that shows greater contrast due to differences among the T2 values, and thus the image is more T2 weighted. Finally, when the signals are sampled at a very long echo time (labeled "TE 3"), an image is generated with "strong" (or "heavy") T2 weighting, which shows tissues with the long T2 values (water, *dashed blue line*) as relatively bright and tissues with shorter T2 values (liver, *dashed brown line*; fat, *dashed yellow line*) as quite dark. (The notes provided for Fig. 2.2 also apply to this figure.)

repetition, just after the excitation RF pulse, and thus each of the echoes following the excitation RF pulse experiences the same amount of phase encoding and corresponds to the same line in k space.

For both T1-weighted and T2-weighted spin-echo acquisitions, the pulse-sequence events, such as shown in Figure 2.1, are repeated as the phase-encoding gradient steps through a series of amplitudes, as described in the section "Phase encoding" in Chapter 1. All spin-echo signals (except the first, which is typically discarded) acquired as the pulse sequence repeats have identical contrast weighting, since the TR and TE associated with each signal are identical. Figure 2.5, which is an extension of Figure 2.2, illustrates the behavior of the longitudinal and transverse components of the magnetization during the first few repetitions of a T1-weighted spin-echo pulse sequence and demonstrates that the contrast weighting is identical for each line of k-space data sampled as the pulse sequence repeats. Similarly, Figure 2.6 illustrates the behavior of the longitudinal and transverse components of the magnetization during the first few repetitions of a dual-echo

spin-echo pulse sequence that generates proton-density and T2-weighted images. Again, the contrast weighting for the respective images is identical for each line of k-space data sampled as the pulse sequence repeats.

2D MULTISLICE IMAGING

For many pulse sequences, such as the T1-weighted and T2-weighted methods described in the previous section, the TR is many times longer than the TE. As a result, the application of RF pulses, gradient pulses, and data sampling occupies only a small fraction of TR; most of TR is spent waiting for the longitudinal magnetization to relax by an amount that provides the desired image contrast. If we want to obtain a series of slices at different positions, we could apply the pulse sequence at a given slice position and collect the associated image data, then apply the pulse sequence at a second slice position and collect the associated image data, and so on. However, this approach would be very inefficient. Instead of just waiting during the period when RF pulses, gradient pulses,

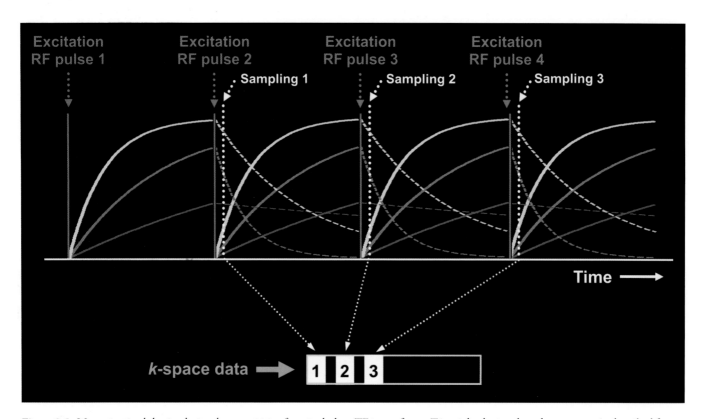

Figure 2.5 *Magnetization behavior during data acquisition for a single short-TE image from a T1-weighted spin-echo pulse sequence.* As described for Figure 2.2, following the initial 90° excitation RF pulse (Excitation RF pulse 1), a second 90° excitation RF pulse (Excitation RF pulse 2) is applied at time TR when the desired differences among longitudinal components of the magnetization vectors have developed due to differences among T1 values. Subsequently, sampling of the transverse magnetization is performed at a short echo time, before significant decay occurs, so that T2 weighting is minimized. Data sampling, labeled "Sampling 1," provides the first line of k-space data for the image slice. (The *yellow box* represents the complete k-space data set and the *first white bar*, labeled "1," represents the first line of data.) Excitation RF pulse 2 brings longitudinal magnetization that was present just before the pulse back to zero, after which the longitudinal magnetization recovers toward thermal equilibrium until the next pulse (Excitation RF pulse 3) is given. Excitation RF pulse 3 again brings the longitudinal magnetization back to zero and creates transverse magnetization, analogous to the effect of Excitation RF pulse 2 on the magnetization. Data sampling (labeled "Sampling 2") is again performed using the same short echo time, creating another line of k-space data (labeled "2" in the yellow box), which has identical contrast weighting as the first line of data since the TR and TE are identical. This process is repeated for the third (right side of figure, Excitation RF pulse 4 and Sampling 3) and subsequent lines of data, until all lines of k-space data for the slice are acquired. The time to complete acquisition of a single slice is given by the product of the time between consecutive 90° excitation RF pulses (TR) and the number of lines (phase-encoding steps) in k space required for the image.

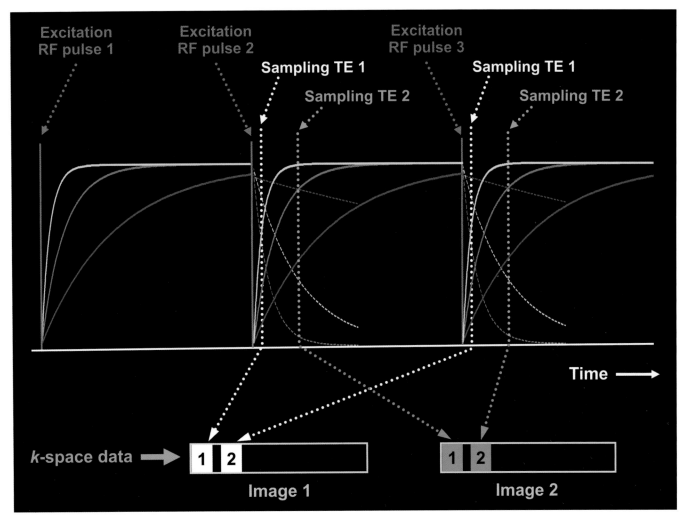

Figure 2.6 *Magnetization behavior during data acquisition for short-TE and long-TE images from a dual-echo spin-echo pulse sequence.* Analogous to Figure 2.3, following the initial 90° excitation RF pulse (Excitation RF pulse 1), a second 90° excitation RF pulse (Excitation RF pulse 2) is applied following a long TR to minimize contributions from differences among T1 values. In this dual-echo pulse sequence, sampling of the transverse magnetization is performed twice after Excitation RF pulse 2 and the subsequent excitation RF pulses, with one line of data obtained shortly after each excitation RF pulse, when there has been little decay of transverse magnetization ("Sampling TE 1," *white dotted line*, at short TE), and the second obtained after some time has elapsed for decay to occur and increase T2 weighting ("Sampling TE 2," *green dotted line*, at long TE). Using these lines of *k*-space data obtained at different TEs, two images can be created, with one image containing the data from sampling at short TE (*white bars* in yellow box for Image 1) and the other containing the data from sampling at long TE (*green bars* in yellow box for Image 2). As described for Figure 2.5, this process is repeated until all lines of *k*-space data are acquired. The acquisition time is determined by the TR and the number of phase-encoding steps, but not by the number of echoes sampled following each excitation RF pulse. Thus, the time to acquire only a single slice having a short TE, or two slices, with one having a short TE and the other having a long TE, is identical.

and data sampling are not applied, we can use this "dead" time for a given slice to collect image data for other slice positions. This process is called *multislice* (or *multisection*) imaging, and is key to the efficiency of routine clinical MRI. Multislice imaging can be performed because slice-selective RF pulses affect the magnetization only within the slice of interest, leaving magnetization outside of the slice essentially unperturbed, as described in the section "Slice selection" in Chapter 1.

Let's discuss multislice imaging in more detail using the T1-weighted spin-echo pulse sequence of Figure 2.1A as an example; Figure 2.7 illustrates the behavior of the longitudinal and transverse components of the magnetization during the first few repetitions of the corresponding multislice acquisition. We will assume that TR is 500 ms and TE is 15 ms and that, for

each repetition, 25 ms elapses from when the first slice-select gradient switches on to when the frequency-encoding gradient switches off. Thus, for a given slice, only relaxation (i.e., no RF pulses, gradient pulses, or data sampling) occurs for 475 ms of TR. A multislice acquisition would proceed as follows. The 90° and 180° RF pulses and associated gradient pulses are applied for slice position #1, and data for the <u>first line</u> of *k* space (first phase-encoding step) for <u>slice position #1</u> are sampled. Immediately after the frequency-encoding gradient associated with data sampling for slice position #1 is switched off, and as the longitudinal magnetization associated with slice position #1 relaxes, 90° and 180° RF pulses and associated gradient pulses are applied for slice position #2, and data for the <u>first line</u> of *k* space for <u>slice position #2</u> are sampled. This scheme is

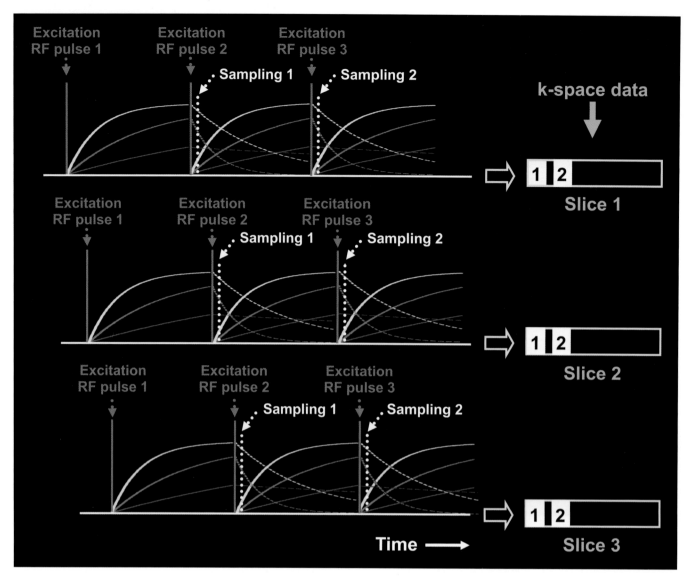

Figure 2.7 *Multislice acquisition for a T1-weighted spin-echo pulse sequence.* Note that the upper, middle, and lower portions of this figure are each directly analogous to Figure 2.5, depicting the acquisition of a single short-TE image. The diagrams are shifted in time relative to one another so that the RF-pulse and sampling events for a given slice occur during the "dead times" of the other slices. For example, for Slice 1, the second 90° slice-selective excitation RF pulse (Excitation RF pulse 2) is applied and first line of data is sampled (Sampling 1), thus generating the first line of *k*-space data (first phase-encoding step) for Slice 1. Immediately after the frequency-encoding gradient (not shown; see Fig. 2.1A) associated with data sampling for Slice 1 is switched off, and as the longitudinal magnetization associated with this slice relaxes, the corresponding 90° slice-selective excitation RF pulse for Slice 2 is applied and sampling is performed, generating the first line of *k*-space data for Slice 2. This scheme is repeated for the remaining slice positions until the first line of *k*-space data is sampled for all slices. When the elapsed time from the application of Excitation RF pulse 2 for Slice 1 equals TR, the process returns to Slice 1, and the next 90° excitation RF pulse (Excitation RF pulse 3) is applied, followed by sampling of the signal, thus generating the second line of *k*-space data (second phase-encoding step) for Slice 1. This is followed by an RF pulse and data sampling to acquire the second line of *k*-space data for Slice 2, and so on for the remaining slices. The process continues to repeat, incrementing through the lines of *k* space, until the last line of *k* space (last phase-encoding step) for each of the slices has been sampled, and the acquisition for all slices is complete.

Note: With reference to the description provided in the text, the 180° refocusing RF pulses are omitted from the diagrams in this figure for simplicity (also see Notes for Fig. 2.2).

repeated for slice positions #3, #4, and so on, until the first line of *k* space is sampled for all slices. Subsequently, once the elapsed time from the application of the 90° excitation RF pulse for slice position #1 equals TR, the process returns to slice position #1. (Although at this point several pairs of 90° and 180° RF pulses have been applied, the magnetization in each slice

has experienced only one pair of RF pulses.) Next, 90° and 180° RF pulses and associated gradient pulses are applied for slice position #1, and data for the <u>second line</u> of *k* space (second phase-encoding step) for <u>slice position #1</u> are sampled, followed by the RF pulses, gradient pulses, and sampling required to acquire the <u>second line</u> of *k* space for <u>slice position #2</u>, and so on for the remaining slices. The process continues to repeat, incrementing through the lines of k space, until imaging is finally completed when the last line of k space (last phase-encoding step) for each of the slices has been sampled.

The temporal order of sampling data for the slices need not match their physical positions. For example, if slices are positioned at –20 mm (#1), –10 mm (#2), 0 mm (#3), and 10 mm (#4), we can acquire data sequentially during each TR—that is, in the order #1, #2, #3, #4—or alternatively we can acquire data in the order #1, #3, #2, #4. (Obviously, there are several other possible combinations.) The latter arrangement, termed an *interleaved* order, is often used to suppress artifacts that arise because the actual slice thickness is somewhat larger than the ideal slice thickness (see the section "Slice selection" in Chapter 1).

The number of slices that can be acquired in a given TR with multislice imaging is determined by the ratio of the TR to the time required to apply the RF pulses, gradient pulses, and data sampling for each slice. Thus, when a long TR is used, more slices can be obtained than when a short TR is used. For our example above, $500/25 = 20$ slices can be acquired within a given TR. Further, the number of slices obtained with multislice imaging does not affect the total scan time, as long as this number does not exceed the maximum allowable number within the TR. For our example, the acquisition time would be the same for 10, 15, or 20 slices. If, however, more than 20 slices were required, for instance to cover a larger region of the body, it would be necessary either to increase the TR to accommodate the greater number of slices, or to perform two concatenated acquisitions. For both of these possibilities, the acquisition time will increase. Further, if the TR is increased, the image contrast will also be affected, and this may affect the diagnostic quality of the images.

Multislice imaging concepts apply equally to multiple spin-echo acquisitions, such as those discussed in the previous section. For example, consider multislice imaging using a pulse sequence that samples echoes at 20 ms and 100 ms following each excitation RF pulse (see Fig. 2.1B). The application of a 90° pulse and two 180° RF pulses samples, for slice position #1, the first line of k space for TE = 20 ms (for the first image at slice position #1) and the first line for TE = 100 ms (for the second image at slice position #1). Subsequently, the application of a 90° and two 180° RF pulses samples the analogous data (first line of k space for the two echo times) for slice position #2, and so on. The process continues in the same fashion as described for the single-TE pulse sequence until all lines of k space are sampled for all slice positions <u>and</u> the two different TE values, yielding two images (TE = 20 and 100 ms) at each slice position. Figure 2.8 illustrates the behavior of the longitudinal and transverse components of the magnetization during the first few repetitions of such a dual-echo multislice acquisition.

Since, for multislice imaging, data collection for all slices is inherently intermingled, anything that occurs during image acquisition that may corrupt the data, such as movement of the tissues being imaged, affects all of the slices. For example, if, during an acquisition of the abdomen, the subject coughs while k-space lines 50 to 55 are being acquired, all of the

images will be affected by the motion. Further, the image degradation, which would likely be image blurring in this example, will have a similar appearance in all images because equivalent lines of k space for each image are acquired during coughing. Multislice imaging is therefore relatively sensitive to the effects of breathing, bowel movement, or other types of motion.

ACQUISITION TIME AND DATA AVERAGING

From our discussion of conventional spin-echo imaging, we can conclude that the overall acquisition time is directly proportional to TR and to the number of phase-encoding steps required to collect all lines of k-space data for a given image. (As discussed above, the acquisition time is the same whether a single MR signal is sampled following each excitation RF pulse, and thus only one line of k-space data is acquired per excitation, or whether MR signals for multiple images, each having a distinct echo time, are sampled following each excitation RF pulse.) Another important factor determining the overall acquisition time is the number of data averages (also commonly called the number of excitations, abbreviated NEX) used for the acquisition. For example, two averages (or NEX = 2) means that all phase-encoding steps are acquired twice. Depending on the configuration of the pulse sequence, a given phase-encoding step may be acquired twice before the acquisition advances to the next phase-encoding step, or all phase-encoding steps may be acquired once, and then acquired again. In either case, the total number of excitation RF pulses for an image with two averages is twice that for an image with only one average. Multiple averages are generally used to increase the signal-to-noise ratio of the image, which varies as the square root of the number of averages. To summarize, we can write the acquisition time as:

$$TR \times N_{PH2D} \times NEX$$

where N_{PH2D} is used to denote the number of phase-encoding steps for a conventional 2D pulse sequence.

For applications in which periodic motion (e.g., breathing) is present, multiple averages are also useful for suppressing the associated image ghost artifacts (see "Artifacts" section below), thereby improving image quality. Multiple-average techniques were commonly used in abdominal imaging before fast imaging techniques, which allow the acquisition to be completed within the duration of a breath hold, became available. However, since the acquisition time is directly proportional to the number of averages, scan times on the order of 10 minutes per pulse sequence were common in the early years of abdominal MR imaging. With the array of breath-hold techniques now available, the use of pulse sequences that employ multiple averages for abdominal MRI has decreased substantially.

As alluded to earlier, the acquisition time for multislice imaging is not affected by the choice of TE or, in multi-echo imaging, the choice of the multiple TE values. However, the (maximum) TE value does affect the maximum number of slices that can be acquired in a given TR. Increasing this value increases

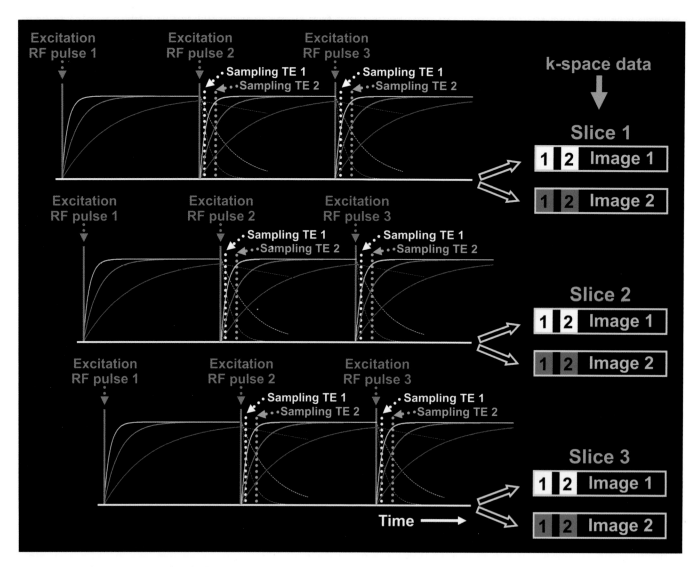

Figure 2.8 *Multislice acquisition for a dual-echo spin-echo pulse sequence.* Analogous to the situation for Figure 2.7, the upper, middle, and lower portions of this figure each directly correspond to Figure 2.6, depicting the acquisition of short-TE and long-TE images from a dual-echo spin-echo pulse sequence. Again, the diagrams are shifted in time relative to one another so that the RF-pulse and sampling events for a given slice occur during the "dead times" of the other slices. Following from the description for Figure 2.6, the transverse magnetization for Slice 1 is sampled twice after each of the second and subsequent 90° excitation RF pulses, with one line of *k*-space data obtained shortly after each slice-selective excitation RF pulse (Sampling TE 1, *white dotted line*, at short TE), and the second obtained after allowing more signal decay to increase T2 weighting (Sampling TE 2, *green dotted line*, at long TE). These data allow creation of two images for Slice 1, with one image containing the data corresponding to a short TE (*white bars* in yellow box for Image 1) and the other containing the data corresponding to a long TE (*green bars* in yellow box for Image 2). As soon as sampling is completed for the second echo following a given excitation RF pulse for Slice 1, the corresponding excitation RF pulse for Slice 2 is applied, after which MR signals at short and long TEs are sampled to yield the first lines of *k*-space data for Image 1 and Image 2, respectively, of Slice 2. This process continues for each subsequent slice position until the elapsed time from the application of a given 90° excitation RF pulse for Slice 1 equals TR, after which the process returns to Slice 1, and the second lines of *k*-space data are acquired at short and long TEs for all slices. The process continues to repeat, incrementing through the lines of *k* space, until the last lines of *k* space for each slice have been sampled and the acquisition is complete.

Note: With reference to the description provided in the text, the 180° refocusing RF pulses are omitted from the diagrams in this figure for simplicity.

the time required to perform the RF pulses, gradient pulses, and data sampling for each slice position, and therefore decreases the number of slices that can be obtained within a given TR.

Based on the formula above, what options do we have for decreasing the acquisition time to fit within a breath hold? For example, consider a T1-weighted spin-echo pulse sequence, with TR = 500 ms, matrix = 256 × 256, and NEX = 1, which has an acquisition time of just over 2 minutes—too long for an

average person to hold his or her breath. We can decrease the number of phase-encoding steps; however, this will in turn decrease the spatial resolution along the phase-encoding direction, which can be done only to a certain degree without resulting in diagnostically inadequate images for assessment of small lesions or structures. Barring a fundamental change to the pulse-sequence structure, the only remaining option is to decrease TR. This is precisely the approach taken for fast

Box 2.1 ESSENTIALS TO REMEMBER

- The magnitude of the transverse magnetization immediately following a 90° excitation RF pulse is equal to that of the associated longitudinal magnetization immediately before the pulse.

- When a 90° excitation RF pulse is applied to tissues whose longitudinal-magnetization components are only partially recovered, these partially recovered longitudinal magnetizations are converted to transverse magnetizations with corresponding magnitudes, and the longitudinal-magnetization components become zero.

- The 180° refocusing RF pulse needed to generate the spin echo for a spin-echo pulse sequence is not essential for sampling of the signals. Hence, an image can be generated without using a refocusing RF pulse, as is done with gradient-echo pulse sequences.

- For a T1-weighted spin-echo image, a relatively short TR is used to accentuate T1-dependent contrast and a short TE is used to suppress T2-dependent contrast. For a T2-weighted spin-echo image, a relatively long TR is used to suppress T1-dependent contrast and a long TE is used to accentuate T2-dependent contrast. A spin-density image is obtained when a spin-echo acquisition is performed using a relatively long TR to suppress T1-dependent contrast and short TE to suppress T2-dependent contrast.

- For most spin-echo pulse sequences, the TE is much shorter than the TR.

- The acquisition time of a conventional spin-echo pulse sequence is the same whether a single MR signal is sampled following each 90° excitation RF pulse, and thus only one line of k-space data is acquired per excitation, or whether MR signals for multiple images, each having a distinct echo time, are sampled following each excitation RF pulse.

- The acquisition time of a conventional spin-echo pulse sequence is also the same independent of whether the acquisition includes a single slice or multiple slices, because, for the latter, the data for the additional slices are collected during the "dead time" between 90° excitation RF pulses for a given slice, during which the longitudinal magnetization corresponding to the slice regrows.

- Multislice imaging is relatively sensitive to motion artifacts because data collection for all slices is intermingled and continues during the entire time of the acquisition. As a result, all slices are affected by motion during the acquisition, and image degradation from motion appears similar in all images.

- The total acquisition time for conventional, 2D pulse sequences is determined by the product of the TR, the number of phase-encoding steps (N_{PH2D}), and the number of excitations (NEX).

T1-weighted methods, as explained in the next section. On the other hand, for T2-weighted imaging, a relatively long TR is required to suppress T1 contributions to the contrast. Thus, for this case, a different pulse-sequence structure, as will be discussed below, is required to achieve a sufficiently short acquisition time for breath-hold imaging.

FAST T1-WEIGHTED IMAGING

Short-TR gradient-echo imaging

As we just discussed, decreasing TR appears to be a straightforward means for achieving breath-hold acquisition times for T1-weighted imaging. For instance, if the TR is decreased to 80 ms or less and if 192 phase-encoding steps are performed, an image can be acquired in a 15-second breath hold. Although such a short TR value can, in principle, be used for spin-echo imaging, the associated signal levels would be very low due to the relatively short time available for T1 relaxation following the 90° excitation and 180° refocusing RF pulses. Therefore, a different pulse-sequence strategy is needed: a *gradient-echo* pulse sequence.

The timing diagram for a basic gradient-echo pulse sequence is shown in Figure 2.9. Comparing this pulse sequence to the single-echo spin-echo method shown in Figure 2.1A, we note that the gradient-echo pulse sequence, by nature, does not include a refocusing RF pulse. As a result,

the prephasing gradient on the frequency-encoding axis is negative instead of positive, leading to the generation of a gradient echo, as discussed in the section "Frequency encoding" in Chapter 1. Also, the echo signal decay is governed by the T2*, as opposed to T2, relaxation time, since inhomogeneity of the static magnetic field is not compensated and thus also contributes to decay of the transverse magnetization (see section "Transverse magnetization and T2 relaxation" in Chapter 1). Note that the T2* relaxation time depends not only on the underlying T2 value, but, in some cases, also on the size and shape of the image voxel. Since T2* values of tissues are often much shorter than the associated T2 values (see Fig. 1.13 in Chapter 1), the TE used for gradient-echo imaging is often much shorter than that used for spin-echo imaging. Because effects of static-field inhomogeneity are not compensated, gradient-echo imaging is much more prone than spin-echo imaging to artifacts from magnetic-susceptibility differences (e.g., air–tissue interfaces), depicted as areas of decreased or absent signal (signal void) in the image. These artifacts become more prominent with longer TE values but are minimized by using the shortest TE possible. In this regard, the absence of a refocusing RF pulse permits a gradient-echo pulse sequence to achieve shorter minimum TE and TR values than a spin-echo pulse sequence.

The most important consequence of not using a refocusing RF pulse is that a "low" or "partial" (i.e., much less than 90°) flip

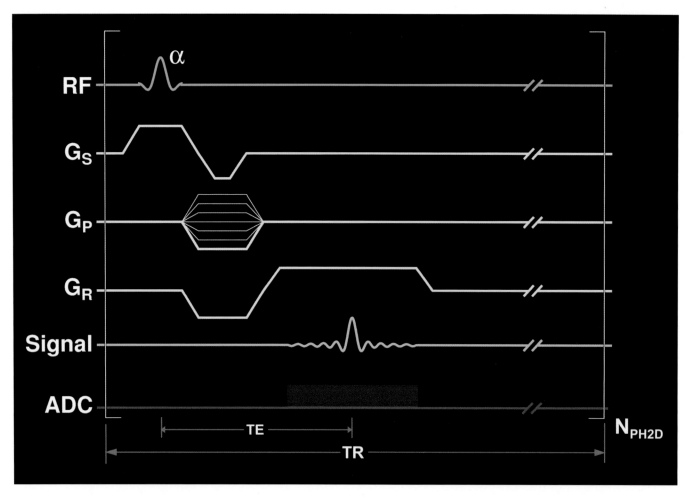

Figure 2.9 *Timing diagram for a gradient-echo pulse sequence.* Analogous to Figure 2.1, the first line of the diagram (in green) shows the radiofrequency (RF) pulse applied in each repetition of the gradient-echo pulse sequence. This type of pulse sequence often uses a flip angle for the excitation RF pulse that is less than 90°, which is denoted by the α symbol. The second, third, and fourth lines (in yellow) illustrate application of the slice-select (G_S), phase-encoding (G_P), and frequency-encoding (G_R) gradients, respectively, as discussed in the section "Spatial localization and *k* space" in Chapter 1. When the positive portion of G_R balances its negative portion (that is, at the time when the area under the positive portion of the G_R waveform exactly matches the area under the negative portion), a gradient echo is formed, as illustrated on the fifth line (in cyan) of the diagram. The last line of the diagram (in magenta) shows when the analog-to-digital converter, or ADC, is turned on to sample the echo signal. The label N_{PH2D} denotes the number of times that the basic pulse-sequence timing events are repeated; N_{PH2D} equals the number of phase-encoding steps. (Adapted from Mugler JP III. Basic principles. In: Edelman RR, Hesselink JR, Zlatkin MB, Crues JV III, eds. *Clinical Magnetic Resonance Imaging*, 3rd ed. Philadelphia: Saunders Elsevier, 2006.)

angle can be used for the excitation RF pulse in gradient-echo imaging. The partial flip angle is denoted by the α symbol next to the RF pulse in the timing diagram (Fig. 2.9). With a partial flip angle, only a portion of the longitudinal magnetization that exists just before the RF pulse is converted to transverse magnetization, and accordingly a large fraction of the magnetization remains on the longitudinal axis. Hence, the time needed for this remaining longitudinal magnetization to recover via T1 relaxation to the desired level is much less than that corresponding to the case when a 90° excitation RF pulse is used, and, as a result, the time period between application of successive partial-flip-angle excitation RF pulses (that is, TR) can be substantially reduced compared to values appropriate for 90° RF pulses. A partial flip angle therefore allows useable levels of longitudinal magnetization to be achieved for relatively short TR values. Consequently, since decreasing the TR leads to a shortening of

the acquisition time, the use of a partial-flip-angle excitation RF pulse makes acquisition of images within a breath hold possible. Note, however, that because a low flip angle converts only a small fraction of the longitudinal magnetization that existed just before the RF pulse to transverse magnetization, and hence signal, while leaving a large fraction of this magnetization along the longitudinal axis, the choice of flip angle represents a tradeoff between achieving a sufficiently high level of longitudinal magnetization, which favors a lower flip angle, and obtaining enough signal for any given excitation from this magnetization, which favors a higher flip angle. Using a simple mathematical formula, the so-called *Ernst angle* can be calculated, which is the flip angle that provides the highest signal level for a given T1 relaxation time and TR.

The rate of longitudinal-magnetization recovery increases as the starting value for the longitudinal magnetization moves away from thermal equilibrium. For example, the rate of T1 recovery just after a 90° RF pulse is faster than that just after a 10° RF pulse. This means that, for a given recovery time, the difference between longitudinal-magnetization vectors associated with tissues having different T1 values will be greater following a 90° RF pulse than following a 10° RF pulse. Stated another way, for a given TR, the T1-weighted contrast generated by a 90° RF pulse is greater than that generated by a 10° RF pulse. In general terms, the flip angle of the excitation RF pulse in a gradient-echo pulse sequence provides control over T1 weighting; increasing the flip angle increases T1 weighting and vice versa. Thus, gradient-echo imaging using a partial flip angle permits breath-hold imaging with a selectable degree of T1 weighting. Gradient-echo imaging is the most commonly used technique for fast T1-weighted imaging of the abdomen, and has completely replaced spin-echo techniques for this application. Both 2D and 3D (see below) implementations of the technique are common.

Because the TR used for breath-hold T1-weighted gradient-echo imaging is shorter than many of the T2 relaxation times of interest, substantial transverse magnetization from a given excitation RF pulse may exist when the next excitation RF pulse is applied. As discussed in the section "Spin echoes" in Chapter 1, two such consecutive RF pulses will then lead to the generation of a spin echo, even if both are intended to function only as excitation RF pulses, as in a gradient-echo acquisition, and even if the flip angles for the first and second consecutive RF pulses are not 90° and 180°, respectively, as is typical for a spin-echo pulse sequence. For T1-weighted imaging using a gradient-echo sequence, we do not want such echoes from the "residual" transverse magnetization, which may exist at the end of a given repetition, to contribute to subsequent repetitions because they would interfere with the desired image contrast. Therefore, short-TR T1-weighted gradient-echo pulse sequences use a process called *RF spoiling* to suppress signal contributions from residual transverse magnetization. The technical details of RF spoiling are not important for our discussion; the important point is that the image contrast created using a so-called RF-spoiled pulse sequence is essentially identical to that which would be achieved if any transverse magnetization remaining at the end of each repetition were to be simply destroyed. There are fast gradient-echo pulse sequences that do not use RF spoiling (e.g., GRASS [gradient-recalled acquisition in the steady state, GE Healthcare] and FISP [fast imaging with steady-state precession, Siemens Healthcare], and so-called "balanced" pulse sequences such as TrueFISP [Siemens Healthcare], FIESTA [fast imaging employing steady-state acquisition, GE Healthcare] and balanced FFE [balanced fast field echo, Philips Healthcare], which are generically termed balanced steady-state free precession [SSFP] methods). In this case, the image contrast depends on both the T1 and T2 relaxation times, sometimes (depending on pulse-sequence type and parameter values) in a complicated fashion. We will not discuss this class of gradient-echo techniques as these are infrequently used for abdominal imaging at this time; however, some of the techniques are widely used for other applications, such as cardiovascular imaging.[2]

Commonly used T1-weighted gradient-echo pulse sequences for breath-hold abdominal MR imaging include FLASH (fast low angle shot, Siemens Healthcare), spoiled GRASS or SPGR (spoiled gradient-recalled acquisition in the steady state, GE Healthcare), or T1-FFE (T1 fast field echo, Philips Healthcare).

Box 2.2 ESSENTIALS TO REMEMBER

- The T2* relaxation time depends not only on the underlying T2 value, but, in some cases, also on the size and shape of the image voxel.

- For all tissues, T1 > T2 > T2*.

- Since T2* values of tissues are often much shorter than the associated T2 values, the TE used for gradient-echo imaging is often substantially shorter than that used for spin-echo imaging.

- Because the effects of static-field inhomogeneity are not compensated in a gradient-echo pulse sequence, this technique is much more prone than spin-echo imaging to artifacts from magnetic-susceptibility differences, such as present at air–tissue interfaces, or due to the presence of iron particles or other metal objects. These artifacts become more prominent with increasing TE and are thus minimized by using the shortest possible TE.

- The most important consequence of the fact that a 180° refocusing RF pulse is not, by nature, used in a gradient-echo pulse sequence is that a low (partial) flip angle can be used for the excitation RF pulse.

- With a partial flip angle, only a portion of the longitudinal magnetization that exists just before the RF pulse is converted to transverse magnetization, and thus a large fraction of the magnetization remains along the longitudinal axis. As a result, the time needed for this remaining longitudinal magnetization to recover via T1 relaxation to the desired contrast level is much less than when a 90° excitation RF pulse is used, and consequently, the time period between successive partial-flip-angle excitation RF pulses (i.e., the TR) can be reduced, which leads to a shorter acquisition time than when 90° excitation RF pulses are used.

- The *Ernst angle* for a gradient-echo pulse sequence is the flip angle that provides the highest signal level for given values of the T1 relaxation time and the TR.

In-phase, opposed-phase gradient-echo imaging

In the section "Effects of chemical shift" in Chapter 1, we saw how the chemical-shift difference between hydrogen nuclei in water-containing tissues and those in fat can affect the slice-selection and frequency-encoding processes, and result in chemical-shift artifacts. There is another effect of this chemical-shift difference that is specific to gradient-echo pulse sequences and important for abdominal imaging.

The difference in resonant frequency between hydrogen nuclei in water-containing tissues and those in fat causes a difference in phase to develop between the associated transverse magnetization vectors as time evolves after the excitation RF pulse. Due to the fundamental cyclic nature of this process, the transverse magnetization vectors associated with water and fat periodically point in opposite directions, and are also periodically aligned with one another (Fig. 2.10).[3] When pointing in opposite directions, water and fat transverse magnetization vectors are said to be "out of phase" or have *opposed phase*, and when aligned, water and fat transverse magnetization vectors are said to be *in phase*. For example, considering the resonant-frequency difference between water and fat of about 224 Hz at 1.5T, it takes approximately 4.5 ms (1/224 Hz) for the transverse magnetization for fat to precess through a complete cycle (360°) relative to that for water. Thus, at 2.25

ms (half of 4.5 ms), 6.75 ms, 11.25 ms, and so on after the excitation RF pulse, the transverse magnetization for water is opposed to that for fat, and at 4.5 ms, 9.0 ms, 13.5 ms, and so on, the two transverse magnetization vectors are aligned. In contrast to the behavior for gradient-echo pulse sequences, a phase difference does not occur between the transverse magnetization vectors for water and fat at a spin echo because the refocusing RF pulse compensates for this effect of the difference in resonant frequency.

Although the transverse magnetization vector is characterized by a magnitude (length) and a phase angle, clinical MR images are typically presented as magnitude images—that is, the signal intensities in the image depict the magnitudes of the transverse magnetization vectors associated with each voxel. Thus, for image voxels containing either all watery tissue or all fat, the relative orientation (phase) of the transverse magnetization is not important. However, the phase of the water and fat transverse magnetization vectors becomes important when water-containing tissue and fat are present in the <u>same</u> voxel. In this case, the signal at <u>opposed-phase</u> times reflects the <u>difference</u> between the transverse magnetizations for water and fat, whereas the signal at <u>in-phase</u> times reflects the <u>sum</u> of the transverse magnetizations for water and fat. So, if TE for the gradient-echo pulse sequence is chosen to match one of these in-phase or opposed-phase times, the image contrast will

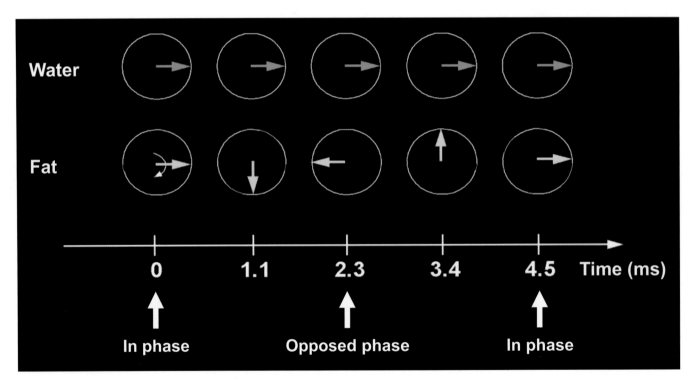

Figure 2.10 *Relationship between water and fat transverse magnetization following an excitation RF pulse.* Immediately following an excitation RF pulse, the transverse magnetization vectors associated with tissues containing water (green) and fat (yellow) are *in phase*—that is, aligned with one another. Since the magnetization for fat precesses at a slightly lower frequency than that for water, the fat transverse magnetization vector gets out of phase with the water transverse magnetization as time progresses following the excitation RF pulse. For example, at 1.5T, the phase difference between the water and fat transverse magnetization vectors is 90° at approximately 1.1 ms after the RF pulse, and 180° (*opposed phase*) at approximately 2.3 ms after the RF pulse. Due to the fundamental cyclic nature of this process, the water and fat magnetization vectors will periodically come back into phase; at 1.5T, this occurs at integer multiples of approximately 4.5 ms.

reflect the corresponding relative orientation of the water and fat transverse magnetization vectors for any voxel containing a mixture of water and fat. As a result, the signal from a voxel containing a mixture of water and fat will periodically decrease and then increase as the TE increases (Fig. 2.11). This effect, called chemical-shift–induced signal modulation or type 2 chemical-shift artifact, leads to a characteristic dark margin artifact in opposed-phase images (also called boundary effect, bounce-point artifact, or India-ink etching) at the interface between muscle (or other water-containing tissues) and fat where the associated voxel contains part muscle (watery tissue) and part fat, as illustrated in Figure 2.12.[4,5]

Most MR scanners include a dual-echo gradient-echo pulse sequence that provides both in-phase and opposed-phase images from the same acquisition. Preferably, the first echo acquires an image at the first opposed-phase time, but, depending on the capabilities of the scanner, the first echo may instead correspond to the first in-phase time. The second echo then collects an image corresponding to the opposite phase relationship. The advantage of using such a dual-echo pulse sequence, as opposed to two separate acquisitions (one for an in-phase image and the other for an opposed-phase image) is that the dual-echo method is faster, requiring only a single breath hold, and that there is perfect spatial registration

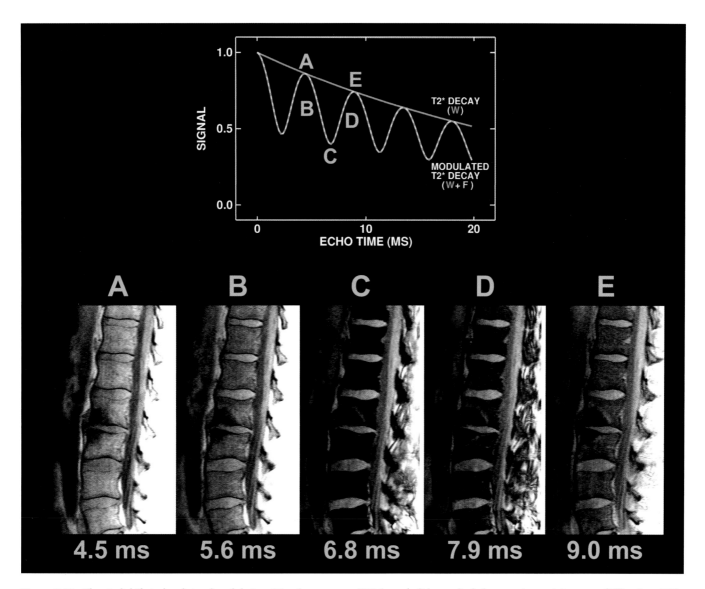

Figure 2.11 *Chemical-shift–induced signal modulation.* The plot compares T2* decay (*solid green line*), for a voxel containing water (W) only, to T2* decay plus chemical-shift–induced modulation (*yellow/green line*), for a voxel containing a mixture of water and fat (F). As described in Figure 2.10, the period of the signal modulation is approximately 4.5 ms at 1.5T. Below the plot are sagittal T1-weighted gradient-echo images (TR/α 500/90°) of the spine in an adult. The images were acquired with TE values of 4.5, 5.6, 6.8, 7.9, and 9.0 ms, corresponding to time points A to E in the plot, and illustrate how the signal intensity in bone marrow first decreases as the phase difference between water and fat magnetization vectors increases (images **A–C**), to a minimum signal at a TE of 6.8 ms when the vectors are opposed. The bone marrow signal then increases as the water and fat magnetization vectors come back into phase (images **C–E**). However, because the echo time for image E is longer than that for image **A**, and hence the decay of transverse magnetization is greater for image E than for image **A**, the overall signal intensities of bone marrow and other structures in image E are less than those in image A, as also shown in the plot. (Adapted from Mugler JP III. Overview of MR imaging pulse sequences. *Magn Reson Imaging Clin North Am.* 1999;7:661-697.)

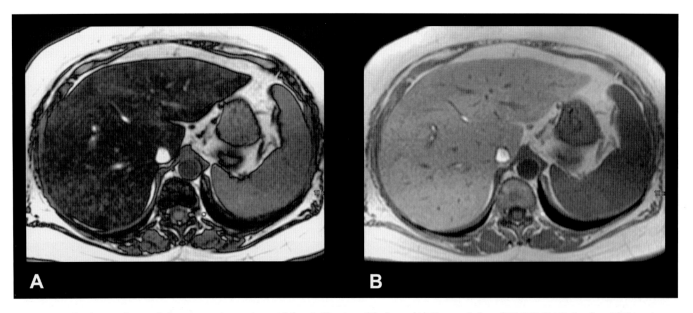

Figure 2.12 *In-phase and opposed-phase images in a patient with fatty infiltration of the liver.* (**A**) Opposed-phase (TR/TE 110/2.4 ms) and (**B**) in-phase (110/4.8) images obtained at 1.5T. In the opposed-phase image **A**, the signal from liver parenchyma is diffusely decreased compared to image **B** because voxels are composed of a mixture of water-containing tissue and fat, with the signal in image **A** reflecting the difference between the transverse magnetizations associated with water and fat. Decreased signal is also present at boundaries between many normal structures (for example, between spleen and surrounding fat) that have a fat–water interface. These boundaries appear as characteristic dark lines, also called boundary effect, bounce-point artifact, or India-ink etching. Compared to image **B**, there is no signal decrease in image A for tissues that contain pure fat, such as the subcutaneous fat, or for pure watery tissues, such as spleen. In the in-phase image **B**, the liver-parenchyma signal intensity is increased compared to that in image **A** because the transverse magnetizations associated with water and fat are aligned and thus the liver signal reflects the sum of the transverse magnetizations associated with fat and water. Tissues that chiefly consist of pure fat, such as the subcutaneous fat, or pure watery tissues, such as spleen, display minimally decreased signal intensity compared to image **A** because of the slightly longer TE associated with image **B**. A dark margin is not seen at the fat–water interfaces.

of the anatomic structures in the in-phase and opposed-phase images.

It is important not to mistake the typical dark margin seen on opposed-phase gradient-echo images between water-containing structures and fat for a capsule or any other anatomic equivalent. Rather, it truly represents an artifact resulting from the associated difference in resonant frequency. As this artifact occurs in voxels that contain signal from both water and fat, and thus at interfaces between water and fat, the distinctness of the dark margin is directly related to the size of the voxel (i.e., the image resolution). Dark margins are more prominent when voxels are large, and less noticeable when small voxels are used.

For clinical application of in-phase, opposed-phase imaging to organs such as the liver or adrenal glands, it is also important to remember that the degree of signal loss on an opposed-phase image reflects only the difference between the associated transverse magnetization vectors, and not the actual degree of fatty infiltration.[3] Hence, the technique should not be used, for instance, to quantify hepatosteatosis. When the transverse magnetization vectors for water and fat are about equal in a given voxel, there will be essentially complete loss of signal on the opposed-phase image and the liver will have a marked low-intensity appearance (Figs. 2.10 and 2.12). However, when the transverse magnetization for fat is greater than that for water, or vice versa, the signal intensity from liver will be greater. Thus, based on the degree of signal loss, one cannot determine whether there is more fat than water in the liver, or vice versa, and hence the degree of fatty infiltration

may be under- or overestimated. The principles associated with in-phase, opposed-phase imaging can also be used to obtain separate water-only and fat-only images. The possibility of obtaining such images was first described by W. Thomas Dixon, and techniques based on this approach are commonly called Dixon methods.[3,6] Such methods allow calculation of the quantity of fat within the liver. The potential of this technique for assessing the degree of hepatosteatosis is not yet determined and is the topic of extensive investigation.

Magnetization-prepared gradient-echo imaging

Magnetization-prepared gradient-echo imaging (MP-GRE) is a gradient-echo–based technique that consists of two independent components: a magnetization-preparation period, composed of some combination of RF pulses, gradient pulses, and time delays, and a data acquisition period that follows the magnetization-preparation period and uses a short-TR gradient-echo pulse sequence, such as those described above. The concept of this technique is to generate the desired image contrast using the magnetization-preparation period, and then acquire image data that reflects the desired contrast using the short-TR gradient-echo pulse sequence. Because contrast generation is performed separately from data acquisition, this method provides contrast behavior that cannot be obtained using a short-TR gradient-echo pulse sequence alone.

Although many types of image contrast can be generated using MP-GRE imaging, the most common type for abdominal imaging is strong T1 weighting. The 2D version of this technique, also called TurboFLASH (Siemens Healthcare), FSGPR-prepared (GE Healthcare), or TurboFFE (Philips Healthcare), has particular advantages for imaging of the upper abdomen, particularly the liver, as it allows characterization of the most common liver lesions (hemangiomas, cysts, and metastases) without the use of intravenous contrast material. To produce strong T1 weighting, the magnetization preparation is typically an inversion-recovery preparation, which consists of a 180° inversion RF pulse followed by a time delay.

To create an image that largely reflects the desired contrast as generated by the magnetization preparation, the total duration of the short-TR gradient-echo pulse sequence must be appropriately limited. To achieve this, the gradient-echo pulse sequence typically uses a TR less than 10 ms, which is much shorter than that used for many other applications of 2D gradient-echo imaging. Further, a relatively low flip angle is used for the gradient-echo pulse sequence so that the contrast contribution from the gradient-echo pulse sequence itself is minimal, and consequently the image contrast is determined primarily by the inversion-recovery preparation. The short TR allows a sufficient number of phase-encoding steps for reasonable spatial resolution to be obtained within an acquisition time of 1 to 2 seconds for each slice, permitting several slices to be collected during a single breath-hold period. Note that with this technique all data for a given slice are acquired before proceeding to the subsequent slice, in contrast to the interleaved nature of data collection used for conventional multislice spin-echo or gradient-echo imaging (see section "2D multislice imaging"). Such an MP-GRE acquisition is thus a so-called *single-slice*, *sequential-slice*, or *single-shot* technique.

Let's review the operation of an MP-GRE acquisition that uses an inversion-recovery preparation (Fig. 2.13). Recall, as described in the section "Manipulating the magnetization using RF pulses" in Chapter 1, that an inversion RF pulse applied to a slice of interest rotates the longitudinal magnetization corresponding to the tissues within the slice from alignment with the positive z axis to alignment with the negative z axis. Following the inversion pulse, the longitudinal magnetization for each tissue grows back toward thermal equilibrium at a rate determined by the corresponding T1 relaxation time (see section "Longitudinal magnetization and T1 relaxation" in Chapter 1). Since, following the inversion RF pulse, the longitudinal magnetization begins aligned along the negative z axis, the magnitude of the magnetization vector must first decrease to zero before growing back along the positive z axis. Thus, during this regrowth, the longitudinal magnetization goes from negative (below the transverse plane) through zero to positive (above the transverse plane). When the gradient-echo pulse sequence is initiated, the signals will reflect the state of the longitudinal magnetization created by the inversion-recovery preparation. That is, depending on the chosen delay after the inversion RF pulse and the T1 for the tissue, the signal could be negative, zero, or positive.

Since, by nature of an MP-GRE acquisition, the longitudinal magnetization is relaxing toward thermal equilibrium when the gradient-echo pulse sequence is initiated, the longitudinal magnetization changes throughout the course of the gradient-echo pulse sequence and so the signal levels, and hence contrast among tissues, varies as the k-space data are collected. So what contrast will the image have? In the section "The Fourier transform and k space" in Chapter 1, we indicated that the data in the central region of k space (the low spatial frequency components) primarily determine the contrast and gross structure in the image. Thus, by adjusting the timing of the MP-GRE technique such that the central region of k space is acquired by the gradient-echo pulse sequence at a particular time during the regrowth of the longitudinal magnetization, we can create image contrast that reflects a chosen T1-dependent relationship among the tissues. This timing can be calculated based on the T1 values of the tissues of interest and the duration of the gradient-echo pulse sequence, as determined by the TR and number of phase-encoding steps. It is our experience that characterization of liver lesions using MP-GRE is best performed by acquiring the central lines of k-space data when the longitudinal magnetization corresponding to hemangiomas passes through zero (Figs. 2.13 and 2.14A).[7] At this time, the signal from hemangiomas is nulled and, consequently, hemangiomas appear black in the image (when using conventional magnitude reconstruction). The normal liver, or lesions with shorter T1 values such as metastases, display intermediate to high signal intensity because their longitudinal magnetization will be positive when the central lines of k-space data are collected (Figs. 2.13 and 2.14B). Because the T1 of fluid in cysts is generally longer than the T1 of hemangiomas, the longitudinal magnetization corresponding to cysts will be negative and, as a result, the signal intensity of cysts may appear similar to that of metastases or the surrounding liver in a conventional magnitude reconstructed image, since such a reconstruction discards the sign of the signal. However, at the interface of the cyst with the surrounding tissue, the signal intensity is low because the voxels at the interface contain tissues having both positive (e.g., liver) and negative (cyst) magnetization, leading to signal cancellation. This creates a dark rim around cysts, also called signal "bounce" effect, giving them a highly characteristic appearance (Fig. 2.14C).

3D gradient-echo imaging

To this point our discussion has focused primarily on 2D imaging techniques—that is, techniques that generate a set of 2D slices. As described in detail in the sections "Slice selection" and "Spatial encoding" in Chapter 1, the excitation RF pulse for 2D imaging affects a single relatively thin slice, typically a few millimeters thick, and 2D spatial encoding is performed on the associated transverse magnetization within the slice. In contrast, for 3D imaging, the excitation RF pulse affects a much larger volume of tissue, and spatial encoding is performed along three, instead of two, dimensions, yielding a 3D image set of the volume. To spatially encode the third dimension, the same phase-encoding process described for the 2D imaging is used; a second phase-encoding gradient table, applied along the slice-select direction, is added to the pulse sequence (Fig. 2.15).

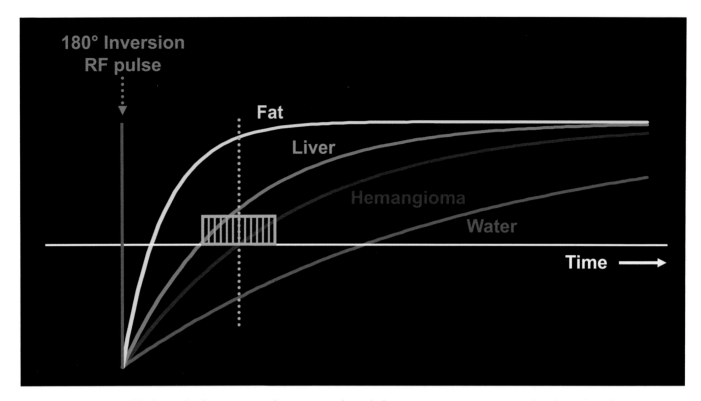

Figure 2.13 *Evolution of the longitudinal magnetization for acquisition of a single slice using a magnetization-prepared gradient-echo pulse sequence.* Conceptually, the magnetization-prepared gradient-echo pulse sequence consists of two independent components: (i) magnetization preparation and (ii) data acquisition using a gradient-echo pulse sequence. The purpose of the magnetization preparation is to create the desired image contrast. In this case, a 180° inversion RF pulse followed by a time delay is used to create strong T1-weighted contrast among the tissues. The purpose of the gradient-echo pulse sequence is to acquire an image that reflects the contrast generated by the magnetization preparation. (The gradient-echo pulse sequence affects the contrast generated by the magnetization preparation to some degree, but this is minimized by appropriate selection of the associated pulse-sequence parameters.) For application to the liver, the timing parameters for the pulse sequence are chosen such that hemangiomas and fluid-filled cysts can be well differentiated. At the start of the pulse sequence for a given slice, the 180° RF pulse "inverts" the longitudinal components of the magnetization associated with the tissues of interest (fat, liver, hemangioma, and fluid in cysts, depicted by *solid yellow, orange, red, and blue lines*, respectively) by rotating them from the thermal equilibrium position, aligned with the positive *z* axis, to the negative *z* axis. Following the inversion RF pulse, the longitudinal magnetization for each tissue relaxes back toward thermal equilibrium from negative (below the transverse plane), through zero, to positive (above the transverse plane) values at a rate determined by its corresponding T1 relaxation time. The gradient-echo pulse sequence (shown as the *green box with vertical lines*) is initiated such that acquisition of the central *k*-space data (represented by the *vertical, dotted white line*) occurs when the longitudinal magnetization associated with hemangiomas passes through zero. Since the transverse magnetization, and hence signal, generated by the gradient-echo pulse sequence for a given tissue is proportional to the corresponding value of the longitudinal magnetization, the signal intensity associated with hemangiomas will be essentially zero and these lesions will appear black in the image (Fig. 2.14A). Likewise, the signal intensity for fat will be relatively high, and that for liver will be lower. Due to its long T1 relaxation time, longitudinal magnetization associated with fluid is negative when the central lines of *k* space are acquired. In a magnitude-reconstructed image (that is, ignoring the sign of the signal), liver and fluid signal intensities will be similar. However, at the boundary between liver and fluid, voxels contain opposing longitudinal magnetizations of roughly the same magnitude and, consequently, signal cancellation occurs. In the image, a characteristic dark rim is seen at the boundary between fluid and liver, as illustrated in Figure 2.14C.

For each value in the second phase-encoding gradient table, the pulse sequence must step through all values in the first phase-encoding gradient table. Thus, the acquisition time for such a 3D pulse sequence is:

$$TR \times N_{PH2D} \times N_{PH3D} \times NEX$$

where N_{PH3D} denotes the number of steps in the phase-encoding gradient table applied along the slice-select direction. As a result, for breath-hold imaging, very short TR values are required to obtain a clinically applicable acquisition time in combination with acceptable spatial resolution.

The image set generated by a 3D acquisition is typically presented as a series of (2D) slices, oriented perpendicular to the slice-select direction. To differentiate these images from those generated by a 2D imaging method, they are often referred to as *partitions*, instead of slices, and the entire volume is referred to as a *slab*. Since the partitions are the result of spatial encoding along the slice-select direction, they are inherently contiguous, in contrast to the slices generated by 2D imaging, which can be separated by gaps. Note that the number of partitions is directly proportional to the number of phase-encoding steps in the slice-select direction (N_{PH3D}), so increasing the number of partitions results in a proportionate increase in the acquisition time.

The additional pulse-sequence repetitions required by using a second phase-encoding gradient table result in a higher signal-to-noise ratio for a 3D acquisition compared to a 2D acquisition that uses the same values for TR, NEX, N_{PH2D},

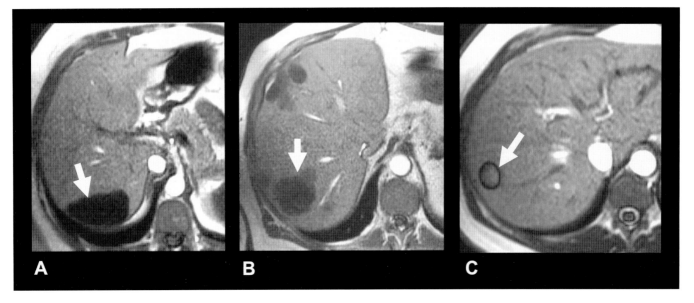

Figure 2.14 *Liver lesion characterization using a magnetization-prepared gradient-echo pulse sequence.* Examples are given of (**A**) a hemangioma, (**B**) a metastasis, and (**C**) a cyst. The images used conventional magnitude reconstruction. Following the 180° inversion RF pulse, the central lines of *k*-space data for image **A** were acquired by the gradient-echo pulse sequence when the longitudinal magnetization corresponding to the hemangioma passed through zero (see Fig. 2.13). As a result, this lesion type displays very low signal intensity, as illustrated in image **A** (*arrow*). The metastasis, shown in **B** (*arrow*), displays signal intensity that is higher than that for hemangiomas because the T1 for metastases is typically shorter than that for hemangiomas and, consequently, the longitudinal magnetization for metastases is positive when the central lines of *k*-space data are collected. The T1 of fluid in cysts is longer than that of hemangiomas, and thus the longitudinal magnetization corresponding to the cyst in image **C** is negative when the central lines of *k*-space data are acquired. However, since the magnitude of the cyst's longitudinal magnetization is similar to that for liver, and because magnitude reconstruction was used, the signal intensity of the cyst appears similar to that of surrounding liver. At the interface of the cyst with adjacent liver, a characteristic dark rim, also called signal "bounce" effect, is seen (*arrow*). This occurs because voxels at the boundary between the two tissues contain transverse magnetization from the liver, which was generated from positive longitudinal magnetization, and transverse magnetization from the cyst, which was generated from negative longitudinal magnetization. As a result, the transverse magnetizations for liver and cyst have opposite phases, leading to signal cancellation, similar to that seen at fat–water interfaces in opposed-phase gradient-echo images (Fig. 2.12A).

and voxel volume. (The relative increase in the signal-to-noise ratio is given by the square root of N_{PH3D}.) As a consequence, the partition thickness used for 3D acquisitions is often much less than the slice thickness used in 2D acquisitions, and 3D acquisitions therefore often provide higher spatial resolution. However, a disadvantage of a 3D acquisition, with its two phase-encoding gradients, is that, depending on the nature of the motion and the details of the pulse sequence, motion artifacts may propagate along both of the phase-encoding directions. Further, compared to a 2D method with equivalent timing parameters, the longer acquisition time associated with the 3D technique may in itself increase the likelihood of motion-related image artifacts.

While 3D gradient-echo acquisitions are commonly used for abdominal MRI, 3D spin-echo–based acquisitions are much less common. Nonetheless, optimized 3D versions of fast T2-weighted spin-echo imaging (see below) are emerging as useful techniques for abdominal MRI.

Contrast-enhanced dynamic imaging and magnetic resonance angiography

Fast 3D gradient-echo pulse sequences are commonly used in the abdomen for breath-hold contrast-enhanced MR angiography (MRA) (Fig. 2.16) and for contrast-enhanced dynamic imaging of organs such the liver, pancreas, and kidneys (Fig. 2.17).[8,9] These sequences provide high temporal resolution

that permits sequential image sets to be obtained during the wash-in and wash-out of a gadolinium-containing contrast agent (Fig. 2.17). Often, these sequences are optimized by using a flip angle that provides the maximum signal-to-noise ratio for the chosen TR and the T1 relaxation time of the gadolinium-containing contrast agent in blood, yielding very strong T1 weighting. Further, the signal from fat is typically suppressed by using FatSat (see section "Fat signal suppression" in Chapter 1). In the resulting images, blood containing the contrast agent demonstrates high signal intensity due to its very short T1 relaxation time, while all other tissues are relatively dark (Fig. 2.16A–E). Multiplanar maximum-intensity-projection images thus clearly depict the architecture of vessels containing the contrast agent (Fig. 2.16F–H). Representative commercially available fast 3D gradient-echo pulse sequences include VIBE (<u>v</u>olumetric <u>i</u>nterpolated <u>b</u>reath-hold <u>e</u>xamination, Siemens Healthcare), LAVA (<u>l</u>iver <u>a</u>cquisition with <u>v</u>olume <u>a</u>cceleration, GE Healthcare), and THRIVE (<u>T</u>1-weighted <u>h</u>igh-<u>r</u>esolution <u>i</u>sotropic <u>v</u>olume <u>e</u>xamination, Philips Healthcare).

To achieve optimal depiction of a given region of interest, intravenous administration of the contrast-agent is typically timed so that arrival of the contrast bolus at the region of interest coincides with acquisition of the central lines in *k* space (i.e., the data that primarily determine image contrast). By doing so, high contrast is obtained between tissues containing the contrast agent and those that do not. For the

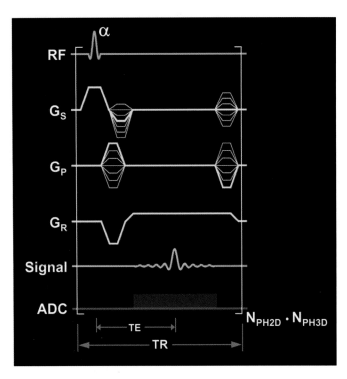

Figure 2.15 *Timing diagram for a 3D gradient-echo pulse sequence.* Most of the features of a 3D gradient-echo pulse sequence are directly analogous to those for its 2D counterpart, illustrated in Figure 2.9. Compared to Figure 2.9, note the second phase-encoding table, applied on the slice-select (G$_S$) gradient axis just after the excitation RF pulse. This timing diagram also shows "rewinder" phase-encoding tables applied on both the G$_P$ and G$_S$ gradient axes, after the MR signal is sampled. For a given repetition of the pulse sequence, such rewinder gradients have the same amplitude, but opposite sign, as the corresponding gradients that occur prior to sampling of the MR signal. These rewinder gradients are part of the RF-spoiling mechanism mentioned above in the section "Short-TR gradient-echo imaging." (Adapted from Mugler JP III. Overview of MR imaging pulse sequences. *Magn Reson Imaging Clin North Am.* 1999;7:661-697.)

abdomen, the region of interest is often at the level of the celiac axis and hepatic arteries, which corresponds to an average bolus arrival time after injection of about 30 seconds. The total acquisition time for routinely available fast 3D gradient-echo pulse sequences used for dynamic or angiographic MR imaging is much less than this, at roughly 10 seconds per 3D image set, while state-of-the-art methods can provide complete 3D image sets in much less than 10 seconds. Nonetheless, since hemodynamic characteristics vary among individuals and are affected by multiple parameters such as cardiac output, blood pressure, and vascular anatomy, the transit time of the contrast-agent bolus from the start of the injection to arrival at the region of interest varies among subjects; consequently, the injection timing required to achieve the desired arrival time needs to be determined separately for each individual.

There are several methods to calculate the time interval between the start of bolus injection and the start of the 3D gradient-echo pulse sequence.[9] The simplest is manual and uses a so-called test (or timing) bolus whereby a small quantity of the contrast material, usually about 1 mL, is injected intravenously into one of the veins in the antecubital fossa while running a separate test pulse sequence that rapidly and repeatedly acquires images at the region of interest. By counting the number of images from the beginning of the test-bolus injection to the moment that the tissues in the target region are seen to enhance, and knowing the duration of the test pulse sequence and the duration and phase-encoding configuration 3D gradient-echo pulse sequence that will be used for dynamic imaging, one can calculate the interval that should be applied between initiation of contrast-agent injection and the start of the 3D gradient-echo pulse sequence (Fig. 2.18). There are also commercially available automated or interactive triggering techniques to detect arrival of the bolus, after which the 3D pulse sequence for dynamic imaging or MR angiography is started. Examples include MR SmartPrep (GE Healthcare) and CARE Bolus (<u>c</u>ombined <u>a</u>pplications to <u>re</u>duce <u>e</u>xposure, Siemens Healthcare).

FAST T2-WEIGHTED IMAGING

As described in the section "Conventional 2D spin-echo imaging," a T2-weighted spin-echo pulse sequence uses a relatively long TR to suppress signal variations arising from differences among the T1 relaxation times of tissues and a relatively long TE to emphasize signal variations arising from differences among the T2 relaxation times of tissues. However, as a consequence of using a relatively long TR (on the order of seconds), the acquisition time for this pulse sequence is much longer than the duration of a breath hold. For example, a conventional T2-weighted spin-echo pulse sequence using a TR of 2,500 ms and 256 phase-encoding steps requires almost 11 minutes. Thus, such an acquisition is not practical for abdominal imaging. Nonetheless, several T2-weighted spin-echo–based techniques have been developed that permit much faster acquisitions, and these currently form the mainstream of T2-weighted imaging of the abdomen. The most commonly used technique is referred to as FSE (<u>f</u>ast <u>s</u>pin <u>e</u>cho, GE Healthcare) or TSE (<u>t</u>urbo <u>s</u>pin <u>e</u>cho, Siemens Healthcare or Philips Healthcare) and includes single-shot versions that are called SS-FSE (<u>s</u>ingle-<u>s</u>hot <u>f</u>ast <u>s</u>pin <u>e</u>cho, GE Healthcare), SS-TSE (<u>s</u>ingle-<u>s</u>hot <u>t</u>urbo <u>s</u>pin <u>e</u>cho, Philips Healthcare), or HASTE (<u>h</u>alf-Fourier <u>a</u>cqui<u>s</u>ition single-shot <u>TSE</u>, Siemens Healthcare).

In the section "Spin echoes" in Chapter 1, we discussed how multiple refocusing RF pulses can be applied following an excitation RF pulse to generate a series of spin echoes, each, of course, having a distinct echo time. The primary difference between the FSE/TSE techniques and a conventional spin-echo pulse sequence is that an FSE/TSE pulse sequence uses such multiple refocusing RF pulses to acquire data corresponding to multiple phase-encoding steps during each sequence repetition (Fig. 2.19), whereas a conventional spin-echo pulse sequence acquires data corresponding to only one phase-encoding step during each repetition.

In terms of acquisition speed, the important consequence of acquiring several phase-encoding steps during each sequence repetition is that the acquisition time is reduced by the same factor (Fig. 2.19). For example, if a "train" of 15 spin echoes is acquired during each repetition and used for 15 phase-encoding

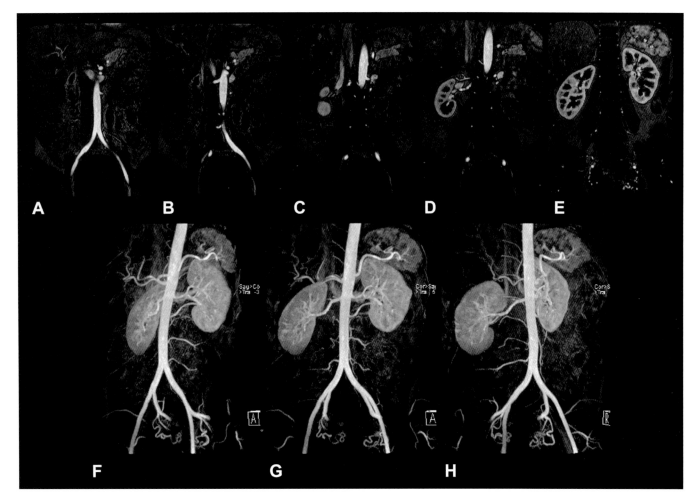

Figure 2.16 *Gadolinium contrast-enhanced magnetic resonance angiography (MRA).* The timing for the start of the pulse sequence was chosen such that arrival of the gadolinium contrast-agent bolus in the volume of interest coincided with the time that the central lines of *k*-space data (i.e., the low spatial frequency components) were acquired. In the resultant images, arteries display very high signal intensity, as demonstrated in the exemplary individual source images **A** through **E** of the 3D data set, which was obtained during a single breath hold. The signal intensities of unenhanced background tissues (for example, liver) and, consequently, contrast among these background tissues, are very low because gadolinium contrast-agent has not yet arrived. Volume rendering of the 3D data set allows calculation of maximum-intensity-projection (MIP) images from selectable viewing angles. These MIP images exhibit high quality independent of the viewing angle due to the approximately isotropic spatial resolution of the source images, and are commonly displayed in a rotating cine presentation. Right-posterior (**F**), frontal (**G**), and left-posterior (**H**) view MIP images generated from the source images of the 3D data set show the major abdominal arteries from different perspectives. Parameters for the 3D gradient-echo pulse sequence included TR/TE 2.6/1.1 ms, matrix 287 × 448 × 128, and voxel dimensions 1.4 × 0.9 × 1.0 mm. A flip angle of 15° was used to provide high signal-to-noise ratio for the chosen TR and the T1 relaxation time of gadolinium-containing contrast material in blood.

steps, the required *k*-space data will be collected 15 times faster compared to a conventional spin-echo pulse sequence that uses the same repetition time. The number of echoes, and hence phase-encoding steps, collected during each sequence repetition of an FSE/TSE pulse sequence is called the echo train length (ETL) or turbo factor (TF). Thus, the acquisition time can be written:

$$\frac{TR \times N_{PH2D} \times NEX}{ETL}.$$

Considering that the phase-encoding steps for an FSE/TSE acquisition correspond to different echo times, which of these echo times determines the contrast in the resulting

image? Recall from our discussion in the section "The Fourier transform and *k* space" in Chapter 1 that the characteristics of the data corresponding to the central region of *k* space primarily determine the contrast for the image. Thus, the echo time corresponding to the phase-encoding steps for the central portion of *k* space determines the image contrast, and therefore the degree of T2 weighting, in FSE/TSE images. For example, if the central phase-encoding steps are acquired at an echo time of 100 ms, then the FSE/TSE image will have contrast that is essentially the same as that for a conventional spin-echo image having an echo time of 100 ms. Since the echo time for the central region of *k* space determines the image contrast, it is called the *effective echo time* for the FSE/TSE pulse sequence, commonly abbreviated TE$_{eff}$ (Fig. 2.19). An associated parameter is the spacing (time interval)

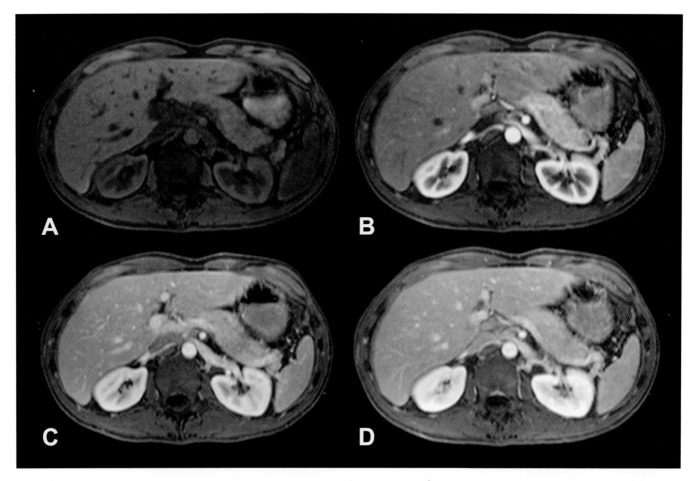

Figure 2.17 *Dynamic contrast-enhanced 3D gradient-echo imaging of the abdomen.* (**A**) Pre-contrast, (**B**) late arterial/early portal-venous phase, (**C**) late portal-venous/early hepatic-venous phase, and (**D**) delayed gadolinium-enhanced images of the abdomen at the level of the liver, pancreas, and kidneys. The 3D data set corresponding to each phase of enhancement was obtained during a breath hold. In image **B** demonstrating early enhancement, high contrast is seen between gadolinium-agent–filled structures and those not yet filled. Signal intensities are further increased in image **C** as the gadolinium agent distributes further into the tissues of interest. However, overall tissue contrast decreases compared to image **B** because all structures of interest have begun to enhance. This effect is even more pronounced in delayed image **D**. Parameters for the 3D gradient-echo pulse sequence included TR/TE 4.9/1.7 ms, matrix 166 × 256 × 60, and voxel dimensions 1.9 × 1.3 × 4.0 mm. A flip angle of 12° was used to provide high signal-to-noise ratio for the chosen TR and the T1 relaxation time of gadolinium-containing contrast material in blood.

between adjacent spin echoes, typically referred to as the *echo spacing* (ESP).

The fact that data in different regions of k space are collected using different echo times does have important consequences. In particular, recall that the characteristics of the data in the outer regions of k space primarily determine the detailed structure of the image. Therefore, if the echo times corresponding to the phase-encoding steps for the outer regions of k space are substantially longer than that corresponding to the phase-encoding steps for the central region of k space, the image may appear blurred because the longer echo times result in lower signal strengths for the high spatial frequency components. (Note that this is particularly an issue when TE_{eff} is relatively short and the train of spin echoes following each excitation RF pulse is relatively long compared to tissue T2 values.) Likewise, if the echo times corresponding to the outer regions of k space are substantially shorter than that corresponding to the central region of k space, the image may appear to have enhanced fine structures. Further, if the echoes are

arranged in k space so that relatively large differences in signal intensity occur among groups of adjacent echoes, ghost artifacts may be generated in the image. Overall, this behavior is in contrast to that for conventional spin-echo imaging, wherein all phase-encoding steps are acquired at a single echo time.

Typically, FSE/TSE pulse sequences are used in a multislice mode (see section "2D multislice imaging") analogous to conventional spin-echo pulse sequences. Thus, even though multiple spin echoes are acquired after each excitation RF pulse, rather than just one or two as in a conventional spin-echo pulse sequence, there is still sufficient "dead time" between sequence repetitions to collect image data for several slice positions. Nonetheless, if TE_{eff} does not occur at the end of the train of spin echoes following each excitation RF pulse, the fraction of TR required for each slice will be larger than that for a conventional spin-echo pulse sequence having an equivalent TE value. As a result, for a given number of slices, the minimum TR required for the FSE/TSE pulse sequence

Box 2.3 ESSENTIALS TO REMEMBER

- Because the magnetization for fat precesses at a slightly lower frequency than that for water, the transverse magnetization for fat gets out of phase with that for water as time progresses following an excitation RF pulse. For voxels containing a mixture of water and fat, this leads to a periodic decrease and increase of the signal in gradient-echo images with increasing TE.

- In opposed-phase gradient-echo imaging, the signal reflects the difference between the transverse magnetizations for water and fat, whereas for in-phase imaging the signal reflects the sum of the transverse magnetizations for water and fat.

- The characteristic dark boundaries between water- and fat-containing tissues in opposed-phase gradient-echo images represent an artifact resulting from the difference in resonant frequencies between water and fat, and should not be mistaken for a capsule or any other anatomic equivalent. These dark margins are more prominent when voxels are large and, conversely, are less noticeable when small voxels are used.

- For liver imaging, the degree of signal loss on opposed-phase gradient-echo images does not reflect the actual degree of fatty infiltration within the organ. Rather, it indicates only the difference between the transverse magnetization vectors of water and fat. Thus, a complete loss of liver signal on opposed-phase images merely indicates that the transverse magnetization vectors for water and fat are about equal; a less dark appearance can indicate that the transverse magnetization for fat is greater than that for water, or that the transverse magnetization for water is greater than that for fat.

- A magnetization-prepared (MP) gradient-echo (GRE) pulse sequence is a single-shot technique that consists of two independent components: the magnetization preparation (typically, a 180° inversion RF pulse followed by a time delay) that creates the image contrast and a short-TR GRE pulse sequence that acquires the data for the image. Because contrast generation is performed separately from the data acquisition, this method provides contrast behavior that cannot be obtained using a gradient-echo pulse sequence alone.

- For a 3D gradient-echo pulse sequence, the acquisition time is determined by the product of the TR, the number of phase encoding steps applied in plane (N_{PH2D}), the number of phase-encoding steps applied along the slice-select direction (N_{PH3D}, which is proportional to the number of partitions), and the number of excitations (NEX).

- In a 3D gradient-echo pulse sequence, the additional pulse-sequence repetitions associated with the second phase-encoding gradient (in the slice-select direction) result in a higher signal-to-noise ratio compared to a 2D acquisition that otherwise uses the same parameters. Compared to the analogous 2D acquisition, the higher signal-to-noise ratio for the 3D acquisition permits acceptable image quality to be obtained for thinner slices (partitions), and thus higher spatial resolution.

- Another advantage of a 3D acquisition is that truly contiguous slices (partitions) are obtained, and thus partial-volume effects are suppressed. A disadvantage is that a 3D acquisition is generally more prone to motion artifacts than a 2D acquisition.

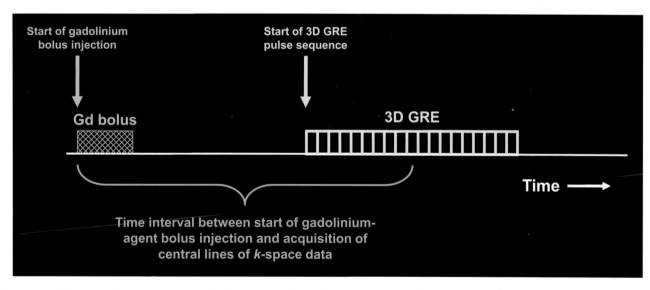

Figure 2.18 *Relationship between contrast-agent bolus injection and MR data acquisition for performing contrast-enhanced imaging.* Intravenous administration of the contrast agent should be timed so that arrival of the contrast-agent bolus at the region of interest coincides with acquisition of the central lines of *k*-space data. For the scenario illustrated in the diagram (that is, when the central lines of *k*-space data are acquired midway through the 3D gradient-echo pulse sequence using a "sequential" phase-encoding order), the time interval between the start of bolus injection and arrival of the contrast material at the region of interest is known prospectively, as determined, for instance, by using a test bolus performed before the actual imaging pulse sequence is executed (see text). Another commonly used configuration acquires the central lines of *k*-space data at the beginning of the 3D gradient-echo pulse sequence ("elliptical centric" phase-encoding order). In this case, determination of the arrival time for the contrast-agent bolus at the region of interest may be performed interactively, as opposed to prospectively, since the central region of *k*-space data is acquired immediately following initiation of the 3D gradient-echo pulse sequence.

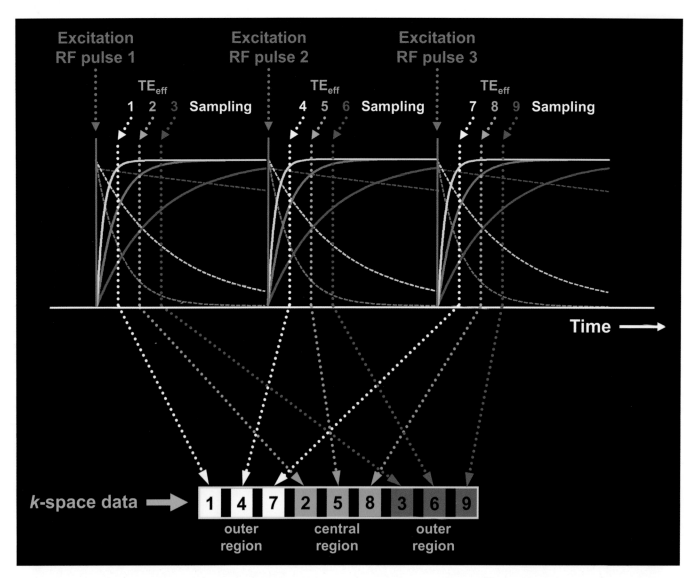

Figure 2.19 *Magnetization behavior during data acquisition for a T2-weighted image from a fast/turbo spin-echo pulse sequence.* Analogous to Figure 2.6, following each excitation RF pulse (except the very first, which is not shown here), multiple refocusing RF pulses are applied to generate multiple spin echoes—two echoes were generated in Figure 2.6 and three echoes are generated in this example. Sampling of the first echo (*white dotted lines*, labeled "1," "4," and "7") occurs when the time after each excitation RF pulse equals the echo spacing (ESP); at this time, the decay of the transverse magnetization is less than that which provides the desired T2 weighting. Sampling of the second echo (*green dotted lines*, labeled "2," "5," and "8") occurs when the time after each excitation RF pulse equals twice the ESP; at this time, the decay of the transverse magnetization equals that which provides the desired T2 weighting and thus this echo is labeled "TE$_{eff}$." Finally, sampling of the third echo (*pink dotted lines*, labeled "3," "6," and "9") occurs at three times the ESP. Also analogous to Figure 2.6, a long TR is used to minimize contributions from differences among T1 values. However, in contrast to the situation illustrated in Figure 2.6 for the conventional spin-echo pulse sequence, wherein two echoes are used to generate two <u>separate</u> images, all echoes collected for the fast/turbo spin-echo pulse sequence are used for the *k*-space data of the <u>same</u> image. Consequently, the acquisition time for this fast/turbo spin-echo pulse sequence is three times less than that for a conventional spin-echo pulse sequence using the same TR. As illustrated by the yellow box at the bottom of the diagram, the phase-encoding gradients are configured so that data associated with the second echo time correspond to the central region of *k* space (low spatial frequencies) along the phase-encoding direction, while data associated with the first and third echo times correspond to the outer regions of *k* space (high spatial frequencies) along the phase-encoding direction. Thus, the contrast in the image is primarily determined by the second echo time, which is why this echo time is called the effective echo time (TE$_{eff}$) for the image. The first and third echoes are used to provide the *k*-space information describing image details. As discussed in the text, certain types of image artifacts may be generated if the signal intensities corresponding to the outer regions of *k* space differ substantially from those corresponding to the central region of *k* space. In practice, a T2-weighted fast/turbo spin-echo pulse sequence would typically use approximately 10 to 20 echoes following each excitation RF pulse, instead of only a small number as shown here; a small number was used to make the illustration simpler while conveying the major points.

will be longer than that required for a conventional spin-echo pulse sequence. Because the collection of data for all slices is inherently intermingled with the multislice approach, FSE/TSE imaging is also relatively sensitive to motion because when the subject moves or breathes, it will affect all images in the data set, yielding artifacts of a similar nature in each image.

In contrast to the repetitive nature of multislice FSE/TSE imaging, the concept of single-shot versions is to acquire a sufficient number of spin echoes (often more than 100) to form an image following a single 90° excitation RF pulse. That is, the k-space data corresponding to one entire image are collected following each excitation RF pulse (Fig. 2.20). Since the transverse magnetization decays throughout the acquisition of the large number of spin echoes, and such signal decay can lead to artifacts such as blurring as described earlier in this section, methods to minimize the required number of echoes are useful for improving image quality of single-shot acquisitions. Therefore, the *half-Fourier* method is often used in conjunction with single-shot FSE/TSE techniques (e.g., in HASTE) to reduce the required duration of the train of spin echoes. The half-Fourier approach takes advantage of the inherent, "conjugate" symmetry relationship between a given component in k space and its partner on the opposite side of k space (e.g., the partner of a component at location k_x, k_y is at $-k_x, -k_y$). Ideally, if the data for one half of k space is measured, the data for the other half can be calculated. In practice, to account for certain non-ideal effects, data for slightly more than one half of

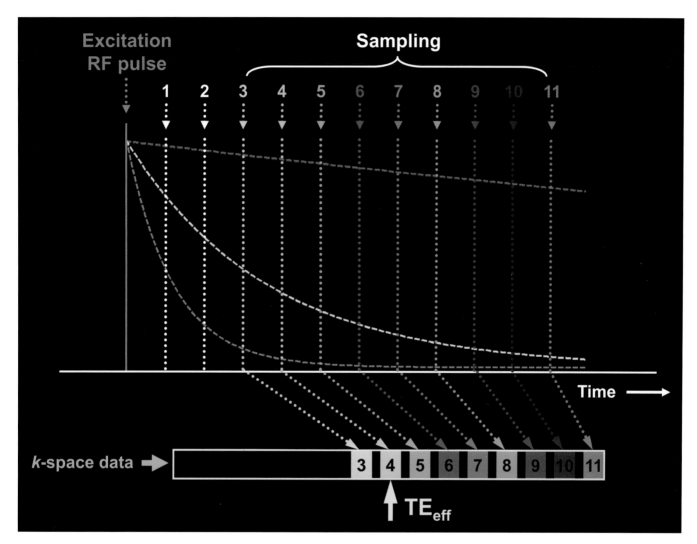

Figure 2.20 *Magnetization behavior during data acquisition for a T2-weighted image from a half-Fourier, single-shot fast/turbo spin-echo pulse sequence.* Following a single 90° excitation RF pulse applied to the longitudinal magnetization at thermal equilibrium, a large number of uniformly spaced 180° refocusing RF pulses are applied, generating an equal number of uniformly spaced spin echoes. These echoes are sampled as the transverse magnetization decays. (For simplicity, only 11 echoes are shown, 9 of which are sampled, while in practice as many as approximately 100 echoes may be used.) Depending on the number of echoes and the echo spacing, and on the desired image contrast, some of the initial echoes may be discarded (that is, not sampled). In this example, the first two echoes are not sampled. As illustrated by the yellow box at the bottom of the diagram, the phase-encoding gradients are configured so that data associated with the echo time (labeled "4") providing the desired T2 weighting (that is, the effective echo time [TE_eff]) are put in the center of k space along the phase-encoding direction (*yellow arrow*), while data associated with the other echoes are used to fill other portions of k space. In this *half-Fourier* acquisition, only slightly more than half of k space is filled with (measured) data; the data corresponding to the remainder of k space (area within the yellow box showing no colored bars) are, in effect, estimated based on the conjugate symmetry properties of the k-space data. Since sufficient data to reconstruct the image are collected following a single 90° excitation RF pulse, the acquisition time for single-shot FSE/TSE is much shorter than that for conventional spin-echo, or multislice fast/turbo spin-echo as depicted in Figure 2.19, since the latter techniques require many excitation RF pulses to collect the data needed for each image. The acquisition time for each single-shot FSE/TSE slice is given by the number of echoes (echo train length [ETL]) times the spacing between echoes (echo spacing [ESP]) as described in the text.

k space are required. Nonetheless, this represents a substantial reduction compared to the complete *k*-space data set.

Since single-shot FSE/TSE methods use only a single 90° excitation RF pulse for each image, there is no repetition time associated with a given slice, or, stated another way, the TR for each slice is infinite. Consequently, the formula provided above is not used to calculate the acquisition time. Rather, the acquisition time <u>per slice</u> is given by the product of the echo train length and the echo spacing. Thus, the acquisition time per slice can be written:

$$\text{ETL} \times \text{ESP}.$$

The acquisition time for single-shot FSE/TSE methods is typically less than 1 second per slice, which is substantially shorter than the acquisition time (on the order of tens of seconds to minutes) for comparable multislice FSE/TSE acquisitions. However, since for clinical imaging multiple slices are usually required to cover a region of interest, single-shot FSE/TSE imaging is commonly used in a *sequential-slice* mode, wherein one complete slice is acquired, followed by a second complete slice at another position, and so on. Thus, in contrast to the fundamentally intermingled nature of data collection for multislice imaging, the acquisition of a given slice is independent of the acquisitions of all other slices, and any effects of subject motion or breathing will not be the same for all slices. For example, if the subject coughs at one point during the acquisition of 15 slices, only the slice being acquired during the cough will be contaminated by associated motion artifacts; the remaining 14 slices will not be affected. Consequently, single-shot FSE/TSE methods are relatively insensitive to motion (Fig. 2.21). In fact, because the time to acquire each slice is shorter than the typical respiratory cycle, single-shot FSE/TSE images show minimal motion-related artifacts (i.e., blurring or ghosting) even when acquired during free breathing. In view of their short acquisition time and relative insensitivity to breathing artifacts, single-shot FSE/TSE methods are commonly used for cross-sectional T2-weighted imaging (TE_{eff} 80 to 100 ms) of the abdomen. At our institution, this technique is included in all of the abdominal protocols.

Since the single 90° excitation RF pulse for each slice is typically applied when the magnetization is at thermal equilibrium, the contrast in single-shot FSE/TSE is determined by differences in T2 relaxation times and proton densities among tissues. To introduce T1 weighting or to permit the signal associated with a particular tissue to be suppressed, a 180° inversion RF pulse (see section "Manipulating the magnetization using RF pulses" in Chapter 1) can be applied before the excitation RF pulse. (Inversion RF pulses are also commonly used with multislice FSE/TSE imaging to permit selective suppression of the signal from fat [STIR, as discussed in the section "Fat signal suppression" in Chapter 1] or fluids.)

Although the contrast for a multislice or single-shot FSE/TSE image with a given TE_{eff} is very similar to that for a conventional spin-echo image with an equivalent TE value, there are important differences that arise due to the large number of closely spaced, high-flip-angle refocusing RF pulses used for FSE/TSE imaging. Probably the most obvious difference is that fat appears relatively bright in T2-weighted multislice or single-shot FSE/TSE images, even for a fairly long TE_{eff} value, whereas it appears relatively dark in T2-weighted conventional spin-echo images acquired with an equivalent

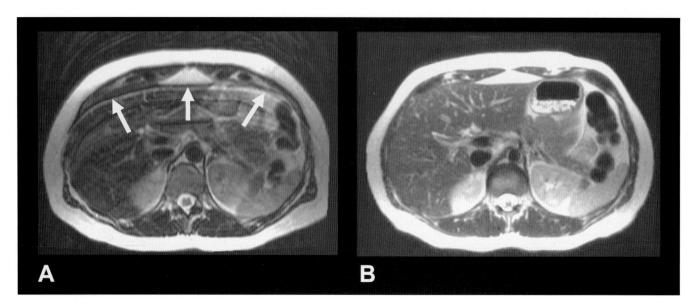

Figure 2.21 *Motion sensitivity of multislice versus single-shot techniques.* (**A**) Image from a multislice FSE/TSE pulse sequence and (**B**) corresponding image from a single-shot FSE/TSE pulse sequence obtained in the same individual who was asked to breath normally while the images were acquired. Each image set consisted of 20 images, acquired in 12 s. In **A**, ghost artifacts (some indicated by *arrow*s) from the moving anterior abdominal wall are seen because filling of *k* space occurred continuously during the entire 12-s period while the subject was breathing. In **B**, ghost artifacts are not seen because the *k*-space data for the entire image were collected in less than 1 sec following a single excitation RF pulse. Even though data collection for image **B** occurred during breathing, movement of abdominal structures was minimal during the short acquisition time and, as a result, there are no noticeable motion artifacts.

TE value (Fig. 2.22). For fat molecules, "J-coupling" (essentially, magnetic crosstalk) among neighboring protons in the molecule plays an important role in the observed decay of transverse magnetization (and hence signal) following the excitation RF pulse. The closely spaced refocusing RF pulses in a multislice or single-shot FSE/TSE pulse sequence suppress the effects of J-coupling, resulting in a slower decay of the fat signal. Since T1-weighted images also display bright fat, the relatively bright fat signal in T2-weighted multislice or single-shot FSE/TSE images can sometimes be a source of confusion, potentially causing T2-weighted images to be mistaken for T1-weighted images.

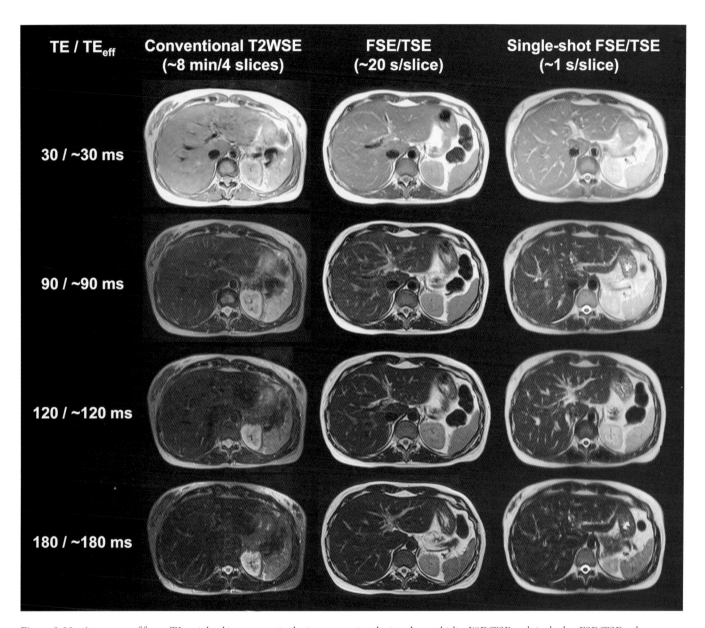

Figure 2.22 *Appearance of fat on T2-weighted images acquired using conventional spin-echo, multislice FSE/TSE and single-shot FSE/TSE pulse sequences.* A four-echo acquisition with TEs of 30, 60, 90, and 120 ms was used for conventional T2-weighted spin-echo (T2WSE) imaging. Approximately the same echo-time values were used as effective TEs for multislice FSE/TSE and single-shot FSE/TSE imaging. All four images of each technique are shown with the same window and center settings. With conventional T2WSE imaging, the fat signal (e.g., in subcutaneous tissues) decreases markedly with increasing TE. However, even at long effective TEs, the signal from fat remains relatively high with both multislice and single-shot FSE/TSE imaging. Note, for example, that fat surrounding the kidney is darker than the kidney at a TE of 90 ms or longer with conventional T2WSE imaging, whereas, even at an effective TE of 180 ms, the fat is brighter than the kidney in the multislice and single-shot FSE/TSE images. Note also that fluid (e.g., cerebrospinal fluid) is brighter in single-shot FSE/TSE images acquired with relatively long effective TE compared to the other techniques because the TR for single-shot FSE/TSE is effectively infinite, and thus even tissues with very long T1 relaxation times, such as fluid, are at thermal equilibrium just before the excitation RF pulse is applied. (In most other T2-weighted spin-echo sequences, the TR is not usually long enough to allow essentially full recovery of the longitudinal magnetization for fluids before each excitation RF pulse is applied.) Other imaging parameters included TR 2,500 ms for both conventional T2WSE and multislice FSE/TSE; ETL 23 for multislice FSE/TSE and 192 for single-shot (half-Fourier) FSE/TSE; NEX 1 for all pulse sequences; and acquisition time ~8 min for conventional T2WSE, 20 s for each multislice FSE/TSE image, and ~1 s for each single-shot FSE/TSE image.

The closely spaced refocusing RF pulses of a multislice or single-shot FSE/TSE pulse sequence also reduce the rate of signal decay for water molecules diffusing through microscopic field inhomogeneities such as those present in the vicinity of hemorrhagic blood products or in the iron-containing nuclei of the brain. Since these entities are characterized in T2-weighted images by relative signal reduction, the contrast between hemorrhagic blood products or iron-containing nuclei and surrounding tissue in a multislice or single-shot FSE/TSE image is less than that in a conventional spin-echo image. For multislice imaging using an FSE/TSE pulse sequence, the large number of closely spaced refocusing RF pulses also cause *magnetization transfer* effects in proteinaceous tissues (e.g., brain tissue or muscle) that result in a relative signal reduction for these tissues compared to those with low protein content.

An important specific application of FSE/TSE imaging, often performed using the single-shot form of the pulse sequence, is magnetic resonance cholangiopancreatography (MRCP). This method, which permits evaluation of the biliary system and pancreatic duct, takes advantage of the very long T2 of fluid within the ducts, and therefore uses a very long TE_{eff}, typically 500 ms or greater, to emphasize signal from fluid. The signal from fat is suppressed using fat saturation (see section "Fat signal suppression" in Chapter 1), yielding images wherein high signal intensities are only from fluid, depicting the ducts in great detail. A common implementation of MRCP entails acquiring multiple thick (40 to 60 mm) slices in coronal/paracoronal orientation using a single-shot FSE/TSE sequence, with each slice collected in approximately 1 second and positioned at a different angle with respect to the common bile duct so that the acquired set of slices "rotate" about the duct (Fig. 2.23A). An advantage of this technique is that because of the short acquisition duration for each slice, images are usually free of breathing artifacts. However, a drawback is that since the slices are relatively thick (40 to 60 mm), fluid-filled structures not related to the bile ducts may be included in the slices and interfere with interpretation (Fig. 2.23A). Another application for the thick-slice MRCP technique is to assess the fluid-filled renal collecting system and ureters (see Chapter 6, Fig 6.22A). Recently, optimized 3D versions of FSE/TSE imaging have become available that are particularly useful for MRCP, providing a large number of contiguous images with high, isotropic spatial resolution (~1 mm or less) in less than 10 minutes and allowing multiplanar maximum-intensity-projection reconstruction (Fig. 2.23B). Since such 3D MRCP acquisitions are much longer than a breath hold, respiratory gating is used to suppress breathing artifacts. For this approach, approximately 1 second of data is acquired each time the abdominal organs reach a point of relatively little

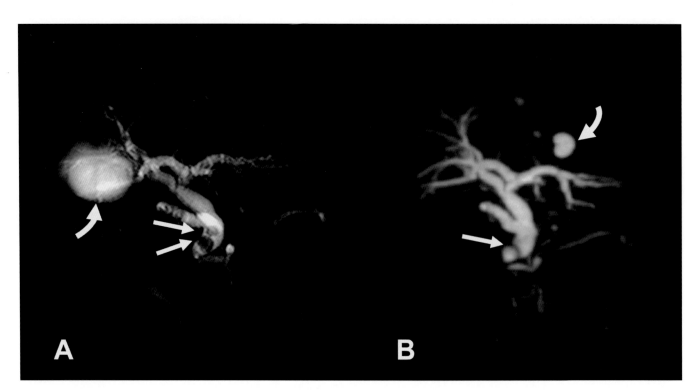

Figure 2.23 *Thick-slice versus multislice MRCP.* (**A**) Paracoronal thick (60 mm)-slice single-shot FSE/TSE (ETL 256, TE_{eff} 750 ms) image of the bile ducts obtained in less than 1 s during a breath hold and (**B**) maximum-intensity-projection (MIP) image from a respiratory-gated 3D FSE/TSE (ETL 128, TE_{eff} 650 ms) acquisition providing thin (1.6 mm) images in approximately 4 minutes. In **A**, two large stones are shown in the distal common bile duct (*straight arrows*). In **B**, the largest of these (*straight arrow*) is seen in the MIP image, but the smaller one is obscured due to the superposition of signals from the multiple slices of the data set. This smaller stone and the larger one were seen on the source images (not shown) of the 3D acquisition. In **A**, part of a large liver cyst (*curved arrow*) is included in the image, as it fell within the thick slice, obscuring part of the bile ducts in the right lobe. This cyst is not seen in the MIP image in **B** as it was not included in the 3D acquisition. However, another small liver cyst is seen in **B** (*curved arrow*), but was not included in the thick slice for the acquisition in **A**.

motion, typically at end expiration. Since the average respiratory cycle is 4 to 6 seconds, respiratory-gated acquisitions usually require several minutes to collect the required k-space data. Although the high spatial resolution with which the images are obtained is an obvious major advantage of the technique, a drawback is that the respiratory-gated acquisition can easily lead to degradation of the images when the patient breathes irregularly, and therefore the technique is not always successful. Further, although maximum-intensity-projection images allow for good 3D assessment of the biliary tree, abnormalities within the ducts, such as stones (Fig. 2.23B), can be easily obscured due to the superimposition of the multiple slices in the data set; therefore, careful evaluation of the individual source images is essential, as otherwise these abnormalities can be overlooked.

FSE/TSE methods are also particularly useful for pelvic imaging, an area where the excursions of the abdominal wall during breathing are less than in the abdomen. High-quality images can thus generally be obtained without breath holding or respiratory gating. A common application is the acquisition images with high spatial resolution for detailed evaluation of the female reproductive organs.

APPEARANCE OF FLOWING BLOOD

The majority of pulse-sequence techniques discussed above, including relatively fast methods that can be completed within a breath hold, have acquisition times that are longer than the cardiac cycle. For these methods, the effect of blood flow during the acquisition plays a primary role in determining the appearance of vessels. Depending on the characteristics of the flow (e.g., speed, direction, and pulsatility) and how these characteristics interact with the particular pulse sequence, flowing blood may appear with low signal intensity (so-called *dark blood* or *black blood*), may appear with high signal intensity (so-called *bright blood* or *white blood*), or may generate ghost artifacts. Either very low (dark blood) or very high (bright blood) signal from flowing blood can be used for MR angiography to assess the vessels. (Bright blood from gadolinium-containing contrast material was discussed above in the section "Contrast-enhanced dynamic imaging and magnetic resonance angiography.") In this section, we will describe briefly several of the basic mechanisms that affect the appearance of flowing blood. The reader is referred to other texts for detailed information on various MR angiographic techniques based on flow.

Box 2.4 ESSENTIALS TO REMEMBER

- The primary difference between FSE/TSE and conventional spin-echo pulse sequences is that, for FSE/TSE, the data from multiple echoes collected during each repetition are used to provide multiple phase-encoding steps, whereas, for conventional spin-echo, the data corresponding to only one phase-encoding step are collected during each sequence repetition. Consequently, the time to complete all phase-encoding steps for a FSE/TSE image is much faster than that for a conventional spin-echo sequence, and is determined by the product of TR, number of phase-encoding steps, and NEX, divided by the number of echoes (echo train length [ETL] or turbo factor [TF]).

- The contrast in a FSE/TSE image is primarily determined by the echo time that corresponds to the central region of k space (low spatial frequencies); this echo time is called the effective echo time or TE_{eff}.

- The major difference between single-shot and multislice FSE/TSE pulse sequences is that, for the former, the k-space data for an entire image are collected following a single 90° excitation RF pulse, whereas, for the latter, multiple 90° excitation RF pulses are required to collect the k-space data for an image. As a result, image acquisition for a single-shot FSE/TSE pulse sequence is much faster than for a multislice FSE/TSE pulse sequence. The imaging time of single-shot FSE/TSE is often further reduced by using a half-Fourier acquisition to shorten the duration of the echo train, thereby reducing artifacts, such as blurring, related to the decay of transverse magnetization during the acquisition of the large number of echoes.

- With appropriate parameters, single-shot and multislice FSE/TSE pulse sequences can be used for both T1- and T2-weighted imaging. In practice, however, the techniques are most commonly used for T2-weighted imaging because of the considerable reduction in acquisition times that can be achieved compared to a conventional T2-weighted spin-echo pulse sequence.

- Because a single-shot T2-weighted FSE/TSE pulses sequence uses only a single 90° excitation RF pulse, the excitation RF pulse is not repeated and, hence, there is no repetition time associated with this technique. In other words, TR for each slice is infinite. Thus, for single-shot FSE/TSE, the acquisition time per slice is determined by the product of the echo train length (ETL) and echo spacing (ESP).

- Single-shot and multislice T2-weighted FSE/TSE images generally show relatively bright fat signal, even when a long effective TE is used, which can be confusing as this potentially causes the images to be mistaken for T1-weighted images. Compared to conventional T2-weighted spin-echo imaging, the high fat signal is related to a reduced decay rate for the transverse magnetization associated with fat, caused by the closely spaced refocusing RF pulses needed to generate the multiple echoes. A conventional T2-weighted spin-echo image obtained with a TE that is the same as the effective TE of a single-shot or multislice T2-weighted FSE/TSE image shows fat with much lower signal intensity than that in the FSE/TSE image.

Dark blood from flow-related signal void

Flowing blood often appears relatively dark in 2D spin-echo-based images when a sizable component of the flow is perpendicular to the slice. The reason for this appearance can be understood as follows. The excitation RF pulse applied each sequence repetition converts longitudinal magnetization for all tissues, including that for flowing blood, into transverse magnetization. Subsequently, in the time interval between the excitation and refocusing RF pulses, a portion of the excited magnetization associated with blood flows out of the slice. As a result, when a given refocusing RF pulse is applied, blood that has flowed out of the slice does not experience this refocusing RF pulse and therefore does not contribute signal to the image. Blood flowing with relatively high velocity thus appears dark, creating a *flow-related signal void*, because most or all of the flowing blood does not experience the refocusing RF pulse(s), while that flowing with relatively low velocity contributes signal to the image (Fig. 2.24). The velocity required for blood to traverse the slice during the time interval between the excitation RF pulse and a given refocusing RF pulse is simply the slice thickness divided by the time interval.

Our discussion of flow-related signal void assumes that the longitudinal magnetization associated with blood has a sufficiently large value for blood to yield measurable signal in the images if it experiences the refocusing RF pulses. However, as described in the next section for blood flowing through a set of slices, the longitudinal magnetization of blood in a given slice may be relatively small due to the effects of the RF pulses associated with slices upstream of the slice of interest. In this case, because the initial longitudinal magnetization for blood is relatively small, blood will appear relatively dark independent of whether it experiences the refocusing RF pulses.

Bright blood from inflow enhancement

The primary reason for flowing blood, in the absence of contrast-agent enhancement, to appear bright is so-called *inflow enhancement* or t*ime-of-flight* (TOF) effect. In abdominal imaging, inflow enhancement is commonly seen with short-TR, gradient-echo pulse sequences, such as those discussed in the section "Fast T1-weighted imaging." For these techniques, excitation RF pulses are applied frequently (short TR) and RF spoiling is used to effectively eliminate transverse magnetization generated by a given RF pulse prior to the following RF pulse. As a result, the size of longitudinal magnetization for each tissue is typically much less than the corresponding thermal equilibrium values because there is relatively little time between RF pulses for T1 relaxation. Further, since the signal produced by an excitation RF pulse is directly related to the amount of longitudinal magnetization that exists just before the pulse, the reduction in longitudinal magnetization translates to correspondingly lower signal intensities relative to those that would be generated from thermal-equilibrium longitudinal magnetization. Therefore, if "fresh" (i.e., having thermal-equilibrium magnetization) blood flows into the slice between applications of the RF pulses, it will, upon experiencing the subsequent excitation RF pulse, generate a relatively high signal compared to other tissues. In other words, the *inflow* of the blood *enhances* its signal, leading to the name *inflow enhancement*. A number of methods specifically designed for MR angiography are based on this phenomenon, and are called time-of-flight MRA techniques because the amount of enhancement of the blood signal depends on the time it takes fresh blood to flow (or "fly") into the volume of interest (an example of TOF MR angiography is shown in Fig. 11.32 in Chapter 11).

Once fresh blood flows into a slice or volume of interest, it will of course experience frequently applied RF pulses, just like stationary tissue, and consequently its longitudinal magnetization and corresponding signal will gradually decrease. Therefore, considering either a series of 2D slices or a 3D volume, the inflow enhancement effect is diminished at locations relatively far from that at which the blood first entered. For example, for a set of axial slices perpendicular to the aorta, blood is very bright (large inflow-enhancement effect) in the first (most cranial) slice, but gradually decreases in signal intensity relative to surrounding stationary tissue in each consecutive slice, as illustrated in Figure 2.25. The inflow-enhancement effect is most pronounced for vessels oriented perpendicular to the slice or volume of interest, and also increases with increasing velocity of blood flow. Thus, inflow enhancement is generally stronger for arteries than for veins.

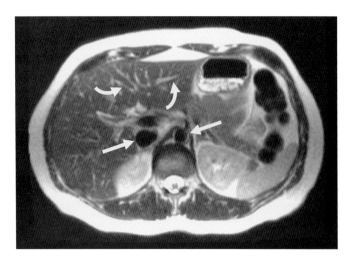

Figure 2.24 *Flow-related signal void.* Axial single-shot FSE/TSE image. The blood in the major vessels, such as the aorta and inferior vena cava (*straight arrows*), flows with relatively high velocity perpendicular to the slice and thus does not experience many of the refocusing RF pulses during data acquisition. As a result, the blood in these vessels appears dark due to the flow-related signal void phenomenon discussed in the text. Blood having a relatively low flow velocity or flowing mostly within the slice, such as that in the small hepatic veins (several indicated by *curved arrows*), contributes signal because it experiences most (or all) of the refocusing RF pulses as it flows through the slice during data acquisition, and appears with intermediate-high signal intensity in the image.

Dark blood from flow-related dephasing

In the section "Spatial encoding" in Chapter 1, we described how magnetic-field gradient pulses are used for frequency and

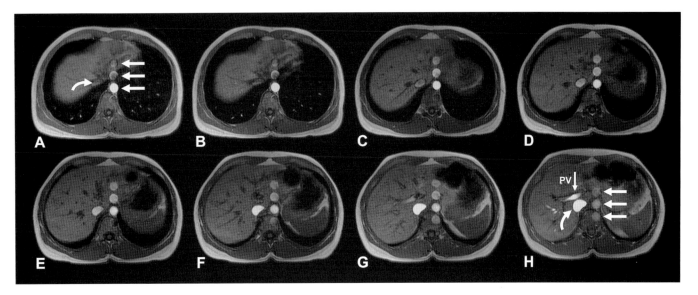

Figure 2.25 *Appearance of inflow (bright blood) relative to slice position.* (**A–H**) Eight contiguous images from the dome of the liver through the level of the main portal vein obtained using a 2D T1-weighted gradient-echo pulse sequence with short TR/TE (115/48 ms). The images were acquired with phase encoding in the anterior-posterior direction. In image **A**, the aorta (*most posterior straight arrow*) shows high signal intensity from strong inflow enhancement effect as blood, with longitudinal magnetization at thermal equilibrium because it has not yet experienced any RF pulses, flows from outside the imaging volume in craniocaudal direction into the first slice. Pulsation (motion) artifacts are also seen along the phase-encoding direction (*other straight arrows*). The signal intensities of the other tissues in the slice are much lower, and thus these tissues appear darker than the inflowing blood, because the associated longitudinal magnetizations are less than the corresponding thermal equilibrium values as there is relatively little time between RF pulses for T1 relaxation. In **A**, the inflow enhancement effect is not seen in the inferior vena cava (IVC, *curved arrow*). In subsequent images (**B–H**) the signal intensity in the aorta decreases gradually, and is the lowest in **H** (*middle horizontal straight arrow*), because the blood in the aorta experiences an increasing number of RF pulses as it flows deeper into the set of eight slices. Pulsation artifacts from the aorta are also less pronounced in **H** (*other horizontal straight arrows*) due to the decreased signal. The reverse is seen in the IVC, in which the blood flows in caudocranial direction. The signal in this vessel is highest in image **H** (*curved arrow*), where the blood enters the set of slices with the longitudinal magnetization at thermal equilibrium. With deeper penetration into the set of slices, and thus from **H–A** and in the opposite direction as the signal changes in the aorta, the signal in the IVC decreases and there is virtually no visible signal in image **A**. Note in **H** that there is also inflow enhancement of the blood in the main portal vein (PV, *vertical straight arrow*).

phase encoding to determine the position of transverse magnetization. The typical configuration of gradient pulses used for such encoding assumes that the transverse magnetization is stationary. However, if the transverse magnetization is moving (e.g., due to blood flow or respiration), it will accumulate an additional phase shift, proportional to velocity, from the encoding process. Depending on the circumstances and design of the pulse sequence, such motion-induced phase shifts can cause signal loss, can cause ghost artifacts, or, on a positive note, can be used to quantitatively measure flow or motion. Here, we are interested in the mechanism for signal loss, causing blood to appear dark.

Many blood vessels exhibit a variation of flow velocity across their lumen. For example, the velocity may peak near the center of the vessel and decrease to zero at the wall. An image voxel within such a vessel will contain blood flowing with a range of velocities. Thus, when the blood within the voxel experiences the spatial-encoding gradient pulses, a

---

Box 2.5 **ESSENTIALS TO REMEMBER**

- Blood flowing within vessels is often dark in 2D spin-echo–based images because it appears as a flow-related signal void when a sizable component of the flow is perpendicular to the slice. This occurs because, in the time interval between the excitation and refocusing RF pulses required for acquisition of the image, a portion of the excited magnetization associated with blood flows out of the slice and does not experience the refocusing RF pulses; hence, it does not contribute signal to the image. Blood flowing with relatively low velocity contributes signal to the image.

- Bright blood, or inflow enhancement, is commonly seen with short-TR, gradient-echo pulse sequences. Blood flowing into a slice from outside the imaging volume has enhanced signal because blood outside of the slice does not experience any of the RF pulses and, consequently, enters the slice with thermal equilibrium magnetization. As a result, its signal is much larger than that for other (stationary) tissues within the slice since these tissues have experienced multiple RF pulses with relatively little time between pulses for T1 relaxation. Hence, for the stationary tissues, the longitudinal magnetizations, and corresponding signal intensities, are substantially reduced compared to inflowing blood.

range of motion-induced phase shifts will result, corresponding to the range of velocities within the voxel. If the range of velocities is sufficiently large, the corresponding magnetization will be dephased over a large range of phase angles, leading to signal reduction or loss (so-called *intravoxel dephasing*). Therefore, *flow-related dephasing* causes blood to appear dark in voxels that contain a sufficiently large range of blood velocities.

Spatial-encoding gradient pulses can be specially designed to compensate for the phase shifts that arise due to motion. In this case, the spatial-encoding gradient pulses have the same effect regardless of whether transverse magnetization is stationary or moving. This is often called gradient moment refocusing (GMR) or flow compensation (for short, *FlowComp*).

PRACTICAL CONSIDERATIONS

We conclude this chapter with a review of several practical issues that are important to remember when performing MR imaging. These include a discussion of common image artifacts and some specific issues related to MR imaging of the abdomen, as well as a brief overview of the effects of changing common imaging parameters. A representative protocol for routine abdominal imaging is provided at the end of the chapter.

ARTIFACTS

An artifact is an undesired alteration of signal intensities in the image arising from a wide variety of possible sources, such as equipment malfunction, RF noise leaking into the scan room, or subject motion. Artifacts are a common problem in MR imaging and there are many distinct types. In this section we focus on the most common artifacts encountered in MR imaging of the abdomen, and discuss strategies for artifact reduction. Our discussion is certainly not all-inclusive; the reader is referred to the literature for more detailed information.

Motion and flow

The most common artifacts in MR imaging of the abdomen arise from movement of the abdominal wall during respiration, and movement (flow) of blood in the vessels. These artifacts, which are generated due to motion of the associated transverse magnetization, are seen primarily along the phase-encoding direction (or possibly both phase-encoding directions in a 3D acquisition) and appear as "ghosts" over the images. As described in Chapter 1, a "ghost" is a replica of a moving structure or a portion of the structure, displaced from the actual structure along the phase-encoding direction.[10]

Fundamentally, motion artifacts occur because the magnetization moves during the spatial-encoding process, and unless the pulse sequence is specifically designed to compensate for effects of this motion, the magnetization will be improperly encoding and thereby cause signals to appear in the wrong location. For the pulse sequences discussed earlier in this chapter, the frequency-encoding process requires only a few milliseconds for a given line of *k*-space data, whereas the phase-encoding process occurs over a period of seconds to minutes. Since the cardiac and respiratory cycles are on the order of seconds, substantial motion may occur over the duration of the phase-encoding process, but not over the duration of the frequency-encoding process. Further, due to the nature of the spatial-encoding process, periodic variations in signal intensity or phase, such as may occur due to respiration or the beating heart, are manifest as periodic signal alterations in the image. Considering these factors, cardiac and respiratory motion can cause multiple ghost artifacts to appear along the phase-encoding direction(s), but not along the frequency-encoding direction. For example, artifacts from breathing often appear as a series of lines propagated along the phase-encoding direction, paralleling the anterior abdominal wall (Fig. 2.26A). As the phase of a ghost signal may differ from that of the underlying stationary tissue, ghost artifacts may appear bright in some locations but dark in others.

Since the entire width of the abdomen, particularly the anterior abdominal wall, moves with respiration, the associated ghosts are seen over the entire abdomen, whereas for flow the ghost artifacts are limited to the width of the vessel. Because the intensity of ghost artifacts is directly related to the signal intensity of the moving structure, artifacts are most severe from tissues that display high signal intensity, such as fat in T1-weighted images, fluid in T2-weighted images, or inflowing blood in gradient-echo images.

There are several ways that ghost artifacts can be suppressed. Obviously, artifacts related to respiration can be eliminated by performing data acquisition during a breath hold. Further, respiratory gating can be used for acquisitions that cannot be completed within a breath-hold period, as discussed in the section "Fast T2-weighted imaging." A limitation of this method is that it is time-consuming, since in most individuals breathing is relatively slow, averaging about 15 cycles per minute, and it may therefore take several minutes to complete a respiratory-gated acquisition. Another approach is to use fat saturation, as discussed in the section "Fat signal suppression" in Chapter 1. This suppresses the bright signal from fat and therefore decreases the associated ghost artifacts (Fig. 2.26B). A downside of fat suppression in abdominal imaging is that it may be more difficult to identify boundaries between some structures because the relatively low signal intensity for fat may parallel that of other structures in the abdomen, such as the liver and pancreas, and therefore fat suppression is not routinely used for several of the pulse sequences in the protocols for abdominal imaging at our institution.

So-called *spatial presaturation* (for short, *spatial presat* or simply *presat*) or *regional inversion* RF pulses can also be used to reduce breathing- or flow-related artifacts.[11] Manipulation of moving (e.g., from respiration) or flowing magnetization using spatial presaturation (90°) or regional inversion (180°) RF pulses is analogous to manipulation of the fat magnetization using 90° or 180° CHESS RF pulses, respectively, as discussed in the section "Fat signal suppression" in Chapter 1. Likewise, the pulse-sequence implementation is analogous to

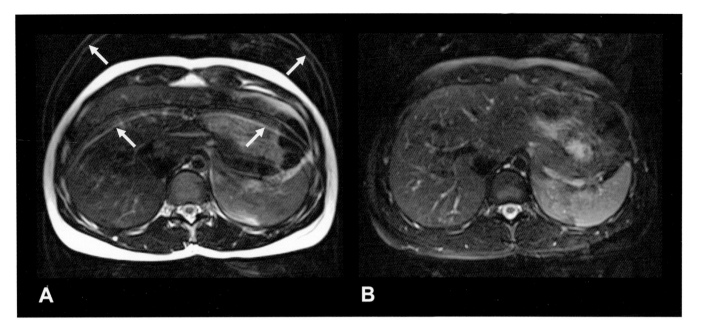

Figure 2.26 *Use of fat suppression to reduce ghost artifacts from breathing.* Axial T2-weighted FSE/TSE images of the abdomen (**A**) without and (**B**) with fat suppression, obtained in a healthy volunteer who was asked to breathe normally while the images were acquired. In **A**, there are pronounced ghost artifacts from breathing that appear parallel to the anterior abdominal wall as *curvilinear lines* propagated along the phase-encoding direction. Representative ghost artifacts are indicated by *arrows*. The ghost artifacts are prominent because their signal intensity is directly related to that of the moving structure, which is the anterior abdominal subcutaneous fat displaying high signal intensity. Acquisition of the images with fat suppression in **B** shows substantial reduction of the ghost artifacts because the signal of the moving anterior abdominal fat is low. However, minor ghost artifacts are still present.

that discussed for CHESS pulses (i.e., the pulses are applied preceding the excitation RF pulse for the pulse sequence of interest). Spatial presaturation and regional inversion RF pulses have the same general disadvantages discussed in Chapter 1 for CHESS and STIR RF pulses: they require additional time within the pulse sequence, which may cause the acquisition time to exceed the breath-hold duration, and they increase the power deposition for the pulse sequence.

For respiratory artifacts arising from the moving anterior abdominal wall when phase encoding is in the anterior-posterior direction (as most commonly used), suppression of the artifacts can be achieved by placing a coronal spatial presaturation region over the anterior abdominal wall so that the associated signal is suppressed (Fig. 2.27). Limitations of this approach are that ghost artifacts may still be present from tissues that are not included in the presaturation region. Further, if not accurately placed, the signal from organs in the anterior abdomen, such as the liver, may be unintentionally suppressed, possibly leading to incomplete visualization of these organs.

An alternative approach for suppressing ghost artifacts from respiration is to obtain images with the subject positioned prone on the scanner table. This reduces movement of the anterior abdominal wall and is particularly helpful for assessing structures within the anterior abdominal wall itself, such as those in the submucosal fat. However, with the subject prone, the posterior wall will of course move more than when the subject is supine, and as a result artifacts will arise from motion of the back of the subject. Another way to diminish the severity of breathing artifacts from the anterior abdominal wall is to change the phase-encoding direction from anterior-posterior to left-right; however, this increases breathing artifacts over the lateral walls of the abdomen and may increase the acquisition time because the left-right dimension of the abdomen is often larger than the anterior-posterior dimension.

Another valuable method for suppressing breathing-related artifacts is to use single-shot rather than multislice pulse sequences. As described in the section "Fast T2-weighted imaging," single-shot techniques are generally robust against ghost artifacts from respiration because the acquisition time per slice is much less than the respiratory cycle. In fact, with typical acquisition times of less than 1 second, these methods do not exhibit ghost artifacts from either breathing or pulsatile blood flow (see Fig. 2.21B), and can even be acquired during free breathing in subjects unable to hold their breath. The most common artifact for single-shot acquisitions related to breathing or other movement by the subject is an apparent irregular spacing of the slice positions resulting from the fact that the position of the anatomy of interest for the acquisition of some slices differs from that for the acquisition of other slices (Fig. 2.28). Changes in tissue contrast between slices can sometimes also be noted on single-shot images acquired without breath holding when tissues move out of the slice during the acquisition, and thus do not experience all of the applied RF pulses of the echo train, or move into the slice after having experienced RF pulses associated with a different slice position.

Ghost artifacts from flow, often seen as high-intensity, vessel-shaped foci along the phase-encoding direction (see Fig. 2.25), can sometimes be a major source of diagnostic

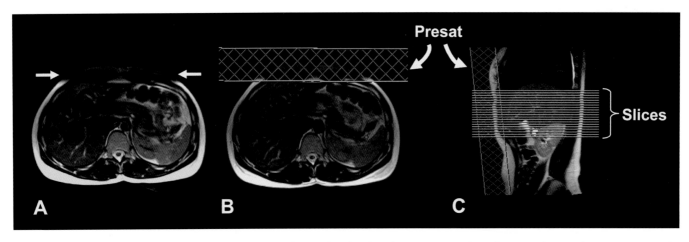

Figure 2.27 *Use of a spatial presaturation RF pulse to suppress ghost artifacts from breathing.* Images are from the same volunteer shown in Figure 2.26. (**A**) By placing a paracoronal spatial presaturation RF pulse over the anterior abdominal wall, the high signal intensity of the abdominal-wall fat is suppressed. The effect of this RF pulse appears as a well-defined band of low signal intensity (between *straight arrows*) through the anterior abdominal-wall fat and muscle. The prominent ghost artifacts demonstrated in Figure 2.26A are substantially reduced because the signal intensity of the anterior abdominal subcutaneous fat is suppressed by the presaturation RF pulse. Screen captures of the planning images show the position of the spatial presaturation RF pulse (*cross-hatched box indicated by curved arrows*) over the anterior abdominal wall in (**B**) an axial view and in (**C**) a sagittal view, which also shows the positions of the slices.

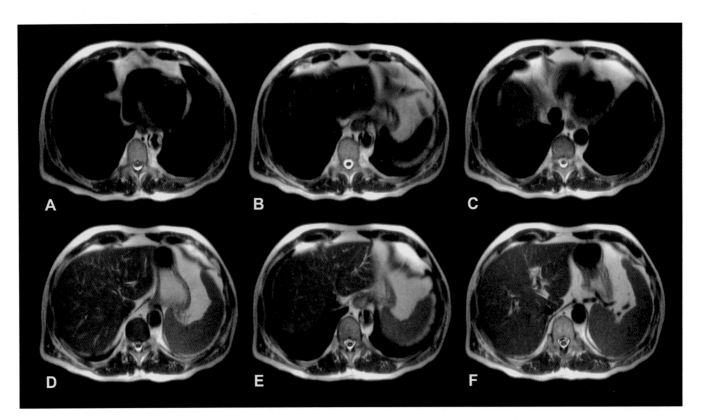

Figure 2.28 *Apparent shifts in slice position when imaging during free breathing using a single-shot pulse sequence.* (**A–F**) Axial images from a single-shot FSE/TSE (TE_eff 84 ms) pulse sequence that provided 20 images in 20 s. The pulse sequence was set up to generate contiguous slices from cranial to caudal positions, and the acquisition order of the slices was interleaved such that odd-numbered slices (1, 3, 5, ...) were obtained first, followed by even-numbered slices (2, 4, 6, ...). (The interleaved acquisition order was used to reduce interference ["crosstalk"] between adjacent slices, which can occur for closely spaced slices when the RF pulses for a given slice have some effect on the magnetization of tissues in immediately adjacent slices as shown in Figure 1.20 in Chapter 1.) In **A–F**, there is apparent irregular spacing of the slice positions. In **A**, the lung above the liver is shown, and the dome of the liver is seen on the next slice, **B**. However, subsequent slice **C** was obtained at a more cranial position than **B**, again showing the lung above the liver. Slice **D** shows a section of the liver that is much more caudal than that in **C**, and a more cranial section of the liver is seen in **E**. Slice **F** was obtained, again, at a much more caudal slice position than **E**. Overall, we see that the positions of the odd slices (**A, C, E**) are fairly consistent with each other, as are the positions of the even slices (**B, D, F**). However, due to the interleaved acquisition order, substantial displacement occurred along the cranial-caudal direction due to breathing between the odd-slice and even-slice portions of the acquisition.

confusion as they can mimic lesions, particularly when projected over other organs such as the liver or lung. Analogous to what was described above for suppressing respiratory artifacts, spatial presaturation or regional inversion RF pulses can be used to make flowing blood appear dark in the image, thereby suppressing the high-signal-intensity artifacts related to pulsatile blood flow. For example, in the common application of using spatial presaturation for suppressing blood signal within the aorta and inferior vena cava in a set of axial images of the abdomen, a spatial presaturation RF pulse is configured to affect a thick slice parallel and immediately cranial to the image set, while a second one is configured to affect a thick slice parallel and immediately caudal to the image set. Since the blood signal affected by these spatial presaturation RF pulses subsequently flows into the slices of interest, the cranial and caudal RF pulses suppress blood signal in the aorta and inferior vena cava, respectively (Fig. 2.29). The frequency of RF-pulse application and flow velocity determine the required thickness for the spatial presaturation region. For example, a relatively thick spatial presaturation region is typically required for the aorta due to its high flow velocity.

Although cardiac gating (or gating to the peripheral pulse) is effective for reducing flow-related artifacts, it has the disadvantage that the timing of the acquisition is dictated by the sub-

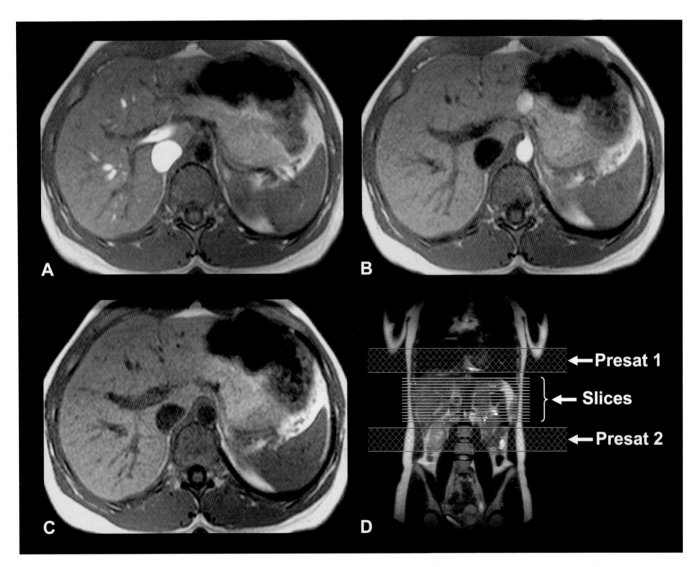

Figure 2.29 *Suppression of flow-related ghost artifacts by using spatial presaturation RF pulses.* (**A**) Representative 2D T1-weighted gradient-echo image from a set of axial slices (see **D**), obtained with a spatial presaturation RF pulse placed cranial to the slices (labeled "Presat 1" in **D**), shows that the signal from flowing blood in the aorta is suppressed, resulting in a signal void. Since a presaturation RF pulse was not placed caudally to the slices for this acquisition, the signal within the inferior vena cava (IVC) is high from "fresh" blood with magnetization at thermal equilibrium, flowing into the slice (inflow enhancement); this blood has not experienced any of the presaturation RF pulses since flow is in the caudocranial direction. (**B**) When a presaturation RF pulse is placed caudal to the slices (labeled "Presat 2" in **D**), and there is not a presaturation RF pulse cranial to the slices, the signal within the IVC is suppressed while the blood in the aorta appears bright from inflow enhancement. Pulsation artifacts associated with the high signal within the aorta propagate along the (anterior-to-posterior) phase-encoding direction, and project over the left lobe of the liver. These artifacts can sometimes be a major source of diagnostic confusion as they can mimic lesions and for this reason spatial presaturation RF pulses are frequently used. (**C**) Application of presaturation RF pulses both cranially and caudally to the set of slices suppresses the signal from flowing blood in both the aorta and IVC.

ject's cardiac cycle. As a result, a gated acquisition may be longer than a similar ungated acquisition. Further, the method does not work well if the subject has an irregular heart rhythm.

Flow-related artifacts can also be observed with single-shot FSE/TSE methods in structures that contain a large volume of fluid, such as ascites in the abdomen or urine in the bladder. In these instances, the artifacts are seen as irregular low-signal-intensity foci within the high-intensity fluid (Fig. 2.30). The appearance can be quite variable and is caused primarily by movement of fluid into or out of the slice during the echo train. The associated magnetization does not experience the full echo train and yields a reduced signal contribution, or essentially no signal if the magnetization does not experience the excitation RF pulse. These artifacts can be reduced by increasing the slice thickness so that the amount of fluid moving into or out of the slice is relatively small compared to the total amount of fluid within the slice. Conversely, the artifact increases as the slice thickness is decreased.

Chemical shift

As described in the section "Effects of chemical shift" in Chapter 1, chemical-shift artifacts occur because hydrogen nuclei in water-containing tissues have a slightly different resonant frequency than those in fat. The most commonly seen manifestation of this situation is spatial misregistration between water-containing tissues and fat along the frequency-encoding direction. The effect is particularly prominent when the signal from fat is relatively high (as in T1-weighted spin-echo or FSE/TSE images) and the receiver bandwidth is low, and appears as bright and dark bands on opposite sides of anatomic structures where fat and water are adjacent.

Since spatial misregistration from chemical shift appears in the frequency-encoding direction at any interface between water-containing tissues and fat, it can sometimes lead to difficulty in determining the margin around a lesion (Fig. 2.31). On the other hand, the chemical-shift artifact can be helpful diagnostically to determine whether fat is present within a lesion such as an adrenal adenoma. Chemical-shift artifacts can be reduced by suppressing the signal from fat using fat saturation, decreasing the field of view, or increasing the receiver bandwidth. (For additional details, refer to the sections on "Effects of chemical shift" in Chapter 1 and "In-phase, opposed-phase gradient-echo imaging" earlier in this chapter.)

Aliasing or wraparound

This common artifact occurs when the extent of the anatomy in the phase-encoding direction is larger than the corresponding dimension of the field of view. Aliasing occurs because the k-space data are sampled at discrete intervals, as opposed to continuously. Discrete sampling leads to a specific field of view for the image, which is inversely related to the spacing between samples in k space. That is, a relatively large spacing between k-space samples corresponds to a relatively small field of view, and decreasing the spacing between k-space samples increases the field of view. If a portion of the anatomy falls outside of the field of view, but within the sensitive volume of the RF coil, it appears to *alias*, or *wrap around*, to the opposite side of the field of view.

For example, suppose we acquire an axial image of the abdomen, with phase encoding in the left-right direction, for a subject lying on the scanner table with arms at his side. If the field of view in the left-right direction is chosen only large enough to accommodate the abdomen itself, then the left arm will alias to appear overlaid on the right side of the abdomen, and similarly the right arm will alias to appear overlaid on the left side of the abdomen (Fig. 2.32A). Obviously, this aliasing can be prevented by choosing a field of view large enough to accommodate both the abdomen and the arms (Fig. 2.32B); increasing the image matrix concurrently maintains the desired spatial resolution.

Most modern scanners provide an option called *oversampling* that permits only the region of interest to appear in the MR image while suppressing aliasing from adjacent structures.

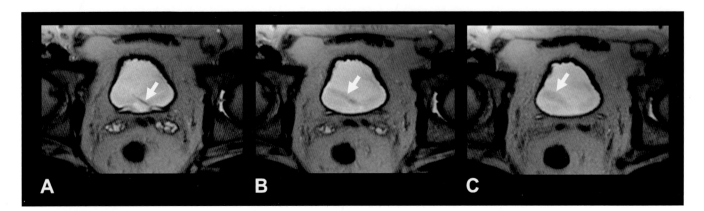

Figure 2.30 *Flow-related artifact in the bladder on single-shot FSE/TSE images.* (**A–C**) Three contiguous axial T2-weighted single-shot FSE/TSE images of the bladder show a linear area of decreased signal intensity (*arrows*) caused by urine flowing (jet phenomenon) from the left ureter into the bladder. The decrease in signal intensity is the result of the fluid moving into or out of the slice during the echo train of the pulse sequence, and hence the magnetization associated with the fluid within the slice volume does not experience the full echo train. As a result, the fluid flowing from the ureter yields a reduced signal contribution and therefore displays decreased signal intensity compared to the surrounding fluid. (An example of a similar flow-related artifact in a patient with a large amount of free intra-abdominal fluid is shown in Chapter 8, Fig. 8.22C.)

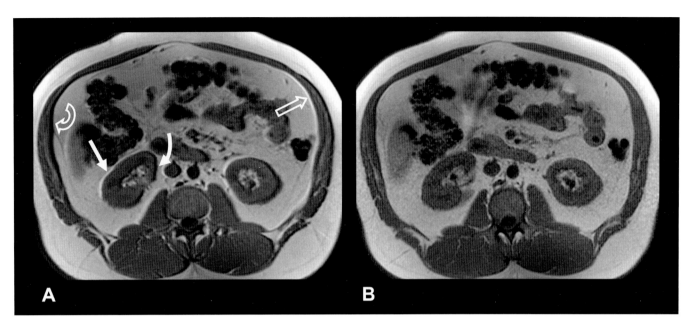

Figure 2.31 *Spatial misregistration artifact from chemical shift.* Axial 2D T1-weighted gradient-echo images obtained with (**A**) low and (**B**) high receiver bandwidth. Images are shown with same window and center settings. Chemical-shift artifact ("Type 1") is seen in A at water–fat interfaces between structures, appearing as a bright line on one side (*straight solid arrow* at the lateral margin of the right kidney and *straight open arrow* pointing to the medial margin of the left abdominal wall muscles) and as a dark line on the other side (*curved solid arrow* at the medial aspect of the right kidney and *curved open arrow* pointing to the medial margin of the right abdominal wall muscles). These artifacts are caused by spatial misregistration between water-containing tissues and fat along the frequency-encoding direction, and are the result of the slight resonant-frequency difference between hydrogen nuclei in water-containing tissues and those in fat. With an increase of the receiver bandwidth, as illustrated in B, the artifacts become less prominent. However, increasing receiver bandwidth leads to a decrease in signal-to-noise ratio due to increased background noise, and thus image **B** looks slightly grainier than image **A**.

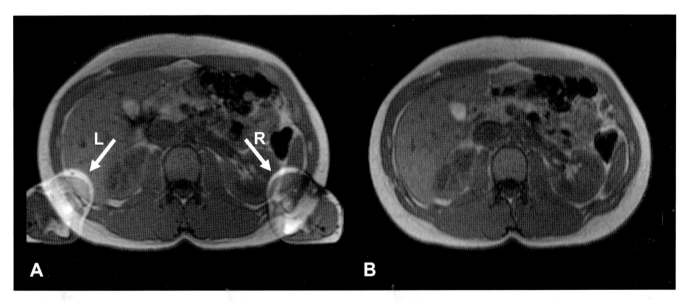

Figure 2.32 *Aliasing or wraparound artifact.* (**A, B**) Axial images of the abdomen acquired with phase encoding in left-right direction. The subject is supine on the scanner table, holding both arms at the side. The right side of the subject is on the left side of the image, and the left side of the subject is on the right. In **A**, the chosen field of view was just large enough to accommodate the abdomen itself. As a result, there is aliasing of the arms: the left arm (*arrow* labeled "L") appears overlaid on right side of the abdomen (left side of image) and the right arm (*arrow* labeled "R") appears overlaid on the left side of the abdomen. In **B**, the field of view was chosen large enough to accommodate both the abdomen (left side of image) and the arms and, consequently, the aliasing artifact is removed and the arms (cropped from image shown) no longer overlap the abdomen. However, because for this example the same image matrix was used for both **A** and **B**, the spatial resolution is decreased in **B**, which is evident from the slightly coarser appearance of the anatomic structures. (For demonstrating the effect of decreased spatial resolution related to the larger field of view, image **B** was magnified to match the size of image **A**.)

When oversampling is activated, additional phase-encoding steps are acquired but the spatial resolution along the phase-encoding direction is held constant. This results in acquisition of data corresponding to a larger field of view than that selected by the user (which thus prevents the aliasing). However, before the MR image is presented on the scanner console, the image-reconstruction software discards the portions outside of the selected field of view. We thus see that activating oversampling, or, alternatively, manually choosing a larger field of view and a larger image matrix, actually accomplish the same thing. The advantage of using oversampling is that only the desired anatomic region is displayed in the MR image. Remember that 3D pulse sequences have two phase-encoding directions, and thus aliasing can occur along either or both directions.

The degree of oversampling is usually specified as a fraction or percentage of the desired field of view. Since oversampling entails collecting additional phase-encoding steps and the acquisition time is proportional to the number of phase-encoding steps, the use of oversampling increases the acquisition time. The principle of oversampling also applies to the frequency-encoding direction, but oversampling along this direction does not affect the acquisition time. As a result, many modern scanners automatically include oversampling along the frequency-encoding direction for all acquisitions. In addition, since oversampling along this direction is "free," the longest dimension of the anatomy of interest should be placed along the frequency-encoding direction unless some other consideration (e.g., motion artifacts) dictates otherwise.

Magnetic susceptibility

Magnetic susceptibility is defined as the tendency of a substance to become magnetized when placed in a magnetic field. Magnetic susceptibility is a property of the material, and can be positive or negative. This means that the magnetic field that is induced within a substance can be greater than the applied field (positive magnetic susceptibility, for example iron) or less than the applied field (negative magnetic susceptibility, for example many biologic tissues). As a result, within the scanner magnet, a magnetic field gradient will exist at the interface between substances with differing magnetic susceptibilities, for example at the interface between air and tissue, potentially leading to image artifacts.

A substance with a negative magnetic susceptibility is called *diamagnetic*. Most tissues in the body are diamagnetic and have relatively small, negative susceptibilities that are similar to that of water. Thus, the susceptibility difference between most tissues in the body (notable exceptions are certain products from the breakdown of blood, discussed further below) is relatively small, and therefore susceptibility-related effects do not substantially alter the image contrast, except at very high field strengths (e.g., 7T). However, when the susceptibility difference is sufficiently large (as, for instance, at the interface between soft tissue and air), the associated artifacts can be pronounced. In the abdomen, the bowel is a common area for artifacts from air–tissue interfaces (Fig. 2.33).

Paramagnetic substances have a relatively small, positive susceptibility, generally resulting from one or more "unpaired" electrons (i.e., an electron that does not have an orbital partner

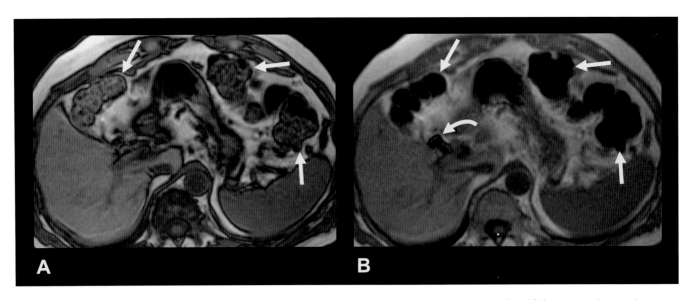

Figure 2.33 *Magnetic-susceptibility artifacts from air and metal.* (**A**) Axial opposed-phase (TR/TE 110/2.4 ms) and (**B**) corresponding in-phase (TR/TE 110/4.8 ms) T1-weighted gradient-echo images obtained at 1.5T. In **A**, the contents of the large bowel (*straight arrows*) are well seen, consisting of stool (intermediate signal intensity within bowel) that contains many small air pockets (low-intensity foci within the stool). Due to the short TE, susceptibility artifacts at air–stool interfaces are limited. In **B**, which was obtained with longer TE, the bowel contents show generally low signal intensity (*straight arrows*) resulting from increased susceptibility artifact at air–stool interfaces within the stool, giving the impression that there is only air within the bowel. Susceptibility artifact from a metal clip (*curved arrow*) placed during a cholecystectomy, which was only minimally apparent in **A**, also becomes more evident in **B**. Note in **A** that there is also signal loss at the interfaces between water-containing tissues and fat, caused by chemical-shift–induced signal modulation (Fig. 2.11). As expected, this effect appears as dark lines around the structures in the opposed-phase image, as also shown in Figure 2.12A.

with opposing spin). Paramagnetic substances of interest in MRI include certain products from the breakdown of blood, molecular oxygen (the source of contrast in oxygen-enhanced lung imaging), deoxyhemoglobin (the source of contrast in functional MRI of the brain), and gadolinium (the "active" ingredient of most MRI contrast agents). In particular, gadolinium has seven unpaired electrons, resulting in its ability to substantially shorten T1 and T2 relaxation times of nearby protons in nearby water molecules.

The undesired field gradient that exists at the interface between substances with markedly different magnetic susceptibilities results in dephasing of transverse magnetization in the vicinity of the interface. Depending on the shape and orientation of the interface, the magnitude of the field gradient, and the type of pulse sequence, this may lead to signal loss and/or geometric distortion in the vicinity of the interface. Signal loss occurs when the dephasing is sufficiently large to result in a wide range of phase shifts within the volume corresponding to a given voxel. This effect, generically referred to as *intravoxel dephasing* (which can also be caused by flow, as described in the section "Dark blood from flow-related dephasing"), is more prominent in gradient-echo images than in spin-echo images because the refocusing RF pulses in spin-echo imaging largely compensate for susceptibility-induced dephasing. Signal loss from intravoxel dephasing can be par-

ticularly pronounced for gradient-echo images in the vicinity of metal clips (Fig. 2.33).

Even in spin-echo images, the signals arising from tissue near a susceptibility interface will be mis-encoded, and appear in the wrong location in the image, if the susceptibility-induced field gradient is relatively large compared to the magnetic-field gradients used for spatial encoding. This spatial misregistration shifts the signal from one location to another along the frequency-encoding direction, leaving a signal void in the original location and "signal pile-up" (a focus of very bright signal) at the location to which the signal is shifted. This form of the artifact is often seen with metallic (particularly *ferromagnetic* [large, positive magnetic susceptibility]) objects and characteristically appears on MR images as bright regions and dark signal voids around these objects (Fig. 2.34). The associated disturbance of the static magnetic field can also compromise the effectiveness of fat saturation, leading to incomplete suppression of the signal from fat. It is important to remember that susceptibility-induced field gradients can cause spatial misregistration along the slice-selection direction in addition to along the frequency-encoding direction. Thus, signal originating from tissue at a given location can appear in a slice that is substantially displaced from that location. In this case, the origin of the artifactual signal may be difficult to ascertain.

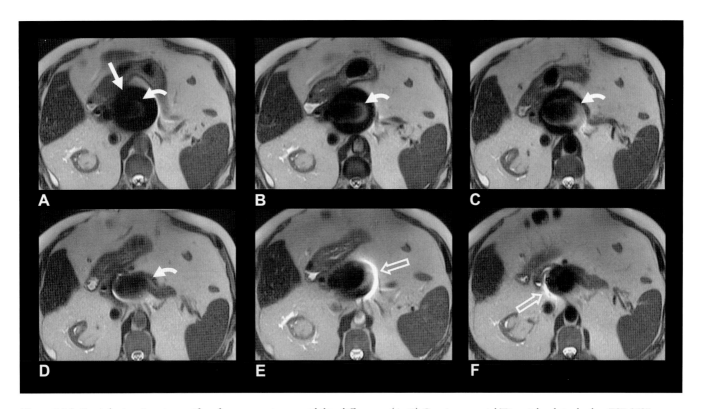

Figure 2.34 *Spatial misregistration artifacts from magnetic-susceptibility differences.* (**A–F**) Contiguous axial T2-weighted single-shot FSE/TSE (TE$_{eff}$ 80 ms) images in a patient who had embolization of the left gastric vein with the use of coils. Images were obtained with frequency encoding in the left-right direction. A large round susceptibility artifact (signal void in **A**, indicated by *straight arrow*) is seen, induced by the presence of the embolization coils. An amorphous structure, representing signal that has been displaced from tissue elsewhere in the abdomen, appears in the slice and "shifts" from right to left (*curved arrows* in **A–D**), parallel to the frequency-encoding direction, on consecutive images. A focus of very bright signal, or "signal pile-up" (*straight open arrows* in E and F), is seen near the most inferior aspect of the artifact and is caused by signal from other locations being displaced along the frequency-encoding and slice-select directions.

Since the magnetic field induced within substances is proportional to the applied field, susceptibility-related artifacts increase with increasing field strength. Other factors affecting the severity of these artifacts include echo time, receiver bandwidth, and type of pulse sequence. Susceptibility-related artifacts increase with increasing echo time (especially for gradient-echo pulse sequences) and decreasing receiver bandwidth, and are typically more prominent on gradient-echo images than on spin-echo images.

Susceptibility-related artifacts can be minimized by prospective selection of the pulse sequence and its parameters. Pulse sequences for abdominal imaging that typically exhibit minimal susceptibility-related artifacts include FSE/TSE and single-shot FSE/TSE methods. If pulse sequences particularly sensitive to susceptibility differences, such as gradient-echo imaging, are required, a short TE should be used to suppress the artifacts. Conversely, if the goal is to emphasize susceptibility effects, for instance to facilitate detection of substances with differing susceptibility values such as blood products in a hematoma, or air within bile ducts, a relatively long TE should be used. Detection of susceptibility-related effects can be easily achieved in routine abdominal imaging using the images obtained from the double-echo gradient-echo pulse sequence that is commonly used for in- and opposed-phase imaging to detect the presence of microscopic fat deposits in organs such as the liver and adrenal glands.[12] By comparing the images obtained with a longer TE with those obtained with the shorter TE, susceptibility effects such as those caused by air in the bile ducts or hemosiderin in the liver become readily evident (Figs. 2.35 and 2.36).

Effect of gadolinium concentration on signal intensity

Although gadolinium-containing contrast agents are best known for their "enhancement" of tissues through T1 shortening (i.e., causing an increase in signal intensity on T1-weighted images), there is also a concomitant T2-shortening effect that is generally less obvious at concentrations typically used in routine clinical practice. However, at high concentrations, the T2 shortening effect becomes more evident, and the T1 and T2 relaxation times converge, as shown in Table 2.1.

A good demonstration of the effect on signal intensity of this convergence of T1 and T2 to relatively small values can be seen in the bladder (Fig. 2.37). Since most contrast agents are excreted through the kidneys, the concentration of gadolinium can become quite high in urine. The T2-shortening effect resulting from high gadolinium concentration can therefore typically be seen in regions where urine accumulates—the bladder and ureters. This can lead to the appearance of three distinct layers in the bladder that correspond to the gravity-dependent variation in the concentration of the gadolinium-containing contrast agent. Since the gadolinium-containing contrast agent has higher density than water, it is concentrated in the most dependent portion of the bladder. Thus, the urine in the nondependent portion of the bladder lacks gadolinium-containing contrast agent and therefore maintains its native, long T1 and T2 relaxation times; on T1-weighted images this urine displays relatively low signal intensity due to the long T1 value (region 1 in Fig. 2.37). In the more dependent portion of the bladder, the signal of the urine increases on T1-weighted images due to the presence of gadolinium-containing contrast agent at concentrations that primarily shorten the T1 relaxation time (region 2 in Fig. 2.37). However, in the most dependent portion of the bladder, where the gadolinium concentration is quite high, both the T1 and T2 relaxation times of urine are very short. When the T2 relaxation time is sufficiently short, the transverse magnetization, and hence signal, decays to a very small value before data sampling occurs. As a result, no signal is measured

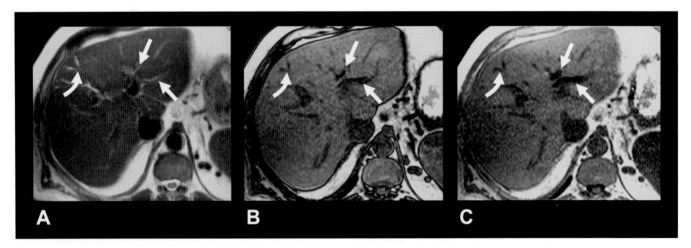

Figure 2.35 *Detecting air in bile ducts using in-phase/opposed-phase gradient-echo imaging.* (**A**) T2-weighted single-shot FSE/TSE (TE_eff 80 ms) image in a patient with primary sclerosing cholangitis who had prior endoscopic retrograde cholangiography with papillotomy. Most bile ducts display intermediate-high signal intensity; two of these in the left lobe are indicated by *straight arrows*. Two small, slightly dilated, fluid-filled ducts are seen at the periphery (*curved arrow*) and show increased signal intensity. (**B**) On the corresponding opposed-phase gradient-echo image (TR/TE 115/2.4 ms), the two ducts in the left lobe (*straight arrow*) show a slight decrease in signal intensity compared to the other ducts, including the two at the periphery (*curved arrow*). (**C**) On the in-phase image (TR/TE 115/4.8 ms), having a longer TE, there is a further decrease in the signal intensity of the two ducts in the left lobe (*straight arrows*) and apparent "enlargement" of the ducts. These findings are consistent with susceptibility artifact from air within the duct. The two ducts at the periphery (*curved arrows*) do not show such an effect, indicating that these ducts do not contain air.

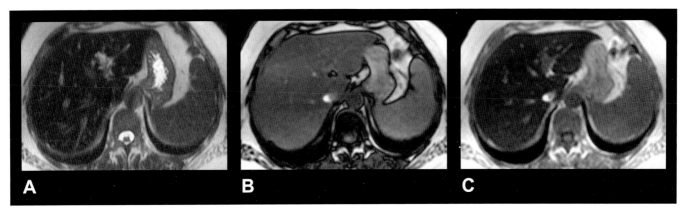

Figure 2.36 *Detecting iron in the liver using in-phase/opposed-phase gradient-echo Imaging.* (**A**) Axial T2-weighted FSE/TSE (TE_eff 80 ms) image obtained at 1.5T in a patient with iron deposition (secondary hemochromatosis) in liver and spleen from repeated blood transfusions. The liver displays marked low signal intensity resulting from T2 shortening induced by the iron. The signal for the spleen is also decreased compared to that for healthy subjects. (**B**) Opposed-phase (TR/TE 110/2.4 ms) gradient-echo image shows that the signal intensity of the liver is lower than that of the spleen. Note signal-loss artifacts at the fat–water interfaces due to chemical-shift–induced signal modulation. (**C**) In-phase image obtained with longer TE (4.8 ms) shows marked decrease of the signal intensity of the liver and spleen compared to **B**, caused by increased susceptibility-related effect from the iron. Note that for the in-phase/opposed-phase gradient-echo pulse sequence, the decrease in liver signal intensity with increase in TE is opposite to the signal change seen in hepatosteatosis (Fig. 2.12). In that case, there was increase in liver signal with increase in TE as shown in Figure 2.12. However, in that case, the decrease of signal at TE 2.4 ms (opposed phase) was from signal cancellation due to chemical-shift differences, when the transverse magnetizations of fat and water are opposed; these magnetizations are essentially aligned at a TE of 4.8 ms. A demonstration of the effect of changing TE to emphasize magnetic-susceptibility artifacts in a patient with Gamna-Gandy bodies in the spleen is given in Figure 8.29 in Chapter 8.

Table 2.1. **RELATIONSHIP BETWEEN GADOLINIUM CONCENTRATION, AND T1 AND T2 RELAXATION TIMES**

GADOLINIUM CONCENTRATION (MMOL/L)	T1 (MS)	T2 (MS)
0.0	1,000	100
0.1	710	95
0.5	330	80
20.0	12	9

even if sampling is performed shortly after application of the RF pulse, as is the case with a T1-weighted sequence that uses a short TE. In these instances, low signal intensity is seen in the most dependent portion of the bladder (region 3 in Fig. 2.37).

HEMORRHAGE AND HEMATOMA

We briefly discuss hematomas as these can appear quite variable, and sometimes confusing, when encountered in MR images. Although the MRI features of hematoma over time have been mostly described for intracranial hematomas, the same MR features are seen in the abdomen and elsewhere.[13] The variability in appearances is predominantly caused by susceptibility effects related to various iron-containing components that occur over time when hemoglobin from the red blood cells breaks down (Table 2.2).[14] This section describes the general sequence of the breakdown of blood into these components, which include *oxyhemoglobin, deoxyhemoglobin, intracellular methemoglobin,*

extracellular methemoglobin, and *hemosiderin.* Some or all of these substances can be present at the same time during the evolution of a hematoma, which explains the often-marked variability of findings on MR images.

When bleeding occurs, the red blood cells containing oxygenated hemoglobin (oxyhemoglobin) extravasate, and the appearance of the hematoma is then essentially similar to that of a collection of proteinaceous fluid. Because oxyhemoglobin in the active, or "hyperacute," hematoma is diamagnetic, there are no substantial relaxivity or susceptibility effects, and the signal intensity of the hematoma is therefore similar to that of any proteinaceous collection, showing relatively low to intermediate signal on T1- and relatively high signal on T2-weighted images, particularly at the periphery. Since the hematoma ages more rapidly at the periphery than at the center, the signal intensity changes observed with aging of the hematoma typically occur from the outside inward.

In the relatively hypoxic environment into which the red blood cells extravasate, the hematoma develops into the "acute" stage, and intracellular oxyhemoglobin is deoxygenized to (intracellular) deoxyhemoglobin. This process takes place within hours to days after the bleeding and may take longer (several weeks) in the center of a hematoma. Deoxyhemoglobin is paramagnetic and its susceptibility leads to hypointensity at the periphery of the hematoma on T2-weighted images. However, because the unpaired electrons in deoxyhemoglobin are not accessible to water protons, there is typically no significant change or a slight decrease in signal intensity on T1-weighted images.

With the subsequent oxidization of deoxyhemoglobin to intracellular methemoglobin (which typically begins a few days after the bleeding), the "early subacute" phase of the

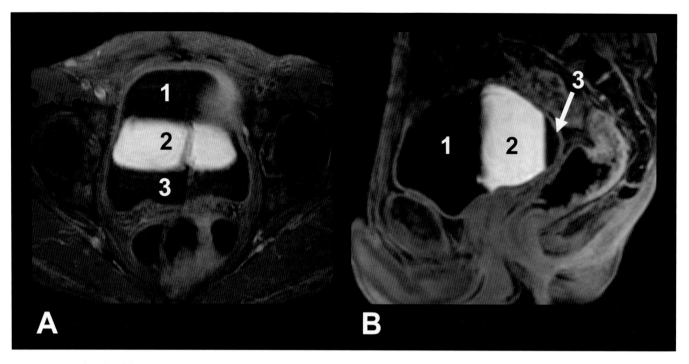

Figure 2.37 *Effect of gadolinium concentration on signal intensity.* (**A**) Axial T1-weighted spin-echo (TR/TE 500/15 ms) image and (**B**) sagittal T1-weighted gradient-echo (TR/TE 49/2.5 ms) image, both obtained with fat saturation and acquired approximately 60 minutes after intravenous administration of gadolinium-containing contrast agent. The subject is supine on the scanner table. Because the gadolinium-containing contrast agent has higher density than water, its concentration is highest in the dependent portion of the bladder. Three layers can be identified within the bladder. In the nondependent portion (labeled "1"), the urine displays low signal intensity because it lacks gadolinium-containing contrast agent and, hence, T1 and T2 relaxation times are long. In the middle layer (labeled "2"), the fluid shows high signal intensity as primarily the T1 relaxation time is decreased. In the most dependent portion (labeled "3"), gadolinium concentration is high and urine shows low signal intensity because the T2 relaxation time is short compared to the echo time, and hence the signal decays to a low value before data are sampled.

Box 2.6 **ESSENTIALS TO REMEMBER**

- With abdominal imaging, ghost artifacts caused by movement of the anterior abdominal-wall fat during breathing can be suppressed by: (1) acquiring images during breath hold, (2) acquiring images with respiratory gating, (3) using fat suppression, (4) using spatial presaturation RF pulses, (5) positioning the patient prone instead of supine, (6) changing the phase-encoding direction from anterior-posterior to left-right, or (7) using a single-shot rather than a multislice pulse sequence.

- Flow-related artifacts can be suppressed by: (1) using spatial presaturation RF pulses, (2) using a single-shot rather than a multislice pulse sequence, (3) acquiring images with cardiac or peripheral-pulse gating, or, for certain situations, (4) increasing the slice thickness.

- Signal-cancellation artifacts due to chemical shift that appear as dark lines at fat–water interfaces can be suppressed by: (1) acquiring in-phase images or (2) using fat suppression.

- Aliasing or wrap-around artifacts can be suppressed by: (1) increasing the field of view or (2) using oversampling.

- Susceptibility-related artifacts are typically more prominent on gradient-echo images than on spin-echo images. The artifacts increase with: (1) increase of field strength, (2) increase of echo time, or (3) decrease of receiver bandwidth.

- Gadolinium has both a T1- and T2-shortening effects. The latter becomes evident with high concentrations, leading to loss of signal that, when severe, can even be observed on images obtained with a short TE, as used in a T1-weighted pulse sequence.

---

hematoma develops. Methemoglobin is also paramagnetic and its unpaired electrons are accessible to water protons, leading to T1 shortening, which, in turn, results in an increase in signal intensity on T1-weighted images (Fig. 2.38). This hyperintensity is often first seen at the periphery of a subacute hematoma, producing a concentric ring. The intracellular methemoglobin also leads to shortening of T2, similar to intracellular deoxyhemoglobin, and may appear as decreased signal intensity on T2-weighted images (Fig. 2.38B).

With additional time, the "late subacute" phase develops, which, on average, takes place between several days to one month after bleeding. During this phase lysis of the

Table 2.2. HEMATOMA AS A FUNCTION OF TIME

	HYPERACUTE	ACUTE	EARLY SUBACUTE	LATE SUBACUTE	CHRONIC
Time Frame	<12 h	Hours to days	Few days	4–7 days to 1 month	Weeks to years
Mechanism	Extravasation	Deoxygenation	Clot retraction	Cell lysis	Macrophages digest clot
State of RBC	Intact	Intact/hypoxic	Intact/↑hypoxic	Lysed	Gone
State of Hb	Intracellular oxy-Hb	Intracellular deoxy-Hb	Intracellular met-Hb	Extracellular met-Hb	Hemosiderin & ferritin
Oxidation state	Ferrous (Fe^{2+}) no unpaired electrons	Ferrous (Fe^{2+}) 4 unpaired electrons	Ferrous (Fe^{3+}) 5 unpaired electrons	Ferrous (Fe^{3+}) 5 unpaired electrons	Ferrous (Fe^{3+}) 2,000 × 5 unpaired electrons
Magnetic properties	Diamagnetic	Paramagnetic	Paramagnetic	Paramagnetic	Super-paramagnetic
T1-weighted signal	≈ or ↓	≈ or ↓	↑↑	↑↑	≈ or ↓
T2-weighted signal	↑	↓	↓↓	↑↑	↓↓

Modified from Parizel PM, et al. *Eur Radiol.* 2001;11(9):1770-1783.

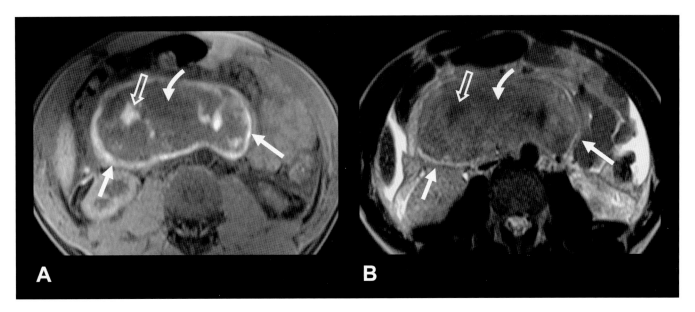

Figure 2.38 *Appearance of subacute hematoma.* (**A**) Axial T1-weighted gradient-echo (TR/TE 115/4.6 ms) image with fat saturation and (**B**) T2-weighted single-shot FSE/TSE (TE$_{eff}$ 118) image obtained in patient who had a blow to the abdomen 8 days prior to imaging. On both T1- and T2-weighted images, the subacute hematoma shows a high-signal-intensity rim (*straight arrows*) on both T1- and T2-weighted images related to the presence of extracellular methemoglobin. The rim appears thicker on the T1-weighted image as an inner layer of intracellular methemoglobin contributes to increased signal on the T1-weighted image, but does not on the T2-weighted image. The remainder of the lesion displays chiefly intermediate signal intensity on both T1-and T2-weighted images (*curved arrows*), primarily from the presence of deoxyhemoglobin. Within this central portion, a few hyperintense foci (one such area indicated with *open arrow*) are shown on the T1-weighted image that display relative low signal intensity (*open arrow*) on the T2-weighted image; this is from intracellular methemoglobin.

methemoglobin-containing erythrocytes occurs and methemoglobin becomes extracellular (Fig. 2.38). At this stage the hematoma remains hyperintense on T1-weighted images, while on T2-weighted images it becomes more heterogeneous and eventually hyperintense. The "chronic" hematoma then develops, a process that can extend over weeks to years. During this phase the red blood cells and hemoglobin, phagocytosed by macrophages, are digested by the lysosomal system and iron is stored as ferric oxyhydroxide in the iron-storage protein called ferritin, with the excess iron stored as hemosiderin. These substances have superparamagnetic properties and cause a decrease in signal intensity, particularly on T2-weighted images (Fig. 2.39). This decrease in signal is often most conspicuous at the margins of the hematoma, and on gradient-echo

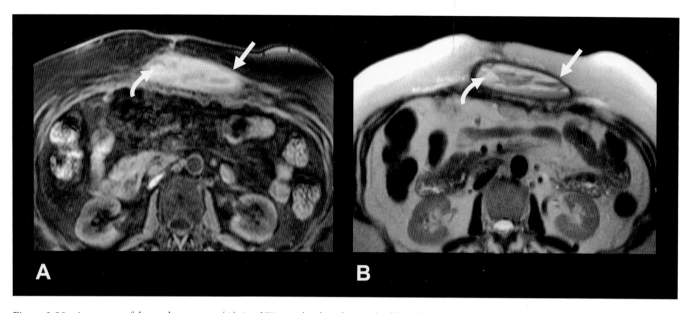

Figure 2.39 *Appearance of chronic hematoma.* (**A**) Axial T1-weighted gradient-echo (TR/TE 115/4.6 ms) image with fat saturation and (**B**) T2-weighted single-shot FSE/TSE (TE$_{eff}$ 118) image of a patient with chronic hematoma who had liver-transplant surgery 9 months earlier. The chronic hematoma shows relatively high signal intensity on both T1- and T2-weighted images (*curved arrows*) from the presence of extracellular methemoglobin, with a few foci of decreased intensity. On the T1-weighted image (**A**) the lesion is surrounded by a rim of relatively high signal intensity (*straight arrow*), which displays marked low signal intensity on the T2-weighted image (*straight arrow*) due to the presence of peripheral hemosiderin and ferritin.

images there may be susceptibility-related artifacts such as "blooming," wherein dark regions appear that are larger than the physical extent of the associated blood products.

IMAGING PARAMETERS

Table 2.3 lists the effects of increasing or decreasing common imaging parameters. When a given parameter is changed, it is assumed that all others are held constant. An increase or decrease in effect is denoted by the symbols ↑ or ↓, respectively; both symbols together (↑↓) indicate that the change may result in either an increase or decrease in effect, depending on the values of other parameters. The designation "↑ and then ↓" indicates that an increase in effect occurs first, and is followed by a decrease in effect with further changes in the parameter value. The following abbreviations are used in the table: SNR, signal-to-noise ratio; M_Z, longitudinal magnetization; M_{XY}, transverse magnetization; M_0, thermal equilibrium magnetization.

REPRESENTATIVE PULSE SEQUENCE PROTOCOL FOR ABDOMINAL MRI

a. Multiplane scout

b. 2D T2-weighted single-shot FSE/TSE without fat saturation (axial, coronal, and sagittal)

c. 2D T2-weighted FSE/TSE with fat saturation (axial)

d. 2D in- and opposed-phase T1-weighted gradient echo (axial)

e. 2D T1-weighted magnetization-prepared gradient echo (axial)

f. 2D single-slice MRCP (single-shot FSE/TSE with fat saturation) obtained in seven to nine paracoronal orientations, centered around the common bile duct, each with 40- to 60-mm slice thickness

g. 3D dynamic, contrast-enhanced, T1-weighted gradient echo with fat saturation (pre-contrast plus three post-contrast phases). A test bolus is used to calculate the time interval between the start of the gadolinium-bolus injection and the initiation of the 3D gradient-echo sequence as described on page 47 and shown in Figure 2.18.

 1. Pre-contrast

 2. Late arterial/early portal venous

 3. Portal venous

 4. Hepatic venous

h. 3D respiratory-gated thin (~1 mm) slice MRCP (FSE/TSE with fat saturation) for multiplanar reconstruction and maximum-intensity-projection images

i. Delayed (10 to 15 min) 3D contrast-enhanced T1-weighted gradient echo with fat saturation (same pulse sequence as that used for g). Longer delay times (20 to 30 minutes) are used with a hepato-specific gadolinium-based contrast agent such as gadoxate disodium (Eovist®) or gadoxetic acid (Primovist®).

The pulse-sequence techniques described in this chapter for fast (breath-hold) MR imaging of the abdomen are available on

Table 2.3. **EFFECT OF CHANGING COMMON IMAGING PARAMETERS**

PARAMETER	EFFECT OF INCREASING	EFFECT OF DECREASING
[1]Repetition time, TR (increasing from very short TR or decreasing from very long TR)	T1-dependent contrast ↑ and then ↓ SNR ↑ Acquisition time ↑ No. slices for multislice acquisition ↑	T1-dependent contrast ↑ and then ↓ SNR ↓ Acquisition time ↓ No. slices for multislice acquisition ↓
[1]Echo time, TE (increasing from very short TE or decreasing from very long TE)	T2- or T2*-dependent contrast ↑ and then ↓ SNR ↓ No. slices for multislice acquisition ↓ Susceptibility-related artifact ↑	T2- or T2*-dependent contrast ↑ and then ↓ SNR ↑ No. slices for multislice acquisition ↑ Susceptibility-related artifact ↓
[2]Flip angle, α	T1-dependent contrast ↑ Steady-state value of M_Z ↓ ➡ tends to decrease signal Fraction of M_Z converted to M_{XY} ↑ ➡ tends to increase signal SNR ↑↓	T1-dependent contrast ↓ Steady-state value of M_Z ↑ ➡ tends to increase signal Fraction of M_Z converted to M_{XY} ↓ ➡ tends to decrease signal SNR ↑↓
Field of view, FOV	Anatomic coverage ↑ Spatial resolution ↓ SNR ↑ Wraparound (aliasing) artifact ↓	Anatomic coverage ↓ Spatial resolution ↑ SNR ↓ Wraparound (aliasing) artifact ↑
Slice thickness	Anatomic coverage ↑ Spatial resolution ↓ SNR ↑	Anatomic coverage ↓ Spatial resolution ↑ SNR ↓
Matrix: frequency-encoding steps	Spatial resolution ↑ SNR ↓ Acquisition time unaffected	Spatial resolution ↓ SNR ↑ Acquisition time unaffected
Matrix: phase-encoding steps	Spatial resolution ↑ SNR ↓ Acquisition time ↑	Spatial resolution ↓ SNR ↑ Acquisition time ↓
Number of slices	Anatomic coverage ↑ Acquisition time: 　Multislice unaffected[3] 　Single-shot ↑ 　3D ↑	Anatomic coverage ↓ Acquisition time: 　Multislice unaffected[3] 　Single-shot ↓ 　3D ↓
Receiver bandwidth	Noise ↑ ➡ SNR ↓ Minimum possible TE ↓ Chemical-shift artifact ↓ Susceptibility-related artifact ↓	Noise ↓ ➡ SNR ↑ Minimum possible TE ↑ Chemical-shift artifact ↑ Susceptibility-related artifact ↑
Number of excitations, NEX	SNR ↑ Acquisition time ↑ Motion artifact ↓	SNR ↓ Acquisition time ↓ Motion artifact ↑
Number of echoes for conventional spin echo	Acquisition time unaffected No. slices for multislice acquisition ↓	Acquisition time unaffected No. slices for multislice acquisition ↑
Number of echoes (ETL) for fast/turbo spin echo	Acquisition time ↓ Blurring for short TE ↑ No. slices for multislice acquisition ↓	Acquisition time ↑ Blurring for short TE ↓ No. slices for multislice acquisition ↑
Field strength	M_0 ↑ ➡ SNR ↑ Susceptibility-related artifact ↑ Chemical-shift artifact ↑ T1 relaxation times ↑ T2 relaxation times unaffected[4]	M_0 ↓ ➡ SNR ↓ Susceptibility-related artifact ↓ Chemical-shift artifact ↓ T1 relaxation times ↓ T2 relaxation times unaffected[4]

[1]applies to spin-echo, fast/turbo spin-echo and spoiled gradient-echo pulse sequences

[2]applies to spoiled gradient-echo pulse sequences

[3]assumes selected number of slices fits within current TR

[4]applies up to ~1.5T; T2 relaxation times for some tissues decrease markedly at very high field strengths (e.g., 7T)

Table 2.4. COMMONLY USED FAST PULSE-SEQUENCE TECHNIQUES FOR ABDOMINAL IMAGING, WITH ACRONYMS BY MANUFACTURER

PULSE SEQUENCE TECHNIQUE			MANUFACTURER				
Contrast weighting	Type	2D vs. 3D	Siemens	General Electric	Philips	Hitachi	Toshiba
Fast T1-weighted	Gradient-echo (RF spoiled)	2D	FLASH	SPGR, FSPGR	T1-FFE	RF-spoiled SARGE	Field Echo, Fast FE
		3D	VIBE	LAVA	THRIVE	TIGRE	
	Magnetization-prepared gradient-echo	2D	T1 Turbo FLASH	IR FGR, IR FSPGR	TFE	RGE	Fast FE
Fast T2-weighted	Multislice	2D	TSE	FSE	TSE	FSE	FSE
	Single-shot	2D	HASTE	SSFSE	Single-shot TSE	Single-shot FSE	FASE
	Single-slab	3D	SPACE	CUBE	VISTA	–	–

most modern scanners. However, many of the sequences have been given different acronyms by the various manufacturers, and recognition of the type of pulse-sequence technique can therefore be confusing. Table 2.4 provides commonly used fast pulse sequences and associated acronyms, by manufacturer, compiled from publicly available lists of MRI acronyms.

REFERENCES

1. Mugler JP III. Chapter 2: Basic principles. In Edelman RR, Hesselink JR, Zlatkin MB, Crues JV III, eds. *Clinical Magnetic Resonance Imaging,* 3rd ed. Philadelphia: Saunders Elsevier, 2006:23-57.
2. Carroll TJ, Sakaie KE, Wielopolski PA, Edelman RR. Chapter 7: Advanced imaging techniques, including fast imaging. In: Edelman RR, Hesselink JR, Zlatkin MB, Crues JV III, eds. *Clinical Magnetic Resonance Imaging,* 3rd ed. Philadelphia: Saunders Elsevier, 2006: 187-230.
3. Lee JK, Dixon WT, Ling D, et al. Fatty infiltration of the liver: demonstration by proton spectroscopic imaging. Preliminary observations. *Radiology.* 1984;153(1):195-201.
4. Outwater EK, Blasbalg R, Siegelman ES, Vala M. Detection of lipid in abdominal tissues with opposed-phase gradient-echo images at 1.5 T: techniques and diagnostic importance. *Radiographics.* 1998;18(6): 1465-1480.
5. Mugler JP III. Overview of MR imaging pulse sequences. Magn Reson Imaging Clin North Am. 1999;7:661-697.
6. Dixon WT. Simple proton spectroscopic imaging. Radiology. 1984;153(1):189-194.
7. de Lange EE, Mugler JP 3rd, Bosworth JE, et al. MR imaging of the liver: breath-hold T1-weighted MP-GRE compared with conventional T2-weighted SE imaging—lesion detection, localization, and characterization. *Radiology.* 1994;190(3):727-736.
8. Rofsky NM, Lee VS, Laub G, et al. Abdominal MR imaging with a volumetric interpolated breath-hold examination. *Radiology.* 1999; 212(2):876-884.
9. Zhang H, Maki JH, Prince MR. 3D contrast-enhanced MR angiography. *J Magn Reson Imaging.* 2007;25(1):13-25.
10. Storey P. Chapter 22: Artifacts and solutions. In: Edelman RR, Hesselink JR, Zlatkin MB, Crues JV III, eds. *Clinical Magnetic Resonance Imaging,* 3rd ed. Philadelphia: Saunders Elsevier, 2006:577-629.
11. Finn JP, Deshpande VS, Simonetti OP. Chapter 5: Pulse sequence design. In: Edelman RR, Hesselink JR, Zlatkin MB, Crues JV III, eds. *Clinical Magnetic Resonance Imaging,* 3rd ed. Philadelphia: Saunders Elsevier, 2006:137-173.
12. Queiroz-Andrade M, Blasbalg R, Ortega CD, et al. MR imaging findings of iron overload. Radiographics. 2009;29(6):1575-1589.
13. Thulborn KR. Chapter 6: Biochemical basis of the MRI appearance of cerebral hemorrhage. In: Edelman RR, Hesselink JR, Zlatkin MB, Crues JV III, eds. *Clinical Magnetic Resonance Imaging,* 3rd ed. Philadelphia: Saunders Elsevier, 2006:174-186.
14. Parizel PM, Makkat S, Van Miert E, et al. Intracranial hemorrhage: principles of CT and MRI interpretation. *Eur Radiol.* 2001; 11(9):1770-1783.

3.

LIVER MR IMAGING

Thomas D. Henry, MD

MR imaging provides several distinct advantages for imaging of the liver when compared to the other cross-sectional modalities, computed tomography (CT) and ultrasound. First, with MR the patient is not exposed to ionizing radiation, which is a distinct advantage over CT, though ultrasound also involves no radiation. Another advantage is that most commonly used intravenous contrast agents used in MR imaging, such as those containing gadolinium, are not associated with nephrotoxicity, whereas most iodine-containing agents used in CT are nephrotoxic. Although gadolinium-based contrast agents generally have an excellent safety record, there is a risk of developing nephrogenic systemic fibrosis, particularly when the patient's renal function is compromised. However, it has become clear that this risk can be reduced by judicious selection of patients, using the lowest necessary dose, and avoiding certain gadolinium compounds.

The fundamental advantage of MR imaging is that the image contrast between the various tissues is intrinsic to the tissues and determined by the differences in concentration and behavior of the water protons within those tissues. With CT, on the other hand, the image contrast is determined by differences in x-ray absorption of the tissues, and there may be significant overlap in the imaging appearance of very different types of soft tissue. For example, with CT a solid liver metastasis may have similar image density as the surrounding normal liver parenchyma and may therefore go undetected. The use of multiphasic contrast-enhanced CT improves detection of lesions; however, the information provided by the enhanced images is unidimensional, answering only the question of how the tissue accumulates and releases the contrast material. Contrast-enhanced MR imaging provides comparable information regarding the vascularity of the tissues, and has the advantage that dynamic post-contrast enhanced imaging can be performed without the need for ionizing radiation.

Ultrasonography, a relatively inexpensive and readily available imaging modality, uses no ionizing radiation and has been valuable for evaluating the liver. Cystic lesions are well characterized in most cases. The major drawbacks of the technique are that the results are operator dependent, the field of view is

limited, there is reduced sensitivity in the setting of diffuse liver disease or in large patients, and characterization of solid lesions is difficult. Thus, although ultrasonography is considered a useful screening tool as well as a problem-solving modality in certain situations, it is regarded as inferior to CT and MR imaging in the thorough evaluation of the liver, and for characterizing solid liver masses.

MR IMAGING TECHNIQUE

Other than performing the imaging study to best answer the clinical question raised by the referring clinician, an important goal in protocoling a liver MRI examination is also to obtain high-quality images in the shortest amount of time possible. This need to perform examinations quickly is driven by the economic realities of owning a very expensive piece of equipment and (more importantly in our discussion here) by the general deterioration of image quality with greater elapsed time. This deterioration can occur as a result of respiratory or other motion, or may be from the patient becoming fatigued or unable to remain still for other reasons. Below, the basic pulse sequences used in liver imaging are presented and their relative merits discussed. Details of these sequences are further described in Chapter 2.

T1-weighted imaging. Breath-hold gradient-echo (GRE) sequences have become the standard T1-weighted technique for imaging of the abdomen, allowing much faster image acquisition than possible with conventional spin-echo sequences. GRE images can be obtained as a single slice or multislice sequence. In-phase (IP) and out-of-phase (OP) GRE imaging takes advantage of the differences in precession of protons in lipid relative to protons in water, allowing detection of hepatic steatosis as well as microscopic lipid within liver lesions; the latter can be useful in lesion characterization.

GRE can also be performed with addition of a magnetization-prepared (MP) pulse preceding the GRE sequence, which allows for fast imaging with high tissue contrast. MPGRE is used as a single-slice technique with each slice obtained in less than 1.5 s, which is useful when a patient is uncooperative.

At our institution, we set the parameters for this sequence such that signal from a liver hemangioma is nulled, thus appearing nearly black in the image. This reference can then be applied to other liver lesions, with cysts typically appearing iso-intense to liver with a characteristic "bounce" artifact producing a dark peripheral ring at the interface between the cyst and surrounding liver, and the signal intensity of most solid lesions such as metastases falling between that of normal liver and hemangioma.

T2-weighted imaging. The development of fast (single slice obtained in less than 1 sec) T2-weighted single-shot fast/turbo spin-echo (FSE/TSE) pulse sequences with half-Fourier reconstruction represent a major advance in abdominal imaging. As images are acquired over a fraction of a second, these techniques are remarkably motion-insensitive.

MR Cholangiopancreaticography (MRCP). We routinely acquire heavily T2-weighted MRCP sequences in all liver protocols as bile duct abnormalities are often encountered in patients with liver disease. These include thin (3 to 4 mm) and thick (40 to 60 mm) slab breath-hold coronal/paracoronal images obtained within a breath hold, as well as a 3D multislice sequence acquired with respiratory gating while the patient breathes quietly. Besides allowing for a thorough study of the biliary tree, the longer TE with which these images are obtained also provides additional information useful for evaluation of liver lesions.

Diffusion-weighted imaging (DWI). With diffusion-weighted MR imaging the mobility of water protons in tissues can be assessed, and determination of DWI as a potential method for identifying and characterizing small liver lesions without the use of intravenous contrast material is a topic of active investigation. On diffusion-weighted images true lesions are seen as bright foci due to restriction of the normal motion of water molecules compared to normal liver tissue. However, because the role of this technique in routine liver imaging is yet to be determined, we will not be further discuss DWI in this chapter.

Gadolinium chelates are the workhorse of intravenous contrast-enhanced MR imaging. Gadolinium chelates are nonspecific extracellular contrast agents with imaging enhancement characteristics similar to those of iodine-based CT agents. The paramagnetic qualities of gadolinium cause shortening of the T1 relaxation time of surrounding protons, resulting in markedly increased signal intensity on T1-weighted images. In contrast to iodine-based CT contrast agents, it is this indirect effect of gadolinium on neighboring molecules that is imaged, rather than the gadolinium itself. Using gadolinium contrast enhancement, image sets are typically acquired in the late hepatic arterial phase (15 to 30 seconds after contrast-material bolus injection), the portal venous phase (45 to 75 seconds), and the hepatic venous (or interstitial) phase (90 seconds to 5 minutes), with additional phases obtained as desired. A high-quality hepatic late arterial phase is indispensable for lesion characterization. Proper timing can be confirmed when contrast material enhances the arteries and main portal vein but with no enhancement of the hepatic veins. Dynamically enhanced image sets that allow coverage of the entire liver in a single breath hold using T1-weighted 3D (volumetric) GRE sequences with fat saturation provide high signal-to-noise images with thin slices.

Hepatocyte-specific agents are chelates excreted into the hepatobiliary system using the bile salt pathway (as well as being excreted via kidneys, pancreas, and gastric mucosa). Traditionally, these compounds were manganese based (manganese dipyridoxyldiphosphate-MnDPDP [Teslascan®]). Like gadolinium, manganese is a T1-shortening agent, generating high signal on T1-weighted images, with non-hepatocyte–containing tissue rendering relatively low signal intensity. As a result, contrast between non-hepatocyte–containing lesions and surrounding liver is increased and lesions become more conspicuous. A minimum delay of 20 minutes is generally advisable to allow for adequate uptake of manganese agents by hepatocytes.[1] Unfortunately, certain benign and malignant tumors have been shown to also take up manganese: focal nodular hyperplasia, well-differentiated hepatocellular carcinoma, and metastatic pancreatic islet cell tumors.[1] More recently, newer gadolinium-based compounds such as gadoxetate disodium (Eovist®) have been developed that combine the advantages of a nonspecific extracellular agent and a hepatocyte-specific agent. These contrast agents have a high T1 relaxativity and are lipophilic, resulting in biliary as well as renal excretion.[1] Normally functioning hepatocytes take up the contrast agent and excrete it into the bile ducts, increasing the conspicuity of non-hepatocyte tissue embedded in the liver[1] (Fig. 3.1). Delayed, contrast-enhanced imaging (typically performed after 20 minutes or greater delay) with these agents has been shown to be helpful in lesion detection and characterization, for example for differentiating focal nodular hyperplasia from hypervascular metastases.[1,2,3,4]

Reticuloendothelial system-specific compounds typically use super-paramagnetic iron oxide. The iron oxide is taken up by functioning Kupffer cells and is cleared by the liver (80%) and spleen. The concentrated intracellular iron oxide has the effect of decreasing the signal in normal liver parenchyma on T2-weighted images as well as gradient-echo images because of increased susceptibility artifact with increasing TE (increased T2* decay effects). Lesions that do not contain Kupffer cells appear as relatively bright islands of tissue against a dark background of normal parenchyma.[1,5] Iron oxide is typically used in conjunction with gadolinium contrast material combining the improved lesion-detection properties of the reticuloendothelial-specific agent with the superior lesion-characterization properties of the nonspecific extracellular agent.

LIVER ANATOMY

The dual blood supply of the liver has important implications in MRI of the liver, just as it does in contrast-enhanced CT. Most of the blood flow to the normal liver comes from the portal venous system, with the remaining approximately one third coming from the hepatic artery. With diffuse liver disease, most importantly cirrhosis leading to portal hypertension, this balance is tipped with the artery assuming a larger role. In gadolinium-enhanced MRI, the effect of the changing blood supply is similar to that seen with contrast-enhanced

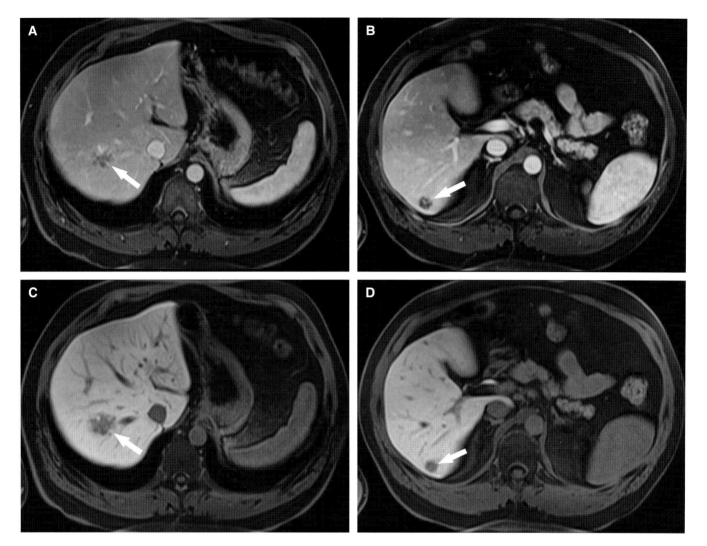

Figure 3.1 *Colorectal mtastases: improved visualization with hepatocyte-specific agent.* Two metastases (*arrows*) from colorectal carcinoma are seen on axial arterial phase T1-weighted gradient-echo images (**A, B**) of the liver after intravenous administration of the hepatocyte-specific agent Gd-EOB-DTPA (gadoxetic acid, Primovist®). Image **A** is obtained at a more cranial level than image **B**. Images **C** and **D** are obtained after a 20- minute delay. Image **C** is obtained at the same level as image **A** and image **D** is obtained at the same level as image **B**. Though these lesions are hypovascular and therefore well -visualized on arterial phase contrast-enhanced images due to gadolinium's inherent nonspecific extracellular kinetics, lesion conspicuity increases over time, as demonstrated in **C** and **D**, as the normally functioning hepatocytes accumulate the contrast agent and excrete it into the bilary system. Since the metastatic tissue contains no hepatocytes or bile ducts, the lesions remain low in signal intensity.

Box 3.1 ESSENTIALS TO REMEMBER

- Gradient-echo techniques allow for rapid single-slice or multislice imaging of the liver, producing high-quality images minimally affected by motion if obtained during breath hold.

- T1-weighted chemical-shift in- and out-of-phase gradient-echo sequences allow for detection microscopic fat such as in hepatic steatosis and fat-containing neoplasms including hepatic adenoma and hepatocellular carcinoma.

- Heavily T2-weighted images are obtained to image the biliary system and to detect focal lesions within the liver.

- Dynamic post-gadolinium contrast-enhanced T1-weighted sequences with fat suppression are important for accurate characterization of liver lesions.

- Hepatocyte-specific contrast agents allow identification of lesions lacking in functional hepatocytes as low-signal-intensity foci on contrast-enhanced T1-weighted images against a background of the higher-signal-intensity liver parenchyma.

CT, with sharply defined boundaries between segments revealing relative arterial and portal inflow. Additionally, altered hemodynamics lead to changes in the microenvironment of segments and entire lobes of the liver as they are exposed to different sources of blood, manifesting as different signal intensities on MR sequences. Many hepatic tumors are primarily fed by arterial branches, so dynamically enhancement sequences are extremely useful in lesion characterization. MRI allows for multiple consecutive post-contrast enhanced sequences without subjecting the patient to increasing doses of ionizing radiation as is the case with multiphasic CT.

The Couinaud system of segmental anatomy has the same use in liver MRI as elsewhere. This system divides the liver into segments based upon predictable vascular boundaries that are particularly relevant to surgical planning. This anatomy is well depicted without the need for contrast agents.

On unenhanced T1-weighted images the normal liver is hyperintense to spleen and most other abdominal tissues other than fat and pancreas due to its relatively short T1 relaxation time (Fig. 3.2). This signal intensity has been postulated to be related to the protein synthesis in the liver. Protein is a known cause of T1 shortening.[6] Its T2 relaxation time is also relatively short, the result being that normal liver is hypointense to spleen on T2-weighted images. The appearance of the normal liver has important implications on the conspicuity of solid lesions on unenhanced images. Most solid lesions appear slightly hypointense to normal liver parenchyma on T1-weighted images and hyperintense to parenchyma on T2-weighted images.

DIFFUSE LIVER DISEASE

Infectious processes, vascular abnormalities, and inherited as well as acquired metabolic disorders can have profound effects on the appearance of the liver parenchyma. Hepatic fibrosis is the common end result when left unchecked. MRI is a powerful tool for detecting diffuse liver disease in helping to identify its cause, and in chronic cases providing surveillance for complications such as hepatocellular carcinoma.

Acute Hepatitis. Numerous insults can cause acute hepatitis, among them viruses, hepatotoxins (alcohol, drugs), and biliary tract obstruction. MRI is of limited use in the management of acute hepatitis, but may be performed to exclude other disease processes. In the setting of acute injury, the liver may be normal or diffusely enlarged. The hepatic arterial-phase images are the most sensitive for detecting the subtle heterogeneous enhancement pattern of acute hepatitis. In severe cases, heterogeneous enhancement may persist into the delayed venous phase.[1] Proper timing of arterial phase acquisition is critical if mild cases are to be detected.

Portal vein thrombosis is most commonly encountered in the setting of cirrhosis, but it may also result from other causes of stasis such as an underlying hypercoagulable state, extrinsic compression by a mass, or vascular injury as a sequela of inflammation or infection. Additionally, tumor may directly invade the portal vein, resulting in tumor thrombus. Thrombosis may be complete or non-occlusive, acute or chronic. Depending upon circumstances, the presentation may be clinically dramatic with hemorrhage and pain, or silent with unsuspected thrombosis identified on imaging for other reasons.

On unenhanced spin-echo images, a thrombosed portal vein will appear with intermediate high signal intensity, in stark contrast to the flow voids normally seen in patent vessels. On gradient–echo, "bright blood" images the appearance will be reversed, with decreased or absent signal from the thrombosed vein standing out compared to the high signal intensity of blood flowing into patent vessels. With dynamic gadolinium-enhanced MRI, even small non-occlusive clot can be identified, with the added benefit of the ability to distinguish between bland and tumor thrombus based upon enhancement of the clot itself. In subacute to chronic thrombosis, "cavernous transformation" of the portal vein occurs. Portal blood is diverted through periportal collateral veins to reach the more distal portal branches beyond the thrombosis. Cavernous transformation appears as numerous serpentine vessels in the expected location of the main portal vein. A common associated finding is a transient geographic wedge-shaped area of increased, arterial-phase enhancement in the subtended portion of liver. This occurs as a compensatory increase in arterial blood supplying the affected liver. Geographic areas of increased signal intensity become inconspicuous in later phases.

Budd-Chiari syndrome is manifested acutely as hepatomegaly, ascites, and right upper quadrant pain, and chronically as progressive portal hypertension and liver failure. The syndrome was originally described as acute thrombosis of the hepatic veins or inferior vena cava, but has since been expanded to include cases of subacute and chronic venous occlusion. Causes of hepatic venous outflow obstruction include hypercoagulable states; tumor, such as hepatocellular carcinoma, directly invading or extrinsically compressing the vein; vascular injury; and stasis. Budd-Chiari syndrome is more common in women, an observation at least partially explained by the hypercoagulable state associated with pregnancy, the postpartum period, and the use of oral contraceptives.[7] The presentation may be acute, with rapid intervention required to avoid severe complications, including death. The prognosis depends upon many factors, including the location of thrombus. Treatments include anticoagulation, thrombolysis, and shunt creation.

Hepatic venous outflow thrombosis leads acutely to the dilatation of veins and sinusoids, and chronically to collagenization of sinusoids and atrophy of parenchyma. The thrombosis usually involves the major veins but in cases may be segmental or isolated. Blood is usually shunted to accessory hepatic veins, so outflow from the liver is not completely blocked. Chronic cases show atrophy of the peripheral liver, as that is the level of most severe venous obstruction, associated with relative hypertrophy of the more central liver and the caudate lobe. The caudate lobe is spared by having separate drainage directly into the inferior vena cava.[4]

Dynamic contrast-enhanced MR allows differentiation of acute, subacute, and chronic Budd-Chiari syndrome based on enhancement characteristics (Figs. 3.3 and 3.4). In cases of acute thrombosis of the hepatic veins or inferior vena cava, the

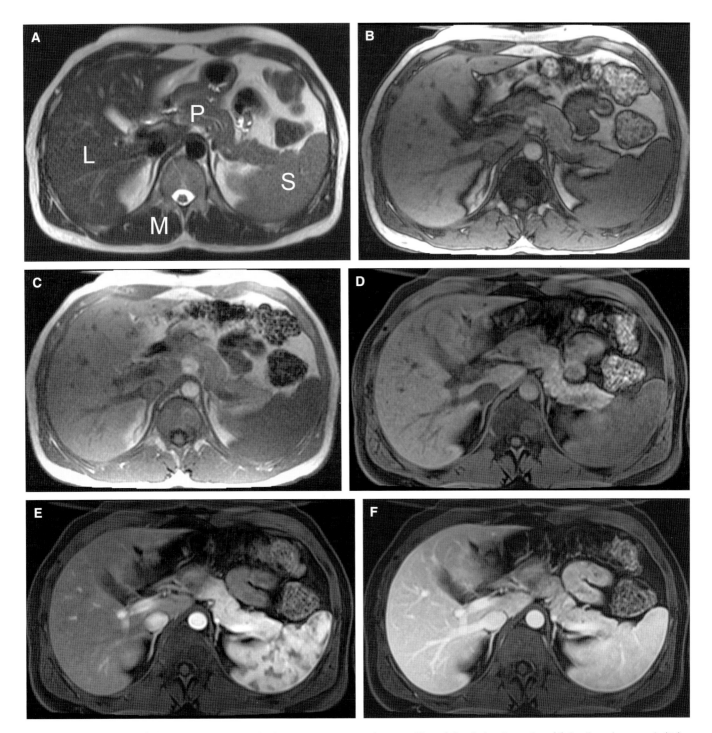

Figure 3.2 *Normal liver.* (**A**) On T2-weighted single-shot FSE/TSE images the normal liver (*L*) is darker than spleen (*S*), brighter than muscle (*M*), and similar in signal intensity to pancreas (*P*). Normal hepatic parenchyma is slightly hyperintense to spleen on both out-of-phase (**B**) and in-phase (**C**) T1-weighted gradient-echo images. Pre-contrast (**D**), hepatic arterial phase (**E**), and portal venous (**F**) phase T1-weighted post-gadolinium contrast-enhanced images illustrate the dual hepatic blood supply. The liver is strikingly hypointense to both pancreas and spleen in the arterial phase and becomes isointense in the portal venous phase, underscoring the dominance of the portal supply.

thrombus results in increased resistance to both hepatic arterial and portal venous inflow. The liver periphery is the area most affected by congestion of the venules and sinusoids, resulting in a lesser degree of enhancement than the central liver, a difference that persists into the delayed venous phase of contrast-enhanced images. On T2-weighted images the peripheral parenchyma will be relatively hyperintense, and

hypointense on T1-weighted images. Hepatomegaly is expected.

With chronicity of thrombosis, this relative increase in enhancement of the liver periphery becomes less conspicuous, particularly on delayed post-gadolinium contrast-enhanced images, although the difference remains apparent in the arterial phase. The caudate lobe hypertrophies, and flow in the

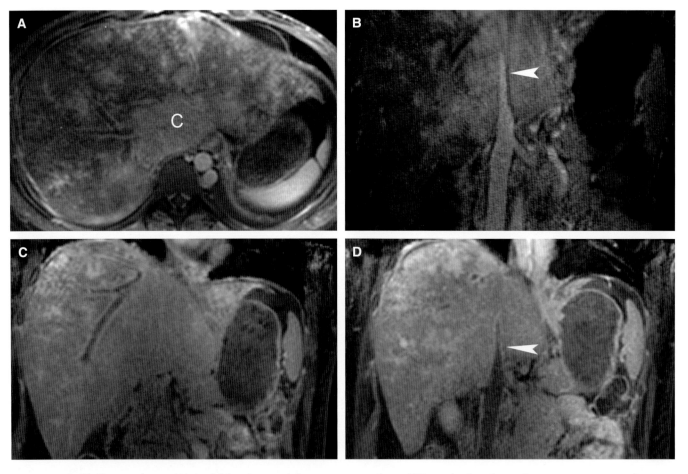

Figure 3.3 *Budd-Chiari syndrome.* (**A**) Axial delayed post-gadolinium contrast-enhanced T1-weighted gradient-echo image in a patient with antithrombin III deficiency demonstrates heterogeneous liver parenchyma with enlargement and relative hyperenhancement of the caudate/central (*C*) liver. Non-filling of the left and right hepatic veins can be seen. (**B**) Coronal venous phase gadolinium-contrast enhanced MRA image offers another view of the same process, with some extrinsic narrowing of the inferior vena cava (*arrowhead*). (**C, D**) Two additional coronal contrast-enhanced MRA images from the portal venous phase demonstrate non-filling of the hepatic veins and inferior vena cava (*arrowhead* in image **D**). The findings indicate acute to subacute Budd-Chiari syndrome.

portal vein reverses. Small extrahepatic venovenous collaterals may be seen, a finding not encountered in other chronic liver diseases. Acute edema is replaced by fibrosis, manifested as increased signal intensity in the liver periphery on both T2- and T1-weighted images. Regenerative nodules may develop on this background of fibrosis, appearing iso- to hypointense on T2-weighted images and hyperintense on T1-weighted images. The enhancement differences between the central and peripheral liver become more subtle, and venous thrombosis may no longer be apparent. Further hypertrophy, sometimes massive, of the caudate lobe is expected. Large bridging curvilinear intrahepatic collaterals as well as extrahepatic collateral vessels and varices are often present. Additional manifestations of portal hypertension such as ascites and splenomegaly usually develop.

Hepatic veno-occlusive disease results from injury to the endothelial lining of the sinusoids, leading to obliteration of the small hepatic venules.[7] The hepatic veins and inferior vena cava are not affected. Chemotherapeutics and radiation are often the cause. The MRI appearance is that of nonspecific

hepatic congestion, with hepatomegaly and third spacing of fluid. Hepatic veins may be compressed by surrounding edema but remain patent.

Passive hepatic congestion secondary to right heart failure is a common cause of hepatomegaly, with characteristic mosaic enhancement of the liver parenchyma. This is differentiated from Budd-Chiari by the patency of the veins, and from veno-occlusive disease by the distention of the hepatic veins with refluxed contrast in the arterial phase.

Peliosis hepatis is a rare benign liver disorder characterized by dilated hepatic sinusoids. It is generally seen in the setting of anabolic steroid and oral contraceptive use, although it is also reported with numerous other associations, including chronic wasting states such as pulmonary tuberculosis, HIV, malignancy, and in the post-transplant population. The dilated intrahepatic sinusoids are small, typically several millimeters to 1 cm, and appear as blood-filled cysts. Histologically, these may be lined by endothelium or may be foci of hepatic necrosis and hemorrhage.[8] On MRI, the dilated sinusoids may diffusely involve the liver or may appear as a more confluent mass,

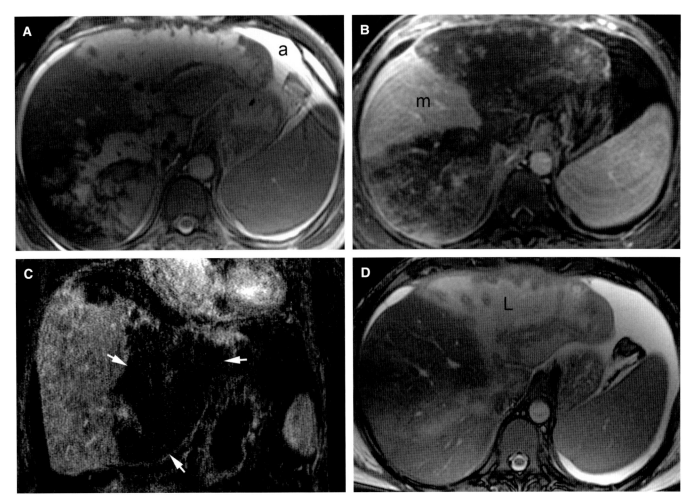

Figure 3.4 *Budd-Chiari syndrome with hepatic necrosis.* (**A**) Axial T2-weighted single-shot FSE/TSE image in a patient following orthotopic liver transplant demonstrates abnormal increased signal intensity throughout the left lobe and posterior segment of the right lobe, sparing a wedge-shaped region centrally. Ascites (*a*) is present. (**B**) On T1-weighted post-gadolinium-enhanced image acquired in the portal venous phase, a similar pattern is seen, indicating occlusion of the left and right hepatic veins and sparing the territory drained by the middle hepatic vein (*m*). (**C**) Coronal contrast-enhanced MRA offers another view, with essentially absent perfusion to those segments drained by the right and left hepatic veins (between *short arrows*). (**D**) T2-weighted image obtained two weeks later shows further increased signal intensity, particularly of the left lobe (*L*), indicating hepatic necrosis. Peripheral areas of relative hypointensity are likely secondary to capsular blood inflow.

with variable signal intensity on T1-weighted and hyperintensity on T2-weighted images. Following contrast material administration, affected regions of liver will initially be hypoenhancing relative to normal parenchyma, with gradual increasing enhancement through the portal and delayed hepatic venous phases as blood enters the dilated spaces.[9] This appearance, when focal, can be mistaken for cavernous hemangioma, but a true mass effect should not be present with peliosis. The condition may regress with withdrawal of the inciting factor, or may progress to portal hypertension and liver failure. Hemorrhage can occur acutely.

Other vascular lesions of the liver include arteriovenous fistulas, arteriovenous malformations, and vascular shunts. Arteriovenous fistulas are commonly seen following liver biopsy and are usually of no consequence. Vascular shunts may occur between branches of the hepatic artery and portal vein, the hepatic artery and hepatic vein, or the portal vein and the systemic circulation. Multiple shunts present as enhancing foci in hereditary hemorrhagic telangiectasia, also known as Osler-Weber-Rendu disease, an inherited syndrome with variable penetrance manifesting with vascular malformations in various organs and tissues.

Hepatic steatosis results from excessive lipid accumulation in hepatocytes, a process that may be driven by both endogenous and exogenous factors. The most common association today is with obesity. Many other contributing factors have been identified, including alcohol abuse, medications (including chemotherapeutic agents and steroids), various metabolic disorders including diabetes, and hepatitis C. The process is reversible with removal of the inciting factor. Unchecked steatosis may progress to inflammation and fibrosis, termed steatohepatitis, which in turn may lead to frank cirrhosis. In addition to steatohepatitis associated with alcohol abuse, there has more recently been increasingly widespread recognition of the burgeoning epidemic of non-alcoholic steatohepatitis (NASH), itself a product of the obesity epidemic. Alcoholic and non-alcoholic steatohepatitis generally cannot be differentiated by imaging or histology.

Hepatic steatosis is commonly discovered incidentally at imaging. Patients may have vague complaints such as abdominal pain and fatigue, or may have more specific signs of hepatocellular injury such as hepatomegaly or elevated liver function tests. Risk factors are generally independent of gender, although certain subtypes may be seen exclusively (acute fatty liver of pregnancy) or disproportionately (alcohol abuse) in one gender. Although the majority of patients is middle aged, it is not uncommon to encounter severe cases of steatosis in patients in their third and fourth decades of life.

Fat deposition in the liver leads to characteristic changes in parenchymal signal intensity on in-phase (IP) and out-of-phase (OP) gradient-echo sequences due to chemical-shift artifact (Fig. 3.5). The presence of lipid and water in the same voxel has the effect of phase cancellation on the OP images, resulting in a decrease in signal intensity of the liver parenchyma. The spleen is a useful reference organ on a single OP image as it does not accumulate lipid, although the spleen signal may be altered in case of iron deposition. When the liver parenchyma shows lower signal intensity than the spleen on the OP sequence, this is diagnostic of steatosis. The diagnosis of hepatic steatosis can also be made by comparing the signal intensity of a region of interest in the liver on both OP and IP slices, whereby a decrease in signal intensity greater than two times the standard deviation on the OP images is generally considered to be diagnositic of steatosis. As the IP and OP slices are acquired simultaneously, quantitative measurements of signal intensity are valid between corresponding slices. These techniques have also been used to calculate hepatic fat fractions.

Fat deposition may be focal or diffuse. Focal areas of steatosis, or of focal fatty sparing, may be mistaken for lesions. Such "lesions" will not show mass effect and tend to occur in predictable locations: adjacent to the gallbladder fossa, adjacent to the falciform ligament, and within the subcapsular liver. The explanation for these preferential sites of focal fat or fatty sparing lies in the "third inflow." Third inflow refers to aberrant systemic venous supply and drainage that alters the amount of portal venous blood supplying focal areas of parenchyma, thus changing the milieu relative to the remainder of the liver.[10] Differential portal flow to the right and left lobes, with a more direct route to the right, leads to preferential regional steatosis based upon the same principles.

Iron Deposition Disease. MRI takes advantage of magnetic susceptibility artifact to reveal excessive hepatic iron deposition, which can be seen in both the primary and secondary forms. The fundamental difference is that primary hemochromatosis involves iron deposition through chelation while secondary hemochromatosis occurs through activities of the reticuloendothelial system. While the secondary form is benign, primary hemochromatosis is a risk factor for progression to cirrhosis and associated increased risk for developing hepatocellular carcinoma.

Primary hemochromatosis (genetic hemochromatosis) is an autosomal recessive disease of persons of northern European descent with a complicated phenotypic expression. The disease causes impairment of the normal regulation mechanism of small bowel iron absorption, resulting in excessive total body iron accumulation via mechanisms of chelation.[11] Clinical presentation is usually in later life, typically the fifth or sixth decade, with nonspecific symptoms generally related to sites and severity of iron deposition. Excess iron is chelated by the hepatocytes and concentrated in the liver sinusoids. With time, iron will also be chelated by the pancreatic acinar cells[12] and to a lesser extent the pituitary gland and heart, as well as diverse other tissues after hepatocytes have been overwhelmed.[13] As this is parenchymal deposition rather than iron overload caused by the reticuloendothelial system, the spleen and bone marrow will not be involved, a helpful imaging feature for differentiating between primary and secondary hemochromatosis. It should be remembered, however, that patients with genetic hemochromatosis may require multiple blood

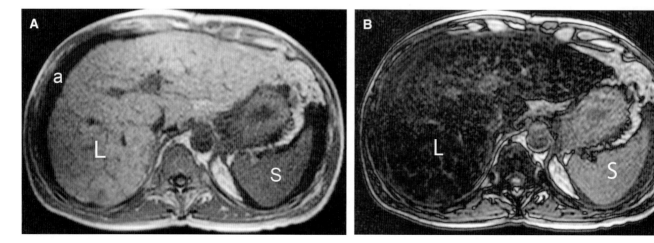

Figure 3.5 *Hepatic steatosis in the setting of cirrhosis.* In-phase (**A**) and out-of-phase (**B**) T1-weighted gradient-echo images show marked loss of signal in the hepatic parenchyma (*L*) on the out-of-phase image due to chemical-shift artifact. Note also that the liver is diffusely hypointense compared to the spleen (*S*) on the out-of-phase image. Ascites (*a*) outlines the liver, which shows mild surface nodularity indicating cirrhosis.

transfusions, which may lead to increased reticuloendothelial iron storage, so imaging features may overlap. As with iron deposition the liver is, in general, homogeneously involved, an iron-free nodule in the setting of primary hemochromatosis should raise suspicion for hepatocellular carcinoma.[4]

Secondary hemochromatosis may result from increased red blood cell turnover in various chronic conditions of ineffective erythropoiesis, including thalassemia major, sideroblastic anemia, megaloblastic anemia, and myelofibrosis. Increased marrow demand spurs increased gastrointestinal tract iron absorption, with similar distribution as with genetic hemochromatosis. Secondary hemochromatosis also occurs as a result of increased exogenous iron exposure in the setting of multiple blood transfusions. Excess iron from damaged red blood cells is taken up in the form of hemoglobin by cells of the reticuloendothelial system, leading to iron accumulation in the liver (Kupffer cells) and spleen (by phagocytosis). However, the spleen may be spared if reticuloendothelial system function is impaired.[4] Patients with anemia generally receive multiple blood transfusions, so features of transfusional iron overload often comingle. As the pancreas is not part of the reticuloendothelial system, lack of pancreatic iron deposition can be used to help differentiate iron deposition disease related to transfusions and conditions of ineffective erythropoiesis from primary (genetic) hemochromatosis.

The paramagnetic effects of iron cause increased $T2^*$ effects resulting in diminished signal intensity on both T2- and T1-weighted images, with the effects becoming more obvious with increasing TE (Fig. 3.6). For this reason, iron deposition causes a reversal of the picture of steatosis seen with in- and out-of-phase gradient-echo images if in-phase images are obtained with the longer TE: the liver will be darker on these images, see also Figure 2.36 of Chapter 1. On T2-weighted images, the signal intensity of the normal liver is approximately midway between that of the relatively dark muscle and relatively bright spleen. In iron overload, the liver will be much lower in signal intensity and iso- or hypointense to muscle. A similarly low-signal-intensity spleen would suggest secondary hemochromatosis as the cause of iron deposition. In mild forms of iron deposition, the liver signal intensity is near normal on T1-weighted images, and susceptibility artifacts from iron deposition are noted only on T2- or $T2^*$-weighted images. When liver and spleen signal is decreased on gradient-echo images with the longest TE, iron deposition is considered moderate; when they approach signal void, iron deposition is considered severe.

Cirrhosis is the end result of chronic hepatocellular injury, characterized by diffuse fibrosis with intervening parenchymal nodules. The most commonly encountered etiologies are chronic hepatitis B and C, and alcohol abuse, often synergistic. Additional important causes are non-alcoholic steatohepatitis (NASH), drug toxicity, autoimmune hepatitis, and genetic metabolic disorders, as well as biliary and vascular diseases.[14] Some cases are idiopathic. Imaging plays a major role in detecting cirrhosis as well as identifying complications such as portal hypertension and hepatocellular carcinoma.

The earliest changes of cirrhosis that are detected by biopsy are not visible by MRI or other imaging modalities, although other indicators of liver abnormality such as hepatomegaly or steatosis may be present (see Fig. 3.5). With further increasing severity and duration of hepatocellular injury, characteristic changes in morphology, signal intensity, and sequelae of portal hypertension are seen. As fibrous parenchymal bands form, the intervening liver parenchyma assumes an increasingly nodular appearance, which may be seen along the capsule or within the deeper parenchyma. Fibrosis leads to segmental and lobar changes influenced by both vascular anatomy and flow dynamics. Compared to the left, the right portal vein has a longer intrahepatic course, and its surrounding parenchymal distortion leads to relatively diminished portal blood flow, resulting in decreased delivery of trophic factors and thus atrophy of the right lobe (segments V–VIII), although the atrophy often involves the medial segment (segments IV a and b) of the left lobe as well.[14] The lateral segment (segments II and III) of the left lobe and caudate lobe (segment I) will hypertrophy to compensate.[4] In the early stages, subtle enlargement of the hilar periportal space and gallbladder fossa is a useful indicator of atrophy.

Fibrotic bands are characteristically mildly hyperintense on T2-weighted images, and may be thin or thick. In advanced cases, confluent fibrosis may result, which should not be mistaken for a mass. Regions of *confluent fibrosis* tend to be wedge-shaped and associated with capsular retraction, both helpful distinguishing features. On dynamic contrast-enhanced sequences, areas of fibrosis will accumulate contrast material in the delayed interstitial phase relative to the remaining parenchyma, just as fibrous tissue of any origin would be expected to do. Intervening nodules may represent islands of relatively normal parenchyma or be true regenerative nodules. As discussed later in this chapter, MRI is quite useful in characterizing these nodules and screening for progression to dysplastic nodules and hepatocellular carcinoma.

With progression of liver fibrosis, the portal venous branches become increasingly compressed and distorted, leading to intrahepatic portal hypertension and its myriad imaging manifestations. Prehepatic portal hypertension, resulting from thrombosis of the main portal or splenic veins, and posthepatic portal hypertension occurring in the setting of inferior vena cava or hepatic vein thrombosis or passive congestion, may also be seen in cirrhotics. The earliest indirect finding is enlargement of the main portal vein, typically considered more than 13 mm in diameter. With time, increased pressure in the portal vein (defined as greater than 10 mmHg) will lead to splenomegaly and shunting of blood away from the liver via portosystemic collateral pathways. Shunting results in decreased delivery of tropic factors to the liver, increased systemic exposure to toxins ordinarily filtered by the liver, and a risk of life-threatening variceal bleeding. Typical findings include (1) splenorenal shunts from the splenic hilum to the left renal vein; (2) enlarged paraumbilical veins, which course within the falciform ligament draining from the left portal vein to the inferior or superior vena cava via abdominal wall pathways; (3) esophageal and paraesophageal varices that arise from the left gastric vein, which extends from the superior aspect of the splenic vein near the portosplenic confluence and drains into the azygos system; and (4) left, posterior or short gastric varices that drain to the left renal vein via phrenic or suprarenal tributaries (Fig. 3.7). Additionally, increased

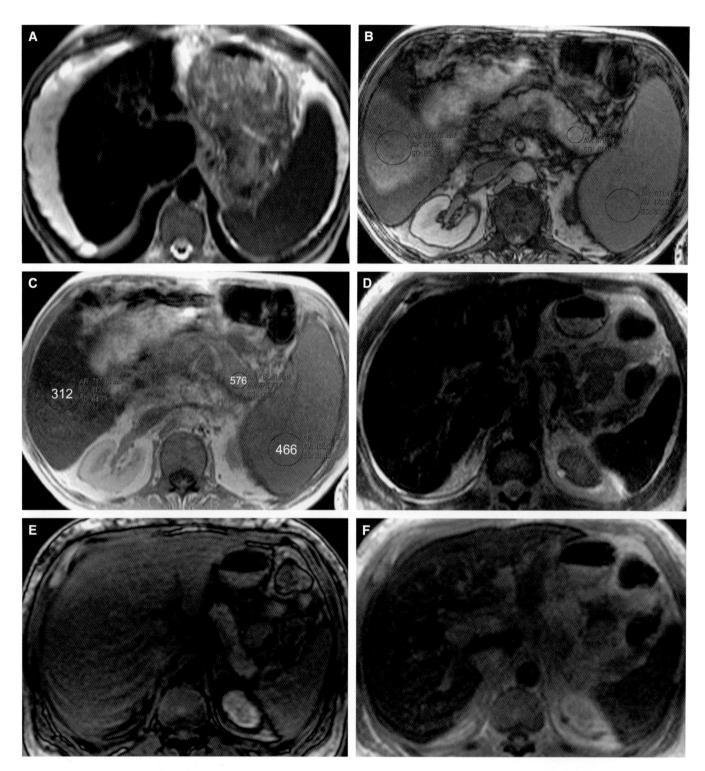

Figure 3.6 *Hemochromatosis.* (**A–C**) **Primary hemochromatosis**. Axial T2-weighted single-shot FSE/TSE images (**A**) and out-of-phase (**B**) and in-phase (**C**) images of a patient with primary (genetic) hemochromatosis. Deposition of iron in the liver and pancreas is confirmed by low signal on the sequences that use a longer echo time (TE), in this case the T2-weighted single-shot FSE/TSE (**A**) and the in-phase gradient-echo image (TE 4.6 ms) shown in C, compared to the out-of-phase (TE 2.3 ms) image shown in B. Region-of-interest measurements (*circles with numbers*) on out-of-phase and in-phase images confirm signal dropout of liver and pancreas but not of spleen, the expected findings in genetic hemochromatosis. The nodular liver contour indicates progression to cirrhosis, the expected natural history of genetic hemochromatosis. (**D–F**) **Secondary hemochromatosis**. T2-weighted (**D**), out-of-phase (**E**), and in-phase (**F**) images depict typical findings in a patient with secondary hemochromatosis. In contrast to primary hemochromatosis, iron deposition in secondary hemochromatois occurs in the spleen but not in the pancreas. The spleen displays low signal intensity on T2-weighted (**D**) and in-phase (**F**) images compared to the out-of-phase image (**E**), while the signal of the pancreas remains relatively high.

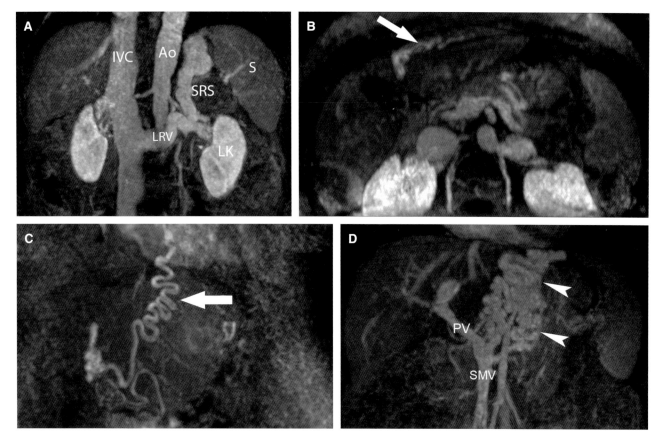

Figure 3.7 *Shunting in portal hypertension.* Four images demonstrate three types of spontaneous shunts occurring in the setting of portal hypertension. (**A**) A coronal MIP from gadolinium contrast-enhanced MRA depicts a large splenorenal shunt (*SRS*) diverting portal blood flow from the high-pressure splenic vein draining the spleen (*S*) to the lower-pressure left renal vein (*LRV*) extending from the left kidney (*LK*). The left renal vein drains directly into the inferior vena cava (*IVC*). *Ao*, aorta. Axial (**B**) and coronal (**C**) MIP images from the same MRA demonstrate a paraumbilical collateral vein (*arrow*) draining from the anterior branch of the left hepatic vein to the anterior abdominal/chest wall. (**D**) Large paraesophageal varices (*arrowheads*) result from collaterals of the left gastric/coronary vein that come off the splenic vein near the portal confluence. *PV*, portal vein. *SMV*, superior mesenteric vein.

pressure within the inferior mesenteric vein may lead to superior hemorrhoidal vein varices that drain into the internal iliac veins via the middle and inferior hemorrhoidals. When markedly enlarged collaterals are present, blood is successfully diverted and the portal venous pressure lowered, and thus the spleen tends to be normal in size. It is not uncommon to see scattered foci of hemorrhage, fibrosis, and hemosiderin, termed *Gamna-Gandy bodies,* in the spleen in the setting of prolonged portal hypertension. These nodules are most conspicuous on GRE sequences with long TE, due to susceptibility artifact related to iron. The signal difference is especially conspicuous on the image of a dual echo, in- and out-of-phase T1-weighted gradient echo sequence obtained with the long TE (often the in-phase image) in comparison to that obtained with a short TE (often the out-of-phase image). Siderotic nodules in the liver have a similar appearance (Fig. 3.8).

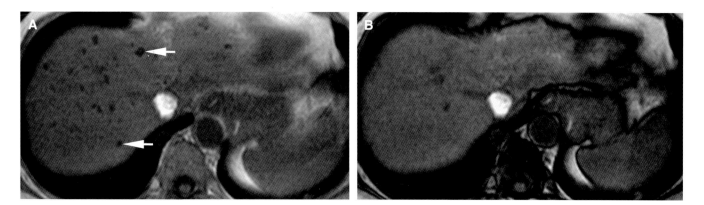

Figure 3.8 *Siderotic nodules.* In-phase (TE 4.6 ms) (**A**) and out-of-phase (TE 2.3 ms) (**B**) images depict siderotic nodules (*short arrows* in image A) in a patient with cirrhosis. Magnetic susceptibility artifact from iron in the nodules shown as low signal foci are best seen on the in-phase (longer TE) image.

Another common finding in cirrhosis is third spacing of fluid, which may be due to hypoproteinemia in the setting of liver dysfunction or portal hypertension.[15] On MRI, third spacing manifests as ascites, pleural effusions, bowel wall thickening, gallbladder wall thickening, and generalized edema of the mesentery, omentum, and even the subcutaneous tissues. The bowel wall thickening particularly affects the right colon and jejunum, postulated to be the result of more limited collateral pathways available to the superior mesenteric vein relative to the richly collateralized inferior mesenteric vein. Third spacing of fluid is seen as increased signal intensity within the fat on T2 fat-suppressed sequences, or as decreased signal intensity on routine T1-weighted images.

Primary biliary cirrhosis is a disease of as yet undetermined etiology causing progressive nonsuppurative inflammation and destruction of the bile ducts.[16] An immunologic basis is suspected.[17] The typical patient is middle-aged and female, and may present with cholestatic symptoms or be asymptomatic. Eventually, cirrhosis and portal hypertension develop.

On MRI, periportal hyperintensity may be seen on T2-weighted images, representing edema, dilated lymph vessels, duct proliferation, and inflammatory infiltrate of the portal tracts.[16] This finding represents active inflammation and is seen in 100% of early cases, diminishing with progression of disease.[18] The periportal halo sign has more recently been identified as a highly specific MRI finding to distinguish end-stage primary biliary cirrhosis from cirrhosis of other causes.[17] The periportal halo appears as 5- to 10-mm round hypointense zones on both T1- and T2-weighted images, surrounding the portal triads in all hepatic segments. No mass effect is evident. Histologically, this finding corresponds to stellate areas of hepatocellular parenchymal extinction around portal branches, encircled by a rosette of regenerating nodules. This process is distinct from the periportal inflammatory infiltrate commonly seen in earlier stages of primary biliary cirrhosis.[17] In distinction, the regenerating nodules of cirrhosis from other causes are of variable sizes and signal intensity, are not centered on portal branches, and may cause mass effect.[17] On dynamic T1-weighted post-contrast-enhanced imaging, small punctate or segmental areas of arterioportal shunting are commonly seen in the hepatic arterial enhancement phase, secondary to inflammation causing occlusion of small portal branches.[16]

Sarcoidosis. The liver is the third most commonly involved organ in sarcoidosis after the lung and lymph nodes, but its involvement is detected by imaging in a minority of cases.[4] The characteristic noncaseating granulomas of sarcoidosis are scattered diffusely throughout the liver. When visible by cross-sectional imaging the granulomas appear as small (less than 15 mm) nodules primarily distributed along the periportal regions. The nodules typically show hypointense signal on T1-weighted images and hypointense signal on T2-weighted images, without enhancement. More often, but still seen in a minority of patients, is generalized hepatomegaly present. Upper abdominal lymphadenopathy and splenic involvement may provide clues to the diagnosis. Though the MRI appearance of the nodules is nonspecific, when seen in the context of thoracic sarcoidosis the diagnosis can be made with a high degree of confidence.

CYSTIC LESIONS OF THE LIVER

Hepatic cysts may be congenital, infectious, neoplastic, or idiopathic in origin. Congenital cystic lesions are believed to arise as a result of malformation of the ductal plate during embryogenesis.[19] The ductal plate is the precursor of the intrahepatic biliary tree. Malformation results in cystic dilatation and fibrosis, causing the MR appearance of multiple cysts seen in various disorders, including autosomal dominant polycystic disease, biliary hamartomas (von Meyenburg complexes), Caroli's disease, mesenchymal hamartomas, and congenital hepatic fibrosis.[4] Acquired cystic lesions include infectious causes such as echinococcal (hydatid) cysts and liver abscesses, as well as both benign and malignant primary neoplasms of the liver, and cystic, necrotic, or mucinous metastases.

Simple hepatic cysts are common and generally asymptomatic, and they increase in incidence with age. Most fall within a range of 5 mm to 5 cm in diameter, and are more likely to be multiple than solitary.[20] Hepatic cysts are thought to arise from cystic dilatation of von Meyenburg complexes and are lined by cuboidal epithelium surrounded by thin fibrous stroma.[21] The MR signal characteristics are that of serous fluid, showing low signal intensity on T1-weighted and high signal intensity on T2-weighted images (Fig. 3.9). The cyst lining is imperceptible except when the cysts are complicated by hemorrhage or infection. In that case the wall may be thickened and the internal signal more complex, indicating proteinaceous fluid and blood. Thin septa may be encountered, but when seen this raises the possibility of the lesion being a cystadenoma. Cysts have no vascular supply and so do not enhance. Differential diagnosis includes hemangioma; biliary cystadenoma; and cystic, necrotic, or mucinous metastasis.

Autosomal Dominant Polycystic Disease. Most individuals with autosomal dominant polycystic kidney disease also have hepatic cysts. Uncommonly, liver cysts may be seen in the absence of renal cysts. Liver cysts are quite variable in size and number, increasing with age and decreased renal function. Women tend to have more extensive involvement than men.[4] Individually, cysts seen in association with autosomal dominant polycystic disease are indistinguishable from simple hepatic cysts both histologically and by imaging. As the cysts become large and confluent they cause mass effect. compressing the vascular structures and bile ducts. Severe cases can lead to liver failure.[22] The cysts contain serous fluid and are lined by cuboidal or columnar epithelium, with or without a fibrous capsule.[22] The MR signal intensity follows that of simple fluid except when the cysts are complicated by hemorrhage or infection. Infected or symptomatic cysts can be percutaneously drained. Large symptomatic cysts can be treated by percutaneous aspiration with sclerosis to prevent reaccumulation of fluid.[23]

Caroli's disease belongs to the spectrum of disorders of ductal plate malformation, in this case resulting in saccular dilatation of intrahepatic ducts. On MRI, Caroli's disease manifests as numerous small fluid signal "cysts" that when carefully inspected can be shown to communicate with the bile ducts (see Fig. 4.11 in Chapter 4). Caroli's disease can be associated with congenital hepatic fibrosis and may progress to cirrhosis with the stigmata of portal hypertension. The disease

Box 3.2 ESSENTIALS TO REMEMBER

- In acute hepatitis, MR imaging of the liver is often normal. Findings, when present, include hepatomegaly and heterogeneous enhancement.

- Portal vein thrombi are seen on MRI spin-echo images as foci of intermediate to high signal replacing the normal signal void within the portal vein. On bright blood gradient-echo images the thrombus will show low signal intensity replacing the high signal of inflowing blood. Cavernous transformation of the portal vein is seen as a network of collateral vessels in the porta hepatis replacing the chronically thrombosed portal vein.

- Budd-Chiari syndrome is caused by acute, subacute, or chronic obstruction of the hepatic veins or inferior vena cava. Acute hepatic venous thrombosis results in edema in the periphery of the liver seen as decreased signal intensity on T1-weighted and increased signal intensity on T2-weighted images. Enhancement is heterogeneously decreased in the liver periphery. Chronic hepatic venous obstruction is characterized by non-visualization of the hepatic veins, hypertrophy of the caudate lobe, and a heterogeneous, mosaic enhancement pattern of the liver. Hepatic venous collaterals appear as comma-shaped enhancing vessels. The liver develops the appearance of cirrhosis with regenerative nodules that may enhance and mimic small hepatocellular carcinomas.

- Passive hepatic congestion, caused by right heart failure, manifests on MR as dilated but patent hepatic veins and inferior vena cava, and with heterogeneous enhancement of the liver parenchyma. Ascites and right pleural effusion are often also present.

- Hepatic steatosis refers to the accumulation of lipids within hepatocytes. Chemical-shift MR imaging is important for the diagnosis of hepatic steatosis as routine T1- and T2-weighted images usually appear relatively normal. Diagnosis of steatosis is made when the liver signal intensity is decreased greater than two standard deviations on out-of-phase images compared to in-phase images. Fat deposition may be diffuse, focal, or diffuse with focal sparing. Fatty infiltration can involve the entire liver or may be geographic in appearance. No mass effect is evident as vessels are seen to course normally through affected parenchyma.

- Iron deposition in liver parenchyma is characterized on MR by a decrease in signal intensity predominantly on T2-weighted images caused by the paramagnetic effect of iron. Decrease in signal can also be observed on the images acquired with the longest TE of an in- and out-of-phase T1-weighted gradient-echo pulse sequence. Although there is overlap, primary hemochromatosis is characterized by involvement of the liver but not of the spleen, whereas secondary hemochromatosis, which is often related to multiple blood transfusions, characteristically involves both liver and spleen.

- Cirrhosis is characterized pathologically by progressive parenchymal destruction, fibrosis, and development of regenerative nodules. MR shows these changes as increased heterogeneity of parenchymal signal intensity, nodularity of the liver, heterogeneous parenchymal enhancement, and reduction in liver size. Associated findings include features of portal hypertension, such as splenomegaly and ascites.

- Portal hypertension can manifest on MR as enlargement of the portal vein (>13 mm), superior mesenteric vein (>10 mm), and splenic veins (>10 mm), splenomegaly, and development of enlarged collateral vessels representing portosystemic shunts. Collateral vessels are seen as esophageal and gastric varices, splenorenal shunts, enlarged paraumbilical veins, and dilated mesenteric and retroperitoneal veins.

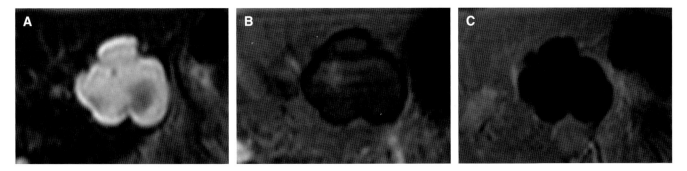

Figure 3.9 *Cyst with septations.* (**A**) T2-weighted axial image shows sharply demarcated lobular high-signal-intensity cyst in hepatic segment 2. (**B**) T1-weighted magnetization-prepared gradient-echo (MP-GRE) image at the same level demonstrates the classic appearance of cyst, iso- to hypointense to liver with black ring at the interface of liver and cyst ("bounce" artifact; see Chapter 2). By imaging alone, the lesion cannot be distinguished from biliary cystadenoma. Hemangioma could display similar high signal intensity on a T2-weighted image but would show marked low signal intensity on MP-GRE (see Fig. 3.13B). (**C**) Delayed post-gadolinium-contrast enhanced image shows no enhancement.

is frequently complicated by biliary stasis resulting in cholangitis, stones, and obstruction. It carries an increased risk of cholangiocarcinoma.

Biliary hamartomas, also known as von Meyenburg complexes, are small (always less than 15 mm and usually less than 10 mm) lesions composed of dilated bile ducts with interspersed fibrous or hyalinized stroma.[4] The origin is a malformation of the ductal plate affecting the small, peripheral, interlobular ducts. The appearance on MRI is that of innumerable tiny cysts throughout the liver. Signal intensity is near that of water, hypointense on T1-weighted images and markedly hyperintense on T2-weighted images, including heavily T2-weighted sequences of the MRCP sequence (Fig. 3.10). Contrast enhancement is absent, but there may be a thin rim of compressed enhancing liver parenchyma. The appearance overlaps considerably with that of Caroli's disease, polycystic disease, microabscesses and, most importantly, cystic or poorly vascularized metastases. In Caroli's disease, communication of cysts with the bile ducts is evident on a good-quality study. When such connections are seen, the diagnosis is made; when they are not, one must decide whether the quality of the examination is such that communications are excluded. Clinical information will help further narrow the differential considerations (e.g., Does the patient have a known malignancy? Is there evidence of autosomal dominant polycystic disease? Is there clinical suspicion for infection?).

Biliary cystadenomas and cystadenocarcinomas are rare neoplasms of biliary tract origin that appear as multiloculated hepatic cysts when they arise from the intrahepatic ducts. The wall of the cyst consists of cuboidal or columnar epithelium, and contents may be serous, mucinous, bilious, hemorrhagic, or any combination.[24] Biliary cystadenoma is considered a precursor to cystadenocarcinoma based upon the presence of rests of benign epithelium in many resected malignant cysts and in documented cases of malignant transformation.[4]

Communication with the biliary tree is occasionally present. These lesions are large, with a mean diameter of 12 cm.[24] Typical presentation is a middle-aged woman with abdominal pain, a palpable mass, elevated liver function tests, jaundice, fever, or weight loss. Smaller lesions may be asymptomatic and discovered incidentally.[24]

Interestingly, biliary cystadenomas and cystadenocarcinomas are closely related to mucinous cystic neoplasms of the ovary and pancreas. Histologically, the lesions are classified according to the presence or absence of ovarian stroma. Lesions with ovarian stroma occur almost exclusively in women and are associated with a more favorable prognosis. This distinction, however, cannot be made by imaging. On MRI, a multiloculated cystic lesion with thin septations is typical, with signal intensity varying from that of water to hemorrhagic or proteinaceous fluid (Fig. 3.11). A fluid–fluid level may be seen. The presence of nodular wall enhancement favors cystadenocarcinoma, but it can be seen with benign lesions as well. Definitive differentiation of benign from malignant cystadenoma is not possible by MRI. Treatment is excision. Aspiration and biopsy carry the risk of peritoneal spillage.

Cystic liver metastases may be seen in three situations: mucinous neoplasms of colorectal or ovarian origin; necrosis of a hypervascular tumor that "outgrows" its vascular supply; and cystic change of a treated metastasis. MR characteristics are nonspecific, with the signal intensity appearance dependent upon fluid components. Fluid–fluid levels may be seen. Walls may be imperceptible or thickened, and may enhance.

Hepatic Abscess. The liver is subject to infection and abscess formation via several pathways, including portal venous and biliary duct transit of bowel pathogens, hepatic arterial delivery of blood-borne pathogens, and direct extension of infection (as with pericholecystic abscess). Hepatic abscesses may be bacterial (pyogenic), fungal, or parasitic (amebic) in etiology, with imaging characteristics typical,

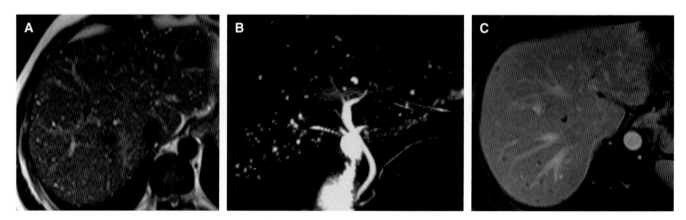

Figure 3.10 *Biliary hamartomas.* Axial T2-weighted single-shot FSE/TSE (**A**) and coronal plane (**B**) MRCP image (MIP from multislice 3D FSE/TSE) demonstrate innumerable bright tiny cysts scattered throughout the hepatic parenchyma, without identifiable communication between cysts and ducts. (**C**) The thin rim of enhancement seen on post-gadolinium-contrast-enhanced T1-weighted image likely represents adjacent compressed parenchyma. Though the differential diagnosis would include polycystic disease, this appearance is characteristic for biliary hamartomas. Both diseases are part of the spectrum of ductal plate malformations. Communication between ducts and cysts would indicate Caroli's disease. However, in Caroli's disease the cysts are characteristically more saccular and peribiliary in location. The clinical importance of identifying biliary hamartomas is in not misdiagnosing them as cystic metastases or infectious foci.

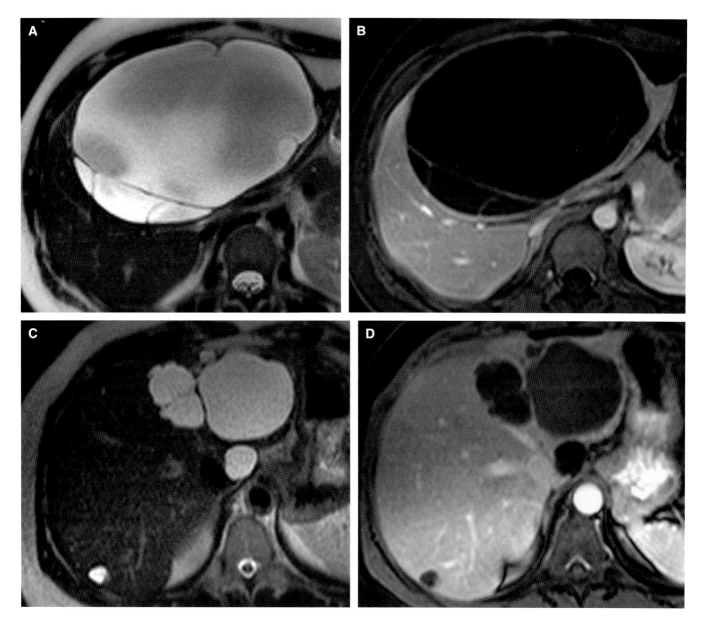

Figure 3.11 *Biliary cystadenomas.* (**A**) T2-weighted axial image depicts a large and homogeneous bright fluid-signal hepatic cyst with thin septations. (**B**) No enhancing components are seen on post-contrast-enhanced T1-weighted gradient-echo image. Benign biliary cystadenoma was confirmed at surgery. (**C**) In a different patient, T2-weighted axial image depicts multiple homogeneous, bright fluid-signal cysts in the liver, the two largest in the anterior left lobe with lobular margins and several thin septations. (**D**) Post-contrast-enhanced gradient-echo axial image demonstrates no evidence of solid or enhancing components. Note that the signal intensity varies between the cysts from black to gray, reflecting the varying fluid composition.

though not specific, for each. Pyogenic abscesses are generally fewer in number and may be quite large and complex in appearance, even mimicking necrotic masses. Amebic abscesses mimic pyogenic abscesses but the patient is usually less toxic. Fungal abscesses tend to be relatively more numerous and smaller (less than 1 cm). The appearance can be expected to change over time.

Pyogenic abscesses are most often seeded by biliary (ascending cholangitis) or gastrointestinal tract infection (diverticulitis or appendicitis). Cultures usually reveal multiple pathogens. Diabetic patients are at particular risk, as are patients with chronic cholestasis. Patients may present acutely with fever, pain, and sepsis, or with more subtle manifestations such as weight loss and laboratory abnormalities. On MR imaging, the appearance of a pyogenic abscess is variable.

Typically, the abscess has a thick wall with intense arterial-phase enhancement that persists on delayed imaging. Enhancing septa are also often present (Fig. 3.12). Perilesional edema is commonly present. The contents of the abscess may follow the signal of simple fluid (low signal intensity on T1-weighted and high signal intensity on T2-weighted images), but more often have a more complex appearance reflecting the presence of proteinaceous material, hemorrhage, and necrotic liver tissue. A non-dependent signal void on all sequences with sharp fluid interface indicates gas, which is highly suggestive of abscess. Pyogenic abscesses of biliary origin will frequently occur in clusters, which coalesce over time.[4] Prompt treatment with antibiotics and percutaneous drainage significantly reduce mortality.

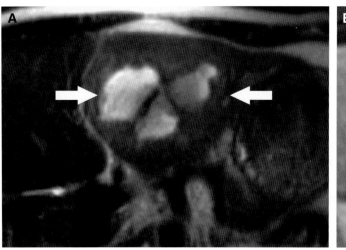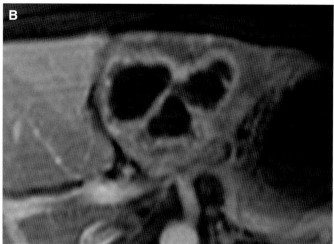

Figure 3.12 *Pyogenic abscess.* 45-year-old man presenting with 2 days of fever and right upper quadrant pain. (**A**) Axial T2-weighted single-shot FSE/TSE image shows a large mass (between *arrows*) in the left lobe with central loculated fluid signal. (**B**) Post-gadolinium-contrast-enhanced axial T1-weighted image demonstrates marked enhancement of the walls. Drainage yielded pus; microbiology confirmed pyogenic abscess.

Amebic abscess occurs in a minority of patients with amebic colitis. Patients present acutely with right upper quadrant pain, fever, leukocytosis, and elevated liver function tests. In endemic areas the causative parasite *Entamoeba histolytica* colonizes the large intestine and gains access to the liver through the portal venous system. The MR appearance of amebic abscess is similar to that of pyogenic abscess, and differentiation is not possible by imaging alone. Concomitant perihepatic ascites, right pleural effusion, intestinal involvement, and contiguous retroperitoneal extension are commonly seen in amebic disease and suggest the diagnosis in the proper clinical context. In contrast to pyogenic abscess, amebic abscesses respond well to antimicrobial therapy alone.[25]

Fungal abscesses of the liver occur in the liver of neutropenic patients and generally also involve the spleen. Typically, the imaging presentation is that of multiple tiny lesions in a cancer patient with a recent course of chemotherapy or recent bone marrow transplantation whose neutrophil count has just started to recover. Fungi from the bowel (most commonly *Candida albicans*) gain access to the bloodstream via breaches in the damaged intestinal mucosa and deposit in the liver and spleen, where they are walled off by the rebounding population of neutrophils. The immune response mounted is ultimately insufficient to eradicate the fungus. The clinical presentation is more insidious than occurs in pyogenic abscess, with persistent fevers despite broad-spectrum antibiotic coverage often the only clue. The MRI appearance is characteristic in the proper clinical setting. Multiple tiny (less than 1 cm) hepatic and splenic lesions will be seen that are hypointense on T1-weighted images and hyperintense to spleen on T2-weighted images, though not as high in signal intensity as water.[4] Many patients will have received red blood cell transfusions on a chronic basis. The resultant transfusional iron overload can aid detection by increasing the conspicuity of the lesions on T2-weighted images relative to the low-signal-intensity spleen and liver. On dynamic contrast-enhanced images, the lesions remain hypointense against the background of enhancing liver and spleen parenchyma. Perilesional rim enhancement may be seen due to inflammatory infiltrate and compressed parenchyma. Differential diagnosis can be effectively managed in most cases based on clinical data and splenic involvement.

Hepatic mycobacterial infection, caused by *M. tuberculosis* or *M. avium-intracellulare*, has various manifestations. The bacilli reach the liver through the portal vein, hepatic artery, or lymphatics. *Hepatic tuberculosis* may present as a localized tuberculoma or abscess, or as numerous small nodules throughout the parenchyma. The latter appearance is seen both in the miliary form of infection and in granulomatous hepatitis. The findings are nonspecific. Differential diagnosis for tuberculoma includes pyogenic abscess and necrotic primary and metastatic malignancies. Differential diagnosis for miliary disease includes sarcoidosis, lymphoma, microabscesses, and metastatic disease.[4]

Hydatid disease results from infection by the tapeworm *Echinococcus granulosus* or *E. multilocularis*. *E. granulosus* infection is much more common and produces a unilocular hydatid cyst. This parasite is endemic in sheep-grazing areas of the world, with humans becoming infected through contact with dogs (the definitive host), sheep (the intermediate host), or infected water. Eggs pass through the bowel wall and reach the liver via the portal venous system. The hydatid cyst consists of three distinct layers—from outer to inner, the pericyst (a thick fibrous layer formed by compressed and modified liver), the ectocyst (a thin acellular membrane that allows nutrients to pass), and the inner endocyst (a germinal layer that produces the scolices).[4] The endocyst also may invaginate, producing characteristic daughter cysts within the mother cyst, a finding that aids in diagnosis. Typical MR appearance is that of a dominant cyst displaying low signal intensity on T1-weighted and high signal intensity on T2-weighted images, with multiple internal daughter cysts, which are slightly less bright on T2-weighted images. The cyst wall may enhance after contrast material administration; however, lack of enhancement should not raise doubt as to the diagnosis. Calcification may be present but is better appreciated on CT. Extensive calcification is usually indicative of death of the parasite.[26] Infected persons may remain asymptomatic for years and come to clinical attention when the cysts rupture or become infected. Although traditionally treated with meticulous surgical resection to reduce the risk of peritoneal spillage, good results are now routinely achieved with combined percutaneous drainage and antimicrobial therapy.[26]

The much less common form of hydatid liver disease, alveolar echinococcal disease, is caused by *E. multilocularis*. A distinct imaging appearance is that of multiple small cysts associated with solid enhancing nodules, which may coalesce into a mass.[26]

Evolving hematomas may appear cystic depending on the stage of breakdown of blood products. Uncommonly, ***pancreatic pseudocysts*** and ***bilomas*** may be (or appear to be) intrahepatic. The MR appearance is nonspecific and images need to be interpreted in clinical context.

BENIGN LIVER LESIONS

Cavernous hemangioma is the most commonly encountered solid benign tumor of the liver. Generally an incidental discovery on imaging studies, most are small and asymptomatic. The tumor consists of blood-filled spaces lined by endothelium on a thin fibrous stroma.[4] It is sharply demarcated from the surrounding liver parenchyma. Most measure less than 5 cm and remain stable in size, although growth has been documented over serial examinations.

Hemangiomas have quite characteristic features on MRI that reflect their internal structure, with round to lobular margins sharply defined against the surrounding liver parenchyma (Figs. 3.13 and 3.14). The tumor shows homogeneous, hypointense signal compared to liver on T1-weighted images and is hyperintense to both liver and spleen on T2-weighted images. The signal intensity on T2-weighted images increases in proportion to the volume of the vascular space within the hemangioma[4] and will be iso-intense to mildly hyperintense to fat on single-shot or multislice fast/turbo spin-echo pulse sequences, approaching the signal of water. This characteristic T2 prolongation can be accentuated by using long TEs on heavily T2-weighted sequences, which can further aid in differentiating hemangiomas from metastases, the majority of which show only mildly increased signal compared to liver. One should be mindful, however, that hypervascular metastases may also be quite bright on T2-weighted images for similar structural reasons. Giant hemangiomas (more than 6 cm in size) may display heterogeneous signal intensity due to thrombosis, hemorrhage, liquefaction, fibrosis, or myxoid degeneration.

Dynamic contrast-enhanced T1-weighted imaging features may be diagnostic on MR, as with multiphasic CT. Three enhancement patterns are described. The most common pattern is clumped nodular, discontinuous, peripheral enhancement that fills centripetally over time, reaching homogeneous signal hyperintensity by the delayed phase from the pooled contrast-enhanced blood. The second pattern is nodular peripheral enhancement with centripetal progression over time but with a persistent central hypointense scar, typically seen in large hemangiomas. The third pattern is the so-called "flash filling" hemangiomas with immediate uniform enhancement, typically seen in smal tumors.

One must be wary of calling all lesions demonstrating nodular peripheral enhancement with gradual centripetal filling hemangiomas, as hypervascular metastases and some primary tumors may also behave in this fashion. A helpful point

---

Box 3.3 ESSENTIALS TO REMEMBER

- Simple hepatic cysts are common, often multiple, and contain serous fluid, which displays low signal intensity on T1-weighted images and very high signal intensity on T2-weighted images. The cyst wall is imperceptibly thin. Uniformly thin septations are often present. Neither the cyst wall nor septa show contrast enhancement.

- Biliary cystadenomas are uncommon cystic neoplasms that are precursors to biliary cystadenocarcinomas. Multiple septations, nodular cyst wall, and enhancement of septa or cyst wall differentiate the lesions from simple hepatic cysts. Fluid is more often proteinaceous, which may cause increased signal intensity on T1-weighted images.

- Cystic liver metastases are characterized by proteinaceous fluid, internal debris, fluid–fluid layers, and nodular thickened walls with enhancement. Some lesions overlap the appearance of benign hepatic cysts and biliary cystadenomas. Cystic liver metastases can be differentiated by clinical history and growth on serial imaging.

- Biliary hamartomas are congenitally malformed bile ducts with focal cystic dilatation. Characteristic MR appearance is a myriad of tiny cystic lesions, low in signal intensity on T1-weighted images and very high in signal intensity on T2-weighted images. Lesions may demonstrate thin rim enhancement on early post-gadolinium-enhanced images that persists on late contrast-enhanced images.

- Hepatic abscesses vary in cause and appearance. Most appear as complex fluid-containing lesions with varying signal intensity on T1- and T2-weighted images, and usually an enhancing wall. Abscesses are further diagnosed by clinical history and ultimately by aspiration.

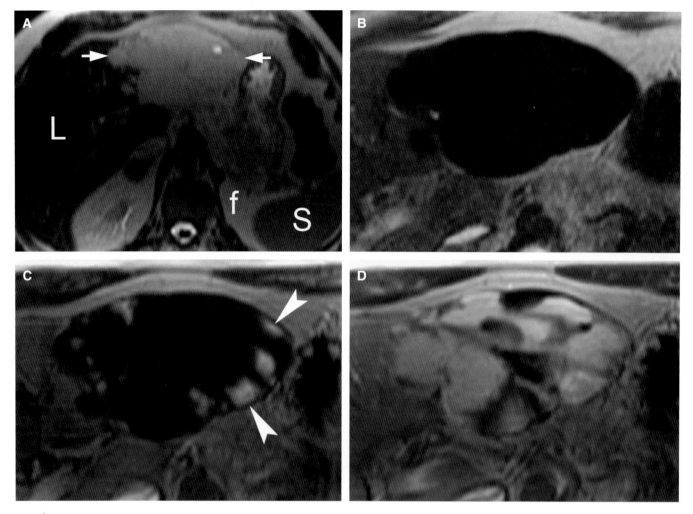

Figure 3.13 *Hemangioma, classic.* Large hemangioma occupying the lateral segments of the left lobe. (**A**) Axial T2-weighted single-shot FSE/TSE image reveals the typical appearance of cavernous hemangioma (*arrows*): lobular, well demarcated, and homogeneously hyperintense relative to liver (*L*). Note that the signal intensity is higher than that of the spleen (*S*) and similar to that of fat (*f*). (**B**) On axial T1-weighted magnetization-prepared gradient-echo image, the hemangioma is characteristically markedly hypointense, approaching signal void (note the difference in appearance compared to that of the cyst in Fig. 3.9B). Hepatic arterial phase (**C**) and 5-minute delayed phase (**D**) post-gadolinium-enhanced gradient-echo images depict characteristic discontinuous, nodular, clumped peripheral enhancement (*arrowheads*) (**C**) and gradual centripetal fill-in with iso-intensity to blood pool (**D**). Note that the enhancing components respect the margins of the lesion as established on pre-contrast enhanced images.

to remember is that once a hemangioma fills with contrast material it should remain iso-intense to the blood pool through all delayed imaging. Never give the benefit of the doubt to a lesion that demonstrates washout on the interstitial phase, no matter how much it looks like a hemangioma otherwise. A second helpful tip to avoid mislabeling a hypervascular malignancy as a hemangioma is to make sure that the nodular, discontinuous peripheral enhancement respects the margins of the lesion established on pre-contrast-enhanced imaging: a hemangioma should not "grow" beyond its borders with further enhancement. Its border with the liver is sharply defined and is never infiltrative. This is not to be confused with the peritumoral enhancement occasionally seen surrounding hemangiomas. This effect has been shown to result from arterioportal shunting in at least some cases, and more often occurs with the small flash-filling variety of hemangiomas.[4]

Finally, "atypical" hemangiomas have been described, though they are not common. These are nonspecific by MRI

(as well as by other imaging modalities) and would be included in an MR report only as one of several possibilities in a differential diagnosis. These varieties include hyalinized or sclerosed hemangiomas, which, as the name implies, are largely thrombosed and fibrosed, presumably resulting from involution of a typical hemangioma. On dynamic T1-weighted post-contrast-enhanced images hyalinized hemangiomas will not demonstrate early enhancement, though they may gradually accumulate contrast material through delayed images. Regardless, these lesions, when seen, cannot be differentiated from hypovascular metastases, so follow-up imaging or perhaps biopsy is necessary.[27]

Focal nodular hyperplasia (FNH) is the second most commonly encountered benign liver tumor after hemangioma (Fig. 3.15).[4] Most are asymptomatic and incidentally discovered, but larger lesions may come to clinical attention as a result of their mass effect. Unlike adenoma, spontaneous hemorrhage is not a complication. FNH is most commonly

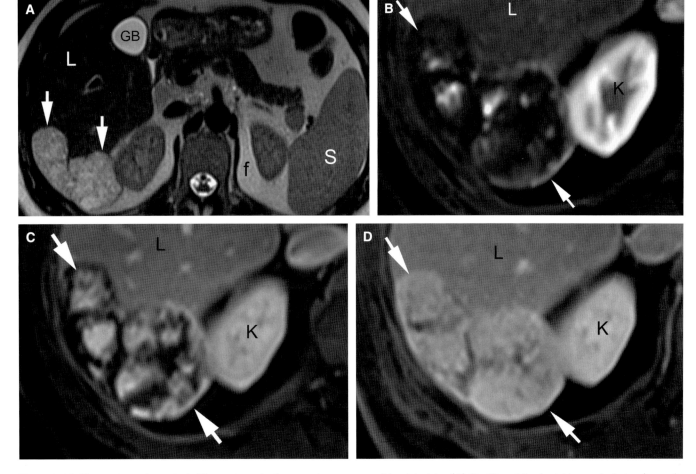

Figure 3.14 *Hemangioma, less typical.* Hemangioma in the posterior segments of the right lobe. (**A**) On T2-weighted axial image the lesion (*arrows*) is not as bright as fluid in the gallbladder (*GB*) but is hyperintense to both spleen (*S*) and liver (*L*) and is iso-intense to fat (*f*). Hepatic arterial phase (**B**) and portal venous phase (**C**) post-gadolinium-contrast enhanced gradient-echo images reveal clumped puddles of enhancement seen initially within the central portion of the lesion (*arrows*), somewhat unusual for hemangioma. (**D**) Persistent enhancement similar to that of the blood pool on the 5-minute-delayed image confirms the diagnosis. *L*, liver. *K*, right kidney.

detected in women of childbearing age, a demographic factor that along with its hypervascular nature leads to its being mistaken for hepatic adenoma. It can also be seen in men and children.[28] Malignant transformation is not known to occur.

FNH is believed to represent a hyperplastic response of the hepatic parenchyma to a preexisting arterial malformation.[28] Hyperplastic hepatocytes, small bile ductules, and Kupffer cells are present surrounding a central fibrous scar, which is considered the hallmark of the lesion, though the central scar is not specific to FNH. In contrast to adenomas, oral contraceptives do not cause FNH. However, there is some conflicting evidence that oral contraceptives may fuel growth of existing lesions.[28]

FNH is almost always solitary, with mean lesion size of 5 cm. Growth occurs in proportion to the tumor's vascular supply.[28] Hemorrhage and necrosis are rare, as is intralesional fat. The MRI features of FNH are those of mass with near iso-intensity to liver on both T1-weighted images (iso-intense to minimally hypointense) and T2-weighted images (iso-intense to minimally hyperintense). The lesions may be easily overlooked without contrast material administration

(Figs. 3.16 and 3.17). When the central scar is visible (reported 75% of lesions), it appears as a central focus that is hypointense to the lesion on T1-weighted images and hyperintense to the lesion on T2-weighted images. The signal characteristics of the scar are the result of the presence of blood vessels, bile ductules, and edema within myxomatous tissue.[4] FNH has no capsule.

On dynamic contrast-enhanced images, FNH demonstrates marked homogeneous enhancement in the arterial phase, becoming isointense by the portal venous phase. Typically, some contrast material is retained through the interstitial phase, so the lesion remains slightly hyperintense to liver on delayed imaging. The central scar is hypointense initially but gradually becomes hyperintense to the lesion on the delayed phase.

Atypical MR findings in FNH include pronounced hyperintensity of the lesion on both T1- and T2-weighted images, hypointensity of the scar on T2-weighted images, absence of enhancement of the scar, and a perceived capsule. It is important to always be conscious of the effect that the surrounding hepatic parenchyma has on the appearance of a liver lesion, as signal intensity features are relative rather than absolute.

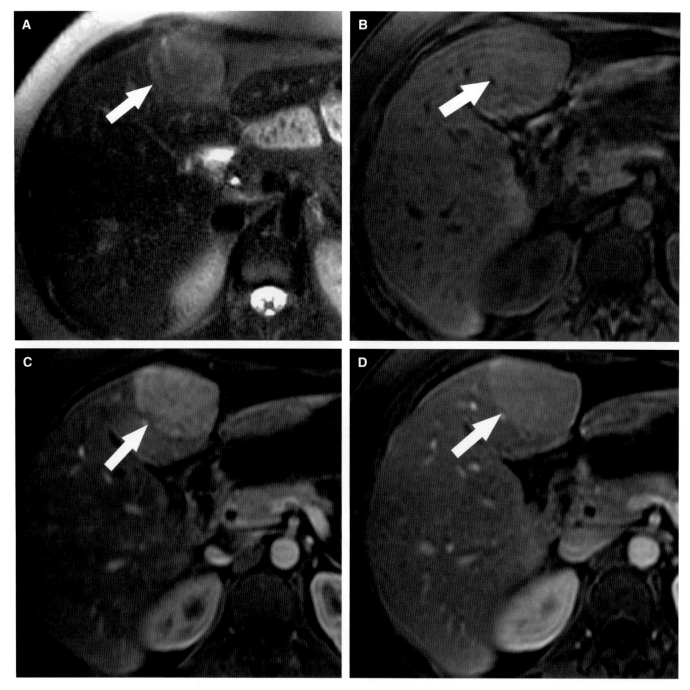

Figure 3.15 *Hepatic adenoma.* (**A**) A hepatic adenoma (*arrow*) displays heterogeneous, slightly hyperintense signal intensity on T2-weighted single-shot FSE/TSE axial image. **B.** On T1-weighted gradient-echo pre-contrast enhanced image with fat saturation, the lesion (*arrow*) is iso-intense to liver. The signal intensity of adenomas is quite variable on both T1- and T2-weighted images, reflecting various components such as fat, hemorrhage, and cystic change. Post-gadolinium-contrast-enhanced images tend to be more predictable. (**C**) Prominent hepatic arterial supply results in the appearance of a hypervascular lesion (*arrow*) on early post-contrast image. (**D**) Adenomas tend to retain gadolinium-based contrast material longer than focal nodular hyperplasia because of leakage into the interstitial spaces. This adenoma (*arrow*) remains relatively bright on the delayed venous phase post-contrast enhanced image. Although the persistent enhancement could suggest the diagnosis of hemangioma, the T2-weighted images allow confident distinction.

In cases with equivocal lesion behavior, a gadolinium-based compound with hepatocyte-specific characteristics (such as Gd-ethoxybenzyl diethylenetriame pentaacetic acid [Primovist®] or gadoxetate disodium [Eovist®]) may be of use. With these contrast agents, FNH will be iso- to hyperintense to liver on 1- to 3-hour delayed images in 96% of cases. This finding differentiates FNH from adenomas, which are hypointense at 1 to 3 hours.[3]

Hepatocellular adenoma is a benign neoplasm of the liver strongly associated with the use of oral contraceptives. Growth of adenomas is driven by both the estrogen dose and duration of use.[29] Individuals using anabolic/androgenic steroids and patients with glycogen storage diseases are also at increased risk. Most adenomas are discovered incidentally, but a only a minority comes to clinical attention because of abdominal pain, a palpable mass, or abnormal liver function tests.

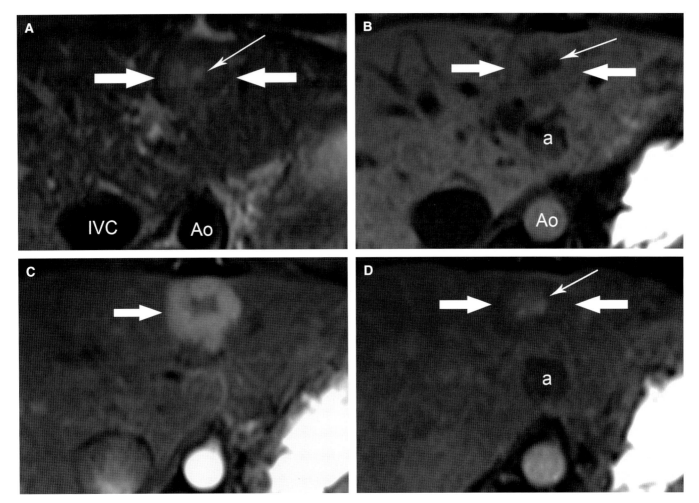

Figure 3.16 *Focal nodular hyperplasia.* MR show sclassic features of a small focal nodular hyperplasia discovered incidentally in 21-year-old female college student. The lesion (*fat arrows*) is iso-intense to surrounding liver parenchyma on unenhanced T2-weighted (**A**) and unenhanced fat-suppressed T1-weighted gradient-echo (**B**) images, reflecting the similarity of the lesion to normal liver. The small central scar (*skinny arrow*) is relatively bright on the T2-weighted and dark on T1-weighted images, characteristic of FNH. However, this finding can be seen in malignant lesions as well. (**C**) The vascular nature of the FNH (*fat arrow*) is revealed on a hepatic arterial phase post-gadolinium-enhanced gradient-echo image, with intense, immediate, and uniform enhancement. (**D**) The late-enhancing central scar (*skinny arrow*) is the dominant feature on the 5-minute-delayed contrast-enhanced image, with the remainder of the lesion (*fat arrows*) washing out to near-liver intensity. *IVC*, inferior vena cava. *Ao*, aorta. *a*, artifact from the aorta.

Hepatic adenomas are vascular lesions composed of benign hepatocytes arranged in large plates or cords separated by dilated sinusoids, without normal acinar architecture. Kupffer cells may be present but are usually nonfunctioning (in contrast to FNH). Bile ducts are notably absent. Adenomas contain intracellular glycogen and lipid, which can be detected with MRI, a feature helpful in making the diagnosis. A fibrous capsule or a pseudocapsule composed of compressed parenchyma may be seen.[29] The importance of identifying hepatic adenomas is related to the propensity of the lesions to hemorrhage, as well as the much rarer possibility of malignant transformation.[29] Hemorrhage is believed to result from infarction as the tumor outgrows its vascular supply.

The imaging characteristics of adenomas have considerable overlap with other benign and malignant vascular lesions of the liver, making the diagnosis challenging. Certainly the presence of known risk factors such as oral contraceptive use can aid in making the diagnosis. Larger lesions are typically quite heterogeneous, reflecting varying degrees of intralesional

hemorrhage, fat, necrosis, fibrosis, and vascularity. On T1-weighted images, adenomas will have portions that are both iso- and hyperintense to liver, which is to be expected given the tumor's hepatocellular origin (see Fig. 3.15). Additionally, areas of fat and hemorrhage within the lesion will be brighter still. On T2-weighted images, heterogeneity is expected due to hemorrhage and necrosis, with the lesion being hyperintense to liver. Intratumoral fat can be confirmed by demonstration of chemical-shift artifact on T1-weighted GRE opposed-phase images, or with fat suppression. On dynamic gadolinium-contrast-enhanced images adenomas will enhance heterogeneously in the arterial phase, though to a lesser degree than FNH. Some washout of contrast material is expected in the delayed phase, another feature helpful in discriminating from FNH. As contrast material washes out of the tumor, the fibrous capsule or pseudocapsule may be revealed.[4]

A lesion with the imaging findings described here, discovered in a woman using oral contraceptives, can be called a hepatic adenoma with a high degree of confidence. However,

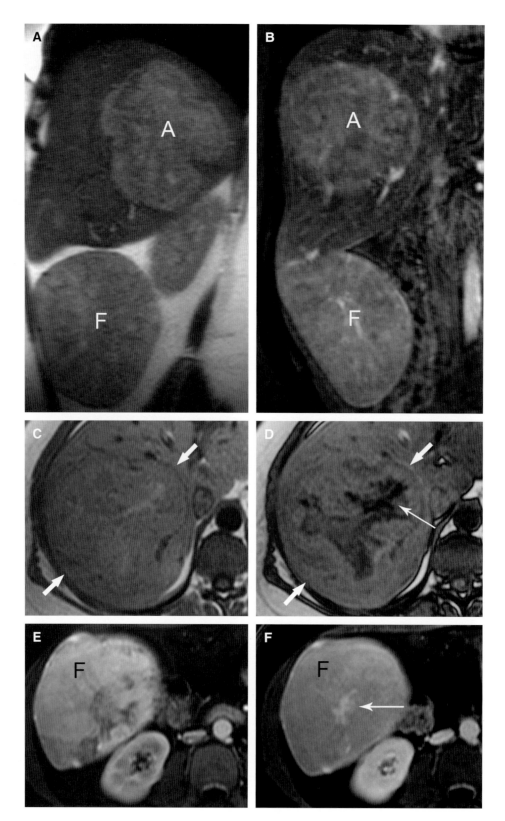

Figure 3.17 *Adenoma and focal nodular hyperplasia.* T2-weighted sagittal image (**A**) and coronal gadolinium-contrast-enhanced MRA obtained in the hepatic venous phase (**B**) demonstrate two large masses (*A, F*) in the right lobe of the liver, similar in size and appearance at first glance but with important differences on MRI. Both masses are heterogeneously and mildly hyperintense to liver parenchyma on T2-weighted images (**A**), and both enhance heterogeneously (**B**). Note that the intervening parenchyma is normal, with no evidence of cirrhosis. Axial in-phase (**C**) and out-of-phase (**D**) images through the more cephalad mass (between *fat arrows*) show an irregular central area of signal dropout (*skinny arrow* in image **D**), confirming the presence of fat and suggesting the diagnosis of hepatic adenoma. Hepatocellular carcinoma may contain fat as well and would still be a consideration. FNH virtually never contains fat. Axial T1-weighted gadolinium-enhanced images through the exophytic inferior mass (*F*) acquired in the hepatic arterial (**E**) and delayed venous (**F**) phases reveal a late-enhancing central scar (*skinny arrow* in image **F**) that corresponds to a mildly hyperintense region on the T2-weighted image shown in A. This appearance is characteristic (though not specific) of FNH. The right lobe was resected, with pathologic confirmation that the more cephalad mass (*A*) was hepatic adenoma and the more caudad mass (*F*) was FNH.

many smaller lesions may be relatively homogeneous without confirmed lipid, and thus in these cases the diagnosis will be equivocal. If the other consideration is FNH, it may be acceptable to simply monitor the lesion with follow-up imaging. In the setting of chronic liver disease this becomes more problematic as adenoma and hepatocellular carcinoma may have an identical appearance. Correlation with serum alpha-fetoprotein can be helpful.

Management depends upon the size of the lesion and coexisting factors. Most adenomas are between 3 and 5 cm in size, but they can be much larger. A lesion less than 5 cm in a patient with normal serum alpha-fetoprotein can be managed by cessation of oral contraceptives, with resolution of the lesion expected but not certain. Resolution of the lesion, however, does not nullify the risk of transformation to hepatocellular carcinoma, as liver cell dysplasia is an irreversible event.[29] In some cases, adenomas may be multiple. When more than three lesions are present, a patient can be said to have *liver adenomatosis*, which can be further divided into multifocal and massive subsets. Most of the lesions in adenomatosis are not estrogen-dependent. Surgical resection or even transplantation may be indicated in adenomatosis.

Differential diagnosis of hepatic adenoma includes FNH, hepatocellular carcinoma, hemangioma (generally included only when small), and solitary hypervascular metastasis.

PRIMARY HEPATIC MALIGNANCY

Hepatocellular carcinoma (HCC) most commonly develops as the end result of progressive dysplasia in the setting of cirrhosis. Incidence and prevalence vary regionally, but in some areas, such as Southeast Asia and tropical Africa, HCC is among the most common malignancies encountered. In the Western world, HCC is less prevalent, but the incidence continues to rise along with infection rates of hepatitis B and C. Additional risk factors include exposure to aflatoxins and alcohol abuse. Metabolic disorders such as genetic hemochromatosis, Wilson's disease, and glycogen storage diseases are also associated with an increased risk. Men are disproportionately affected. Although cases of HCC developing in non-cirrhotic livers occur, these are rare and tend to occur in association with nonspecific hepatocellular injury, including steatosis, hepatitis, NASH, and inflammation.[4]

As a regenerative nodule undergoes progressive dysplasia, a hemodynamic shift occurs resulting in a decrease in blood supply from the portal vein and a gradual compensatory increase in blood arriving via the hepatic artery. The net result of this alteration is that the lesion becomes increasingly hypervascular as dictated by this altered blood supply, enhancing in the arterial phase and washing out in the venous phase. Though differentiation of small (less than 2 cm) lesions can be very difficult and sometimes impossible, a lesion that enhances homogeneously in the arterial phase, becomes iso- to slightly hypointense in the portal venous phase and then hypointense in the delayed interstitial phase is highly concerning for HCC. Neither regenerative nor dysplastic nodules typically display this behavior.

On T1-weighted images HCC may be hypo-, iso-, or hyperintense to liver, depending on its internal components (Figs. 3.18 and 3.19). T1 prolongation in HCC can be due to the presence of lipid, glycogen, or copper, and is most

---

Box 3.4 ESSENTIALS TO REMEMBER

- Cavernous hemangiomas are common, benign, variable in size, and often multiple. The lesions are sharply demarcated from surrounding parenchyma and consist of a network of blood-filled spaces through which blood slowly flows. Because of the slow blood flow, hemangiomas are prone to central thrombosis. Chronic thrombi become fibrotic. Imaging findings reflect the nature of the lesion, displaying low signal on T1-weighted and high signal intensity on T2-weighted images. MPGRE sequences with image parameters set to null the signal from hemangioma show the lesions as signal voids. Dynamic post-contrast-enhanced T1-weighted sequences show discontinuous nodular enhancement at the periphery. In most cases delayed images show complete uniform contrast enhancement. If the lesion has foci of fibrosis resulting from chronic thrombosis, the fibrotic portions will not enhance. Atypical lesions may not be definitively characterized by MR as hemangioma and may require follow-up or additional imaging.

- Focal nodular hyperplasia (FNH) is a benign tumor containing hepatocytes, reticuloendothelial (Kupffer) cells, and malformed bile ducts. Because the tissue makeup is similar to that of normal liver parenchyma, FNH follows closely the signal characteristics of normal hepatic tissue on unenhanced T1-and T2-weighted MR sequences. Early dynamic gadolinium contrast-enhanced T1-weighted sequences reveal characteristic avid uniform enhancement of the lesions with rapid contrast washout to become iso-intense to liver parenchyma on later enhanced images. The stellate central scar, if present, shows no enhancement on early post-contrast-enhanced images but characteristically enhances on delayed images.

- Hepatic adenoma is a benign lesion that is a precursor to hepatocellular carcinoma. Similar to FNH, adenoma contains hepatocytes; however, there is a reduced number or absence of Kupffer cells, and there are no bile ducts. The lesion characteristically occurs in women using oral contraceptives. While there is considerable overlap with other benign and malignant lesions, several characteristic MR features suggest the diagnosis. Adenomas may contain intracellular fat, detected on MR by chemical-shift imaging revealing a distinct drop in signal intensity on out-of-phase compared to in-phase gradient-echo images. On dynamic contrast-enhanced images adenomas usually show moderate heterogeneous enhancement on early images. Enhancement is occasionally as intense as that seen with FNH.

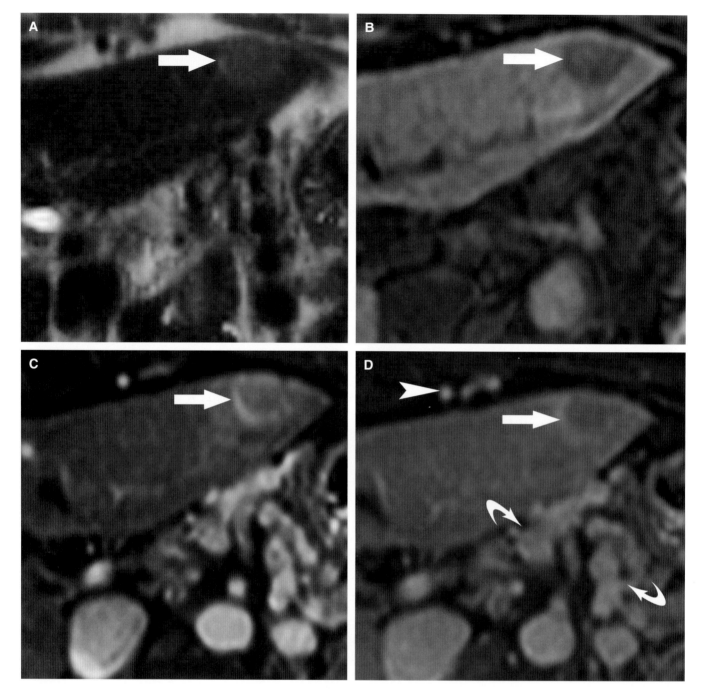

Figure 3.18 *Hepatocellular carcinoma, small.* (**A**) Axial T2-weighted image reveals typical mildly hyperintense lesion (*arrow*) in the left lobe. T1-weighted pre-contrast (**B**), arterial (**C**), and portal venous phase (**D**) post-gadolinium-enhanced images demonstrate the peripheral early arterial enhancement and rapid washout classic for hepatocellular carcinoma (*straight arrows*). Paraumbilical (*arrowhead*) and perigastric (*curved arrows*) portosystemic collateral vessels are also evident in this patient with cirrhosis.

commonly seen in lesions less than 3 cm.[4] Lesions less than 1.5 cm are usually iso-intense on T1-weighted images. T2 prolongation is mild relative to normal liver, but T2-weighted images can be quite useful in the triage of small lesions in cirrhosis. A hyperenhancing lesion that is iso-intense to spleen on T2-weighted images is highly concerning for HCC.

HCC has a characteristic fibrous capsule, or a pseudocapsule of compressed parenchyma, that may be seen on both unenhanced and enhanced imaging. The fibrous capsule is typically thin and discontinuous, becoming more conspicuous in tumors of large size. The fibrous capsule is usually hypointense on T1- and T2-weighted images and shows delayed enhancement. Tumor invasion through the capsule is seen as a protruding nodule or as satellite nodules. Multifocal HCC is relatively common.[2] Given our understanding of the pathway of hepatocarcinogenesis and the volume of cirrhotic liver at risk, this is not surprising. A second pathway to multifocal HCC is by spread of tumor via venous invasion.

The portal vein is frequently invaded by HCC, resulting in tumor thrombus. Less frequently, the tumor enters the hepatic

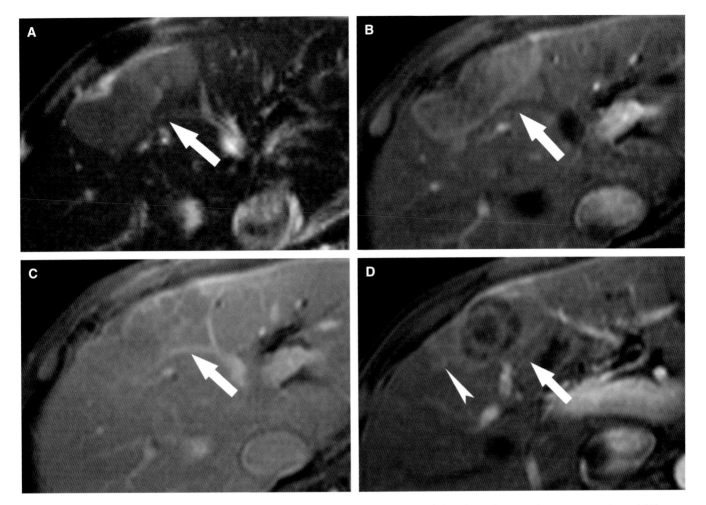

Figure 3.19 *Hepatocellular carcinoma with satellite nodule.* Axial T2-weighted (**A**), arterial (**B**), and portal venous phase contrast-enhanced (**C**) images through a lesion (*arrows*) in the right lobe reveal classic mildly increased signal on T2-weighted image, and early arterial enhancement and rapid washout relative to surrounding parenchyma. (**D**) Arterial phase image at the inferior margin of the dominant mass depicts a hypervascular satellite lesion (*arrowhead*).

veins, with direct access to the right heart. Dynamic, contrast-enhanced images are extremely valuable, allowing detection of bland thrombus and tumor thrombus based on enhancement characteristics already discussed.

HCC will eventually develop in the cirrhotic liver, with a stepwise progression of dysplasia from regenerative nodule to low-grade and then high-grade dysplastic nodule and finally to HCC. The challenge is to differentiate these steps in hepatocarcinogenesis to optimize management, using (radiofrequency) tumor ablation, chemoembolization, surgical resection, and ultimately transplantation as indicated. Large tumors are easily recognized; it is the small lesions (less than 2 cm) that are difficult to detect. MRI offers a decided advantage over CT in that it not only examines the vascularity of the lesion but also allows lesion characterization based on intrinsic tissue contrast based on T1 and T2 relaxation.

Regenerative nodules represent the more normal parenchyma in the cirrhotic liver and should not be mistaken for HCC.[1] They are usually less than 1 cm in diameter and are outlined by fibrous bands. On MRI, regenerative nodules are iso-intense to liver on T1-weighted images and on T2-weighted images and are generally inconspicuous on dynamic contrast-enhanced

images since they receive their blood supply from the portal vein.[4] Siderotic regenerative containing iron is characteristically hypointense on gradient-echo images due to magnetic susceptibility effect (see Fig. 3.8).

Dysplastic nodules become more similar to HCC as they become progressively more dysplastic with increasing recruitment of the hepatic artery. Dysplastic nodules are generally slightly hyperintense compared to surrounding liver on T1-weighted images, though their appearance is variable. T2-weighted images can be quite helpful. Dysplastic nodules are characteristically hypointense on T2-weighted images in contrast to the mild but definite hyperintensity of HCC. The "nodule within a nodule" appearance has been used to describe a focus of HCC developing in a dysplastic nodule. This appears on T2-weighted images as a hyperintense nodule (the HCC) within a larger hypointense nodule (the dysplastic nodule).[4] Clinically the distinction between a high-grade dysplastic nodule and a well-differentiated HCC has little relevance as both lesions are managed identically.

Hypervascular metastases tend to be hypointense on T1-weighted images, which can be helpful, although hemorrhage within the lesion will result in T1 shortening. More useful are T2-weighted images, with hypervascular metastases characteristically appearing quite hyperintense and easily distinguishable from the subtle hyperintensity of HCC.[2] On dynamic arterial-phase contrast-enhanced images there may be a peripheral homogeneous, or heterogeneously appearing rim. On delayed images obtained 0.3 to 3.0 hours after administration of Gd-based hepatocyte-specific compounds, metastases are hypointense relative to liver or demonstrate "target" appearance, regardless of whether they are characterized as hyper- or hypovascular (see Fig. 3.1). Hypervascular metastases include neuroendocrine (islet cell, pheochromocytoma, carcinoid), renal cell, thyroid, choriocarcinoma, melanoma, and sarcoma sources.[2]

Benign hypervascular lesions including hepatic adenoma, FNH, and hemangiomas have been previously discussed. Small flash-filling hemangiomas can be indistinguishable from HCCs on arterial phase, but are differentiated on 5-minute delayed phase contrast-enhanced images. The hemangioma will remain similar in intensity to the blood pool while the other HCC will typically, at least partially, wash out. Additionally, T1-weighted MP-GRE pulse sequences can be helpful. Parameters may be set so that hemangiomas will be maximally nulled and thus showing marked low signal intensity. HCC and metastasis show intermediate decreased signal intensity compared to surrounding liver.

Pseudolesions: The term *transient hepatic intensity difference* (THID) describes a non-tumorous region of enhancement, seen only in the arterial phase (Fig. 3.20). These are typically small, peripheral, wedge-shaped, and without mass effect, and are the result of arterioportal shunts or distal portal vein obstruction resulting in increased arterial supply.[2] When small, the appearance may not be definitive with respect to the nature of the finding, necessitating follow-up imaging to exclude a well-differentiated HCC.

Another potential source of confusion is the decreased portal venous-phase enhancement seen with *third inflow*, when systemic veins empty into hepatic sinusoids, causing altered venous inflow and drainage. In some instances focal flow is altered sufficiently to mimic a lesion. The predictable location of third inflow, near the gallbladder fossa, adjacent to the falciform ligament, and in the porta hepatis, suggests this etiology. Like THIDs, third-flow lesions show no mass effect. Focal fat deposition and focal fatty sparing also occur at the common sites for third inflow.[10]

Confluent fibrosis appears mildly hyperintense on T2-weighted images with slight enhancement in the arterial phase, features that can create the appearance of a lesion. The presence of parenchymal atrophy with capsular retraction and persistence of enhancement on delayed-phase contrast-enhanced images argue against HCC. In these cases, one must instead be wary of cholangiocarcinoma and look for dilated ducts converging on a apical mass.

Fibrolamellar hepatocellular carcinoma, an exceedingly rare and distinct variant of HCC, arises in younger individuals without underlying liver disease. Men and women are affected equally, with clinical presentation usually in the second to

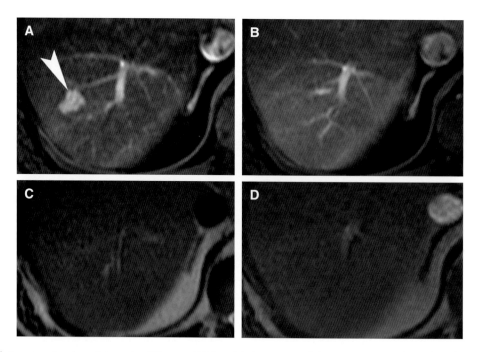

Figure 3.20 *Pseudolesions: transient hepatic intensity difference.* (**A**) Arterial phase post-gadolinium-contrast-enhanced gradient-echo image demonstrates well-defined, homogeneously enhancing focus (*arrowhead*) in the right lobe. This becomes iso-intense to liver parenchyma on subsequent dynamic post-gadolinium-enhanced image (**B**) and is not visible on either T2-weighted (**C**) or T1-weighted magnetization-prepared gradient-echo image (**D**). While not entirely conclusive, a hypervascular "lesion" that is seen on the arterial phase and not on any other sequences is suggestive of transient hepatic intensity difference (THID), a simple vascular flow phenomenon. The enhancement was intermittently seen on contrast-enhanced MRI examinations over years, without change. Benign hypervascular lesions such as FNH, hemangioma, and adenoma are considerations, but each of these lesions should be also visible on the other sequences.

third decade. As the tumor is usually large and infiltrative when discovered (reported mean diameter of 13 cm), presenting signs and symptoms are often due to mass effect and include pain and a palpable abdominal mass. In contrast to conventional HCC, serum alpha-fetoprotein is usually normal.[30]

Pathologically the tumor consists of malignant hepatocytes separated by fibrous sheets, with the capsule of conventional HCC notably absent.[30] Internally, hemorrhage and necrosis are often present, resulting in a heterogeneous appearance by MR. The presence of lipid has not been reported. A central fibrous scar is a common feature.[30]

The MRI appearance reflects the underlying tumoral architecture. On T1-weighted images the tumor is relatively hypointense to liver. On T2-weighted images it is markedly heterogeneous and hyperintense (Fig. 3.21). The central scar is hypointense on both T1- and T2-weighted images, differentiating it from the hyperintense scar of FNH seen on T2-weighted images. Enhancement is pronounced and heterogeneous in the arterial and portal venous phases, becoming homogeneous in delayed phases. The scar typically does not enhance and is thus best seen against the background of homogeneous tumor enhancement in the delayed venous phase.[30] Venous invasion and lymph node metastases are reportedly common.

Treatment is surgical, with either resection or transplantation depending upon total liver and vascular involvement. The prognosis is better than for conventional HCC.

Angiosarcoma is an exceedingly rare, highly vascular mesenchymal tumor of the liver, accounting for fewer than 2% of all primary liver tumors.[31] Chemical carcinogens such as polyvinyl chloride, Thorotrast, and arsenic have been implicated as causative factors and are detected in up to one third of all cases.[31] In most of cases, however, no identifiable (or avoidable) chemical cause can be found. Thus, even as regulations limiting the use of known carcinogens will ultimately lead to a decreased incidence of hepatic angiosarcoma, cases will continue to occur. Patients are more commonly male, regardless of exposure risk,

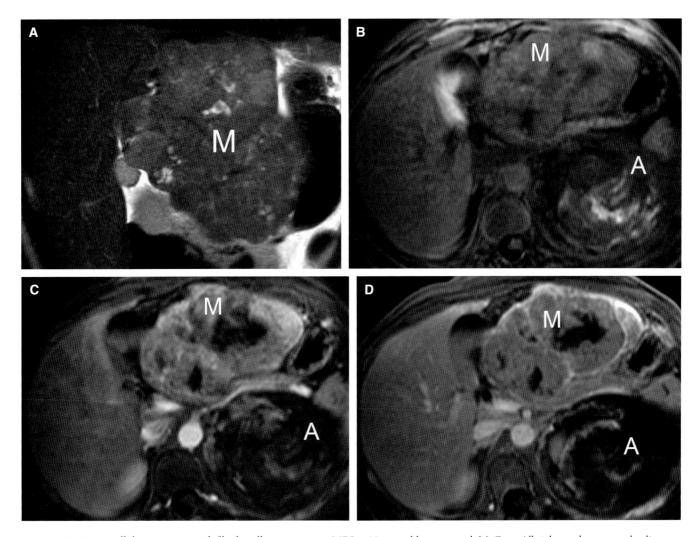

Figure 3.21 *Hepatocellular carcinoma with fibrolamellar components.* MRI in 30-year-old woman with McCune-Albright syndrome reveals a liver lesion. (**A**) Coronal T2-weighted image shows a large heterogeneous mass (*M*) in the left lobe. The underlying liver parenchyma is normal. Axial pre-contrast (**B**) as well as arterial (**C**) and portal venous phase (**D**) post-contrast enhanced images through the mass (*M*) demonstrate marked enhancement of solid portions of the tumor with areas of central liquefaction showing low signal centrally. Additionally, tumor replacing the left adrenal gland (*A*) shows signal intensity indicative of evolving hemorrhage. Resection of the left lobe of the liver revealed hepatocellular carcinoma with fibrolamellar components.

and usually middle-aged to elderly.[31] Presenting complaints include fever, abdominal pain, hepatomegaly, jaundice, and weight loss. Notably, spontaneous hemorrhage may occur, leading to acute clinical presentation. Serum alpha-fetoprotein is usually negative.

On MRI, solitary or multiple masses may be seen, typically sharply demarcated from surrounding parenchyma (Fig. 3.22). The appearance is dominated by the vascular nature of the lesion, with nodular peripheral early enhancement and centripetal filling on subsequent phases, an appearance that can be easily mistaken for hemangiomas. Angiosarcomas may not fill completely because of internal hemorrhage. The appearance

on T1-weighted imaging is nonspecific, but T2-weighted imaging can be quite helpful because angiosarcomas may be heterogeneously hyperintense, compared to the strikingly homogeneous hyperintensity of hemangiomas. Rapid growth is also expected and close follow-up imaging should make this clear. Beware of "atypical" hemangiomas; when there is incomplete filling and heterogeneity on T2-weighted images this should raise concern for angiosarcoma.

Peripheral intrahepatic cholangiocarcinoma, although arising from the bile duct, manifests as a liver mass. Approximately 10% of all cholangiocarcinomas arise peripherally within the liver, distal to the second-order ductal branches.[32]

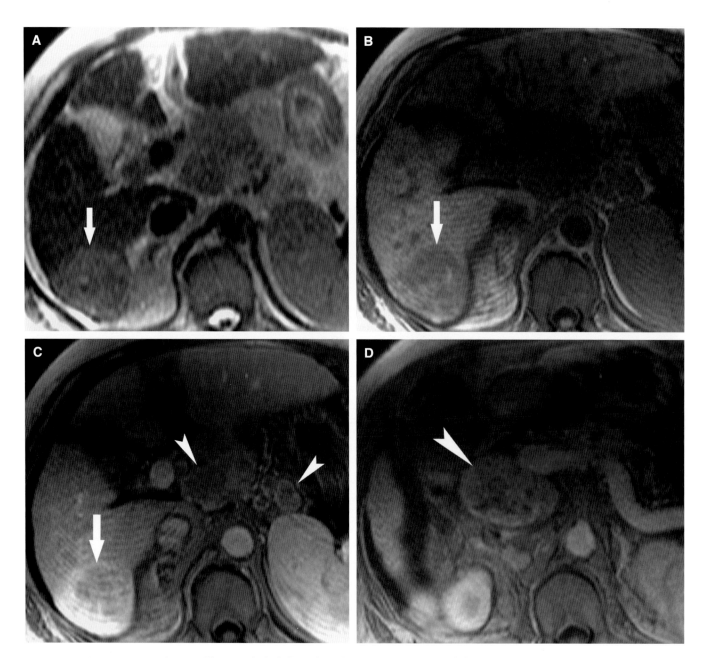

Figure 3.22 *Angiosarcoma.* A 62-year-old man with alcoholic cirrhosis has liver masses on MRI. (**A**) The dominant, relatively well demarcated lesion (*arrow*) is seen in the right lobe, displaying slightly increased signal intensity on the axial T2-weighted image. Several smaller lesions (not shown) had a similar appearance. Pre-contrast (**B**) and post-contrast-gadolinium-contrast-enhanced (**C**) T1-weighted images show a heterogeneous hypervascular mass (*arrow*) with prominent lymphadenopathy (*arrowheads* in C). (**D**) Periportal/peripancreatic lymphadenopathy (*arrowhead*) seen more inferiorly is striking. Biopsy revealed epithelioid angiosarcoma.

With growth, extension of tumor occurs through the ducts, sinusoids, vascular channels, perineural spaces, and periportal tissue. The tumor is variable in composition and may contain mucin, fibrosis, and areas of hyalinization and coagulative necrosis. Signal is hypointense on T1-weighted images and heterogeneously hyperintense to liver parenchyma on T2-weighted images. The rare mucin-containing variant is predictably more hyperintense on T2-weighted images.[4] A helpful finding in both detecting lesions and suggesting the diagnosis is biliary dilatation proximal to the lesion associated with capsular retraction. On dynamic gadolinium-enhanced imaging, mild to moderate rim enhancement with gradual heterogeneous and incomplete centripetal progression and delayed enhancement is common but nonspecific.[4] Differential diagnosis includes the sclerosing variant of HCC, colorectal carcinoma metastases, and fibrolamellar HCC. Biopsy may be necessary to distinguish the lesions. Prognosis is poor with all types of cholangiocarcinoma.

METASTATIC DISEASE AND LYMPHOMA

Liver metastases are traditionally characterized as hyper- or hypovascular with regard to their enhancement relative to normal liver parenchyma. This distinction is made with both MRI and CT. The advantage MRI offers is the ability to acquire multiple phases of contrast enhancement without ionizing radiation, as well as the ability to use inherent tissue contrast to both detect and characterize lesions.

The appearance of a liver metastasis is determined by cell of origin, effects upon surrounding liver parenchyma, and tumor vascularity (Figs. 3.23, 3.24, and 3.25). Although the appearance

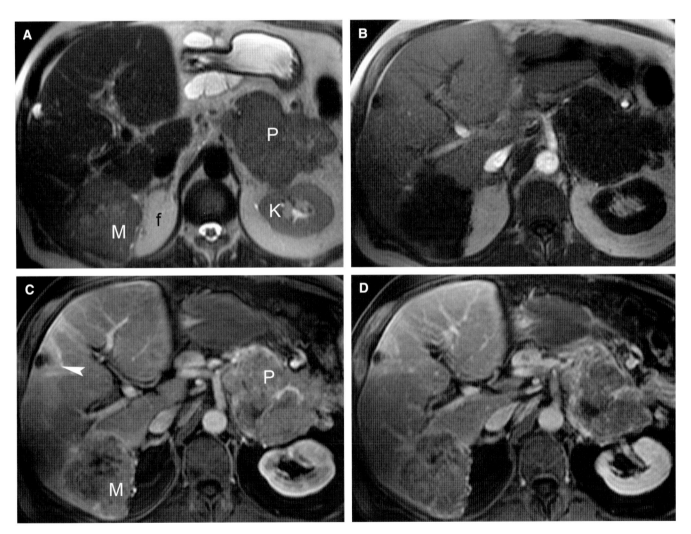

Figure 3.23 *Hypervascular metastasis.* Large, lobulated masses of the pancreatic tail (*P*) and the posterior segments of the right lobe liver (*M*) show similar imaging characteristics. (**A**) On an axial T2-weighted single-shot FSE/TSE image, the masses are heterogeneously hyperintense to liver parenchyma, are similar in signal intensity to the adjacent kidney (*K*), and are not as bright as adipose tissue (*f*). (**B**) The lesions are even more conspicuous on the T1-weighted magnetization-prepared gradient-echo image. (**C**) On the arterial phase post-gadolinium-contrast-enhanced image, the lesions are markedly hypervascular relative to liver. An additional liver metastasis (*arrowhead*) is identified. (**D**) The lesions retain contrast material into the 5-minute-delayed phase post-contrast enhanced image. Though the appearance of the liver mass is nonspecific, only confirming underlying highly vascular architecture, the nearly identical appearance of the mass in the pancreatic tail suggests that the tumors possess the same tissue. Subsequent histopathologic assessment confirmed neuroendocrine tumor of the pancreas with metastases to the liver.

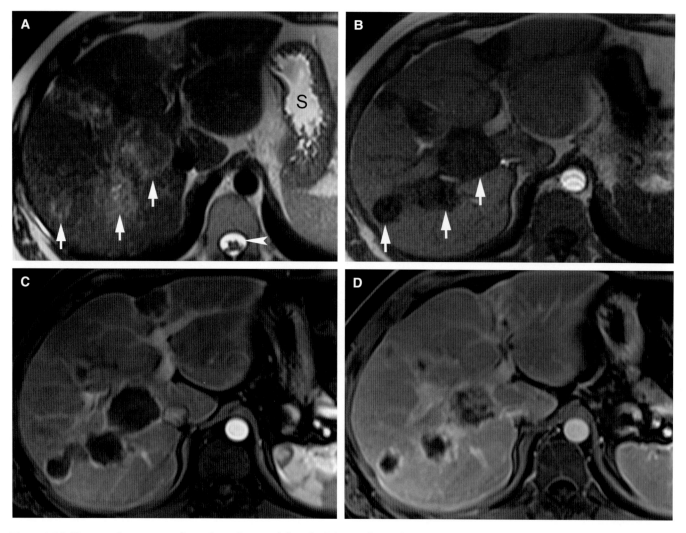

Figure 3.24 *Hypovascular metastases from colorectal cancer.* (**A**) Multiple lesions (*arrows*) of varying sizes are seen throughout the liver parenchyma, showing heterogeneous hyperintensity to liver on T2-weighted single-shot FSE/TSE images, though much less bright than the fluid seen in the stomach (*S*) and thecal sac (*arrowhead*). (**B**) T1-weighted magnetization-prepared gradient-echo image shows the lesions (*arrows*) to good advantage against the background normal liver parenchyma. Though the lesions are hypointense, they are not the near-signal-void black of classic hemangiomas, providing important differential information. Arterial phase (**C**) and 5-minute-delayed phase (**D**) post-gadolinium contrast-enhanced T1-weighted gradient-echo images show relatively hypovascular lesions with a thin rim of peripheral enhancement, highly specific for metastases. Furthermore, the "cauliflower" morphology, seen here best on the delayed image (**D**) is nearly pathognomonic for colorectal metastases.

of individual metastatic lesions varies widely, certain cell types do have predictable enhancement patterns. In general, similar vascularity will be observed in both the primary tumor and its metastases. Except for the rarely encountered completely cystic or necrotic lesions, all metastases have vascular supply and thus will have some degree of enhancement.

On unenhanced images, most metastatic lesions are mildly hypointense on T1-weighted images and moderately to markedly hyperintense on T2-weighted images, with the brightest areas representing necrosis or cystic change. While characteristic of metastasis, this morphologic pattern has not been particularly useful in suggesting tumor origin, although hypervascular metastases tend to be brighter on T2-weighted images (Fig. 3.23).[33] Importantly, this high signal on T2-weighted images does allow differentiation from the typical, mildly hyperintense appearancing HCC. Hemangiomas are markedly bright on T2-weighted images and may be indistinguishable from hypervascular metastases. For this reason, employing a T1-weighted

magnetization-prepared GRE pulse sequence can be invaluable to distinguish between the two lesions. Image acquisition for this sequence occurs at a specific set time after application of the crontrast-creating preparatory pulse so that signal from hemangioma will be maximally nulled, appearing nearly black in contrast to the intermediate signal intensity of a metastatic lesion (compare Figs. 3.24B and 3.13B).

Common hypervascular liver metastases include those from renal cell and thyroid carcinoma, neuroendocrine tumor and carcinoid, and sarcomas, with those from breast cancer somewhat less common. Rare hypervascular metastases from colon, gastric, and pancreatic adenocarcinoma have also been reported.[33] Common hypovascular metastases include those from colon, gastric, and small bowel adenocarcinoma, lung cancers, pancreatic adenocarcinoma, breast carcinoma, and prostate and transitional cell carcinoma. It is important to remember the effects of the surrounding liver parenchyma and contrast timing on both the lesion and one's perception of

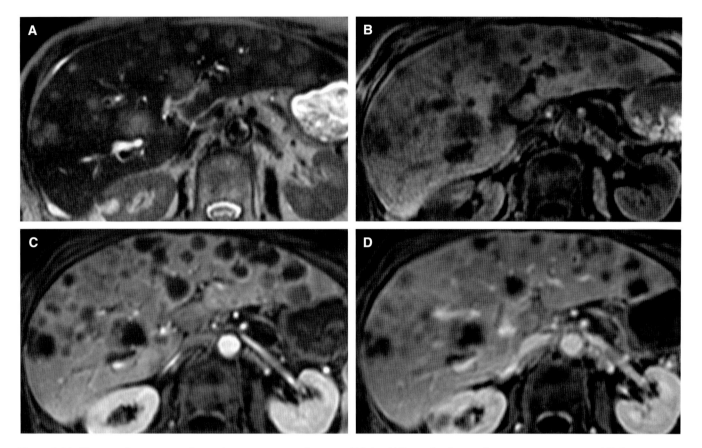

Figure 3.25 *Hypovascular metastases from unknown primary malignancy.* (**A**) Axial T2-weighted image demonstrates numerous mildly hyperintense lesions throughtout the liver parenchyma, appearance characteristic for metastases. Pre-contrast (**B**) as well as arterial phase (**C**) and 5-minute-delayed (**D**) post-contrast-enhanced images provide confirmation, showing hypovascular lesions with rim enhancement.

relative enhancement. For this reason, some have advocated using the pancreas as a reference tissue for a more accurate and objective comparison. The pancreas is a highly vascular organ and lies in close proximity to the liver, allowing easy comparison, often on the same slice. A lesion enhancing similarly to pancreas in the hepatic arterial phase can reliably be considered hypervascular.[33]

Several specific patterns of enhancement have been described that can help differentiate metastases from benign liver lesions. The classic nodular discontinuous peripheral enhancement with centripetal filling seen with large hemangiomas has been discussed. Cysts have no vascularity and no enhancement and can be confidently distinguished. Four major patterns of hepatic arterial-phase enhancement for liver metastases have been described:[33] peripheral ring enhancement, homogeneous enhancement, heterogeneous enhancement, and negligible enhancement.

The *peripheral ring enhancement* pattern is the most common in both hyper- and hypovascular metastases, seen in 72% of lesions in one series.[33] This pattern is considered relatively specific for metastases, though HCC can appear similar. This appearance is generally seen once a metastasis reaches a threshold size. It reflects continued parasitization of small hepatic arterial branches at the periphery of the lesion as the central portion becomes more distanced from blood supply, with resultant fibrosis and necrosis.[33]

Homogeneous arterial enhancement is typical for small hypervascular lesions (less than 1.5 cm). It is these lesions that are particularly problematic as they can appear very similar to flash-filling hemangiomas, FNH, hepatic adenomas, and small HCC. Additionally, transient arterial flow phenomena (THIDs) appear as focal arterial-phase enhancing lesions. Behavior on subsequent phases of contrast enhancement as well as features on T1- and T2-weighted imaging can clarify, but specific diagnosis may not be possible. In these situations follow-up imaging to assess for change, or biopsy, is required.

Heterogeneous arterial enhancement is usually seen in lesions larger than 3 cm, and is not a specific pattern indicating the tumor of origin for the metastasis as it is also commonly seen in HCC.

Negligible arterial enhancement is common, seen in one third of metastases.[33]

In portal venous and delayed venous phases, incomplete central progression, presumably reflecting the relative paucity of vessels reaching the central portion of the tumor, is the most common pattern in both hyper- and hypovascular metastases. Progression to iso-intensity on delayed-phase images, likely secondary to leakage of gadolinium into the interstitial spaces, occurs in a minority of both hyper- and hypovascular lesions.[33]

Like arterial-phase ring enhancement, delayed peripheral washout is considered a highly specific feature of liver metastases, approaching 100% specificity.[33] This appearance is more

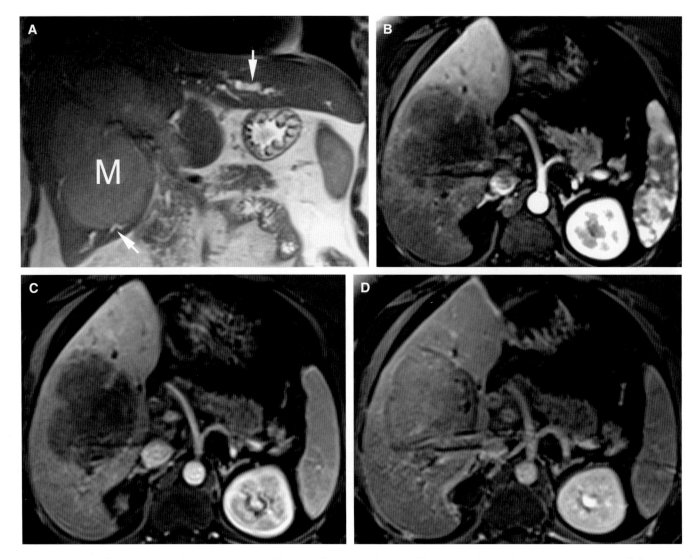

Figure 3.26 *Lymphoma.* Liver involvement in non-Hodgkin's lymphoma can take several forms, including a solitary mass, as in this case. (**A**) On coronal T2-weighted image, the central right lobe mass (*M*) is homogeneously hyperintense in signal intensity compared to the surrounding parenchyma. Mass effect causes obstruction of the bile ducts (*arrows*). Arterial phase (**B**), portal venous phase (**C**), and 5-minute-delayed (**D**) post-gadolinium contrast-enhanced images demonstrate a nonspecific, relatively hypovascular mass, which accumulates some contrast material as seen in the 5-minute-delayed images. Alternative appearances of hepatic lymphoma include hypervascularity and, less commonly, an infiltrative mass.

common in hypervascular metastases, and likely reflects the better-developed arterial supply and venous drainage in the periphery of the lesions abutting the normal hepatic parenchyma. This finding does not predict tumor of origin.

With the notable exception of colorectal carcinoma metastases, enhancement patterns are less useful for predicting the cell or organ of origin, as there is considerable overlap. Metastases from colon carcinoma produce two distinctive and specific features. The "cauliflower" pattern (Fig. 3.24) describes scalloped margins and enhancing internal septations. The second feature is a marginal ring of strong enhancement in the hepatic arterial phase that persists through the delayed venous phase.[33] The cauliflower pattern corresponds histologically to fibrosis and inflammatory strands surrounding tumor islets. The marginal ring enhancement pattern represents a tumoral zone of fibrous tissue and inflammatory cells.

A small but very important subset of metastases will appear as primarily fluid-signal lesions on MRI and must not be mistaken for benign cysts. This appearance can be a related to the architecture of the tumor of origin (mucinous primary tumors such as ovarian or colorectal carcinoma), necrosis (aggressive hypervascular lesions that "outgrow" or have poorly constructed vascular supply), or to therapy (treated gastrointestinal stromal tumors and testicular teratomas). Careful attention will often reveal some enhancement, and the clinical information should help guide the diagnosis.

Treated Metastases: Chemotherapeutic agents may alter the appearance of liver metastases, resulting in a less aggressive appearance of the lesion. Characteristically, early nodular peripheral enhancement and delayed retention of contrast material may be seen, features mimicking hemangioma. Careful inspection will reveal that the rim of the treated metastasis is nodular but intact, differentiating it from the hemangioma's discontinuous nodular peripheral enhancement.[33]

Lymphoma: Primary hepatic lymphoma is extremely rare. Secondary involvement in both Hodgkin's and non-Hodgkin's

Box 3.5 ESSENTIALS TO REMEMBER

- Detection of small HCCs in the setting of cirrhosis with a myriad of nodules demonstrated on MR remains a diagnostic challenge. Typically small HCCs (<2 cm) appear as hypointense nodules with internal foci iso-intense to liver parenchyma on T1-weighted images. On T2-weighted images, HCCs show heterogeneous foci of increased signal intensity. Fat, if present, demonstrated by chemical-shift imaging raises the likelihood of HCC. Increased signal intensity on T2-weighted images differentiates small HCC from dysplastic nodules, which typically show decreased signal. The hallmark finding is intense enhancement on early enhanced images with washout on later phase images.

- Extensive HCC may appear as a large solitary mass, as multiple nodules, or as diffuse infiltration. Signal intensity is variable on T1- and T2-weighted images. Increased signal intensity on unenhanced T1-weighted images may reflect the presence of fat, glycogen, or copper within the tumor. Moderate- to high-signal-intensity foci within a heterogeneous tumor are typical on T2-weighted images. Early phase intense gadolinium-contrast enhancement, which may be heterogeneous or focal, is characteristically seen in HCC. A fibrous capsule or a pseudocapsule consisting of compressed liver parenchyma may be seen on unenhanced images and may show enhancement on delayed contrast-enhanced images, a highly sensitive and specific feature.

- Fibrolamellar HCC is typically seen as a solitary, lobulated mass in the noncirrhotic liver of a young person. On T1-weighted images the signal intensity is slightly low and heterogeneous compared to surrounding parenchyma. On T2-weighted images the tumor is variably hyperintense. Enhancement is early, intense, and heterogeneous. The presence of a central stellate scar is characteristic. The scar shows low signal intensity on T1- and T2-weighted images. Enhancement of the scar is weak on early post-contrast-enhanced images and is seen to increase on delayed images.

- Peripheral intrahepatic cholangiocarcinomas appear as intrahepatic masses, commonly with satellite lesions and bile duct dilatation proximal to the tumor. Tumor signal intensity is lower than that of the surrounding normal liver parenchyma on T1-weighted images and mildly hyperintense to parenchyma on T2-weighted images. Early peripheral gadolinium-contrast enhancement may occur but maximal enhancement on delayed post-contrast-enhanced images is characteristic.

- Metastases are a consideration for nearly every hepatic mass lesion. Appearance is variable. Typical lesions show hypointense to iso-intense signal compared to normal liver on T1-weighted images and show intermediate high intensity on T2-weighted images. High-signal-intensity foci on unenhanced T1-weighted images suggest the presence of hemorrhage or melanin. On T2-weighted images metastases typically show iso-intense to hyperintense signal. Very high signal intensity on T2-weighted images suggests a cystic, necrotic, or mucinous lesion. Early peripheral rim enhancement with progressive, incomplete central fill-in is most characteristic. Hypervascular metastases, typical of neuroendocrine tumors, renal cell carcinoma, and melanoma, show intense early enhancement mimicking HCC. Adenocarcinomas are typically hypovascular and show weak enhancement.

lymphoma occurs more commonly. Furthermore, the liver is a common site of lymphoproliferative disorder (PTLD) occurring after liver transplantation. Hodgkin's disease infiltrates the portal tracts and manifests as diffuse nodular disease more often than as a focal mass or masses.[34] The liver may be enlarged. Diagnosis requires identification of the pathognomonic Reed-Sternberg cells histologically. Non-Hodgkin's lymphoma more commonly involves the liver than Hodgkin's lymphoma, with focal involvement also occuring more commonly in the former than the latter.[34] Manifestations differ somewhat depending on the causative cells, with small nodules in low-grade B-cell lymphoma and larger masses with high-grade B-cell lymphoma.[4] Primary lymphoma of the liver usually manifests as a discrete mass or multifocal lesions rather than as an infiltrative process. Primary lymphoma is often large at discovery but has a better prognosis than secondary hepatic lymphoma.[34] Tumor markers such as alpha-fetoprotein and carcinoembryonic antigen will often be normal.

Focal lymphomatous lesions are typically well defined and are hypointense to liver on T1-weighted imaging and hyperintense on T2-weighted imaging (Fig. 3.26). T2 signal intensity may vary from mildly hypointense to moderately hyperintense with increasing amounts of extracellular fluid and vascularity.[34]

Large lesions commonly have central necrosis. Focal lesions are more readily identified by imaging than is diffuse lymphomatous involvement. Lymphoma may mimic metastasis. With gadolinium administration, both ring enhancement and transient perilesional enhancement are commonly seen in the arterial phase. Heterogeneous enhancement and hypovascular lesions reflect variable vascularity.[34] Generally, arterial-phase enhancement is seen with lesions that are more hyperintense on T2-weighted images.[34] Primary non-Hodgkin's lymphoma is aggressive but potentially resectable and responsive to chemotherapy and radiation.

The liver is the most frequently involved solid organ in post-transplant lymphproliferative disease (PTLD). PTLD is most commonly seen in the setting of liver transplantation, but also occurs following pancreas, kidney, heart, and lung transplantations. Involvement may manifest as discrete nodules, infiltrative disease, or a heterogeneous mass in the porta hepatis. Lesions are typically mildly hypointense on T1-weighted images and hyperintense on T2-weighted images and display variable patterns of enhancement. The imaging characteristics are generally not distinguishable from those seen with opportunistic infection, the major differential consideration in this patient population.

REFERENCES

1. Martin DR, Semelka RC. Magnetic resonance imaging of the liver: review of techniques and approach to common diseases. *Semin Ultrasound CT MRI.* 2005;26:116–131.
2. Silva AC, Evans JM, McCullough AE, et al. MR imaging of hypervascular liver masses: a review of current techniques. *Radiographics.* 2009;29:385–402.
3. Grazioli L, Morana G, Kirchin MA, Schneider G. Accurate differentiation of focal nodular hyperplasia from hepatic adenoma at gadobenate dimeglumine-enhanced MR imaging: prospective study. *Radiology.* 2005;236:166–177.
4. Fisher A, Siegelman ES. Body MR Techniques and MR of the liver. In: Siegelman s, ed. *Body MRI,* 1st ed. Philadelphia: Elsevier Saunders, 2005:1–53.
5. Helmberger T, Semelka RC. New contrast agents for imaging the liver. *Magn Reson Imaging Clinic North Am.* 2001;9:745–766.
6. Cameron IL, Ord VA, Fullerton GD. Characterization of proton NMR relaxation times in normal and pathological tissues by correlation with other tissue parameters. *Magn Reson Imaging.* 1984;2:97–106.
7. Wanless IR. Vascular disorders. In: MacSween RMN, Burt AD, Portmann BC, et al., eds. *Pathology of the Liver,* 4th ed. Churchill Livingstone, 2002:539–573.
8. Savastano S, San Bartolo O. Pseudotumoral appearance of peliosis hepatis. *AJR Am J Roentgenol.* 2005;185:558–559.
9. Yekeler E, Dursun M, Tunaci A, et al. Diagnosing of peliosis hepatis by magnetic resonance imaging. *J Hepatol.* 2004;41:351.
10. Macari M, Yeretsian R, Babb J. Assessment of low signal adjacent to the falciform ligament on contrast-enhanced MRI. *AJR Am J Roentgenol.* 2007;189:1443–1448.
11. Mitchell DG. Chemical shift magnetic resonance imaging: applications in the abdomen and pelvis. *Top Magn Reson Imaging.* 1992;4:46–63.
12. Torres CG, Lundby B, Sterud AT, et al. MnDPDP for MR imaging of the liver. Results from the European phase III studies. *Acta Radiol.* 1997; 38:631–637.
13. Semelka RC, Lee JK, Worawattanakul S, et al. Sequential use of ferumoxide particles and gadolinium chelate for the evaluation of focal liver lesions on MRI. *J Magn Reson Imaging.* 1998;8:670–674.
14. Crawford JM. Liver cirrhosis. In: MacSween RMN, Burt AD, Portmann BC, et al., eds. *Pathology of the Liver,* 4th ed. Churchill Livingstone, 2002:539–573.
15. Guingrich JA, Kuhlman JE. Colonic wall thickening in patients with cirrhosis: CT findings and clinical implications. *AJR Am J Roentgenol.* 1999;172:919–924.
16. Kobayashi S, Matsui O, Gabata T, et al. MRI findings of primary biliary cirrhosis: correlation with Scheuer histologic staging. *Abdom Imaging.* 2005;30:71–76.
17. Wenzel JS, Donohoe A, Ford, III KL, et al. *Primary biliary cirrhosis. AJR Am J Roentgenol.* 2001;176:885–889.
18. Matsui O, Kadoya M, Takashima T, et al. Intrahepatic periportal abnormal intensity on MR images: an indication of various hepatobiliary diseases. *Radiology.* 1989;171:335–338.
19. Desmet VJ. Ludwig symposium on biliary disorders. 1. *Pathogenesis of ductal plate abnormalities. Mayo Clin Proc.* 1998;73:80–89.
20. Gaines PA, Sampson MA. The prevalence and characterization of simple hepatic cysts by ultrasound examination. *Br J Radiol.* 1989;62:335–337.
21. Craig JR, Peters RL, Edmondson HA. Tumors of the Liver and Intrahepatic Bile Ducts. Washington DC: Armed Forces of Institute of Pathology, 1989.
22. Mortele KJ, Ros PR. Cystic focal liver lesions in the adult: differential CT and MR imaging features. *Radiographics.* 2001;21:895–910.
23. Ferris JV. Serial ethanol ablation of multiple hepatic cysts as an alternative to liver transplantation. *AJR Am J Roentgenol.* 2003;180: 472–474.
24. Buetow PC, Buck JL, Pantongrag-Brown L, et al. Biliary cystadenoma and cystadenocarcinoma: clinical-imaging-pathologic correlations with emphasis on the importance of ovarian stroma. *Radiology.* 1995;196:805–810.
25. Murphy BJ, Casillas J, Ros PR, et al. The CT appearances of cystic masses of the liver. Radiographics. 1989:9:307–322.
26. Pedrosa I, Saiz A, Arrazola J, et al. Hydatid disease: radiologic and pathologic features and complications. *Radiographics.* 2000;20: 795–817.
27. Kato H, Kanematsu M, Matsuo M, et al. Atypically enhancing hepatic cavernous hemangiomas: high-spatial-resolution gadolinium-enhanced triphasic dynamic gradient-recalled-echo imaging findings. *Eur Radiol.* 2001;11:2510–2515.
28. Leconte I, Van Beers BE, Lacrosse M, et al. Focal nodular hyperplasia: natural course observed with CT and MRI. *J Comput Assist Tomogr.* 2000;24:61–66.
29. Tao LC. Oral contraceptive-associated liver cell adenoma and hepatocellular carcinoma: cytomorphology and mechanism of malignant transformation. *Cancer.* 1991;68:341–347.
30. McLarney JK, Rucker PT, Bender GN, et al. Fibrolamellar carcinoma of the liver: radiologic-pathologic correlation. *Radiographics.* 1999; 19:453–471.
31. Molina E, Hernandez A. Clinical manifestations of primary hepatic angiosarcoma. *Dig Dis Sci.* 2003;48:677–682.
32. Soyer P, Bluemke DA, Sibert A, Laissy JP. MR imaging of intrahepatic cholangiocarcinoma. *Abdom Imaging.* 1995;20:126–130.
33. Danet IM, Semelka RC, Leonardou P, et al. Spectrum of MRI appearances of untreated metastases of the liver. *AJR Am J Roentgenol.* 2003; 181:809–817.
34. Kelekis NL, Semelka RC, Siegelman ES, et al. Focal hepatic lymphoma: magnetic resonance demonstration using current techniques including gadolinium enhancement. *Magn Reson Imaging.* 1997; 156:625–636.

4.

BILIARY SYSTEM MR IMAGING

Juan Olazagasti, MD

The biliary tree has historically been studied with invasive cholangiographic methods (T- tube, intra-operative, percutaneous transhepatic or endoscopic retrograde cholangiopancreatography) as well as noninvasive methods (conventional radiography, ultrasound, CT, and scintigraphy). Pancreatic and biliary MR imaging largely came from "their inclusion on hepatic MR images and the goal seemed to be the imitation of the cross sectional anatomy seen on radiographs and computerized tomography."[1]

Technical advances, including the introduction of echo planar imaging, short scan times, the widespread use of gadolinium chelates, the development of fast heavily T2-weighted technique, and magnetic resonance cholangiopancreatography (MRCP), have allowed MR to become a clinically important imaging tool in the diagnosis and treatment planning of biliary pathology. Together with standard abdominal MR imaging sequences of related organ systems, mainly the liver, pancreas, stomach and duodenum, the porta hepatis and retroperitoneum, MRCP provides a comprehensive and thorough assessment of the biliary system not possible with any other diagnostic technique. It serves as a road map prior to invasive therapeutic procedures, provides high-quality images of postoperative or post-traumatic complications, and is excellent for the staging of tumors. MRI, in combination with MRCP, allows in-depth evaluation of the biliary tree with a large field of view, excellent patient tolerance, multiplanar images, and 3-dimensional (3D) capabilities specifically tailored to the biliary diagnosis in question.

Endoscopic retrograde cholangiopancreatography (ERCP) and percutaneous transhepatic cholangiography offer the ability to diagnose, biopsy, and even treat some disease processes. However, these are invasive, operator-dependent procedures that carry a significant level of risk.[2] Recent studies indicate a significant (3% to 9%) incidence of adverse events for invasive biliary procedures, including acute pancreatitis, perforation, hemorrhage, bacteremia, and sepsis.[3]

MRCP in combination with multiplanar MRI has become an important noninvasive diagnostic tool for the evaluation of the biliary tree. In this chapter we will discuss the MR techniques used to perform an adequate evaluation of the biliary system, and provide an overview of the accompanying imaging pitfalls and artifacts. We will review the normal anatomy and common variants, and discuss frequently occurring disease entities with their clinical features and imaging characteristics. The role of biliary tree MR imaging following trauma will be addressed, as well as the use of the technique for perisurgical "road-mapping" before or after liver transplantation. We will also discuss the role of hepatocyte-specific MR contrast agents, such as gadoxetic acid, or gadoxetate disodium (Eovist® in the United States, Primovist® in the European Union and Australia), in assessing the biliary ducts. These agents are excreted, for a large part, with the bile and accumulate in the bile duct system.

MR TECHNIQUES

Prior to the biliary investigation using MRI, we recommend that our patients fast for 4 to 6 hours to decrease the fluid content within the stomach and duodenum, reduce peristalsis, and promote filling of the gallbladder. Overlying or superimposed high-signal-intensity fluid in the gastrointestinal tract on heavily T2-weighted MRCP images (Fig. 4.1) can be removed with use of a so-called "negative" oral contrast agents such as oral ferrous sulfate. Intramuscular glucagon aids in decreasing bowel peristalsis. Overlying hepatic and renal cysts, motion artifacts, and changes from previous instrumentation can bring about interpretation problems. Careful evaluation of the source images of a 3D thin-slice MRCP sequence as well as assessment of multiplanar T2-weighted images may help avoid difficulties with interpretation caused by superimposed structures. Comparison with prior imaging and careful attention to significant clinical history are vital for best interpretation of MRI and MRCP. We also recommend that MR imaging be performed *before* endoscopic instrumentation and/or stent placement, whenever possible, to decrease the

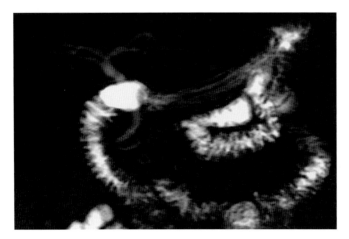

Figure 4.1 *Obscuration of pancreatic and biliary ductal system by overlying bowel.* A nonfasting patient has a significant amount of overlying bowel contents, obscuring the pancreaticobiliary ductal system and making it difficult to assess the ducts.

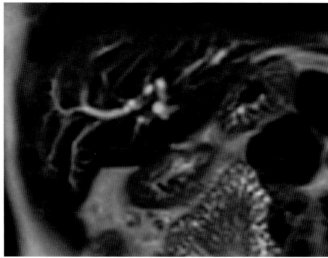

Figure 4.2 *Dilated intrahepatic bile ducts.* Dilated intrahepatic biliary system is well seen on a T2-weighted coronal image given the normal high signal intensity of bile against the background of normal liver.

chance that postprocedural inflammation is misinterpreted as tumor extension or cholangitis.

MRCP is usually performed by using heavily T2-weighted imaging to optimize visualization of the high water content (97%) of the normal bile, rendering its high signal intensity against the low signal intensity of the surrounding soft tissues. Standard T2-weighted or contrast-enhanced MR imaging is also highly accurate for the detection of bile duct dilatation[3] (Fig. 4.2).

Late arterial-phase and portal venous-phase contrast-enhanced T1-weighted images may improve the detection of hypovascular tumors that involve the biliary system, including cholangiocarcinoma, gallbladder cancer, pancreatic adenocarcinoma, and metastatic disease. When cholangiocarcinoma is clinically suspected, delayed imaging (10 to 20 minutes after contrast administration) often reveals contrast material accumulation within the tumor and improves visualization against the nearby normal liver parenchyma, from which most of the contrast material has by then cleared.[3]

MRCP is generally performed with both 2D and 3D heavily T2-weighted single-shot or multislice fast/turbo spin-echo (FSE/TSE) sequences, providing complementary information. At our institution we include a single-slice thick-slab breath-hold (4 to 6 cm in thickness) 2D sequence (Fig. 4.3A) with which 7 to 9 slices are obtained, a multislice thin-section (4 mm) breath-hold 2D sequence, both obtained within a single breath hold, and a heavily T2-weighted, respiratory-gated, 3D FSE/TSE sequence that generates a large number (~60) of very thin (1 mm) slices with isotropic voxels, allowing reconstruction of the images in any orientation without distortion. The images for all of the aforementioned sequences used for MRCP are generally acquired in coronal or paracoronal orientation. Use of appropriate centering and a larger field of view minimizes wraparound artifact.[3]

With the thick-slab single-section sequence, most of the biliary ducts as well as the pancreatic duct are included in the

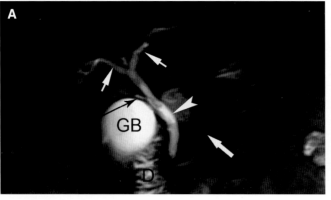

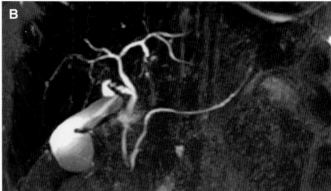

Figure 4.3 *Normal MRCP.* (**A**) Thick-slab MRCP image shows normal intra- and extrahepatic bile duct system. *GB*, gallbladder; *D*, duodenum; *arrowhead*, common bile duct; *short arrows*, right and left hepatic bile ducts; *long black arrow*, segment of the cystic duct; *fat arrow*, pancreatic duct. (**B**) Maximum-intensity-projection (MIP) image of a 3D thin-slice FSE/TSE sequence for MRCP shows normal intrahepatic, extrahepatic, and pancreatic ductal systems.

tissue volume that is included in the slice, providing an overview of biliary and pancreatic ductal anatomy (Fig. 4.3B). In our experience this sequence is particularly useful for identifying obstruction and strictures of the ducts. The thin-section multislice sequence helps with visualizing intraductal disease such as stones. The very thin slice sections of the 3D data set can be reconstructed to create rotational images similar to ERCP. However, since small areas of signal void, such as those caused by stones, may be obscured on postprocessed images, the original thin-section source images should be carefully reviewed individually for detection of these abnormalities.[3]

Isotropic 3D MRCP has recently caught the attention of imagers as it offers the advantage of obtaining thinner sections without intersection gaps.[4] Several studies have shown that 3D MRCP outperforms 2D thick-slab imaging in depicting the biliary anatomy.[4,5] However, a disadvantage of the 3D MRCP technique is that the overall acquisition time is generally greater than that of most 2D techniques that acquire the data within a breath hold. The acquisition of the data of the 3D MRCP sequence is therefore often performed with respiratory gating, a technique whereby each time during a certain phase of the respiration, usually at end-expiration, a few data points are obtained. Since the normal respiration is relatively slow (~15 breaths/min), it can take several minutes until all data are acquired, and therefore the 3D MRCP technique is relatively slow. However, this is favored by patients who have difficulty holding their breath.[4]

PITFALLS

Pitfalls of MRCP include missing a calculus when stone size is 3 mm or less, or when the stone is not surrounded by enough fluid to be visible. The latter can occur when a stone is impacted at the ampulla of Vater. Similarly, when a segment of the biliary tree is impacted with stones and there is little bile surrounding the stones, this can be easily misinterpreted as a segmental stricture.

Sources for incorrectly diagnosing the presence of a stone include a signal void created by a vessel crossing the duct, a surgical clip, for instance from cholecystectomy, or an air bubble within the duct (Fig. 4.4). Typically, air bubbles are located in the nondependent portion of the duct and show with air–fluid levels. When there is air within the duct there is often a history of recent instrumentation or surgery, and the findings can be further corroborated with those of plain radiographs and CT. Susceptibility artifact can be seen with increase of the TE on a dual-echo, in/out-of-phase, gradient-echo sequence, resulting from the increased signal loss due to excessive T2* decay caused by the presence of air. Recognition of this artifact can be used to confirm the presence of air bubbles.

The pseudocalculus effect due to sphincter spasm is more commonly seen during ERCP due to manipulation, forceful contrast medium injection, and analgesics. This artifact is much less often seen on MRI and MRCP. Additionally, the time it takes to perform the MR examination proves helpful in allowing enough time to clear an intermittent spasmodic sphincter, as spasm may be seen to resolve on later image sequences.

NORMAL ANATOMY

The gallbladder is a pear-shaped hollow viscus located in the right upper quadrant, lodged on the visceral surface of the liver between segments IV and V, and connected to the common hepatic duct by the cystic duct to form the common bile duct. It is approximately 7 to 10 cm long and 2.5 cm wide. Normal wall thickness is less than 3 mm. The gallbladder serves as the repository for bile produced in the liver, with an average intraluminal volume of 30 to 50 mL.[2] Bile within the gallbladder may become supersaturated with cholesterol, leading to crystal precipitation and gallstone formation (Fig. 4.5).[6]

The normal cholangiographic anatomy is well displayed with MRCP as a branching-pattern ductal system with the intrahepatic bile ducts (IHBDs) measuring less than 2 mm. Normal extrahepatic bile ducts (EHBDs) measure 7 mm or less. EHBDs increase in diameter with age at a rate of 1 mm per decade.[3] After cholecystectomy, a common bile duct size up to 12 mm with subtle smooth tapering is accepted as within normal range.

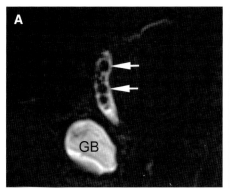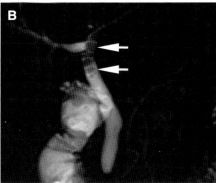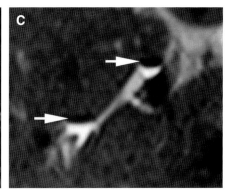

Figure 4.4 *Air bubble artifact.* 3D free-breathing MRCP (**A**) and thick-slab MRCP (**B**) show "filling defects" (*arrows*) from air bubbles appearing as possible stones in the common bile duct. Note how they lie nondependently and how they produce air–bile levels (*arrows*) on the axial T2-weighted single-shot FSE/TSE image (**C**). In-phase and opposed-phase gradient-echo imaging (not shown) can help differentiate air from true stones, see also Figure 2.35 of Chapter 2. The presence of air and absence of stones was proven at subsequent ERCP (not shown). *GB*, gallbladder.

Box 4.1 ESSENTIALS TO REMEMBER

- T2-weighted and post-gadolinium-contrast-enhanced multiplanar T1-weighted images are very good for demonstrating biliary ductal dilatation.

- Late post-contrast enhanced arterial or portal venous phase T1-weighted images are the images of choice for detecting gallbladder carcinoma and metastases.

- Early post-contrast enhanced arterial phase T1-weighted images are best for revealing hepatocellular carcinoma.

- Delayed (10 to 20 minutes) post-contrast enhanced images are best for detection of cholangiocarcinoma.

- Thick-slab single-section MRCP images give a high-quality overall picture of the anatomy of the pancreatico-biliary tree and display obstruction and biliary strictures.

- Thin source multisection MRCP images are better for visualizing intraductal disease such as stones.

- Calculi smaller than 3 mm may be missed on MRCP, especially when not surrounded by bile, such as when the small stone is impacted at the ampulla of Vater.

- Surgical clips, air bubbles, and crossing vessels may mimic the presence of stones.

The normal biliary tree follows the Couinaud segmental anatomy of the liver and runs parallel to the portal venous supply of the liver (Fig. 4.6). Anatomic variants are common. The "normal" pattern is seen in approximately 60% of the population.[2] The *right hepatic duct* drains the segments of the right hepatic lobe (V–VIII) and has two major branches: the *right posterior duct*, which drains the posterior segments (VI and VII), and the *right anterior duct*, which drains the anterior segments (V and VIII).[7] The right posterior duct dives behind the right anterior duct and joins it from the left side to form the right hepatic duct. The *left hepatic duct* is formed by segmental tributaries draining segments II to IV. These unite and receive the duct from segment I, the caudate lobe, to form the left hepatic duct. Right and left ducts then join to form the *common hepatic duct*, which further downstream receives the *cystic duct* from the gallbladder. At this point it becomes the *common bile duct* (CBD). The CBD courses caudally and medially to join the pancreatic duct for a short (4 to 5 mm) segment. At this level, and within the sphincter of Oddi, muscular fibers surround this common channel, limiting pancreatic and biliary fluid reflux. Narrowing of duct diameter at the sphincter is a normal finding.

The most common anatomic variant of intrahepatic biliary branching is drainage of the right posterior duct into the left hepatic duct before its confluence with the right anterior duct. This occurs in 13% to 19% of the population.[2]

Another common variant of the main intrahepatic branches is the so-called "trifurcation" (11% of the population). This anomaly is characterized by a three-way confluence with simultaneous emptying of the right posterior duct, right anterior duct, and left hepatic duct to form the common hepatic duct (Fig. 4.7). Variants at the level of the confluence are important in patients being considered as potential donors for right hepatic lobe transplantation.[7]

Extrahepatic variants of the bile ducts account for most of the clinically important cases, presenting with a variety of symptoms ranging from nonspecific abdominal pain to jaundice and nausea. These anatomic variants are also associated with recurrent pancreatitis, cholangitis, choledocholithiasis, and even some malignancies.[3] Prompt diagnosis and treatment may be vital.

CONGENITAL VARIANTS

Anomalous pancreaticobiliary junction refers to junction of the biliary and pancreatic duct outside the duodenal wall to form a long common channel, defined as more than 15 mm in length. This anomalous junction is associated with acute pancreatitis, choledochal cysts, cholangitis, stones, and biliary tract malignancy (as high as 30%).[3,4,8,9] The long common channel is present in up to 60% of patients in the United States

Figure 4.5 *Gallstones in the gallbladder.* Sagittal T2-weighted single-shot FSE/TSE image clearly depicts gallstones (*arrow*) layering within the gallbladder (*GB*). *RK*, right kidney.

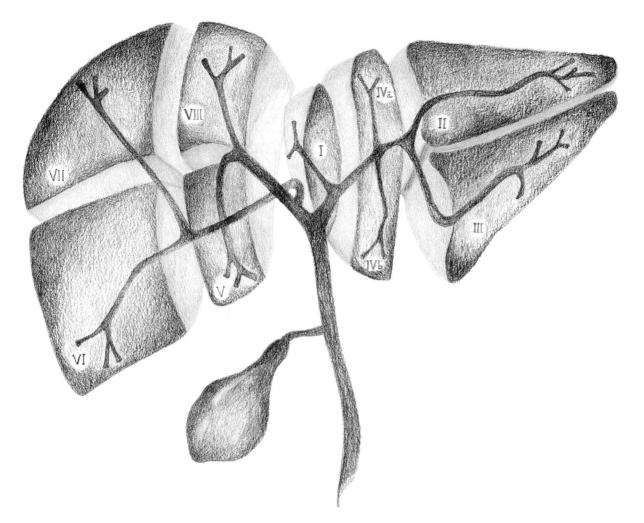

Figure 4.6 *Segmental anatomy of the liver with corresponding intrahepatic biliary segments.* Line drawing by Brooke Olazagasti, adapted from Mortele KJ, Ros PR. Anatomic variant of the biliary tree MR cholangiographic applications. *AJR Am J Roentgenol.* 2001;177:389-394.

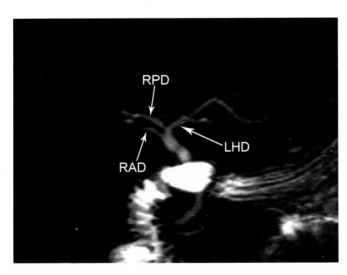

Figure 4.7 *Trifurcation: common normal variant of the IHBD anatomy.* Thick-slab MRCP clearly shows a trifucation of the IHBDs with the simultaneous emptying of the right posterior duct (*RPD*), the right anterior duct (*RAD*), and the left hepatic duct (*LHD*) into the common hepatic duct to form a three-way confluence. These variants are important in patients being considered as potential donors for right hepatic lobe transplantation.

and 90% of patients in Japan with type 1 choledochal cysts.[3] An anomalous junction should be recognized and treated surgically before pancreaticobiliary complications or biliary tract carcinomas develop.[9] ERCP has typically been the diagnostic tool of choice. In a year 2000 study of 120 patients, CT cholangiography was able to accurately diagnose the aberrant ducts in all patients. MRI, then performed on a 1.5T magnet, lagged behind. A 2006 study from Duke University has demonstrated a higher contrast-to-noise ratio and a higher level of confidence in identifying intrahepatic congenital variants with 3.0T than with 1.5T MRI.[10]

Congenital cystic lesions of bile ducts may involve IHBDs or EHBDs. Intrahepatic abnormalities include five different entities: congenital hepatic fibrosis, Caroli's syndrome, von Meyenburg complexes, simple cyst of the liver, and polycystic liver disease. Congenital hepatic fibrosis and von Meyenburg complexes are secondary to ductal plate malformation affecting the smallest IHBDs. Cystic dilatations are of small size and are most apparent at histologic examination of the liver. The main clinical manifestations of congenital hepatic fibrosis result from portal hypertension. Caroli's syndrome is secondary to ductal plate malformation affecting the largest IHBDs.

Cystic dilatations are macroscopic, result in cholangitis, and may lead to biliary stones and carcinoma developing within cystic dilatations.

Simple hepatic cysts and cysts occuring in polycystic liver disease are characterized by cystic dilatations that, in contrast to the preceding entities, do not communicate with the biliary tree. As a result, they have few clinical consequences. Renal malformations are associated with biliary malformations in congenital hepatic fibrosis and polycystic liver disease. Ectasia of the renal collecting tubules is associated with two thirds of the cases of congenital hepatic fibrosis, which is transmitted as an autosomal recessive trait. Polycystic disease of the kidneys is associated with half of the cases of polycystic liver disease, which is transmitted as an autosomal dominant trait.[3,7]

Choledochal cysts are usually defined by the Todani classification (Fig. 4.8). Embryologic errors during involution and remodeling of the ductal plate that surrounds the portal vein lead to multiple fibrocystic abnormalities, including chole-

dochal cysts, Caroli's disease, and biliary hamartomas. These are rare disorders with either cystic or fusiform dilatation of the intrahepatic and or extrahepatic duct branches.[3,7] Eighty percent are diagnosed during childhood, and they have a strong female tendency (4:1). Most adult patients have nonspecific symptoms, which may cause a delay in diagnosis. Others present with bile stasis, gallstones, sludge, or cholangitis.[3,7]

Type I choledochal cysts are confined to the EHBD. Type I cysts result from an anomalous pancreaticobiliary junction. These account for the vast majority (85%) of cases of choledochal cysts and have a higher correlation with malignancy. Malignancy risk is believed to be related to bile stasis and pancreatic fluid reflux secondary to the long common channel that lies outside the boundaries of the muscular sphincter of Oddi. When a large choledochal cyst is present, MRCP thin slice source images and MIP reconstructions should be carefully evaluated so as not to miss the long channel connection. *Type Ia* refers to cystic or saccular dilatation of part of or the

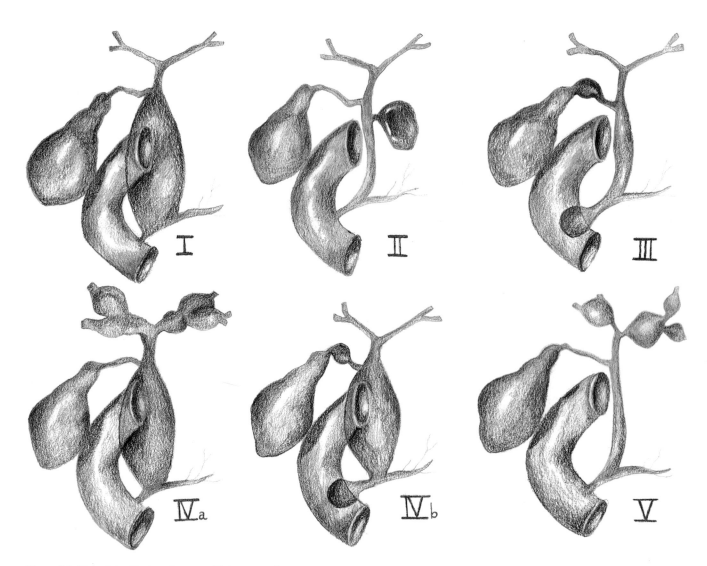

Figure 4.8 *Todani classification of congenital biliary cystic disease. Type I:* cystic or saccular dilatation of part of or the entire EHBD. *Type II:* represents true diverticula of the EHBD. *Type III: al*so known as *choledochocele,* represents focal dilatation of the intramural distal-most CBD segment *Type IV:* there are multiple and segmental dilatations that can have both intrahepatic and extrahepatic components. *Type V (Caroli's disease):* uneven cystic dilatation of the IHBDs with normal EHBD. Line drawing by Brooke Olazagasti, adapted from Federle MP, Jeffrey RB, Woodward PJ, Borhani A. *Diagnostic Imaging—Abdomen, Part II, Section 2, Biliary System.* Philadelphia: Lippincott Williams & Wilkins, 2009.

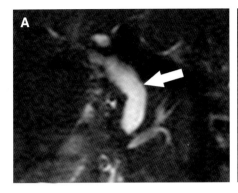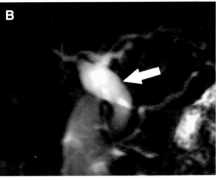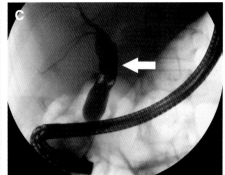

Figure 4.9 *Choledochocal cyst, type Ia.* Coronal T2-weighted image (**A**) and thick-slab MRCP (**B**) and corresponding ERCP (**C**) images demonstrate dilatation of the entire extrahepatic biliary duct (*arrows*), indicative of a type Ia choledochal cyst.

entire EHBD (Fig. 4.9). *Type Ib* refers to segmental saccular dilatation involving a limited segment of the duct. *Type Ic* refers to diffuse fusiform dilatation that involves most or all of the EHBD.

Type II choledochal cysts represent true diverticula of the EHBD and have the second highest cancer risk.[3]

Type III choledochal cysts, also known as *choledochoceles*, represent focal dilatation of the intramural distal-most CBD segment (Fig. 4.10). These are analogous to ureteroceles and have a high association with choledocholithiasis.[3] Most frequently in the 1- to 2-cm size range, the cysts can be large enough to cause biliary obstruction. The lesions are not embryologically related to the other choledochal cysts. Patients present with intermittent biliary colic, jaundice, and pancreatitis.

Type IV choledochal cysts are multiple and segmental and can have both intrahepatic and extrahepatic components. *Type IVa choledochal cysts* involve both the IHBD and the EHBD. *Type IVb cysts* involve saccular dilatation of the EHBD only.

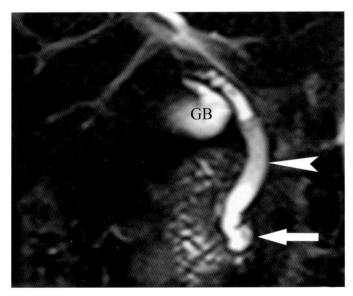

Figure 4.10 *Choledochocele.* Coronal MRCP image depicts a cystic dilatation (*arrow*) of the distal-most CBD (*arrowhead*) at the level of the ampulla, indicative of a choledochocele or Todani type III choledochal cyst. *GB*, gallbladder.

Type V choledochal cysts (Caroli's disease) represent a rare autosomal recessive disorder characterized by uneven cystic dilatation of the IHBDs with normal EHBDs (Fig. 4.11). The embryologic deviation results in remodeling, producing varying degrees of destructive inflammation and dilatation. If the larger IHBDs are affected, the result is Caroli's disease. Alternatively, if the small interlobular bile ducts are affected, the result is congenital hepatic fibrosis. If both small and large levels of the intrahepatic biliary tree are involved, features of both congenital hepatic fibrosis and Caroli's disease will be present. The latter condition has been termed *Caroli's syndrome*.[7] Clinical features include recurrent bouts of cholangitis due to bile stasis with recurrent attacks of right upper quadrant pain, fever, and rarely jaundice. Imaging studies show intrahepatic saccular or fusiform dilated cystic structures of varying sizes that communicate with the biliary tree. The presence of a tiny dot within the dilated IHBD (termed "central dot sign") seen on post-contrast enhanced images is considered highly indicative of Caroli's disease.[7] The central dot sign is produced by enhancing portal vein branches, surrounded by the cystic alterations of the IHBD.[7] Intraluminal biliary calculi may be present as well.

Differential diagnosis of cystic lesions of the intrahepatic biliary system includes primary sclerosing cholangitis, recurrent pyogenic cholangitis, autosomal dominant polycystic liver disease, biliary hamartomas, multiple microabscesses, and rarely obstructive biliary dilatation.[3,7] Associated conditions include choledochal cysts, cholangiocarcinoma, and renal cystic disease such as medullary sponge kidney with tubular ectasia.

STONE DISEASE, CHOLECYSTITIS, AND COMPLICATIONS

Cholecystectomy is the most frequently performed elective abdominal surgery in the United States and is most commonly prompted by gallstones. Gallstones are seen in about 10% of the general population, are twice as common in women, and become more prevalent with advancing age. Risk factors for developing gallstones include obesity, rapid weight loss, pregnancy, and the hormone estrogen. Cholesterol stones (containing at least 50% cholesterol) are the most frequently encountered,

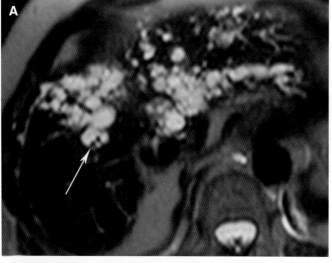

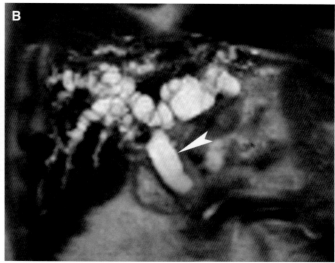

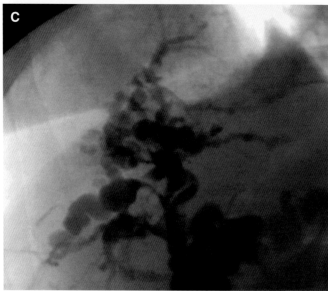

Figure 4.11 *Caroli's disease.* Axial (**A**) and coronal (**B**) T2-weighted single shot FSE/TSE images and ERCP (**C**) image of a patient with Caroli's disease show multiple saccular and fusiform dilatations of the IHBD. The axial image (**A**) shows the "central dot sign" (*arrow*) representing portal branches surrounded by cystic alterations of the dilated IHBDs. This patient has had a cholecystectomy. Note that this patient also has a dilated CBD (*arrowhead*, **B**) measuring 12 mm. This finding was caused by a stricture in the distal CBD at the ampulla. The CBD is characteristically normal in Caroli's disease. Liver biopsy confirmed the diagnosis.

accounting for over 80% of cases in the United States. Pigment stones contain lesser amounts of cholesterol and higher percentages of calcium bilirubinate and glycoproteins.[6]

Although most gallstones remain asymptomatic throughout life, some are responsible for clinical symptoms, the most common being biliary colic. Laboratory blood values (Table 4.1) are often nonspecific, and imaging plays a vital role in diagnosis and management. The cumulative risk of gallstone complications is 1% per year. Complications of cholelithiasis include cholecystitis, pancreatitis, biliary fistula, gallstone

---

Box 4.2 **ESSENTIALS TO REMEMBER**

- Clinically significant biliary tract variants predispose patients to recurrent pancreatitis, cholangitis, choledocholithiasis, and biliary tract malignancies.

- The most clinically significant variants include:

  - Anomalous pancreatico-biliary junction: >15-mm common channel, commonly associated with type I choledochal cysts. When a large choledochal cyst is present, MRCP source images and MIP reconstructions must be carefully evaluated so as not to miss the long channel and its connection.

  - Types I and II choledochal cysts have the highest correlation with cancer.

  - Choledochoceles are associated with common bile duct stones.

  - Caroli's disease, Caroli's syndrome, and autosomal recessive polycystic disease affect the IHBD. Important features include right upper quadrant pain, fever, hepatic fibrosis, and cholangiocarcinoma.

Table 4.1 LABORATORY VALUES ASSOCIATED WITH BILIARY DISEASE

	LABORATORY VALUES				
DIAGNOSIS	ALANINE TRANSAMINASE (ALT)	ASPARTATE AMINOTRANSFERASE (AST)	GAMMA-GLUTAMYL TRANSPEPTIDASE (GGT)	SERUM BILIRUBIN	ALKALINE PHOSPHATASE (ALP)
Gallstones/ biliary colic	Normal to elevated	Normal to elevated	Normal	Normal	
Obstructive jaundice					
Intrahepatic	Elevated	Elevated	Elevated	Elevated	Elevated
Extrahepatic	Elevated	Elevated	Elevated	Elevated	Markedly elevated
Cholecystitis (uncomplicated)	Normal to elevated	Normal to elevated	Normal to elevated	Normal to elevated	

ileus, and Mirizzi syndrome. Cholelithiasis is found in two thirds of patients with gallbladder carcinoma, suggesting that chronic irritation may be a causative factor.[11]

Ultrasound is the most commonly used modality in the evaluation of gallstone disease, with a high specificity (>95%) and sensitivity (95%) for stones larger than 2 mm.

MRI shows gallstones best on T2-weighted images and MRCP. Stones appear as signal voids on both T1- and T2-weighted images. On T2-weighted images stones are visualized as "filling defects," areas of low signal intensity, within the high-intensity bile (Figs. 4.5 and 4.12). MRCP has reported sensitivity and specificity in the range of 89% to 100% and 83% to 100%, respectively, for detecting bile duct stones, and overall best results are obtained with careful examination of the thin source images.

Calculi are missed on MRCP most commonly when the stone caliber is 3 mm or less, or when the stones are not surrounded by enough bile to stand out in the high-signal-intensity fluid to be visualized. Stones impacted in the fluid-devoid ampulla of Vater are easily overlooked. A bile duct segment of impacted stones with little surrounding bile may be misinterpreted as a segmental stricture.

Differentiation between the type of stone may be important for determining treatment. The soft pigmented stones may be removed endoscopically, while cholesterol stones usually require surgery. Both cholesterol and pigment stones are shown as hypointense structures on T2-weighted sequences. However, pigment stones regularly have increased signal intensity on T1-weighted images, while cholesterol stones show with low signal intensity on these images.[9]

Stones presenting with biliary obstruction are most often found in the CBD and are easily seen on MRCP sequences (Fig. 4.13). MRCP has a 81% to 93% sensitivity and 91% to 98% specificity in detecting CBD stones, significantly higher than ultrasound and comparable to CT cholangiography.[3,12] Additionally, MRCP has comparable sensitivity and specificity to ERCP in the evaluation of choledocholithiasis and is superior to ERCP for detecting intrahepatic biliary ductal stones. MRCP is important in determining the presence of stones in the CBD prior to laparoscopic cholecystectomy. Patients at high risk for choledocholithiasis include those with symptomatic cholelithiasis, acute cholecystitis complicated by cholangitis, gallstone pancreatitis, a dilated CBD, and jaundice.

Differential diagnosis of "filling defects" in the biliary tree on MRCP images include stones, blood clot, air bubbles, neoplasm, sludge, and post-instrumentation debris. Other sources that can mimic stones include crossing vessels, nearby surgical clips from cholecystectomy, and vascular pulsation artifacts.

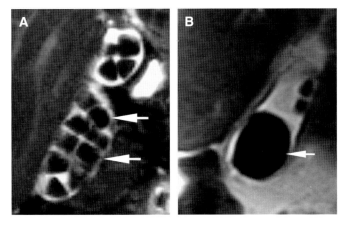

Figure 4.12 *Gallstones.* Single shot FSE/TSE T2-weighted images (**A**, **B**) of the gallbladder in two patients show gallstones (*arrows*) of varying size as foci of signal void surrounded by high-intensity bile. The faceted shape of gallstones is common and characteristic.

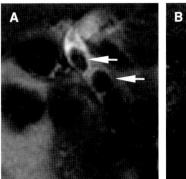
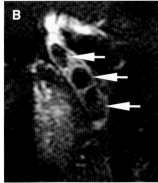

Figure 4.13 *Choledocholithiasis.* Coronal single shot FSE/TSE T2-weighted image (**A**) and source image from an MRCP sequence (**B**) demonstrate multiple gallstones (*arrows*) within the CBD against the high-signal-intensity, biliary fluid background in a man with colicky abdominal pain.

Biliary stones are commonly lamellated, oval, circular, or angular in shape and usually lie in the dependent portion of the duct. Neoplasms and blood clots, sometimes indistinguishable from calculi, tend to have irregular margins, and show different signal intensities on T1- and T2-weighted images than stones. In case of a neoplasm, tumor enhancement may be shown on post-contrast images.

Acute cholecystitis is by far the most common acute complication of gallstone disease. The clinical presentation is characterized by abdominal pain, classically in the right upper quadrant, fever, and leukocytosis. In 90% of cases, the cause is an impacted gallstone obstructing the cystic duct. Differential diagnosis of acute right upper quadrant pain includes pancreatitis, hepatic flexure diverticulitis, liver abscess, and peptic ulcer disease.

Acalculous cholecystitis occurs in the absence of stones and accounts for 5% to 10% of acute cholecystitis cases. Acalculous cholecystitis is usually seen in critically ill patients; is secondary to ischemia, inflammation, or infection (AIDS cholangitis); and carries higher morbidity and mortality rates than cholecystitis caused by stones. *Emphysematous cholecystitis* is an acalculous cholecystitis caused by gas-forming bacteria, usually in diabetic patients or in patients with cystic artery atherosclerotic disease.

Ultrasound is the usual modality of choice for the diagnosis of acute cholecystitis. It is, however, significantly limited in patients with a large body habitus. When sonographic findings are equivocal, MRI proves valuable in detecting stones in the gallbladder neck and cystic duct and associated gallbladder wall abnormalities. On T2-weighted images the gallbladder wall may show thickening and increased signal intensity due to inflammation, pericholecystic fluid, and edema surrounding the gallbladder.[6] Periportal hyperintensity, also seen with cholangitis, may be observed as well. Hyperemic enhancement of the hepatic parenchyma adjacent to the inflamed gallbladder, seen on dynamic contrast-enhanced images, is a specific sign for acute cholecystitis and is reported in up to 75% of patients.

Gallbladder empyema, or suppurative cholecystitis, refers to a pus-filled, distended gallbladder. Usually occurring in diabetic patients, it can progress quickly and behave like an intra-abdominal abscess. Heavily T2-weighted images show dependent low signal intensity of viscous pus resembling sludge and a thickened inflamed gallbladder wall.[13] Definitive diagnosis may require percutaneous needle aspiration or cholecystostomy.

Gangrenous cholecystitis is suggested by inhomogeneous or asymmetric wall thickening with focal disruption of the gallbladder wall enhancement, the "interrupted rim sign." The focally decreased enhancement represents areas of necrosis, intramural hemorrhage, or microabscess.[6]

Pericholecystic and liver abscesses result from perforation of the gallbladder and appear on contrast-enhanced images as localized rim-enhancing fluid collections. These complications of cholecystitis carry significant morbidity and mortality, so early diagnosis is crucial.

Chronic cholecystitis is the most common form of clinically symptomatic gallbladder disease and is almost always associated with gallstones.[14] Vague and sometimes equivocal signs and symptoms including abdominal distention, epigastric discomfort, and nausea are frequent.[14] On MR the gallbladder is found to be small and contracted, sometimes with irregular and thick walls.

Adenomyomatosis of the gallbladder is a fairly common (up to 9% of cholecystectomy specimens) non-inflammatory and benign condition that has a female predilection.[12] It may be asymptomatic or present with right upper quadrant pain. It is associated with gallstones in 90% of patients. Adenomyomatosis is characterized by excessive proliferation of surface epithelium with deep and branching invaginations (Rokitansky-Aschoff sinuses) into the thickened tunica muscularis. At gross pathologic examination adenomyomatosis manifests as diffuse, segmental, or focal disease. Diffuse adenomyomatosis manifests as circumferential wall thickening and overall luminal narrowing. In the segmental form, there is focal circumferential thickening in the midportion of the gallbladder, sometimes producing an hourglass appearance. The localized form of adenomyomatosis manifests as a focal, frequently semilunar or crescentic solid mass, usually in the fundus of the gallbladder.[6]

MR imaging demonstrates mural thickening and may be difficult to distinguish from gallbladder malignancy. Multiple intramural cystic components, which correlate with the bile-filled Rokitansky-Aschoff sinuses, characteristically demonstrate high signal intensity on T2-weighted images. It is this typical "string of beads" pattern that is most specific (92%) in differentiating adenomyomatosis from cancer. Contrast-enhanced T1-weighted images of the diffuse type show early mucosal and subsequent serosal enhancement. The focal type usually shows linear wall enhancement and a fundal semilunar or crescentic solid mass.[6]

Xanthogranulomatous cholecystitis is an uncommon inflammatory disease of the gallbladder that is characterized histologically by a focal or diffuse destructive inflammatory process with xanthoma-like foam cells, scarring, and nodules. Xanthogranulomatous cholecystitis is thought to be induced by intramural extravasation of bile from the Rokitansky-Aschoff sinuses or from superficial mucosal ulcerations, leading to an inflammatory response.[6] The disease usually manifests as acute episodes of cholecystitis in women in the sixth and seven decades and may persist for years. Gallstones are present in most patients. Gross macroscopic examination demonstrates a nodular gallbladder with thick and ill-defined walls with associated inflammatory change. The adjacent liver may be infiltrated by the inflammatory process. Rare complications include extension into nearby organs such as colon or duodenum and development of fistulous tracts or abscess formation.[6] At cross-sectional imaging, xanthogranulomatous cholecystitis closely resembles gallbladder carcinoma, with diffuse or focal gallbladder wall thickening, heterogeneous wall enhancement, and intramural nodules. MR imaging demonstrates intramural lesions with markedly elevated signal intensity on T2-weighted images. Preservation of linear mucosal enhancement on post-contrast enhanced T1-weighted MR is suggestive of xanthogranulomatous cholecystitis rather than carcinoma.[6] This is a helpful though not a specific differentiating finding.

Functional MRCP is an emerging technique that has the potential to provide a comprehensive anatomic and functional evaluation of the gallbladder and biliary tree. It is performed with hepatobiliary-specific contrast agents that are taken up by hepatocytes and are excreted in the bile. These agents shorten the T1 of bile, converting bile from low signal to high signal intensity on T1-weighted images. Contrast-enhanced functional T1-weighted MRCP is performed using a high-resolution T1-weighted 3D gradient-echo sequence. In practice, T1-weighted 3D gradient-echo often affords a smaller voxel size than that achieved by conventional single shot FSE/TSE. Enhancement of the bile is seen at 10 minutes or 20 minutes following intravenous contrast injection, depending upon the agent used. Demonstrated are anatomic abnormalities, strictures, stones, and subtle ductal as well as functional abnormalities such as cholecystitis, ductal obstruction, and biliary extravasation.

Acute cholecystitis may show a delay of greater than 4 hours in contrast enhancement of the gallbladder on contrast-enhanced functional T1-weighted MRCP images, in addition to the characteristic findings shown by conventional T2-weighted MRCP. Research concerning the diagnosis of chronic cholecystitis with functional MRCP thus far is very limited, but suggestive findings include delayed gallbladder filling, delayed gallbladder emptying, and decreased gallbladder response to intravenous cholecystokinin. Functional MRCP may help to rule out obstruction in a dilated but unobstructed biliary tree.

Mirizzi syndrome, a potential mimicker of cholangiocarcinoma, occurs when a calculus becomes impacted in the gallbladder neck or cystic duct, causing extrinsic narrowing of the common hepatic duct and obstruction (Fig 4.14).[15]

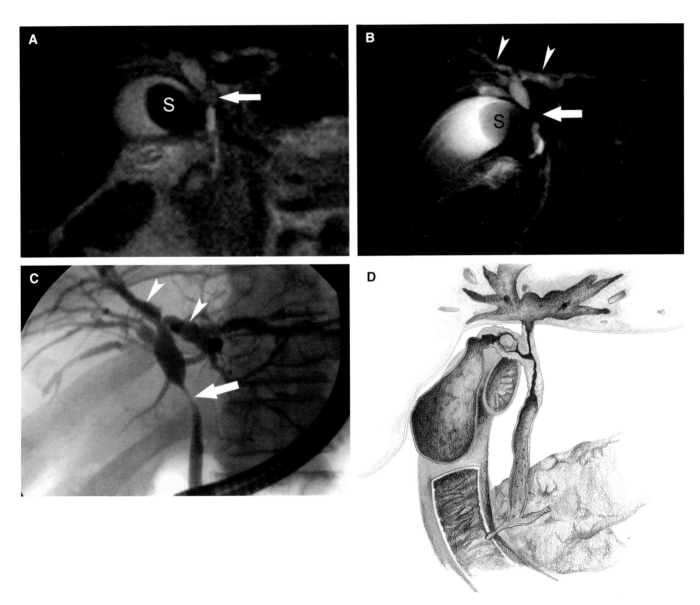

Figure 4.14 *Mirizzi syndrome.* Coronal single shot FSE/TSE T2-weighted (**A**), MRCP (**B**), and ERCP (**C**) images illustrate a large stone (*S*) impacted in the neck of the gallbladder and causing narrowing of the common hepatic bile duct (*arrow*) with upstream dilatation of the IHBD (*arrowheads*). (**D**) Schematic drawing of Mirizzi syndrome shows the gallstone impacted at the gallbladder neck with surrounding inflammation of the cystic and common hepatic ducts creating the findings of Mirizzi syndrome. Line drawing by Brooke Olazagasti, adapted from Federle MP, Jeffrey RB, Woodward PJ, Borhani A. *Diagnostic Imaging—Abdomen, Part II, Section 2, Biliary System.* Philadelphia: Lippincott Williams & Wilkins, 2009.

Box 4.3 **ESSENTIALS TO REMEMBER**

- Acute calculous cholecystitis, caused by a stone impacted in the cystic duct, is by far the most common acute complication of gallstone disease. MRI shows stones, gallbladder wall thickening with increased signal intensity on T2-weighted images, and hyperemic enhancement of the pericholecystic hepatic parenchyma on dynamic post-gadolinium-contrast enhanced images.

- Contrast-enhanced MRI improves detection of the serious complications of acute cholecystitis, including suppurative, emphysematous, and gangrenous cholecystitis and abscess formation.

- Complications of cholelithiasis include cholecystitis, pancreatitis, biliary fistula, gallstone ileus, and Mirizzi syndrome. Cholelithiasis is found in two thirds of patients with gallbladder carcinoma.

- T2-weighted images and thin-slice as well as thick-slab MRCP images are best to depict either cholelithiasis or choledocholithiasis. MRCP has significantly higher sensitivity and specificity in the diagnosis of choledocholithiasis than ultrasound and is comparable to CT cholangiography.

- MRCP has comparable sensitivity and specificity to ERCP in the diagnosis of choledocholithiasis and is superior to ERCP in the diagnosis of intrahepatic biliary ductal stones.

- Chronic cholecystitis is the most common form of clinically symptomatic gallbladder disease and is almost always associated with gallstones.

- Contrast-enhanced functional T1-weighted MRCP using hepatobiliary-specific contrast agents shows great promise in high-resolution functional evaluation of the biliary system.

This condition is facilitated by a low insertion of a long cystic duct that runs parallel to the common hepatic duct. A characteristic finding of Mirizzi syndrome is a large non-mobile stone in the neck of a shrunken gallbladder in association with dilatation of the IHBD. Repeated contractions of the gallbladder attempting to empty produces inflammation of the cystic and common hepatic ducts, which leads to further increase of the obstruction.

MRCP shows the typical features of Mirizzi syndrome: a gallstone within the cystic duct, dilatation of the IHBD and proximal common hepatic duct with extrinsic narrowing of the common hepatic duct, and a normal CBD.[15] Preoperative identification of this condition changes the surgical approach to an open procedure to avoid bile duct injury.

BILIARY DILATATION AND OBSTRUCTION

Obstructive jaundice results from blockage of the bile duct (Fig. 4.15). Causes include impaction of a calculus, postinflammatory or postsurgical strictures, and malignant tumors.[13] Laboratory values provide clues to diagnosis (see Table 4.1). The role of imaging is to determine the level and severity of the bile duct obstruction and to identify the cause of obstruction (Fig. 4.16).

MRI with MRCP can diagnose biliary ductal dilatation and obstruction with a very high degree of accuracy. Sensitivity of 91% to 96% and specificity of 99% to 100% have been reported. Since the entire biliary tract is included in the MR imaging volume, biliary evaluation is not limited by the ability to inject contrast material past an obstruction, as is the case with ERCP.[3] Associated abnormalities of the liver, pancreas, and retroperitoneum are clearly visualized and allowing a more complete differential diagnosis. Both standard T2-weighted or contrast-enhanced T1-weighted images are used to demonstrate ductal dilatation.[4] MRI with MRCP delineates the level and quantifies the degree of obstruction while characterizing the process causing the obstruction as benign or malignant (Fig. 4.17).

Obstructions of the bile duct caused by malignant tumors are characterized by abrupt margins with associated shouldering,

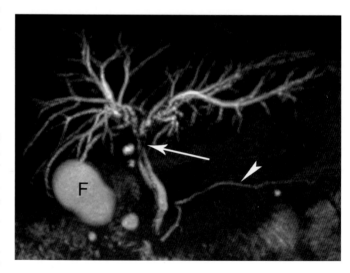

Figure 4.15 *Biliary obstruction caused by benign stricture.* In a patient with a liver transplant, thick-slab MRCP image shows a benign stricture (*arrow*) at the confluence causing mild dilatation of the IHBD. The gallbladder is absent, as is usual with a liver transplant. A postoperative fluid collection (*F*) is present in the gallbladder fossa. The pancreatic duct (*arrowhead*) is normal.

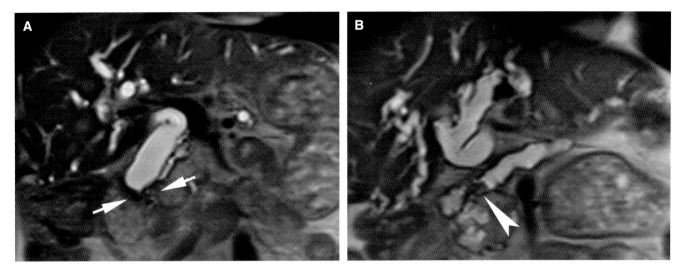

Figure 4.16 *Head of pancreas mass causing dilatation of biliary and pancreatic ducts.* (**A, B**) Coronal T2-weighted images show massive dilatation of both biliary and ductal pancreatic systems caused by a mass at the head of the pancreas. Notice the significant shouldering (*arrows* in image A) of the distal CBD at the level of the tumor and the abrupt irregular cutoff (*arrowhead* in image B) of the pancreatic duct.

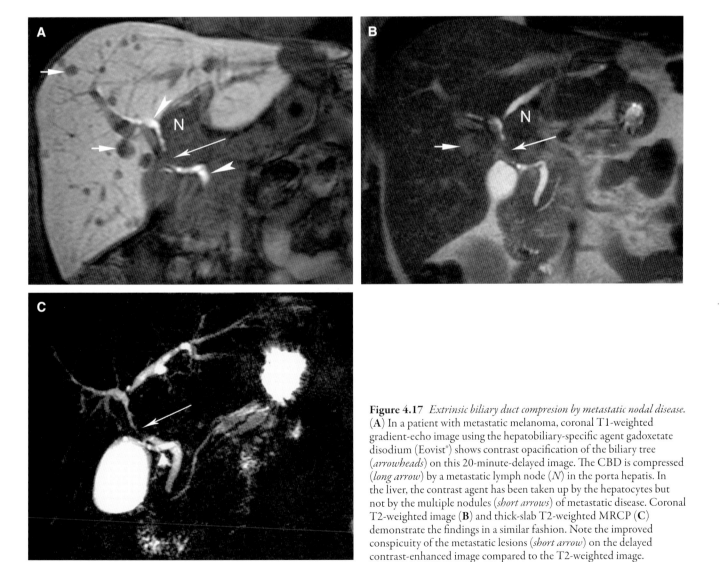

Figure 4.17 *Extrinsic biliary duct compresion by metastatic nodal disease.* (**A**) In a patient with metastatic melanoma, coronal T1-weighted gradient-echo image using the hepatobiliary-specific agent gadoxetate disodium (Eovist®) shows contrast opacification of the biliary tree (*arrowheads*) on this 20-minute-delayed image. The CBD is compressed (*long arrow*) by a metastatic lymph node (*N*) in the porta hepatis. In the liver, the contrast agent has been taken up by the hepatocytes but not by the multiple nodules (*short arrows*) of metastatic disease. Coronal T2-weighted image (**B**) and thick-slab T2-weighted MRCP (**C**) demonstrate the findings in a similar fashion. Note the improved conspicuity of the metastatic lesions (*short arrow*) on the delayed contrast-enhanced image compared to the T2-weighted image.

Box 4.4 ESSENTIALS TO REMEMBER

- Obstructive jaundice results from impeded bile flow caused by impacted calculi, strictures, and malignant tumors.

- MRI with MRCP delineates the level and severity of biliary obstruction while characterizing the cause as benign or malignant with very high degree of accuracy. Intrinsic biliary abnormalities are most commonly stones, while extrinsic abnormalities include primary tumors or enlarged lymph nodes.

- Thin-slice source images and heavily T2-weighted images should always be reviewed carefully to detect subtle "filling defects" (foci of low signal intensity) that may be caused by stones and to recognize artifacts that simulate pathology.

- Typical malignant strictures have abrupt margins with shouldering, are eccentric, and may extend over a long segment. Benign strictures usually have smoother, concentric, and tapered narrowing.

eccentric wall thickening, mucosal irregularity, and extension over a long segment of the duct (see Fig. 4.16). Etiologies of malignant obstruction in the porta hepatis include cholangiocarcinoma, central hepatoma, liver metastases, lymphadenopathy, and direct extension from adjacent cancers. Extrahepatic causes of malignant obstruction of the bile duct include pancreatic adenocarcinoma, ampullary cancer, and distal cholangiocarcinoma.

Benign strictures produce a more smooth, concentric, and tapered narrowing of the duct compared to strictures caused by malignancy.[3] Benign strictures can occur after passage of a stone or after surgery or trauma, or can be associated with chronic pancreatitis or infectious cholangitis. Careful inspection of thin-slice source images should alert the interpreter to crossing vessels, surgical clips, and to misregistration artifacts that mimic stone disease (see Fig. 4.4).

CHOLANGITIS

Cholangitis is classified as primary sclerosing, secondary sclerosing, and secondary non-sclerosing (Table 4.2).[16] Imaging differentiation between these entities is sometimes difficult because the MRI findings overlap. Differentiation is important, however, because some conditions require urgent intervention with surgical or percutaneous decompression to avoid serious complications. Familiarity with the classic imaging findings of each entity and careful correlation with clinical and laboratory findings establish the correct diagnosis.

Primary sclerosing cholangitis is characterized by chronic, progressive inflammation of the biliary tract that ultimately leads to fibrosis and destruction of the IHBDs and EHBDs.[16] This sequence of events leads to portal hypertension, hepatic failure, and cirrhosis within a median time frame of 12 years after the diagnosis of primary sclerosing cholangitis is made (Fig. 4.18). Most (75%) patients also suffer from inflammatory bowel disease, with 80% to 90% of these having ulcerative colitis and 10% to 20% having Crohn's disease (Fig. 4.18). Primary sclerosing cholangitis is associated with cholangiocarcinoma, which develops in 5% to 15% of the cases.[16]

Diagnostic findings on MRCP reach sensitivity and specificity of 88% and 97% respectively.[12] Together with conventional MRI, MRCP provides assessment of the bile duct proximal and distal to high-grade strictures and shows hepatic lobar atrophy and cirrhosis. The classic imaging findings of primary sclerosing cholangitis include multifocal strictures,

Table 4.2 CLASSIFICATION OF CHOLANGITIS

DIAGNOSIS	CLINICAL FEATURES/ETIOLOGY	MR IMAGING FINDINGS
Primary sclerosing	75% patients have inflammatory bowel disease. Progression to cirrhosis. 5–15% develop cholangiocarcinoma.	"String of beads," multifocal short strictures, pruning, diverticula
Secondary sclerosing		
Recurrent pyogenic cholangitis	Biliary parasites, clonorchis, ascaris, Southeast Asia descent. 2–6% of cholangiocarcinoma	Dilated IHBD/EHBD gallstones
Ascending cholangitis	Gallstones and infection in industrialized countries Poor nutrition and parasites in underdeveloped countries	Irregular borders, dilated bile ducts, thickened walls
AIDS	Opportunistic cytomegalovirus, Cryptosporidium, acalculous cholecystitis	IHBD strictures, ampullary stenosis, thick gallbladder wall; lack of EHBD involvement
Chemotherapy-induced	Iatrogenic after intra-arterial chemotherapy for liver tumors	Common hepatic duct strictures sparing distal CBD

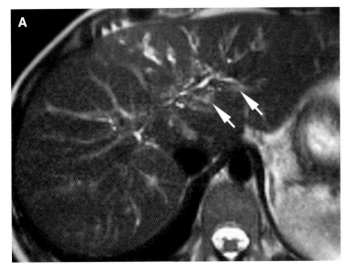

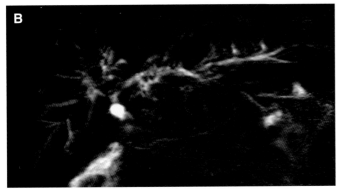

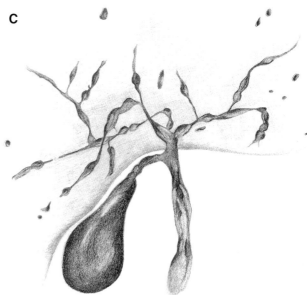

Figure 4.18 *Primary sclerosing cholangitis.* (**A**) Axial T2-weighted single shot FSE/TSE image of a young woman with Crohn's disease shows periportal edema (*arrows*) as focal areas of high signal intensity surrounding the portal triads. (**B**) MRCP thick-slab image shows interrupted appearance of IHBD with associated beading. (**C**) Schematic representation of primary sclerosing cholangitis with diffusely beaded appearance and alternating areas of stricture and normal ducts involving both the IHBD and the EHBD. Line drawing by Brooke Olazagasti, adapted from Johns Hopkins Medicine Gastroenterology and Hepatology website (www.hopkins-gi.org).

usually alternating with segments of normal ducts, segmental ectasia, ductal wall thickening, and irregular beading of the IHBD and EHBD. Pruning of peripheral ducts with isolated appearance of an ectatic duct may also be present. Periportal edema, best seen on T2-weighted images, and portocaval and periportal lymphadenopathy, commonly reactive, are frequently encountered. The strictures associated with cholangiocarcinoma are difficult to differentiate from inflammatory strictures, so serial imaging is usually needed. The presence of an enhancing periductal or intraductal mass with contiguous liver involvement is characteristic of cholangiocarcinoma.

Ascending cholangitis is secondary to complete or partial biliary obstruction (most commonly by gallstones) in conjunction with ascending infection from the bowel.[12] Inflammation of the IHBD and EHBD occurs secondary to ductal obstruction.

MRI findings classically demonstrate hypointense gallstones and thickened and enhancing bile walls coupled with ductal dilatation and strictures. Biliary dilatation in ascending cholangitis predominantly occurs in the central liver, as opposed to the peripheral third-ductal involvement commonly seen with primary sclerosing cholangitis. The pruning and alternating multifocal strictures seen in primary sclerosing cholangitis are not frequently seen in ascending cholangitis.[12] Specific MR imaging findings of ascending cholangitis include pus-filled IHBDs shown as low signal intensity structures on heavily T2-weighted images and intermediate signal intensity on fat-suppressed T1-weighted sequences.[13] Periportal edema

is shown with high signal intensity on T2-weighted images along the intrahepatic and extrahepatic portal veins.[13]

Acute suppurative cholangitis is a potentially life-threatening complication of stone disease with bacterial infection, acute cholecystitis, liver abscess, and sepsis.[13,16] The acute obstruction produces increased pressure within the hepatobiliary tree, which leads to hepatovenous bacterial reflux and sepsis.[13] Prompt intervention with surgical or percutaneous cholecystostomy and gram-negative antibiotic coverage is required as this suppurative disease carries a near-100% mortality rate if left untreated.[16]

AIDS cholangiopathy prevalence has decreased dramatically after widespread use of antiretroviral drugs.[15] Affected patients usually have cluster of differentiation 4 (CD4) cell counts below 135/mm^3. Patients present with fever, right upper quadrant pain, and jaundice. Typically affecting the large intrahepatic ducts, AIDS cholangiopathy is characterized by fibrotic strictures of the IHBD and the CBD. The cholangiopathy is caused by *Cytomegalovirus* and *Cryptosporidium* organisms, herpes simplex virus, *Mycobacterium avium complex*, and *Microsporidium*. No definite pathogen can be identified in almost half of patients. Sphincterotomy provides pain relief but does not alter the intrahepatic disease. MRI findings include irregular mural thickening of IHBD, thickening of the gallbladder wall, pericholecystic fluid, and ampullary stenosis. The lack of involvement of the EHBD is important in differentiating AIDS cholangiopathy from primary sclerosing cholangitis.

Box 4.5 ESSENTIALS TO REMEMBER

- Cholangitis is most commonly caused by a bile duct obstruction with an intraluminal stone.

- With this disease MRI classically demonstrates hypointense stones and thickened and enhancing bile duct walls associated with dilatation and strictures.

- Classic imaging findings of primary sclerosing cholangitis include multifocal strictures alternating with normal ducts, segmental dilatation, thickening of bile duct walls, and irregular beading of the IHBDs and EHBDs. Primary sclerosing cholangitis is strongly associated with ulcerative colitis and development of biliary cirrhosis and cholangiocarcinoma.

- Clinical history, laboratory values, and careful interpretation of MR images are vital for differentiating the various types of cholangitis.

- The strictures of cholangiocarcinoma are difficult to differentiate from benign inflammatory strictures and require careful comparison on serial imaging.

Recurrent pyogenic cholangitis, also known as "Oriental cholangiohepatitis," is characterized by repeated attacks of acute pyogenic cholangitis that occur in the setting of biliary obstruction associated with pigmented calculi and biliary strictures.[15] Patients present with recurrent abdominal pain, fever, and jaundice. The disease is common between the third and fifth decades and shows no sex predilection. Linked pathogens include *Ascaris lumbricoides*, *Clonorchis sinensis*, *Opisthorchis viverrini*, *O. felineus*, and *Fasciola hepatica*. Infestation incites cholangiocyte injury that leads to inflammatory strictures with chronic recurrent pyogenic infections, development of pigmented calculi, and cholangitic abscesses.[12,15] Patients with recurrent pyogenic cholangitis have an increased risk (2% to 6%) of developing cholangiocarcinoma.

Imaging manifestations include biliary strictures, ductal wall thickening secondary to fibrosis, and intraductal stones. The imaging hallmark of recurrent pyogenic cholangitis is complete obstruction of the IHBD secondary to a stricture or impacted stones.[3] The disease shows particular predilection for the lateral segment of the left lobe, the posterior segment of the right lobe, and the extrahepatic ducts.[15]

PREOPERATIVE AND POSTOPERATIVE BILIARY IMAGING

Preoperative anatomic assessment, "road-mapping" the biliary tree, is an invaluable tool in preventing surgical complications during laparoscopic cholecystectomy, liver transplantation, and biliary-enteric anastomosis.[6,17] Anatomic variants of the biliary tree are seen in up to 30% of patients and are known risk factors for bile tract injury during surgical intervention. The most common anomalies include a low and medial-sided insertion of the cystic duct (Fig. 4.19), a parallel course of the cystic duct alongside the common hepatic duct, and an aberrant right hepatic duct.[17] MRCP is a noninvasive, safe, and rapid way to demonstrate the anatomic variations of the biliary tract. Hepatic vascular variants are well demonstrated by concomitant contrast-enhanced MR angiography and venography.

Postoperative biliary complications increase with the frequency of hepatobiliary surgery. Biliary tract complications after liver transplantation occur in 13% to 35% of patients and endanger allograft survival in a significant portion of these. Complications include anastomotic leak, biloma, stricture with obstruction, and stone disease. Bile duct strictures (see Fig. 4.15) are the most common late complications of liver transplantation and can develop a few months or years after the procedure.[6,17] Additional complications of hepatobiliary surgery include bile duct injury caused by a misplaced surgical clip, inadvertent cutting or ligation of a bile duct, periductal bile leakage with resultant edema, fibrosis and secondary stricture, and ischemia.[17] Calculi may remain within the cystic duct remnant, the intrahepatic ducts, or the extrahepatic biliary tree after a laparoscopic cholecystectomy, sphincterotomy, or biliary–enteric anastomosis. Retained CBD calculi lead to continued pain, or signs and symptoms of

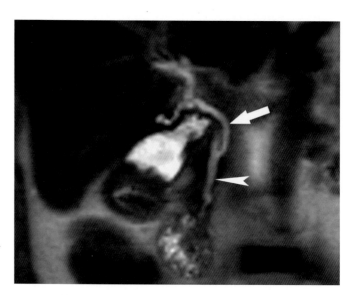

Figure 4.19 *Variant anatomy of the cystic duct.* Coronal T2-weighted single shot FSE/TSE image depicts a low and medial insertion of the cystic duct (*arrow*) into the CBD (*arrowhead*). This anomaly requires a different surgical approach when performing cholecystectomy to avoid complications

Box 4.6 ESSENTIALS TO REMEMBER

- Preoperative anatomic assessment of the biliary tree with MRCP and of the hepatic vascular anatomy with MRA and MRV has become invaluable in preventing complications of hepatobiliary surgery.

- During the past decade, the increasing number of hepatobiliary surgical procedures has increased the frequency of postoperative biliary complications.

- Postsurgical fluid collections are identified and characterized by MR so management can be decided based on imaging without invasive intervention.

- Contrast-enhanced T1-weighted MRCP using hepatobiliary-specific contrast agents may provide higher-resolution imaging of the biliary tree than conventional T2-weighted MRCP and adds functional information with regard to the biliary excretion.

biliary obstruction.[17] Prompt and accurate diagnosis is crucial for treatment planning.

Percutaneous transhepatic cholangiography and ERCP are invasive techniques that may lead to further complications. Both studies are limited by nonvisualization of ductal structures beyond a complete obstruction. MRCP and contrast-enhanced MR provide both anatomic and functional information to identify bile leaks, dropped stones, calculus retention, and fluid collections such as hematoma, seroma, biloma, and abscess. Fluid collections are extremely common in the postoperative hepatobiliary patient and require characterization for adequate treatment. Characteristic extracellular blood signal intensity on MR images suggests hematoma, while enhancement after contrast material administration suggests abscess.

PROBLEM SOLVING WITH HEPATOBILIARY-SPECIFIC AGENTS

Three contrast agents recently developed for hepatobiliary imaging are mangafodipir trisodium (Mn-DPDP), gadobenate dimeglumine (Gd-BOPTA or MultiHance®), and gadoxetic acid (Gd-EOB-DTPA or Eovist®). Only the latter two are approved by the Food and Drug Administration for use in the United States. These agents are taken up by functioning hepatocytes and excreted in the bile. Thus, they are particularly useful in determining whether a lesion contains hepatocytes or is not hepatocellular in origin.[18] Biliary excretion allows assessment of the biliary tract. Inherent paramagnetic properties of the contrast agents cause T1 shortening of the liver and bile, making the agent useful for contrast-enhanced T1-weighted MRCP in combination with routine T2-weighted MRCP. Contrast-enhanced T1-weighted MRCP offers potential for high resolution imaging and functional assessment of biliary excretion not possible with conventional T2-weighted MRCP. However, fluid collections that may obscure important findings on T2-weighted MRCP are less conspicuous on contrast-enhanced T1-weighted MRCP.[18]

In the normal liver, Gd-BOPTA and Gd-EOB-DTPA are excreted in the bile at approximately 20 minutes and 10 minutes, respectively, after the start of contrast agent injection. Delay in appearance of contrast agent in the bile is evidence of impaired biliary excretion or obstruction. Delayed imaging is required to visualize the contrast-enhanced biliary tree if significant obstruction is present. Acute cholecystitis is diagnosed by scintigraphy if the gallbladder does not fill at 4 hours (or at 90 minutes following morphine or cholecystokinin stimulation). The same criteria may apply for diagnosis of acute cholecystitis by contrast-enhanced T1-weighted MRCP. If severe hepatic dysfunction or high-grade biliary obstruction is present, no excretion of the contrast agent into the bile may occur.

GALLBLADDER CARCINOMA

Gallbladder carcinoma is a rare but aggressive malignancy. It predominantly affects females (3:1 ratio) and has an incidence of 2.5 new cases per 100,000 population per year. Average age of presentation is 65. These tumors present with vague and nonspecific symptoms of right upper quadrant abdominal pain, weight loss, and fever. Obstructive jaundice develops when the tumor involves the CBD or the common hepatic or right hepatic duct. Most (90%) gallbladder malignancies are adenocarcinomas, with the remainder being small cell and squamous cell carcinomas. Risk factors include gallstones, found in 90% of cases; porcelain (calcified wall) gallbladder; a long common pancreatic biliary channel, which allows pancreatic juice reflux; and chronic typhoid carrier state.[6]

Because of the thinness of the muscular layer and the continuity of the connective tissue of the gallbladder wall with the interlobular connective tissue of the liver, gallbladder carcinoma can easily invade the liver and gain access to the lymphatic and vascular channels (Fig. 4.20). Lymphatic spread usually involves the cystic and pericholedochal nodes initially, with subsequent extension into the posterior pancreaticoduodenal, retroportal, and celiac nodes. Involvement of the interaortocaval nodes occurs later and is considered tumor stage M1 (Table 4.3). Once it has penetrated the serosa, the tumor can also spread to the peritoneal cavity.[6] Most tumors are advanced at presentation, with direct extension to the liver and regional or distant lymph nodes. The median survival time is 3 months and the 5-year survival rate a dismal 5%.[12] Newer more radical operations, including removal of the gallbladder and hepatic segments IVb and V (sometimes with

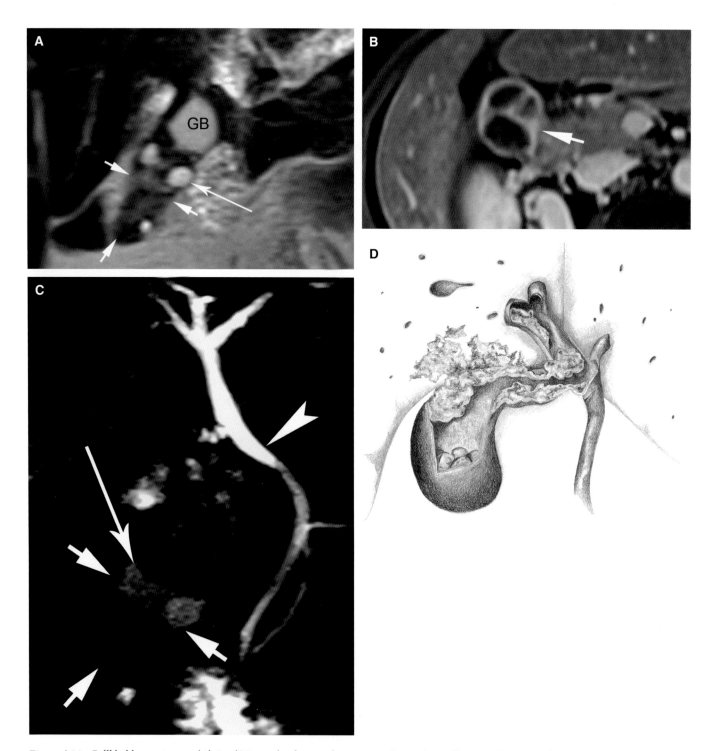

Figure 4.20 *Gallbladder carcinoma.* (**A**) Axial T2-weighted image shows an intraluminal mass (between *short arrows*) replacing a large portion of the gallbladder (*GB*). Prominent cystic areas (*long arrow*) are present within the mass. Multiple tiny (1 to 2 mm) gallstones found are embedded within the mass and are seen as tiny areas of signal void. (**B**) Post-gadolinium-contrast-enhanced axial T1-weighted image shows enhancement of the irregular wall (*arrow*). (**C**) Thick-slab MRCP shows an irregular "filling defect" (between *short arrows*) replacing the normal high-signal bile within the gallbladder lumen. The complex cystic areas (*long arrow*) within the tumor are lower in signal intensity on T2-weighted images than the bile filling the CBD and cystic duct. Surgery confirmed moderately differentiated adenocarcinoma of the gallbladder. The CBD (*arrowhead*) is not affected by the tumor. (**D**) Schematic representation of advanced gallbladder carcinoma shows an advanced, infiltrating tumor with invasion of adjacent liver and bile ducts. Unfortunately, this is a typical presentation. Line drawing by Brooke Olazagasti, adapted from Federle MP, Jeffrey RB, Woodward PJ, Borhani A. *Diagnostic Imaging—Abdomen, Part II, Section 2, Biliary System.* Philadelphia: Lippincott Williams & Wilkins, 2009.

extended right hepatectomy) and regional lymphadenectomy, are achieving significantly better results than previously possible, increasing the 5-year survival rate up to 50%.[6]

At macroscopic examination, gallbladder cancer typically manifests as:

- *Focal or diffuse mural thickening* of more than 1 cm. Wall enhancement is usually irregular, early, and prolonged. In chronic cholecystitis, an important clinical differentiation, wall enhancement is usually smooth, slow, and prolonged.

- *Intraluminal polypoid mass* (25% of cases) (Fig. 4.20) tends to have a better overall prognosis and is sometimes found incidentally. Polypoid lesions larger than 1 cm are more likely cancers. Malignant intraluminal polypoid lesions demonstrate early and prolonged enhancement. Benign lesions usually demonstrate early enhancement with subsequent washout.[6]

- *Soft tissue mass replacing the gallbladder* with invasion of the liver is the most common manifestation (more than 68% of cases).

Non-visualization of the gallbladder and the presence of gallstones within the mass are helpful in making the diagnosis. The mass demonstrates intermediate signal intensity on T1-weighted and heterogeneously hyperintense signal intensity on T2-weighted images. Enhancement is early and prolonged after gadolinium-based contrast material administration.[1,6,12]

Gadolinium-enhanced fat-suppressed T1-weighted images are useful in diagnosing tumor extent, direct invasion of surrounding organs, liver metastases, and involvement of critical vascular structures such as the portal vein and hepatic artery.[3] MRI has high sensitivity (up to 92%) for the detection of lymphadenopathy. MRCP facilitates identification of the site of biliary obstruction, which may be caused by bile duct compression or invasion by the tumor or by lymphadenopathy. MRI and MRCP are not as effective in detecting bile duct invasion, with a reported 69% sensitivity. Microscopic invasion should be suspected in cases of tumor contiguity with a duct, even if a biliary obstruction is not present. Small metastatic peritoneal implants are better appreciated on delayed gadolinium-contrast-enhanced fat-suppressed T1-weighted images. Staging of gallbladder carcinoma is reviewed in Table 4.3.

Other gallbladder malignancies are relatively rare and include lymphoma, typically non-Hodgkin's, and metastatic lesions from melanoma and breast primaries. Melanoma presents as a focal nodule with high signal intensity on T1-weighted images, dependent on the amount of melanin content of the lesion (Fig. 4.21).[12]

BILE DUCT NEOPLASMS

Biliary hamartomas, also known as von Meyenburg complexes, are small congenital biliary cysts (less than 1.5 cm). These lesions are composed of dilated bile ducts with interspersed fibrous stroma. The appearance on MRI is that of

Table 4.3 TNM STAGING OF GALLBLADDER CARCINOMA

STAGE	FINDINGS
T stage	**Size and location of the tumor**
TX	The primary tumor cannot be assessed (information not available)
T0	No evidence of primary tumor
Tis	Carcinoma in situ
T1	Tumor invades lamina propria or muscle layer
T1a	Tumor invades lamina propria
T1b	Tumor invades muscle layer
T2	Tumor invades perimuscular connective tissue; no extension beyond serosa or into the liver
T3	Tumor perforates the serosa (visceral peritoneum) and/or directly invades the liver and/or adjacent organ or structure, such as the stomach, duodenum, colon, pancreas, omentum, or extrahepatic bile ducts
T4	Tumor invades main portal vein or hepatic artery or invades two or more extrahepatic organs or structures
N stage	**Involvement of lymph nodes**
NX	Regional lymph nodes cannot be assessed (information not available)
N0	No spread to regional lymph nodes
N1	Metastases to nodes along the cystic duct, common bile duct, hepatic artery, and/or portal vein
N2	Metastases to periaortic, pericaval, superior mesenteric artery, and/or celiac artery lymph nodes.
M stage	**Distant metastases**
M0	No metastatic disease
M1	Distant metastases are present (distant lymph nodes, lung, bones, brain, etc.)

Reprinted with permission from American Joint Committee on Cancer. *AJCC Cancer Staging Manual*, 7th ed. Springer, 2010. Effective with the 2010 edition, this staging system now includes the cystic duct.

innumerable tiny cysts throughout the hepatic parenchyma (see Fig. 3.10). Biliary hamartomas display low signal intensity on T1-weighted and high signal intensity on T2-weighted images. Wall enhancement is sometimes visible. The differential diagnosis includes multiple cysts as in polycystic liver disease, Caroli's disease, microabscesses, and most importantly, cystic or poorly vascularized metastases.

Biliary cystadenoma is a rare benign cystic neoplasm lined by mucin-secreting epithelium. The lesions are thought to represent the premalignant form of biliary cystadenocarcinoma; therefore, resection is usually recommended. Typical presentation is that of a middle-aged woman with abdominal pain, a palpable mass, elevated liver function tests, jaundice,

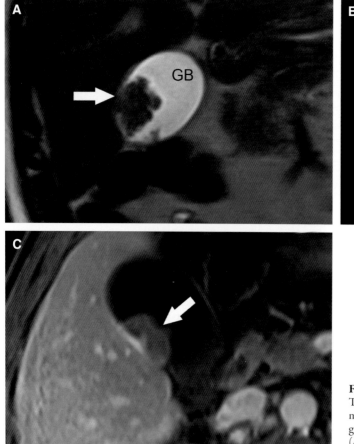

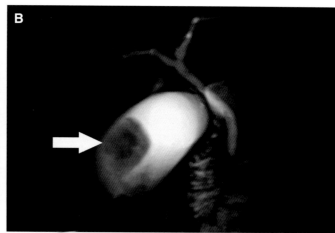

Figure 4.21 *Melanoma metastasis to the gallbladder.* Coronal T2-weighted image (**A**) and thick-slab MRCP (**B**) show a polypoid mass (*arrow*) within the lumen of the gallbladder (*GB*). (**C**) Post-gadolinium-contrast-enhanced image shows enhancement of the mass (*arrow*) and irregularity of the wall. This patient had widely spread melanoma with metastatic disease in multiple other organs.

and fever, with or without weight loss. Smaller lesions are asymptomatic and are incidentally discovered by imaging. Biliary cystadenomas are frequently large, with lesions reported up to 12 cm in diameter. On MRI, the tumors are multilocular cystic lesions (Fig. 4.22) and can mimic simple cysts. Internal septa and mural nodularity may be identified, resulting in considerable overlap with the imaging appearances of cystadenocarcinoma. Although the presence of mural nodules does not allow distinction between cystadenoma and cystadenocarcinoma, the absence of mural nodules suggests the diagnosis of cystadenoma.

Cholangiocarcinoma is a malignant tumor arising from the biliary tract and is the second most common hepatobiliary malignancy after hepatoma.[12] Tumors show no gender predilection and the peak incidence is in the sixth to seventh

decade. Presenting symptoms include abdominal pain, pruritus, anorexia, and obstructive jaundice. Most cholangiocarcinomas are adenocarcinomas with abundant fibrous stroma, which causes characteristic delayed hyperenhancement in 40%.[19,20]

Risk factors for cholangiocarcinoma share the common features of chronic biliary inflammation, including infection with liver flukes (*Clonorchis sinensis*, *Opisthorchis* viverini), hepatolithiasis, and association with nitrosamine compounds (found in tobacco, latex products, beer, and fish).[19] Thorotrast, a contrast agent no longer in use, is a known highly potent carcinogen with a significantly increased risk for the development of liver and biliary tumors. Gallstones in the IHBD, commonly associated with recurrent pyogenic cholangitis, are found in up to 70% of cholangiocarcinomas in

---

Box 4.7 **ESSENTIALS TO REMEMBER**

- The classic presentation of gallbladder carcinoma is a soft tissue mass that replaces part or the entire gallbladder and demonstrates intermediate signal intensity on T1-weighted and heterogeneous, hyperintense signal intensity on T2-weighted images.

- Enhancement in gallbladder carcinoma is early and prolonged after gadolinium-based contrast material administration. Dynamic gadolinium-contrast-enhanced fat-suppressed T1-weighted images are useful in determining tumor extent, direct invasion of surrounding organs, liver metastases, lymphadenopathy, and involvement of the portal vein and hepatic artery.

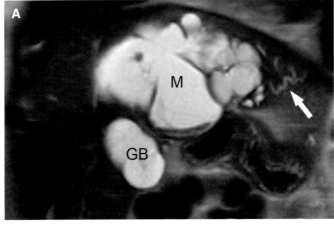

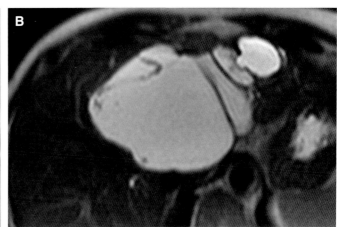

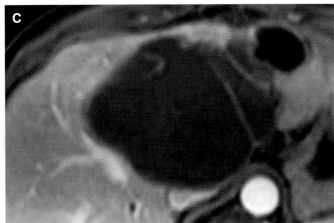

Figure 4.22 *Biliary cystadenoma.* Axial (**A**) and coronal (**B**) T2-weighted single shot FSE/TSE images demonstrate a large multilocular, septated mass (*M*) within the left hepatic lobe intimately associated with the biliary system. The bile ducts (*arrow* in image A) peripheral to the mass are dilated and tortuous. *GB*, gallbladder. (**C**) Post-gadolinium-contrast-enhanced T1-weighted image shows enhancement of the sepatations. Patient was symptomatic and the lesion was resected, revealing a benign biliary cystadenoma.

endemic areas.[20] In Western countries, cirrhosis, chronic hepatitis C, heavy alcohol consumption, primary sclerosing cholangitis, and chronic inflammatory bowel disease are risk factors for cholangiocarcinoma.[19,20] Cholangiocarcinoma can develop in a congenital choledochal cyst, with a lifetime risk of 10% to 15%.[20]

Cholangiocarcinoma is categorized into three types on the basis of gross morphologic features (mass-forming [the most common], periductal infiltrating, and intraductal growth) and on anatomic location: *hilar*, arising at the confluence (Klatskin tumor) (60%) (Figs. 4.23 and 4.24); *distal*, arising from the common hepatic duct or the CBD (30%) (Fig. 4.25); and *intrahepatic*, arising from the peripheral bile ducts within the liver (10%) (Figs. 4.25 and 4.26).[17,18]

MR has become an invaluable tool in the diagnosis, staging, and treatment planning of malignant biliary disease (Tables 4.4, 4.5, 4.6).[21] Hilar and extrahepatic cholangiocarcinomas tend to spread along the circumference of the bile ducts and are sometimes difficult to visualize adequately on T1- and T2-weighted images. These tumors present with secondary signs of upstream ductal dilatation with abrupt shouldering and irregular strictures. MRCP shows the dilatation proximal and the normal duct distal to the site of obstruction. Ductal wall thickening is not a defining characteristic for cholangiocarcinoma since cholangitis can also present in

this fashion. However, irregular wall thickening of 5 mm or more, and prolonged delayed enhancement of the duct wall suggest malignancy. Smoother, concentric thickening with tapered narrowing and early enhancement suggest benign etiologies.

The tumors demonstrate hypo- or iso-intensity to liver parenchyma on T1-weighted images and iso- to slight hyperintensity to liver on T2-weighted images (Fig. 4.26). They are typically hypovascular, showing little enhancement on early post–contrast enhanced images and progressive heterogeneous enhancement on delayed-phase images.[12] Irregular enhancement may be accompanied by capsular retraction and satellite nodules.[20] These lesions can be fairly well circumscribed and manifest vascular encasement without visible tumor thrombus.[20] More prominent ductal dilatation and associated segmental hepatic atrophy are seen when the tumor occupies one of the first-order ducts (Fig. 4.27).

Intraductal biliary cancers display several imaging patterns, including diffuse and marked ductal ectasia with or without a visible papillary mass; an intraductal polypoid mass within localized ductal dilatation; intraductal cast-like lesion within a mildly dilated duct; and focal stricture-like lesion with mild proximal ductal dilatation.[20,21]

The TNM classification of cholangiocarcinoma has been recently (2010) revised by the American Joint

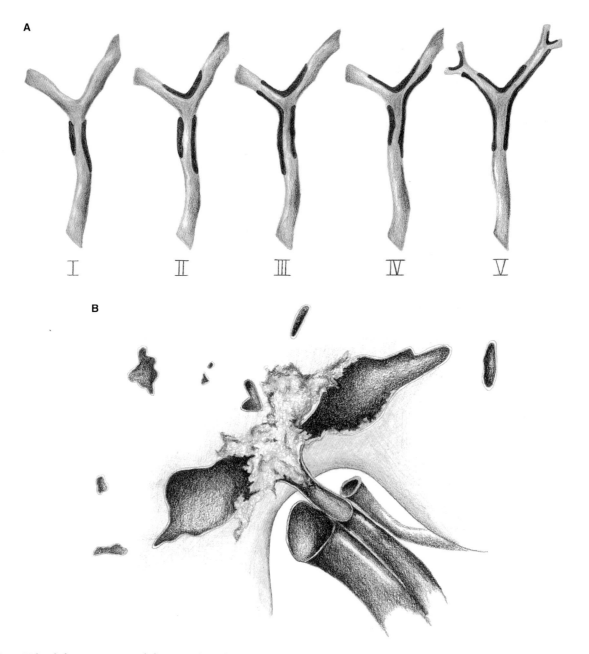

Figure 4.23 *Hilar cholangiocarcinoma.* (**A**) Staging depends on tumoral involvement at the hilum and its intrahepatic extension into the right and left IHBD system, as well as vascular invasion. Shaded areas represent tumor involvement. Typically resectable tumors include stages I–III. Line drawing by Brooke Olazagasti, adapted from Nisha I, Sainani O, Catalano A, et al. Cholangiocarcinoma: Current and Novel Imaging Techniques. *Radiographics.* 2008;28:1263-1287. (**B**) Schematic drawing demonstrates an infiltrative hilar cholangiocarcinoma with involvement of both left and right IHBDs and upstream dilatation of the biliary ductal system. This lesion would be at least a Bismuth IV lesion, with further staging dependent on the vascular invasion. Line drawing by Brooke Olazagasti, adapted from Federle MP, Jeffrey RB, Woodward PJ, Borhani A. *Diagnostic Imaging—Abdomen, Part II, Section 2, Biliary System.* Philadelphia: Lippincott Williams & Wilkins, 2009.

Committee on Cancer (Tables 4.4, 4.5, and 4.6). The revised Bismuth-Corlette classification of perihilar cholangiocarcinomas is as follows:

- *Type I* involves the common hepatic duct.

- *Type II* involves the common hepatic duct, and the junction of the right hepatic duct and left hepatic duct, without involvement of the secondary intrahepatic ducts.

- *Type IIIA* involves the CBD, biliary junction, and the right hepatic duct including its secondary intrahepatic ducts.

- *Type IIIB* involves the CBD, biliary junction, and the left hepatic duct including its secondary intrahepatic ducts.

- *Type IV* involves the CBD biliary junction, with extension to the secondary intrahepatic ducts on both the right and left side, or there is a multifocal bile duct tumor (see Fig 4.23A).[22]

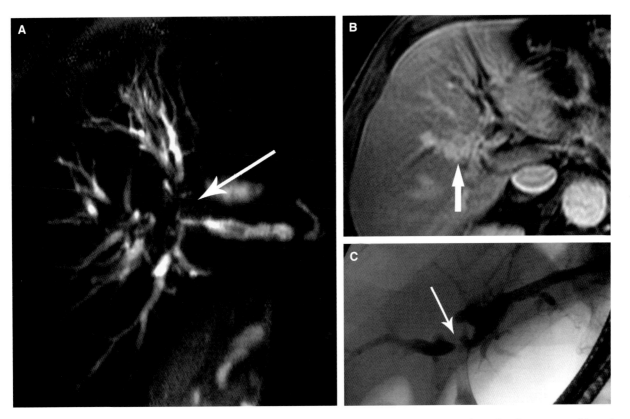

Figure 4.24 *Hilar cholangiocarcinoma, unresectable.* (**A**) MRCP thick-slab image shows an irregular stricture (*arrow*) at the junction of the right and left bile ducts involving the secondary intrahepatic ducts on both sides and the proximal common hepatic duct. (**B**) Delayed post-contrast-enhanced images show an enchancing perihilar soft tissue mass (*arrow*). (**C**) ERCP confirms the findings (*arrow*) and guided biopsy, which showed cholangiocarcinoma. The extent of involvement makes this tumor a Bismuth type IV, unresectable lesion.

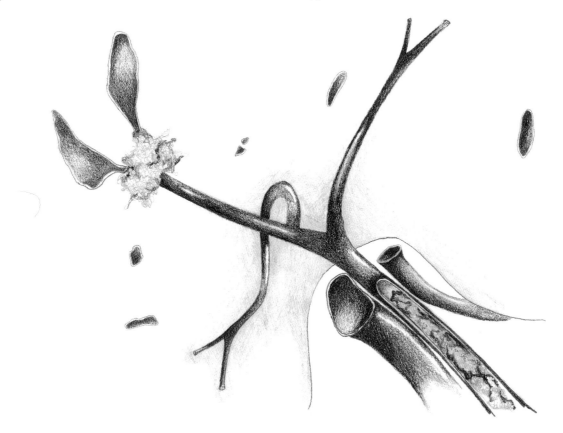

Figure 4.25 *Peripheral and infiltrating ductal cholangiocarcinoma.* Drawing shows two separate kinds of cholangiocarcinoma by anatomic location: the peripheral mass-forming type and the extrahepatic type arising from the CBD. Line drawing by Brooke Olazagasti, adapted from Federle MP, Jeffrey RB, Woodward PJ, Borhani A. *Diagnostic Imaging—Abdomen, Part II, Section 2, Biliary System.* Philadelphia: Lippincott Williams & Wilkins, 2009.

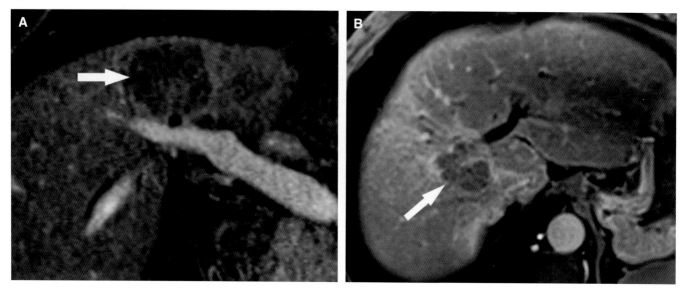

Figure 4.26 *Peripheral cholangiocarcinoma.* Post-gadolinium-contrast-enhanced coronal (**A**) and axial (**B**) T1-weighted gradient echo images show an intrahepatic tumor (*arrow*), which was proven by histopathologic examination to be cholangiocarcinoma. These tumors arise from the intrahepatic bile ducts in the periphery of the liver and do not involve the hilar region or the common hepatic or common bile duct.

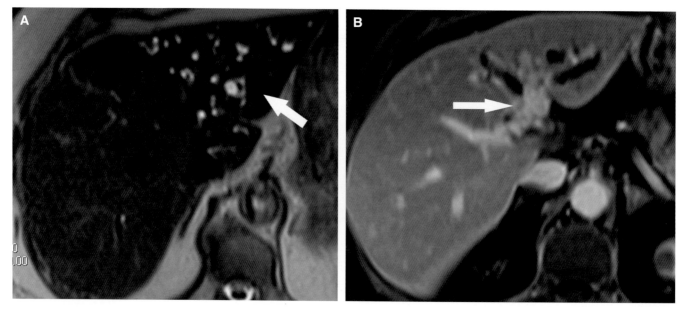

Figure 4.27 *Cholangiocarcinoma with hepatic atrophy.* (**A**) Axial T2-weighted image demononstrates asymmetric dilatation of IHBD in the left lobe (*arrow*). The parenchyma of the left lobe shows mild atrophy. (**B**) Delayed post-gadolinium-enhanced T1-weighted image demonstrates a mass (*arrow*) along the intrahepatic ducts with asymmetric involvement of the left-sided ductal system. At surgery, the mass involved the left hepatic duct and extended to the confluence with the right hepatic duct, with involvement of the first-degree radicles just beyond the confluence. The lesion proved to be unresectable, a Bismuth IV lesion.

Table 4.4 TNM STAGING OF PERIHILAR BILE DUCT CANCER

STAGE	FINDINGS
T stage	**Primary Tumor (T)**
TX	The primary tumor cannot be assessed (information not available)
T0	No evidence of primary tumor
Tis	Carcinoma in situ
T1	Tumor confined to bile duct, with extension up to the muscle layer or fibrous tissue
T2a	Tumor invades beyond the wall of the bile duct to surrounding adipose tissue
T2b	Tumor invades adjacent hepatic parenchyma
T3	Tumor invades unilateral branches of the portal vein or hepatic artery
T4	Tumor involves the main portal vein or its branches bilaterally; or the common hepatic artery; or the second-order biliary radicals bilaterally; or unilateral second-order biliary radicals with contralateral portal vein or hepatic artery involvement
N stage	**Involvement of Regional Lymph Nodes (N)**
NX	Regional lymph nodes cannot be assessed (information not available)
N0	No spread to regional lymph nodes
N1	Regional lymph node metastases (includes nodes along the cystic duct, common bile duct, hepatic artery, and portal vein
N2	Metastases to periaortic, pericaval, superior mesenteric artery, and/or celiac artery lymph nodes
M stage	**Distant metastases**
M0	No metastatic disease
M1	Distant metastases are present

Reprinted with permission from American Joint Committee on Cancer. *AJCC Cancer Staging Manual*, 7th ed. Springer, 2010. Effective with the 2010 edition extrahepatic bile duct tumors are now separated into perihilar and distal groups, with separate staging classifications for each.

Table 4.5 TNM STAGING OF DISTAL BILE DUCT CANCER

STAGE	FINDINGS
T stage	**Primary Tumor (T)**
TX	The primary tumor cannot be assessed (information not available)
T0	No evidence of primary tumor
Tis	Carcinoma in situ
T1	Tumor confined to bile duct histologically
T2	Tumor invades beyond the wall of the bile duct
T3	Tumor invades the gallbladder, pancreas, duodenum, or other adjacent organs without involvement of the celiac axis or the superior mesenteric artery
T4	Tumor involves the celiac axis or superior mesenteric artery
N stage	**Involvement of Regional Lymph Nodes (N)**
NX	Regional lymph nodes cannot be assessed (information not available)
N0	No spread to regional lymph nodes
N1	Regional lymph node metastases
M stage	**Distant metastases**
M0	No metastatic disease
M1	Distant metastases are present

Reprinted with permission from American Joint Committee on Cancer. *AJCC Cancer Staging Manual*, 7th ed. Springer, 2010. Effective with the 2010 edition extrahepatic bile duct tumors are now separated into perihilar and distal groups, with separate staging classifications for each.

Box 4.8 ESSENTIALS TO REMEMBER

- MRI with MRCP has become a crucial noninvasive tool in the diagnosis, staging, and treatment planning of malignant biliary disease.

- Bile duct wall thickening is a common finding for both cholangiocarcinoma and cholangitis. Thickening of 5 mm or more, irregular wall thickening, and prolonged delayed wall enhancement suggest malignancy, while smoother, concentric thickening with tapered narrowing and early enhancement suggest a benign etiology.

- Cholangiocarcinoma typically demonstrates hypo- or iso-intensity to liver parenchyma on T1-weighted images and is iso-intense to slightly hyperintense to liver on T2-weighted images. Tumors are typically hypovascular on early post-contrast enhanced images and show progressive hyper-enhancement on delayed post-contrast enhanced images.

- Surgical resection remains the only chance for cure of cholangiocarcinoma. Tumors that extend into the left and right second-order intrahepatic biliary radicles, that have vascular involvement with encasement or occlusion of the portal vein, or that have concomitant involvement of both the contralateral hepatic artery and portal vein are not surgically resected.

Table 4.6 TNM STAGING OF INTRAHEPATIC BILE DUCT CANCER

STAGE	FINDINGS
T stage	**Primary Tumor (T)**
TX	The primary tumor cannot be assessed (information not available)
T0	No evidence of primary tumor
Tis	Carcinoma in situ (intraductal tumor)
T1	Solitary tumor without vascular invasion
T2a	Solitary tumor with vascular invasion
T2b	Multiple tumors, with or without vascular invasion
T3	Tumor perforating the visceral peritoneum or involving the local extrahepatic structures by direct invasion
T4	Tumor with periductal invasion
N stage	**Involvement of Regional Lymph Nodes (N)**
NX	Regional lymph nodes cannot be assessed (information not available)
N0	No spread to regional lymph nodes
N1	Regional lymph node metastases
M stage	**Distant metastases**
M0	No metastatic disease
M1	Distant metastases are present

Reprinted with permission from American Joint Committee on Cancer. *AJCC Cancer Staging Manual*, 7th ed. Springer, 2010. Effective with the 2010 edition, this staging system is now independent of the staging system for hepatocellular carcinoma, hilar bile duct cancers, and extrahepatic bile duct malignancy. This staging system includes the rare mixed hepatocholangiocarcinomas.

REFERENCES

1. Stark DD, Bradley WG Jr. *Magnetic Resonance Imaging*, 3rd ed., vol. 1. Philadelphia: CV Mosby, 1999.
2. Hirao K, Miyazaki A, Fujimoto T, et al. *Evaluation of aberrant bile ducts before laparoscopic cholecystectomy: helical CT cholangiography versus MR cholangiography. AJR Am J Roentgenol.* 2000;175:713–720.
3. Yeh B, Liu P, Soto J, et al. MR imaging and CT of the biliary tract. *Radiographics.* 2009;29:1669–1688.
4. Nandalur KR, Hussain HK, Weadock WJ, et al. Possible biliary disease: diagnostic performance of high-spatial-resolution isotropic 3D T2-weighted MRCP. *Radiology.* 2008;249:883–890.
5. Sodickson A, Mortele KJ, Barish MA, et al. Three-dimensional fast-recovery fast spin-echo MRCP: comparison with two-dimensional single-shot fast spin-echo techniques. *Radiology.* 2006;238:549–559.
6. Catalano OA, Sahani DV, Kalva SP, et al. MR imaging of the gallbladder: a pictorial essay. *Radiographics.* 2008;28:135–155.
7. Mortelé KJ, Rocha TC, Streeter JL, Taylor AJ. Multimodality imaging of pancreatic and biliary congenital anomalies. *Radiographics.* 2006;26:715–731.
8. Hirao K, Miyazaki A, Fujimoto T, et al. Evaluation of aberrant bile ducts before laparoscopic cholecystectomy: helical CT cholangiography versus MR cholangiography. *AJR Am J Roentgenol.* 2000; 175:713–720.
9. KimuraK, Ohto M, Saisho H, et al. Association of gallbladder carcinoma and anomalous pancreaticobiliary ductal union. *Gastroenterology.* 1985;89:1258–1265.
10. Merkle EM, Haugan PA, Thomas J, et al. 3.0- versus 1.5-T MR cholangiography: a pilot study. *AJR Am J Roentgenol.* 2006;186:516–521.
11. Bortoff GA, Chen MYM, Ott DJ, et al. Gallbladder stones: imaging and intervention. *Radiographics.* 2000:20:751–766.
12. Siegelman ES. *Body MRI*. Philadelphia: Elsevier, 2005:63–89.
13. Watanabe Y, Nagayama M, Okumuru A, et al. MR Imaging of acute biliary disorders. *Radiographics.* 2007;27:477–495.
14. Sherlock S, Dooley J. Gallstones and inflammatory gallbladder diseases. *In:* Sherlock S, Dooley J, eds. *Diseases of the Liver and Biliary System*, 11th ed. Malden, MA: Blackwell, 2002:597–628.
15. Menias CO, Surabhi VR, Prasad SR, et al. Mimics of cholangiocarcinoma: spectrum of disease. *Radiographics.* 2008;28:1115–1129.
16. Federle MP, Jeffrey RB, Woodward PJ, Borhani A. *Diagnostic imaging, abdomen*, 2nd ed. Philadelphia: Lippincott Williams & Wilkins, 2009.
17. Hoeffel C, Azizi L, Lewin M, et al. Normal and pathologic features of the postoperative biliary tract at 3D MR cholangiopancreatography and MR imaging. *Radiographics.* 2006;26:1603–1620.

18. Seale MK, Catalano OA, Saini S, et al. Hepatobiliary-specific MR contrast agents: role in imaging the liver and biliary tree. *Radiographics*. 2009;29:1725–1748.

19. Khan SA, Thomas HC, Davidson BR, Taylor-Robinson SD. Cholangiocarcinoma. *Lancet*. 2005;366:1303–1314.

20. Chung YE, Kim M-J, Park YN, et al. Varying appearances of cholangiocarcinoma: radiologic-pathologic correlation. *Radiographics*. 2009;29:683–700.

21. Park HS, Lee JM, Choi J-Y, et al. Preoperative evaluation of bile duct cancer: MRI combined with MR cholangiopancreatography versus MDCT with direct cholangiography. *AJR Am J Roentgenol*. 2008; 190:396–405.

22. Sainani N, Catalano O, Holalkere N-S, et al. Cholangiocarcinoma: current and novel imaging techniques. *Radiographics*. 2008;28: 1263–1287.

5.

PANCREAS MR IMAGING

Marc Sarti, MD

MR TECHNIQUES

State-of-the-art magnetic MR imaging of the pancreas requires a high-field-strength system (1.5 to 3.0T) with rapid gradients. With such systems, images with high signal-to-noise ratios, fine resolution, and uniform fat suppression can be obtained in a single breath hold.

The pancreas is best evaluated with T1-weighted fat-suppressed images. On these images, the normal pancreas appears as the organ with the highest signal intensity in the abdomen. The intrinsic high signal of pancreatic parenchyma is caused by the high concentrations of aqueous protein and manganese in the pancreatic acinar cells (Fig. 5.1). Consequently, on T1-weighted fat-suppressed images, virtually all pancreatic pathology will appear as focal or diffuse decreased signal against the background high-signal normal pancreatic tissue.

Chemical-shift, or phase-opposed, T1-weighted images are of limited value for pancreatic evaluation but may be useful for defining regions of focal fatty infiltration within the pancreas and liver, and for characterizing incidentally discovered adrenal adenomas.

T2-weighted images, with or without fat suppression, are essential for characterizing cystic pancreatic lesions, assessing peripancreatic inflammation, and defining the pancreatic ductal system. The pancreatic ductal system is best depicted on heavily T2-weighted magnetic resonance cholangiopancreatography (MRCP) sequences. MRCP imaging is preferably performed after the ingestion of substances such as ferrous sulfate to suppress the high signal intensity of the fluid within the stomach and duodenum, which may otherwise obscure the pancreatic duct.

There are several MRCP techniques available. One is a breath-hold thick-slab 2D single shot FSE/TSE sequence, acquired in coronal or oblique-coronal planes. With this sequence a single 40- to 60-mm-thick slice is obtained in approximately 1 second; by repeating the sequence multiple times at different obliquities, high-temporal-resolution images of the entire pancreatic duct can be obtained. Another MRCP technique is a multislice sequence in which multiple thin 2D T2-weighted images are obtained in coronal orientation during a single breath hold. A more recent technique is a respiratory-gated 3D FSE/TSE volume acquisition of a large number of very thin (1 mm), high-resolution slice sections obtained during quiet respiration. As with this technique the images are typically acquired with isotropic voxels, assessment can be performed by using multiplanar reconstruction, a method that is particularly useful for determining the presence or absence of communication between a cystic pancreatic lesion and the pancreatic duct. Intravenous administration of secretin, a hormone that stimulates pancreatic exocrine secretion, may improve visualization of the pancreatic duct but is not necessary in routine imaging of the pancreas.

Dynamic, contrast-enhanced images using a gadolinium-based agent are obtained to improve characterization of cystic and solid pancreatic masses, and to adequately characterize incidentally discovered hepatic lesions. (In general, the entire liver should be included in a pancreatic imaging examination, as pancreatic malignancies have a tendency to metastasize to the liver.) Modern techniques for dynamic, contrast-enhanced imaging of the abdomen begin with a test bolus injection or use of triggering software to determine the time required for the contrast material to reach the abdominal aorta. The first series of contrast-enhanced images should be obtained approximately 15 seconds after the agent reaches the abdominal aorta, as this corresponds to maximal parenchymal enhancement of the pancreas. These early-phase enhanced images are essential for defining the arterial anatomy, vessel patency, and vessel involvement by tumor (if present). Hypervascular neuroendocrine tumors are occasionally visualized only during this phase of contrast enhancement; hypovascular lesions, such as adenocarcinoma, will best appear as regions of decreased signal intensity against avidly enhancing normal parenchyma. Abdominal and retroperitoneal lymph nodes are often best delineated on this sequence as well. Subsequent dynamic acquisitions are obtained every 30 seconds for a total of three or four acquisitions. These delayed enhancement phases are valuable for assessing peripancreatic and hepatic veins, and provide an additional opportunity to characterize pancreatic lesions. A delayed image obtained more than 10 minutes after contrast material administration may be

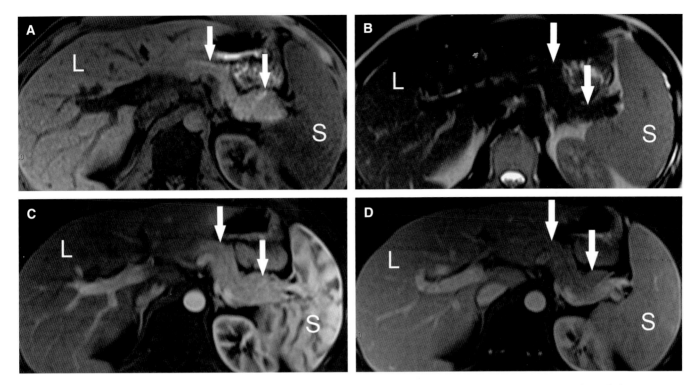

Figure 5.1 *Normal pancreas signal and enhancement characteristics.* (**A**) Axial T1-weighted fat-saturated gradient-echo image through the pancreatic tail (*arrows*) shows the inherent high signal of the pancreatic parenchyma compared to spleen (*S*) and liver (*L*) on T1-weighted images. (**B**) Axial T2-weighted single-shot FSE/TSE image at a similar level; the signal intensity of the normal pancreas (*arrows*) is similar to that of the liver (*L*) and less than that of the spleen (*S*). Following the administration of gadolinium contrast material, the pancreas (*arrows*) shows greater enhancement than the liver (*L*) in the pancreatic parenchymal phase (**C**) and similar enhancement to the liver (*L*) during the portal venous phase (**D**). The spleen (*S*) enhances heterogeneously during the parenchymal phase and becomes homogeneous during the portal venous phase.

obtained to better characterize incidental hepatic lesions, which may affect management of the pancreatic abnormality (i.e., differentiating hemangiomas and metastases in a patient with pancreatic cancer).

Additional dedicated magnetic resonance angiography (MRA) sequences are particularly valuable for evaluating the pancreas in the setting of pancreatic adenocarcinoma. 3D MRA acquisitions may be reconstructed in any plane to assess the presence of vascular involvement by tumor, thereby aiding in the staging of pancreatic adenocarcinoma.

EMBRYOLOGY, ANATOMY, AND ANATOMIC VARIANTS

During the embryonic period two pancreatic buds (dorsal and ventral) form at the foregut/midgut junction, along what will become the duodenum. The buds fuse at 7 to 8 weeks of gestation. The dorsal bud gives rise to the anterior pancreatic head, the body, and the tail; the ventral bud gives rise to the posterior head and uncinate process. The mature pancreas is a retroperitoneal organ within the anterior pararenal space. It is bound anteriorly by the peritoneal surface of the lesser sac and the transverse mesocolon, and posteriorly by the anterior renal fascia. The head conforms to the concavity of the duodenum; the uncinate process, in the posterior head, is the only portion of the pancreas posterior to the superior mesenteric vessels. The gastroduodenal and superior pancreaticoduodenal arteries mark the junction of the head and neck. The neck is a focal constriction of the gland that extends 2 to 3 cm between the antero-superior gastric pylorus and the postero-inferior commencement of the portal vein. The neck joins the body at a focal anterior prominence of the gland known as the omental tuberosity. For purposes of tumor location, the body is also

---

Box 5.1 ESSENTIALS TO REMEMBER

- The pancreas is initially best evaluated on T1-weighted fat-suppressed images, as any focus of pathology will have relatively low signal compared to the intrinsic high signal intensity of the normal pancreatic parenchyma.

- The pancreatic ductal system is best depicted on heavily T2-weighted MRCP sequences.

- Dynamic, gadolinium-contrast-enhanced images improve characterization of cystic and solid masses.

- MRCP images obtained with intravenous administration of secretin may improve visualization of the pancreatic duct.

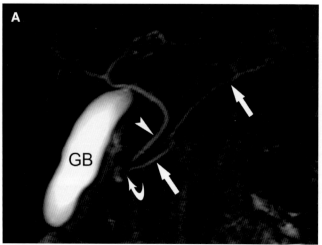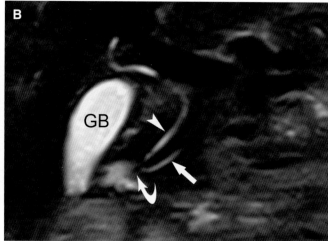

Figure 5.2 *Normal pancreatic ductal anatomy.* (**A**) On the thick-slab MRCP image, the main pancreatic duct (*arrows*) courses inferiorly through the pancreatic head and drains via the duct of Wirsung into the duodenum at the major papilla/ampulla of Vater (*curved arrow*) with the CBD (*arrowhead*). (**B**) Thin-section coronal single-shot FSE/TSE image shows the main pancreatic duct (*arrow*) and the CBD (*arrowhead*) converging within the inferior pancreatic head and draining at the ampulla of Vater (*curved arrow*). *GB*, gallbladder.

defined as extending from the left edge of the superior mesenteric–portal vein confluence to the left edge of the aorta. Along the anteroposterior line demarcated by the left edge of the aorta, the body merges with the tail, which extends leftward as far as the splenic hilum.

Fusion of the pancreatic buds is accompanied by fusion of the ducts. In normal development the main duct of the ventral pancreatic bud fuses with the main duct of the dorsal pancreatic bud at the junction of the pancreatic head and neck. This becomes the main pancreatic duct, which drains via the duct of Wirsung through the large-caliber major papilla at the ampulla of Vater; the accessory duct of Santorini remains small and drains through the small-caliber minor papilla, approximately 2 cm superior and anterior to the major papilla. On MRCP images, the normal pancreatic duct courses posteriorly and inferiorly through the head to join the common bile duct (CBD) at the major papilla (Fig. 5.2).

Blood supply to the pancreas is complex. The head is supplied by the anterior and posterior pancreaticoduodenal arcades. The anterior arcade courses along the anterior head and is formed superiorly by the anterior superior pancreaticoduodenal artery, one of the two terminal branches of the gastroduodenal artery (GDA), and inferiorly by the anterior inferior pancreaticoduodenal artery, which arises from the inferior pancreaticoduodenal artery, the first branch of the superior mesenteric artery (SMA). The posterior arcade courses along the posterior head and is formed superiorly by the posterior superior pancreaticoduodenal artery, the first branch of the gastroduodenal artery, and inferiorly by the posterior inferior pancreaticoduodenal artery, also a branch of the inferior pancreaticoduodenal artery. The body is primarily supplied by the dorsal pancreatic artery, which usually arises from the splenic artery but less commonly arises from the proximal hepatic artery or the SMA, or directly from the celiac axis. The splenic artery courses along the posterior pancreas and supplies the tail, primarily via the proximal

pancreaticomagna artery and to a lesser extent via a small distal branch called the caudal pancreatic artery. Of note, the GDA and splenic artery provide most of the blood flow to the pancreas and course along the surface of the gland; the SMA and celiac axis are separated from the gland by a layer of retroperitoneal fat.

Venous drainage is via the portal venous system. The pancreaticoduodenal veins drain the head and join the superior mesenteric vein (SMV) or the caudal aspect of the main portal vein. The splenic vein drains the body and tail. The SMV, main portal vein, and splenic vein course along the surface of the gland without an intervening layer of fat.

The pancreatic ductal anatomy is subject to many variations, but the most common and clinically significant congenital variant is ***pancreas divisum*** (Fig. 5.3). The reported incidence of pancreas divisum ranges from 3% to 14% in ERCP, MRCP, and autopsy series. A pancreas divisum results from failure of fusion of the duct systems of dorsal and ventral pancreatic buds. Consequently, the ventral pancreas, which constitutes the bulk of the pancreas, drains via the duct of Santorini through the small-caliber minor papilla. The duct of Wirsung remains short and narrow, and drains only the posterior head and uncinate process via the major papilla. On MRCP images, the main pancreatic duct takes a relatively straight course through the anterior-superior head, passes anterior to the distal CBD, and drains via the minor papilla. Although rarely necessary, MRCP with intravenous secretin administration may improve the sensitivity of diagnosing pancreas divisum, or reveal a "Santorinicele," a focal dilatation of the dorsal duct just proximal to the minor papilla, the presence of which suggests relative obstruction. Pancreas divisum can also be easily diagnosed on axial T2-weighted images: in this case the pancreatic duct courses anterior to the CBD and drains into the duodenum through the papilla minor a few slice sections higher (superior) than the slice demonstrating drainage of the CBD into the duodenum through the papilla major.

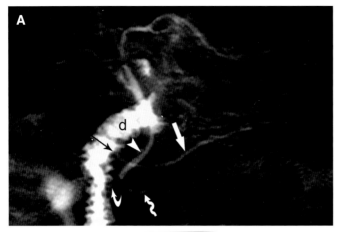

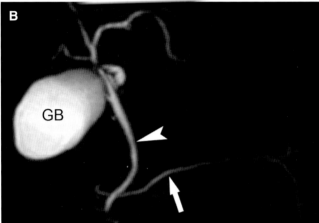

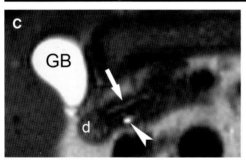

Figure 5.3 *Pancreas divisum.* (**A**) Thick-slab MRCP image and (**B**) reconstructed image from a respiratory-gated 3-D FSE/TSE acquisition show the main pancreatic duct (*arrow*) and the CBD (*arrowhead*) crossing within the pancreatic head. The pancreatic duct drains into the duodenum (*d*) superiorly via the duct of Santorini at the minor papilla (*skinny black arrow*); the CBD drains inferiorly at the major papilla (*curved arrow*). The small duct of Wirsung (*squiggly arrow*), best seen on image A, takes a horizontal course in the inferior pancreatic head and drains via the major papilla. (**C**) Axial T2-weighted single-shot FSE/TSE image through the pancreatic head (from a different patient) shows the duct of Santorini (*arrow*) crossing anterior to the common bile duct (*arrowhead*) and entering the duodenum (*d*) at the minor papilla. *GB*, gallbladder.

The clinical relevance of pancreas divisum is controversial, as most affected individuals are asymptomatic. However, among patients with idiopathic recurrent pancreatitis, pancreas divisum is present in 12% to 26%, a higher prevalence than seen in the general population. Episodes of recurrent pancreatitis are presumably caused by outflow obstruction of pancreatic exocrine secretions at the functionally stenotic minor papilla; as such, affected patients may benefit from endoscopic sphincterotomy or stenting of the minor papilla.[1]

CONGENITAL PARENCHYMAL ANOMALIES

Total pancreatic agenesis is rare and usually associated with other severe malformations incompatible with life. *Agenesis of the dorsal pancreas* is rare and can occur in otherwise normal individuals, or in association with other congenital abnormalities. Dorsal agenesis is usually asymptomatic, but may present with abdominal pain, diabetes, or pancreatitis. Dorsal agenesis may be partial or complete. In partial dorsal agenesis, the minor papilla, the terminal duct of Santorini, and a portion of the pancreatic body are present; in complete dorsal agenesis, the dorsal ductal system and the body and tail of the pancreas are absent. Dorsal agenesis may be simulated by complete atrophy of the body and tail secondary to chronic pancreatitis, a condition known as pseudo-agenesis; in such cases, the complete absence of a dorsal duct and demonstration of a short ventral duct (Wirsung) indicates agenesis.

Annular pancreas is a rare congenital anomaly, occurring in approximately 1 in 20,000 individuals, and is characterized by a band of pancreatic tissue that partially or completely surrounds the second portion of the duodenum. Annular pancreas is often clinically evident in infancy with symptoms of duodenal obstruction; when symptoms are present at infancy, there is a high association (70%) with other anomalies, including duodenal atresia, tracheoesophageal fistula, or trisomy 21. However, as half of individuals with annular pancreas remain undiagnosed until adulthood; presenting symptoms include upper abdominal pain, nausea/vomiting, peptic ulcer disease, and pancreatitis. Adult presentation is less commonly associated with other congenital anomalies (20% to 25%).

At MR imaging, annular pancreas is well appreciated on fat-suppressed T1-weighted images as a ring of high-signal-intensity pancreatic tissue that surrounds the second portion of the duodenum. MRCP may show an aberrant pancreatic duct surrounding the duodenum, but this finding is not necessary in establishing the diagnosis.

Ectopic pancreatic tissue is found in 2% of individuals at autopsy series. The most common sites of ectopia are the submucosa of the gastric antrum and the proximal duodenum; less common sites include the jejunum, Meckel's diverticula, and the ileum. Although usually an incidental finding, foci of ectopic tissue may cause inflammation or give rise to primary pancreatic neoplasms. On MRI, the signal intensity and enhancement pattern of ectopic tissue is similar to that of the normal pancreas.

HEREDITARY CONDITIONS AFFECTING THE PANCREAS

Cystic fibrosis (CF) is an autosomal recessive disorder of ion transport that causes abnormally viscous secretions in exocrine glands and the epithelial lining of the respiratory,

Box 5.2 **ESSENTIALS TO REMEMBER**

- The pancreas is retroperitoneal, bounded anteriorly by the lesser sac and transverse mesocolon, and posteriorly by the anterior renal fascia.

- The GDA and splenic artery course along the surface of the gland and provide most of the blood flow to the pancreas.

- The SMA and celiac axis are separated from the gland by a layer of retroperitoneal fat.

- The pancreas has portal venous drainage, via the SMV and splenic vein, which course along the surface of the gland.

- The most common congenital variant is pancreatic divisum, best depicted at MRCP, in which the main pancreatic duct courses anterior to the CBD and drains via the duct of Santorini through the small-caliber minor papilla.

gastrointestinal, and reproductive tracts. Occurring in 1 in 2,500 live births, it is the most common lethal genetic disease among Caucasians. Clinically apparent pancreatic exocrine insufficiency is present in 85% to 90% of CF patients and leads to protein and fat malabsorption with associated poor weight gain, fat-soluble vitamin deficiency, and hypoproteinemia. Obstructive mucus in small pancreatic ducts leads to progressive fibrosis and fatty degeneration of the gland.

The appearance of the pancreas at MR imaging varies depending on the amount of fat or fibrosis present. The most common appearance is complete fatty replacement of the gland; in this case the gland displays high signal intensity on T1-weighted images and low signal intensity on fat-suppressed images (Fig. 5.4). If fibrosis is present, the pancreas will show decreased signal on both T1- and T2-weighted images. A rare manifestation of CF is pancreatic enlargement with multiple nodular fatty masses, known as lipomatous pseudo-hypertrophy.

Pancreatic duct dilatation and calcifications are present in up to 8% of patients; calcifications are better seen on CT. Small cysts, usually 3 mm or less in size, are commonly present.

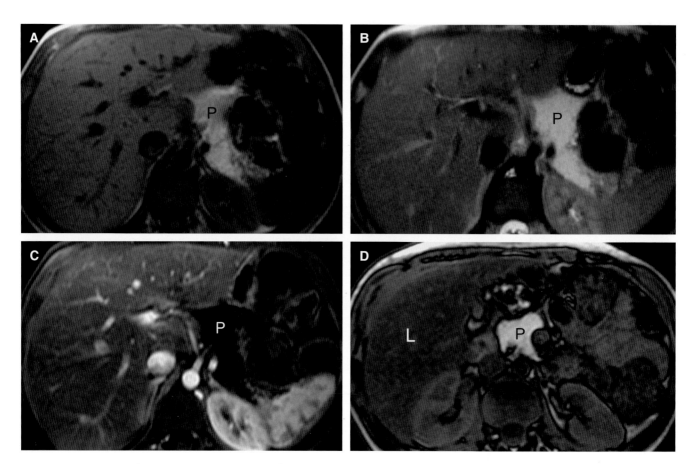

Figure 5.4 *Cystic fibrosis.* (**A**) Axial T1-weighted in-phase gradient-echo, (**B**) axial T2-weighted single-shot FSE/TSE, and (**C**) post-gadolinium-contrast-enhanced fat-saturated T1-weighted images through the pancreatic tail (*P*) show the signal intensity of the tail parenchyma to follow that of fat on all sequences. (**D**) Axial T1-weighted out-of-phase gradient-echo image through the pancreatic head (*P*) shows fatty replacement of the head and diffuse loss of signal within the liver (*L*) indicating concomitant hepatic steatosis.

Rarely, the pancreas will undergo extreme cystic change, known as pancreatic cystosis, with multiple cysts more than 1 cm in size or complete replacement of the pancreas by large cysts.[2]

Hemochromatosis (also called primary hemochromatosis or hereditary hemochromatosis) is an autosomal recessive disorder characterized by excessive accumulation of body iron. Most of the iron accumulates in parenchymal organs, including the liver, pancreas, and heart. Although both sexes are affected, the disorder is more common in males (1.8:1); also, hemochromatosis is clinically evident at a younger age in men, as physiologic iron loss in women delays accumulation of iron in the pancreas. Hemochromatosis is distinct from hemosiderosis (also called secondary hemochromatosis or acquired hemochromatosis), a condition caused by parenteral administration of iron, usually blood transfusions. Excess iron in hemosiderosis is predominantly deposited in the reticuloendothelial system of the liver, spleen, and bone marrow.

Iron ions are superparamagnetic; this property shortens the longitudinal relaxation time (T1) and distorts the local magnetic field, shortening the transverse relaxation time (T2). The increased magnetic field inhomogeneity is most sensitively appreciated as an increased T2* effect, manifested by loss of signal on gradient-echo images. The T2* effect increases with the echo time, and thus the loss of signal becomes more evident using a gradient-echo sequence with a relatively long echo time. Iron deposition within a particular organ is proportional to the degree of signal loss; algorithms exist that use gradient-echo images to estimate the quantity of iron deposition.

The pattern of signal loss on gradient-echo images follows the distribution of iron deposition. In hemochromatosis, iron initially accumulates in the periportal hepatocytes and then spreads to the remainder of the liver, the pancreas, and the thyroid gland. In advanced disease, the myocardium is affected. Excessive pancreatic iron is found in the acinar cells, islet cells, and the interstitium. Excess acinar cell and interstitial iron may lead to parenchymal atrophy and interstitial fibrosis; excess islet cell iron may lead to diabetes mellitus ("bronze diabetes") late in the course of hemochromatosis. In contradistinction, hemosiderosis does not result in abnormal iron accumulation in the pancreas.[3]

Von Hippel-Lindau (VHL) disease is a rare multisystem disorder caused by a mutation of the VHL gene, a tumor suppressor gene. Most cases are inherited in an autosomal dominant pattern, with high penetrance but variable expression. Approximately 1% to 3% of cases occur sporadically. Men and women are affected equally. Mean age at diagnosis is 25 years; however, diagnosis may occur from infancy to late adulthood.

Morbidity and mortality are most commonly related to renal or central nervous system manifestations of the disease. Renal cell carcinoma is the main cause of death, and the reported prevalence ranges from 24% to 75%; other tumors causing significant morbidity include central nervous system hemangioblastomas and pheochromocytomas. Pancreatic involvement is frequent but rarely of clinical significance, as the most common lesions, seen in 50% to 91% of patients, are simple cysts (Fig. 5.5). These cysts are homogeneously hyperintense on T2-weighted images and may be single or multiple or virtually replace the entire gland. Benign serous cystadenomas, described in detail below, occur in 12% of patients. In general, cystic pancreatic lesions in VHL are asymptomatic or associated with only mild symptoms.[4]

Neuroendocrine tumors of the pancreas occur in only 5% to 17% of patients with VHL but may cause significant morbidity or mortality. Unlike sporadic neuroendocrine tumors, the majority of neuroendocrine tumors in VHL are nonfunctional. One study suggests that despite the fact that neuroendocrine tumors in VHL are nonfunctional, they are malignant in only 10% of cases;[5] this rate of malignancy is far less than the 60% to 92% seen in sporadic nonfunctioning neuroendocrine tumors. At MR imaging, the appearance of neuroendocrine tumors in VHL is similar to the appearance in sporadic disease. However, tumors are more likely to be multiple in VHL.

Hereditary pancreatitis is an autosomal dominant disease with an equal sex distribution and 80% penetrance. Hereditary pancreatitis accounts for approximately 1% of cases of chronic pancreatitis. Over 25 mutations in the gene encoding cationic trypsinogen lead to enhanced activation of trypsinogen to trypsin, or prevent prematurely activated trypsin from being inactivated by autolysis; this deregulation of trypsin leads to inflammation and autodigestion of the pancreas.

Genetic testing establishes the diagnosis of hereditary pancreatitis. Prior to genetic testing, however, the clinical criteria required to establish the diagnosis were as follows: recurrent episodes of acute pancreatitis or signs of chronic pancreatitis often beginning in the first two decades of life, a family history of at least two other affected members, frequent presence of intraductal calcified stones, and the absence of known etiologic factors (e.g., alcohol, gallstones).[6]

The appearance of hereditary pancreatitis at MR imaging is indistinguishable from that of pancreatitis caused by other common etiologies. However, hereditary pancreatitis is characterized by the early appearance of imaging findings of chronic pancreatitis, described in detail below. When evaluating a patient with known hereditary pancreatitis, keep in mind that affected patients have a more than 50-fold increased risk of developing pancreatic cancer after age 50 compared to the general population.

PANCREATITIS

Acute pancreatitis is the result of inflammation of the pancreas, characterized by sudden abdominal pain with elevation of pancreatic enzymes in the blood. Excessive alcohol or gallstones cause pancreatitis in up to 75% of cases; less common causes include hypertriglyceridemia, hypercalcemia, trauma, drugs (azothioprine, chemotherapeutic agents, antiretrovirals), iatrogenesis (endoscopic retrograde cholangiopancreatography), pancreas divisum, and pancreatic cancer. Twenty percent of cases are idiopathic. Clinical and laboratory criteria establish the diagnosis. Imaging aids in the assessment of disease severity, reveals complications, and may detect a cause.

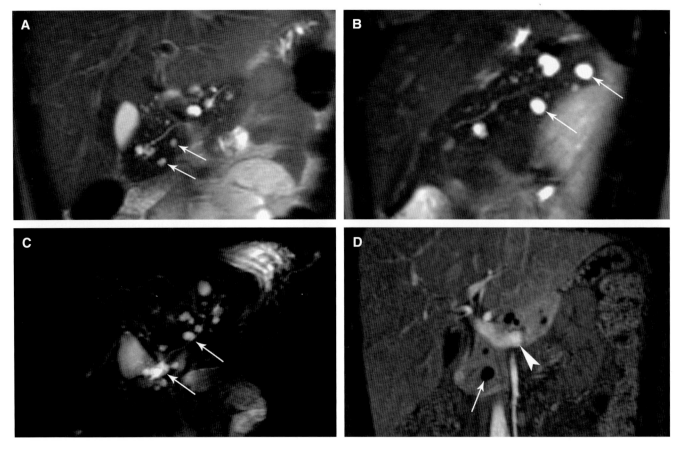

Figure 5.5 *Von Hippel-Lindau disease.* (**A**) Coronal, (**B**) sagittal T2-weighted single shot FSE/TSE, and (**C**) thick-slab MRCP images through the pancreatic body and tail show numerous simple cysts (*arrows*) with bright signal throughout the gland in this patient with VHL. (**D**) Coronal gadolinium-contrast-enhanced T1-weighted fat-suppressed image from a MR angiography sequence shows that the cysts (*arrow*) remain low in signal and do not contain enhancing components. A subcentimeter focus of early enhancement (*arrowhead*) in the lateral pancreatic head likely represents a small islet cell tumor.

The spectrum of pathologic changes precipitated by the release of pancreatic digestive enzymes ranges from mild inflammation to parenchymal necrosis. In very mild cases the gland retains its normal size, shape, and signal intensity characteristics. In more advanced cases, inflamed portions of the pancreas are best seen as regions of decreased signal intensity on fat-suppressed T1-weighted images, with glandular enlargement and loss of definition of its normal boundaries (Fig. 5.6). Peripancreatic edema may be present, causing stranding of adjacent fat, best seen as linear bands of decreased signal intensity on T1-weighted or increased signal intensity on T2-weighted images. Severe pancreatitis occurs in 20% of cases and is associated with focal or diffuse necrosis. Gadolinium contrast material administration is essential in detecting necrosis, as the signal intensity of nonviable parenchyma may be similar to that of inflamed tissue; however, necrotic tissue does not enhance and is sharply demarcated from regions of viable pancreatic tissue on contrast-enhanced MR images.[7]

Fluid collections frequently develop in cases of moderate to severe pancreatitis and commonly occur within the pancreas, the anterior retroperitoneal space, the lesser sac, or paracolic gutters. Acute fluid collections lack a defined wall

---

Box 5.3 ESSENTIALS TO REMEMBER

- Cystic fibrosis, the most common lethal genetic disease among Caucasians, may affect the pancreas in various ways but most commonly causes complete fatty replacement of the gland.

- Primary and secondary hemochromatosis are characterized by specific patterns of abnormal iron deposition, best depicted on gradient-echo sequences obtained with a relatively long TE.

- VHL most commonly affects the pancreas by causing simple cysts, which occur in 50% to 91% of patients. Neuroendocrine tumors, usually solitary in the general population, are often multiple in patients with VHL and occur in 5% to 17% of patients with the disease.

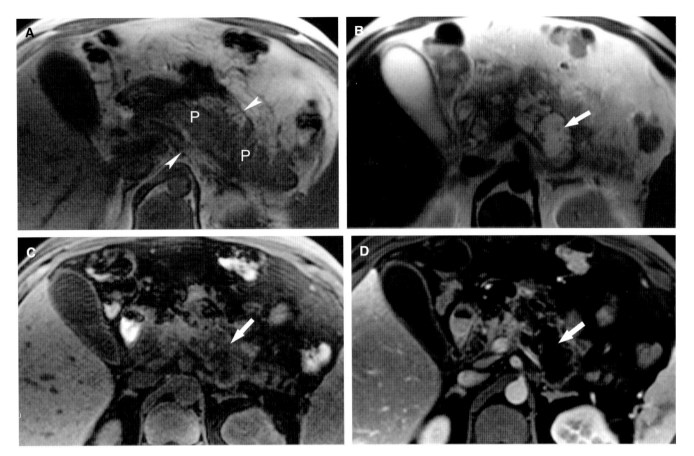

Figure 5.6 *Acute pancreatitis.* (**A**) Axial T1-weighted gradient-echo image through the pancreatic body and tail (*P*) shows an enlarged gland with loss of definition of its normal boundaries. Edema appears as low-signal-intensity bands (*arrowheads*) in the peripancreatic fat. (**B**) Axial T2-weighted single-shot FSE/TSE image obtained slightly below image A shows a complex pseudocyst (*arrow*) with heterogeneous, predominantly increased signal, replacing portions of the body and tail. (**C**) Axial T1-weighted fat-saturated gradient-echo image through the pseudocyst (*arrow*) shows heterogeneous internal signal due to the presence of hemorrhage or necrotic debris. (**D**) Axial T1-weighted post-contrast-enhanced fat-saturated image through the pseudocyst (*arrow*) shows irregular enhancing walls and lack of internal enhancement, due to necrosis of this portion of the pancreas.

and contain serous fluid, displaying low signal on T1-weighted and homogeneous high signal intensity on T2-weighted images. Acute collections may spontaneously resolve, but if a collection persists for 4 to 6 weeks and a wall of fibrous or granulomatous tissue develops, the diagnosis of an acute pseudocyst can be made. Because the walls of pseudocysts have a fibrous component they show minimal enhancement on early post-gadolinium contrast-enhanced images, with progressive enhancement on delayed images. If complicated by hemorrhage, infection, or necrotic debris, the contents of a pseudocyst may show increased signal on T1-weighted images and heterogeneous signal on T2-weighted images. Superinfection is suggested if gas is present within a pseudocyst. MR pancreatography aids in pseudocyst characterization as it may show communication with the pancreatic ductal system, with sensitivities between 70% and 92% compared to ERCP. Treatment of such pseudocysts is usually performed with transpapillary drainage.

Therapeutic intervention for pseudocysts is considered when the collections are complex or if adverse symptoms persist despite conservative management, or in cases of persistent large asymptomatic collections. Complications include

infection, gastric or duodenal obstruction, biliary obstruction, or pancreaticopleural fistula. Symptoms include pain, nausea and vomiting, or upper gastrointestinal bleeding. Asymptomatic collections are usually drained if they are larger than 5 cm and have not changed in size for more than 6 weeks, or are larger than 4 cm in patients with chronic alcoholic pancreatitis. Drainage may be performed via an endoscopic transpapillary or transmural approach, or a percutaneous approach. However, if at imaging solid necrotic debris is detected within a pseudocyst, minimally invasive drainage procedures are inadequate in the prevention of infection and surgical debridement is indicated.[8]

In patients with acute pancreatitis MRI is particularly useful in demonstrating the presence of hemorrhagic peripancreatic fat necrosis, depicted as high signal intensity in the peripancreatic fat on fat-suppressed T1-weighted images. Severe hemorrhagic fat necrosis is associated with increased complications and mortality.[9]

The most common vascular complication in acute pancreatitis is venous thrombosis. The splenic vein is most frequently involved, followed by the SMV, portal confluence, and main portal vein. Acute thrombosis is best appreciated on contrast-enhanced MR as enhancement of the vessel wall with low-signal-intensity thrombus within the lumen. Distention of perigastric collaterals is an indirect sign of splenic vein thrombosis.

An uncommon but potentially fatal complication of acute pancreatitis is severe intraperitoneal hemorrhage. Autodigestion of the arterial walls by pancreatic enzymes may result in pseudo-aneurysm formation in up to 10% of patients. A pseudo-aneurysm appears as a circumscribed structure in contiguity with a peripancreatic vessel, showing enhancement similar to that of the abdominal aorta. Pseudo-aneurysms most frequently involve the splenic, gastroduodenal, and pancreaticoduodenal arteries.

Chronic Pancreatitis. Recurrent inflammation of the pancreas leads to irreversible morphologic changes of the gland. As in acute pancreatitis, the most common cause of chronic pancreatitis is excessive alcohol. Obstructive chronic pancreatitis may be caused by papillary stenosis, tumors, ductal scars, or cysts and may improve following removal of the obstructive cause. Less common etiologies include hereditary pancreatitis and autoimmune pancreatitis. In 30% of patients, no cause is found.

The pathologic hallmark of chronic pancreatitis is parenchymal fibrosis and sclerosis, which leads to stricture and dilatation of the ductal system and diffuse glandular atrophy. Parenchymal fibrosis causes loss of aqueous protein in the pancreatic acini, which results in low signal intensity on T1-weighted images in the affected portions of the gland. Fibrosis also causes decreased and delayed peak enhancement of the pancreas on gadolinium contrast-enhanced images. Prolonged disease results in glandular atrophy.

Parenchymal changes may precede or occur simultaneously with ductal changes. Ductal pathology is best depicted on MRCP images. Focal side-branch dilatation occurs early in the disease, followed by more extensive stricture formation and beading of the main duct. Early ductal abnormalities may be very subtle, and diagnostic sensitivity can be improved by obtaining MRCP images following intravenous administration of the hormone secretin, which stimulates exocrine function and improves ductal visualization. Furthermore, assessment of small bowel filling following secretin administration allows a subjective assessment of exocrine function. Late in disease, extensive side-branch and main-duct dilatation may result in a characteristic "chain-of-lakes" appearance. Ductal calcification also occurs late in disease and is better appreciated on CT than MRI (Fig. 5.7). Fibrosis in the pancreatic head may also lead to biliary ductal pathology, including stricture and dilatation of the CBD and choledocholithiasis.[10]

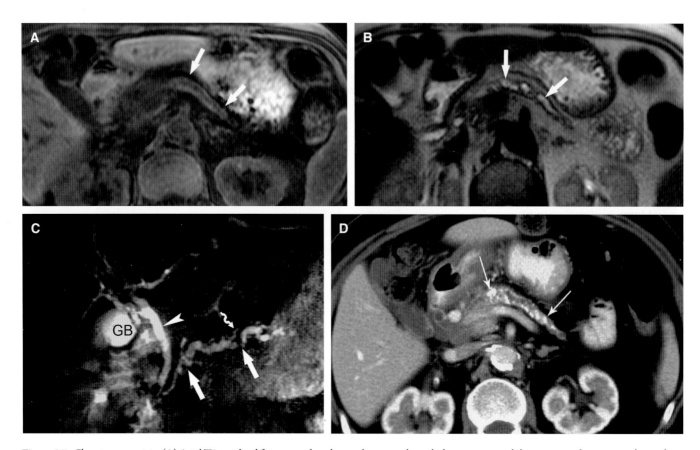

Figure 5.7 *Chronic pancreatitis.* (**A**) Axial T1-weighted fat-saturated gradient-echo image through the pancreatic tail shows an atrophic pancreas (*arrows*) with decreased inherent signal intensity, secondary to parenchymal fibrosis and calcification. (**B**) Axial T2-weighted and (**C**) thick-slab MRCP single-shot FSE/TSE images show multifocal stricture and dilatation of the main pancreatic duct (*arrows* in images B and C) with multifocal side-branch dilatation (*squiggly arrow* in image C). The CBD (*arrowhead* in image C) and a portion of the gallbladder (*GB*) are shown on the MRCP image. (**D**) Contrast-enhanced CT image through the pancreatic tail shows that parenchymal calcification (*arrows*) is much better appreciated on CT than MRI.

Chronic pseudocysts may arise in chronic pancreatitis without a preceding episode of acute pancreatitis. The appearance and potential complicating features of chronic pseudocysts are similar to those seen in acute pancreatitis.

Chronic pancreatitis can cause a focal inflammatory mass that is difficult to differentiate from pancreatic adenocarcinoma because both processes lead to a decrease in signal intensity on T1-weighted images, decreased contrast enhancement, and an increase in ductal diameter from obstruction (Fig. 5.8). Features favoring chronic pancreatitis include diffuse distribution of the pancreatic changes, ductal irregularity, intraductal or parenchymal calcifications, and/or a smoothly stenotic pancreatic duct penetrating the mass ("duct penetrating sign"). Features favoring carcinoma include a smoothly dilated duct with abrupt tapering, dilatation of both biliary and pancreatic ducts, and obliteration of perivascular fat planes. Regardless, because differentiation between carcinoma and a benign inflammatory mass in a patient with chronic pancreatitis is difficult, biopsy is usually required for definitive diagnosis.

Groove pancreatitis is an uncommon form of chronic pancreatitis affecting the groove between the pancreatic head, duodenum, and CBD. Symptoms are similar to those of chronic pancreatitis, with recurrent vomiting caused by impaired duodenal mobility and stenosis. In the pure form, the inflammation and subsequent fibrosis exclusively affects the groove; in the segmental form, both the groove and the superior portion of the pancreatic head are affected. In groove pancreatitis MRI reveals a sheet-like mass between the pancreatic head and duodenum. The abnormal tissue is hypointense on T1-weighted images, has variable intensity on T2-weighted images dependent on chronicity, and shows gradually increased and progressively homogeneous enhancement with delayed gadolinium contrast-enhanced imaging (Fig. 5.9). Associated findings include cysts in the duodenal wall or groove, duodenal wall thickening and stenosis, and widening of the space between the distal pancreatic duct and CBD. Regular tapering of the distal pancreatic duct and CBD is often present as well. If portions of the pancreatic head are involved, as in the segmental form, differentiation from carcinoma may be difficult, as is the case of focal chronic pancreatitis. Other differential considerations include duodenal cancer and cholangiocarcinoma of the distal common bile duct.[11]

Autoimmune pancreatitis is a form of chronic pancreatitis and has been variably termed primary sclerosing pancreatitis, lymphoplasmacytic pancreatitis, and nonalcoholic duct-destructive pancreatitis. There is an association between autoimmune pancreatitis and other autoimmune disorders such as Sjögren syndrome, primary sclerosing cholangitis, primary biliary cirrhosis, ulcerative colitis, and systemic lupus erythematosus. MRI features include focal or diffuse enlargement of the gland (Figs. 5.10 and 5.11); if focal, the appearance may be mass-like and difficult to distinguish from adenocarcinoma. Affected portions of the gland are shown as foci of decreased signal intensity on T1-weighted images, moderately increased signal intensity on T2-weighted images, and homogeneous enhancement on delayed images. The gland may have a capsule-like rim of abnormal parenchyma that is hypointense on T2-weighted images and shows delayed

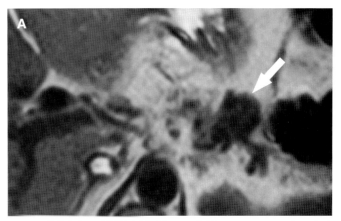
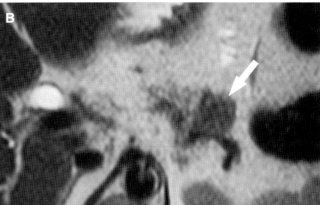
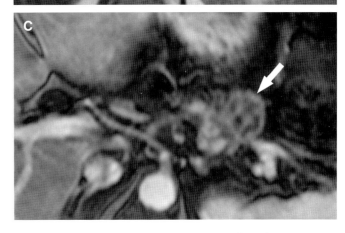

Figure 5.8 *Chronic pancreatitis.* Focal 2-cm mass (*arrow*) within the pancreatic tail has decreased signal intensity on both the axial T1-weighted (**A**) and axial T2-weighted (**B**) images. (**C**) Axial T1-weighted fat-suppressed post-gadolinium-contrast-enhanced image obtained during the pancreatic parenchymal phase shows decreased enhancement of the lesion (*arrow*) compared to the adjacent normal pancreatic tissue. No ductal dilatation was appreciated, but the distal tail showed complete atrophy (not shown). As imaging features were concerning for pancreatic carcinoma, the lesion was resected. The specimen showed chronic pancreatitis with focal fat necrosis.

enhancement, with relative paucity of peripancreatic inflammation and absence of peripancreatic fluid collections compared to acute pancreatitis. MRCP shows diffuse irregular narrowing of the main pancreatic duct that resolves following steroid therapy.[12]

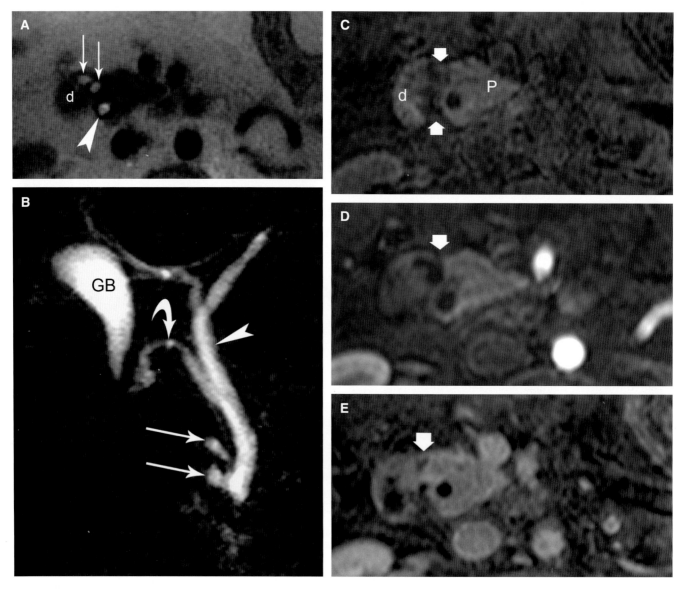

Figure 5.9 *Groove pancreatitis.* (**A**) Axial T2-weighted single-shot FSE/TSE image through the pancreatic head shows two subcentimeter cysts (*arrows*) along the anterior groove between the pancreatic head and duodenum (*d*), anterior to the distal CBD (*arrowhead*). Cysts (*arrows*) are also visible lateral to the distal CBD (*arrowhead*) on the (**B**) thick-slab MRCP single-shot FSE/TSE image. Also seen on this image are the gallbladder (*GB*) and the cystic duct (*curved arrow*). (**C**) Axial T1-weighted fat-saturated image at the same level as image A shows decreased signal intensity (between *arrows*) within the medial wall of the duodenum (*d*) and the affected portion of the lateral pancreatic head (*P*). The affected portion of the pancreas (*arrow*) shows decreased enhancement on the (**D**) pancreatic parenchymal-phase post-gadolinium-contrast-enhanced image and progressive enhancement on the (**E**) delayed post-contrast-enhanced image, consistent with fibrosis.

CYSTIC LESIONS OF THE PANCREAS

Cystic pancreatic lesions are commonly encountered at cross-sectional imaging (Table 5.1). Most (75% to 85%) are pseudo-cysts, and the remainder are cystic pancreatic neoplasms. It is the role of the radiologist to differentiate between these entities. MRI is ideally suited for characterizing the various cystic pancreatic lesions because of its potential for characterizing cyst contents. Furthermore, with MRCP, the presence of communication between the cyst and the pancreatic ductal system can be determined, a feature that is essential for developing a differential diagnosis. Pre- and post gadolinium-contrast-enhanced fat-saturated T1-weighted images are required for the detection of any solid, nodular, enhancing component associated with the cystic lesion, a finding strongly suggestive of malignancy.

Pseudocyst. As discussed in the previous section, pseudo-cysts occur in the setting of acute and chronic pancreatitis and represent acute inflammatory fluid collections or tissue necrosis encapsulated by granulation tissue and a fibrous capsule. The fibrous wall shows progressive enhancement on contrast-enhanced images. Pseudocysts are usually unilocular and may contain simple serous fluid or may be complex (i.e., have internal components including blood, proteinaceous fluid, or necrotic debris). With increasing complexity, pseudocyst contents may show higher signal on T1-weighted images and

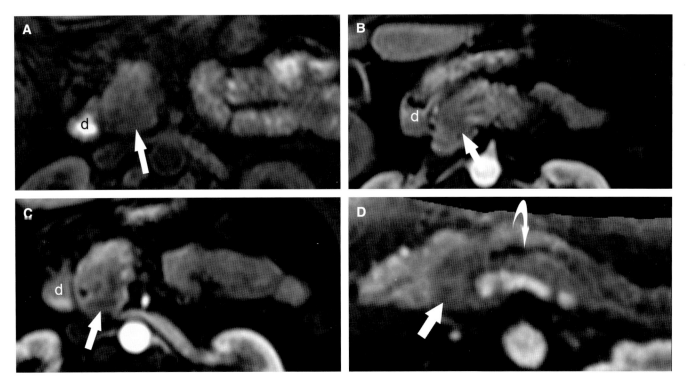

Figure 5.10 *Autoimmune pancreatitis, focal.* (**A**) Axial T1-weighted fat-saturated gradient-echo image through the pancreatic neck shows a transition between normal pancreatic parenchyma (high signal) and affected parenchyma (low signal) (*arrow*). Axial T1-weighted fat-saturated gradient-echo images through the pancreatic neck (**B**) and head (**C**) show a focal, mass-like region of decreased enhancement (*arrow*) corresponding to lymphoplasmacytic infiltrate of autoimmune pancreatitis. *d*, duodenum. (**D**) Para-axial reconstruction from a contrast-enhanced MRA acquisition shows the affected parenchyma as a focus of decreased enhancement (*arrow*), which causes mild proximal ductal dilatation (*curved arrow*).

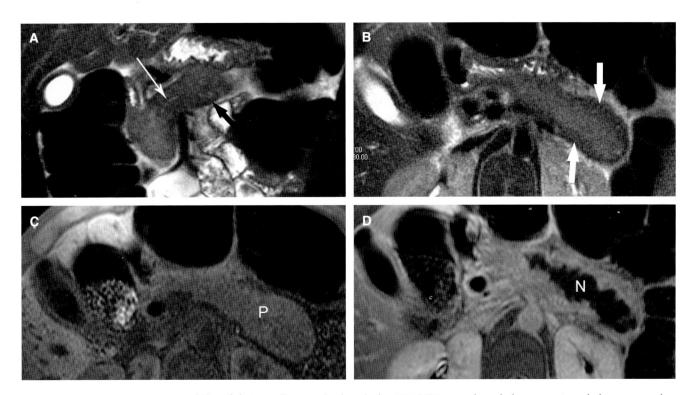

Figure 5.11 *Autoimmune pancreatitis, diffuse.* (**A**) Coronal T2-weighted single shot FSE/TSE image through the pancreatic neck shows a normal-caliber pancreatic duct (*white arrow*) and a subtle capsule-like rim of decreased signal at the periphery of the gland (*black arrow*). (**B**) On the axial T2-weighted image through the tail, the capsule-like rim of decreased signal (*arrows*) is more apparent. There is a relative paucity of peripancreatic inflammation. (**C**) Axial T1-weighted fat-saturated gradient-echo image through the tail shows diffuse decrease signal within the gland (*P*). (**D**) Late-phase T1-weighted fat-saturated post-gadolinium-contrast-enhanced image shows delayed peripheral enhancement. Central gland necrosis (*N*) is evident from absent enhancement in the central portion of the gland; necrosis may occur in severe cases of autoimmune pancreatitis.

Box 5.4 ESSENTIALS TO REMEMBER

- In acute pancreatitis, affected portions of the gland are best appreciated as regions of decreased signal intensity on fat-suppressed T1-weighted images.

- In the setting of acute pancreatitis, it is necessary to obtain gadolinium contrast-enhanced images to differentiate inflamed pancreatic parenchyma from necrosis, as only the latter will show absent enhancement.

- The peripancreatic fluid collections of acute pancreatitis often resolve. Persistence for 4 to 6 weeks and development of a wall of fibrous tissue or granulation tissue confirms the presence of a pseudocyst.

- If solid necrotic debris is present in a pseudocyst, minimally invasive drainage procedures are generally not effective and surgical debridement may be necessary.

- Always assess for the vascular complications of acute pancreatitis, which include peripancreatic venous thrombosis or less commonly arterial pseudo-aneurysm formation with or without intraperitoneal hemorrhage.

- The pathologic hallmark of chronic pancreatitis is parenchymal fibrosis or sclerosis, which appears as low signal intensity on T1-weighted images in the affected portions of the gland.

- Early ductal abnormalities of chronic pancreatitis may be subtle; visualization of these abnormalities, which include ductal stenosis and side-branch dilatation, can be improved if MRCP images are obtained during intravenous administration of the secretin.

- Chronic pancreatitis may cause a focal inflammatory mass that has signal and enhancement characteristics similar to those of pancreatic adenocarcinoma. In such cases, biopsy is usually required for differentiation.

decreased or heterogeneous signal on T2-weighted images. Adjacent inflammation strongly favors the diagnosis of a complicated pseudocyst. Cyst communication with the pancreatic ductal system narrows the differential diagnosis to pseudocyst and intraductal papillary mucinous neoplasm (IPMN), as the remaining cystic pancreatic neoplasms do not communicate with the ducts. These tumors will be further discussed below. Pseudocysts evolve over relatively short time intervals compared to cystic neoplasms. If solid and vascularized soft tissue elements are present within the cyst, evidenced by contrast enhancement of these tissues, the lesion is not a pseudocyst but neoplastic.[13]

Serous cystadenoma is a benign neoplasm that occurs in older individuals (median age 62 years) with a female-to-male

Table 5.1 CYSTIC LESIONS OF THE PANCREAS: DIFFERENTIAL DIAGNOSIS

LESION	COMMUNICATION WITH PANCREAS DUCTAL SYSTEM	DEFINING FEATURES
Pseudocyst	May be present	Associated findings of pancreatitis Fibrous wall Often unilocular May contain extensive debris
Serous cystadenoma	Absent	Most common in elderly women Multiple small cysts, usually <1 cm Larger lesions have central scar.
Mucinous cystic neoplasm	Absent	Almost exclusively in women Typically in distal body or tail Composed of a few large (>2 cm) cysts, separated by prominent septa
Intraductal papillary mucinous neoplasm (IPMN)	Present	Pseudoseptations Alternate duct narrowing and dilatation without stricture Bulging ampulla may be present in main duct lesions.
Lymphoepithelial cyst	Absent	Rare
Duodenal diverticulum	Duct may empty into diverticulum	Communicates with duodenum Often changes morphology during imaging Air–fluid level Usually within 2 cm of ampulla along medial C-loop

prevalence ratio of approximately 2:1. Serous cystadenomas are incidentally discovered and asymptomatic in up to one third of patients. Common symptoms include abdominal pain, nausea, and weight loss; jaundice and pancreatitis are rare.

At presentation, serous cystadenomas range in size from 1 to 20 cm, with an average size of 5 to 6 cm. They can occur in all portions of the pancreas, with a slight predilection for the pancreatic head. The tumor is composed of a cluster of multiple small cysts ranging from 0.1 to 2.0 cm, but typically less than 1 cm; this appearance originally led to the descriptive name "microcystic adenoma," a term that is no longer used. The cysts in serous cystadenomas are lined with a uniform layer of glycogen-secreting cuboidal cells and separated by fibrous septa. As tumors enlarge, fibrous tissue retraction occurs, producing a central scar, which may calcify. The rare oligocystic variant of serous cystadenoma has larger and fewer cysts and may only contain a single cyst, mimicking a mucinous cystic neoplasm or pseudocyst. Serous cystadenomas slowly enlarge over time.

At MR imaging, the simple fluid within the cysts displays high signal intensity on T2-weighted images, separated by low-signal fibrous septa; this leads to the classic "cluster of grapes" appearance (Fig. 5.12). The fibrous septa and central scar display low signal on T2-weighted images and may show variable enhancement that persists on delayed contrast-enhanced imaging. If central calcification is present, it will produce a signal void on all sequences. Serous cystadenomas do not communicate with the pancreatic ductal system.

If characteristic imaging findings of a serous cystadenoma are present in an asymptomatic patient, these lesions can be safely followed with serial imaging and without intervention. Lesions with an atypical appearance may require aspiration of the fluid from the cysts to confirm the presence of serous fluid. Resection is reserved for symptomatic lesions, as the risk for malignant degeneration is exceedingly rare.

Mucinous cystic neoplasm is an uncommon primary cystic lesion of the pancreas with malignant potential. The premalignant form is often termed mucinous cystadenoma, and the malignant form is called mucinous cystadenocarcinoma; however, as of 2000, both lesions fall under the single WHO classification of mucinous cystic neoplasm (MCN). MCNs affect comparatively young individuals, in the fourth and fifth decades, and over 95% are women. Affected individuals may be asymptomatic or complain of abdominal pain and fullness; anorexia and weight loss may indicate malignancy.

MCNs are generally large at presentation, usually between 6 and 10 cm, and show a strong predilection for the tail of the pancreas and for the body of the pancreas near the tail. The lesions may be unilocular or more commonly multilocular, composed of a few large cysts (more than 2 cm) separated by prominent septa. Because the cysts are relatively large the lesion was originally called a "macrocystic adenoma," a term that is no longer used. The fluid within the cysts is viscous, contains mucin, and may be hemorrhagic. The histologic hallmark of MCNs is the presence of ovarian-type stroma in the cyst wall, a feature not seen in any other pancreatic neoplasm. Calcifications are uncommon and are in the periphery of the

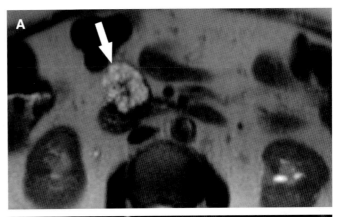

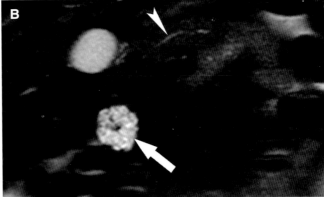

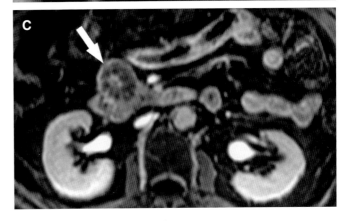

Figure 5.12 *Serous cystadenoma.* (**A**) Axial T2-weighted single-shot FSE/TSE image through the pancreatic head shows a high-signal-intensity cystic lesion (*arrow*) composed of innumerable small cysts, separated by thin, low-signal fibrous bands, and a low-signal-intensity fibrous central scar. (**B**) Coronal thin-section T2-weighted single-shot FSE/TSE image with fat suppression shows numerous small cysts and no communication (*arrow*) with the pancreatic duct (*arrowhead*). (**C**) Axial T1 fat-saturated post-contrast-enhanced image obtained 15 minutes after administration of intravenous gadolinium contrast material shows delayed enhancement of the fibrous septa and central scar in the cystic lesion (*arrow*).

tumor when present. MCNs do not communicate with the pancreatic ductal system.

At MR imaging, the cyst contents often shows homogeneous low signal intensity on T1-weighted and high signal intensity on T2-weighted images. Increasing mucin concentration or hemorrhage may lead to increased signal on T1-weighted and decreased or heterogeneous signal on T2-weighted images. The cyst walls and septations, which display low signal intensity on T1- and T2-weighted images, enhance and are typically thicker than those seen in serous cystadenomas (Fig. 5.13). Features predictive of malignancy include markedly thickened walls or septa, solid or nodular enhancing components, pancreatic ductal obstruction, or invasion of adjacent organs (Fig. 5.14). On MRCP sequences, MCNs will show no communication with the pancreatic ductal system; if ductal communication is present, MCN is excluded and the lesion most likely represents either a pseudocyst or IPMN.

As all MCNs are potentially malignant, surgical resection is generally performed. Unfortunately, the imaging features of

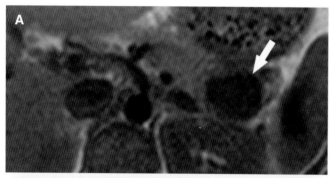

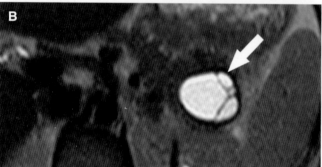

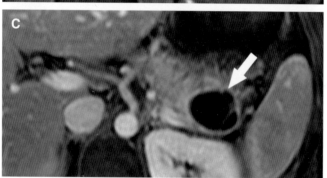

Figure 5.13 *Mucinous cystic neoplasm.* Axial images of the pancreatic tail show a 3-cm cystic lesion (*arrows*). Cyst contents is homogeneous with low signal intensity on T1-weighted gradient-echo (**A**) and high signal on the T2-weighted single-shot FSE/TSE (**B**) image. The cyst wall and internal septations display low signal intensity on the T2-weighted image. MRCP images (not shown) revealed no evidence of communication with the ductal system. (**C**) Axial T1-weighted post-contrast-enhanced gradient-echo image obtained during the portal venous phase shows enhancement of the cyst wall and septations. Absence of thickened septa or solid enhancing components suggests that malignant transformation has not occurred. This was confirmed following resection.

MCNs and pseudocysts may show significant overlap. If MCN is suspected, however, it should not be drained (as is often done in case of a pseudocyst) because this may lead to tumor spread. If a typical lesion is seen in a middle-aged woman with no history or imaging findings of pancreatitis, MCN should be strongly favored. However, with MCNs, peripancreatic inflammatory changes and ductal irregularities are occasionally also seen, making distinction from pseudocysts difficult. Elevation of tumor markers such as serum cancer antigen (CA) 19-9 has a high specificity (96%) in the detection of mucinous tumors or pancreatic adenocarcinoma but is insufficiently sensitive; elevated carcinoembryonic antigen (CEA) within cyst fluid shows higher specificity and sensitivity. Consequently, cyst aspiration may be necessary for differentiation between MCN and pseudocyst. Specifically, the presence of elevated CEA, the presence of mucin, and the absence of elevated amylase support the diagnosis of MCN.[14]

Intraductal papillary mucinous neoplasm (IPMN) is a neoplastic proliferation of intraductal columnar, mucin-secreting cells and is clinically and histopathologically distinct from a MCN. Historical names for IPMN include mucinous ductal ectasia, intraductal mucin-hypersecreting tumor, and ductectatic cystadenoma, but these are no longer used. The current WHO grading system divides IMPNs into benign, borderline, and malignant subtypes. If severe dysplastic epithelial change is present, the lesion is defined as malignant even in the absence of invasion; malignant lesions are designated intraductal papillary mucinous carcinomas. Although malignant, intraductal papillary mucinous carcinoma has a far better prognosis than typical pancreatic adenocarcinoma, with 5-year survival between 36% and 60% for resected invasive carcinoma. IPMNs typically present in the sixth or seventh decades and are seen more commonly in men. Affected individuals may be asymptomatic or experience abdominal pain, jaundice, or worsening diabetes.

IPMN has been divided into main-duct and side-branch subtypes, as the tumor location has been found to correlate with the presence of malignancy. Main-duct involvement is associated with rates of malignancy ranging from 60% to 92%. Isolated side-branch IPMNs show a frequency of malignancy ranging from 6% to 46%.

MR imaging is ideally suited for the characterization of IPMNs, as T2-weighted images and MRCP accurately depict IPMNs as high-intensity tubular lesions distending the ductal system. Isolated side-branch IPMNs may occur in all portions of the pancreas but are more commonly seen in the pancreatic head and uncinate process. Side-branch lesions may assume a rounded and septated appearance similar to MCNs, but careful multiplanar evaluation reveals communication with the ductal system and a lack of complete septations, allowing differentiation (Fig. 5.15). These incomplete septations are often termed "pseudo-septations." Thus, even though IPMN is generally listed as a cystic neoplasm, it is not cystic in origin but shows tubular changes at imaging, indicating its ductal nature. Main-duct involvement is diagnosed when dilatation of the main pancreatic duct is greater than 6 mm (Fig. 5.16). Contrast-enhanced fat-saturated T1-weighted

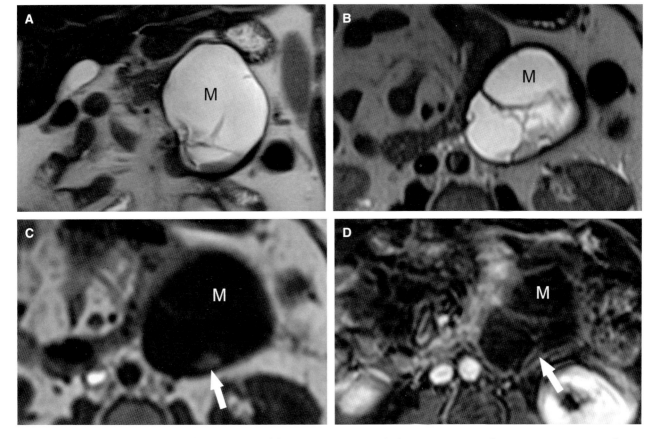

Figure 5.14 *Mucinous cystadenocarcinoma.* (**A**) Coronal and (**B**) axial T2-weighted single-shot FSE/TSE image demonstrates an 11-cm complex cystic mass (*M*) arising from the pancreatic tail. The mass has a thick wall and there are thick septations within the lesion (*M*). Dependent material displays intermediate low signal, which may represent debris or solid tumor. (**C**) Axial T1-weighted gradient-echo image again shows a dependent nodular component (*arrow*) with intermediate signal. (**D**) Axial T1-weighted post-gadolinium-contrast-enhanced gradient-echo image with fat saturation shows enhancement of the nodular component (*arrow*). This confirms the presence of solid tumoral tissue, a finding indicative of malignancy.

images are obtained to evaluate for the presence of solid, enhancing components, a feature of malignancy.

In 2006 an international consensus panel developed guidelines for the management of IMPNs.[15] Indications for resection of IPMN include main-duct involvement or side-branch lesions with any of the following features: overall size more than 30 mm, solid enhancing components, or symptoms attributable to the lesion. Uncomplicated side-branch lesions less than 30 mm may be followed with serial imaging.

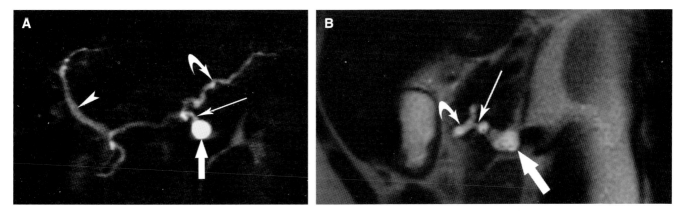

Figure 5.15 *Intraductal papillary mucinous neoplasm, side branch.* (**A**) Thick-slab MRCP single-shot FSE/TSE image demonstrates an approximately 1.5-cm lesion (*arrow*) within the pancreatic tail that appears to communicate (*skinny arrow*) with a normal-caliber main duct (*curved arrow*). CBD, *arrowhead*. (**B**) Sagittal T2-weighted single-shot FSE/TSE image through the pancreatic tail shows the lesion (*arrow*) to have homogeneous high signal content and a single pseudo-septation, found to represent a fold within the dilated side branch on adjacent images. This image also confirms communication (*skinny arrow*) with the normal-caliber main duct (*curved arrow*). Small size and absence of solid components allow this lesion to safely be followed with serial imaging.

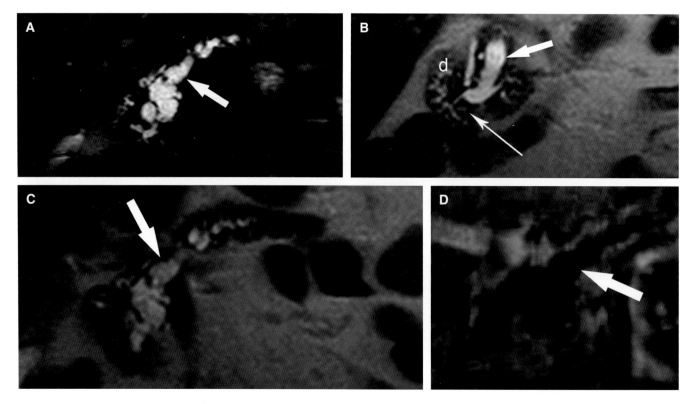

Figure 5.16 *Intraductal papillary mucinous neoplasm, main duct.* (**A**) Thin-section coronal T2-weighted single-shot FSE/TSE image shows marked (more than 15 mm) dilatation of the main pancreatic duct (*arrow*) with a pseudo-septation at the level of the pancreatic head. Coronal T2-weighted images through the (**B**) pancreatic head and (**C**) pancreatic body/tail show the main duct (*arrow*) to be diffusely dilated with regions of narrowing, but no focal stenosis. No ductal stones are seen. The pancreatic parenchymal volume is relatively preserved. Image B also shows mild bulging of the ampulla of Vater (*skinny arrow*) into the duodenum (*d*). All of these findings favor IPMN over chronic pancreatitis. (**D**) Multiplanar reconstructed T1-weighted post-gadolinium-contrast-enhanced gradient-echo image along the main duct (*arrow*) shows no evidence of a solid enhancing nodule. Regardless, main-duct dilatation should prompt resection.

It is well recognized that main-duct IPMNs may be difficult to differentiate from chronic pancreatitis, given the similar clinical and imaging findings. Extensive glandular fibrosis with decreased parenchymal signal intensity on T1-weighted images favors the diagnosis of chronic pancreatitis. Parenchymal and ductal calcification also favors chronic pancreatitis. Both entities result in ductal dilatation, but with chronic pancreatitis tight ductal stenoses are usually present, whereas with IMPN there is diffuse ductal dilatation with regions of relative narrowing, an appearance whimsically compared to a "snake that has swallowed mice." A bulging or patulous ampulla of Vater favors the diagnosis of main-duct IPMN. In many cases, however, endoscopic aspiration of the ductal fluid is required for definitive diagnosis. If imaging features are characteristic of IPMN, confirmatory findings at cyst aspiration include elevated CEA, cytologic staining showing mucin, and the absence of elevated amylase, as in the case of MCNs.

Lymphoepithelial cyst of the pancreas is a rare benign cystic tumor seen most commonly in middle-aged (mean age 54 years) adult men (M:F = 4:1). Half of reported cases were asymptomatic and incidentally discovered; the most common symptoms in the remaining cases were abdominal pain, nausea, vomiting, and diarrhea. Lymphoepithelial cysts are lined by squamous epithelium surrounded by mature lymphoid tissue and are filled with "cheesy" material composed of debris, keratin, and cholesterol crystals. They may be unilocular (40%) or multilocular (60%). They occur in any region of the pancreas and are usually superficial, surrounded only partially by normal pancreatic tissue. Rare reported instances of rupture show an intense desmoplastic reaction in surrounding tissue.[16]

Lymphoepithelial cysts are not well described in the MR literature; however, the reported internal signal intensity on T1- and T2-weighted images varies depending on the nature of the cyst's contents. Fine-needle aspiration is required for definitive diagnosis, as the appearance of this rare lesion may mimic that of other cystic lesions of the pancreas. The cysts are managed either with simple excision or partial pancreatectomy; however, some recommend observation in asymptomatic patients.

Intraluminal duodenal diverticula are rare congenital lesions that result from incomplete canalization of the duodenum, and should not be mistaken for a pancreatic cystic lesion, as they are confined to the duodenal lumen.

Extraluminal duodenal diverticula, however, are extremely common acquired outpouchings of the mucosa and muscularis mucosa; as the majority (90%) occur along the medial aspect of the duodenum, they may distort or appear to be within the pancreatic head and may therefore occasionally be confused with a cystic pancreatic lesion. Extraluminal duodenal diverticula are usually asymptomatic. Fewer than 10% are symptomatic, and complications include obstruction, food impaction, perforation, bleeding, or diverticulitis. The majority of lesions are within 2 cm of the major papilla and may distort the ampulla of Vater; affected patients have an increased frequency of CBD stones.

At MR imaging, extraluminal duodenal diverticula are well depicted on T2-weighted images as cystic lesions with an air–fluid level along the medial aspect of the duodenal C-loop (the C-shaped curve defined by the first three portions of the duodenum), usually in a periampullary location. The dependent fluid component displays high signal on T2-weighted images but may show heterogeneous signal if food products are present; the non-dependent air is seen as a signal void. The presence of air and visualization of communication with the duodenum are characteristic findings of a duodenal diverticulum and differentiate the lesion from a cystic pancreatic neoplasm or pseudocyst. Because a diverticulum moves with the contractions of the duodenum, they change in size and shape during image acquisition and, consequently, their morphology varies on consecutive images, something that is not the case with cystic neoplasm or pseudocysts. However, when the diverticulum contains only fluid and no air is present, differentiation can be difficult. If the finding of a diverticulum is uncertain, the diagnosis can be confirmed if the lesion fills with barium suspension on an upper GI examination.

Incidentally Discovered Simple Cysts. True epithelial cysts of the pancreas are rare and associated with hereditary disorders such as VHL, CF, or (less commonly) autosomal-dominant polycystic kidney disease. However, small (less than 10 mm) pancreatic cysts are seen in as many as 20% of individuals on MRCP; the prevalence is higher in patients with a history of pancreatitis. Many of these cysts represent tiny pseudocysts or retention cysts, particularly in patients with a history of pancreatitis; the majority remain undiagnosed.

Management of simple pancreatic cysts is controversial. Some authors argue that simple cysts as large as 2 or even 3 cm can be managed conservatively with serial imaging, as the vast majority of such cysts show long-term stability or benign pathology.[17,18] Others argue that more aggressive management is indicated, as many of the reported benign cysts represent premalignant lesions such as MCNs and IPMNs.[19]

Box 5.5 **ESSENTIALS TO REMEMBER**

- When evaluating a cystic pancreatic lesion, first assess MRCP images to determine if the lesion communicates with the pancreatic ducts, as only pseudocysts and IPMNs communicate with the ductal system.

- Most (75% to 85%) of cystic pancreatic lesions are pseudocysts. The presence of acute or chronic pancreatitis and inflammation adjacent to the cyst strongly favors the diagnosis of pseudocyst.

- If the cystic lesion contains solid, vascularized soft tissue, the lesion is neoplastic and not a pseudocyst.

- Serous cystadenomas are benign lesions that occur in older individuals and are more common in women. They do not communicate with the ductal system and are composed of multiple small (<2 cm) cysts; however, the rare oligocystic variant has fewer, larger cysts and may therefore mimic a pseudocyst or MCN.

- Mucinous cystic neoplasm (MCN) occurs almost exclusively in women (>95%). MCNs are composed of a few large cysts separated by prominent septa, have a strong predilection for the distal body and tail, and do not communicate with the pancreatic ducts. As MCNs have malignant potential, surgical resection is indicated.

- MCNs may be associated with inflammation and can therefore be misdiagnosed as pseudocysts. However, if MCN is suspected, drain placement is contraindicated; rather, cyst aspiration may be performed to confirm the diagnosis.

- An intraductal papillary mucinous neoplasm (IPMN) is a potentially malignant proliferation of intraductal cells and appears as cystic/saccular dilatation of a portion of the pancreatic ductal system, with or without a soft tissue component. Therefore, even though IPMN is generally listed as a cystic neoplasm, it is not cystic in origin but shows tubular changes at imaging, indicating its ductal nature.

- Indications for resection of IPMN correlate with features that portend an increased risk of malignancy: (1) symptoms attributable to the lesion; (2) main duct involvement (duct >6 mm); (3) a side-branch lesion that is more than 30 mm in diameter; or (4) the presence of a solid enhancing component.

- A duodenal diverticulum may be misdiagnosed as a cystic pancreatic lesion. Features characteristic of a duodenal diverticulum include communication with the duodenal lumen, the presence of an air–fluid level, changing morphology during the examination, and proximity to the ampulla.

- True epithelial cysts of the pancreas are rare, and management of simple pancreatic cysts is controversial. Some argue for conservative management (serial imaging) of simple cysts up to 3 cm in diameter. Others argue that many reported benign cysts actually represent premalignant lesions (e.g., MCNs, IPMNs) and should be considered for removal.

SOLID LESIONS OF THE PANCREAS

The main diagnostic consideration when confronted with a solid pancreatic lesion is primary adenocarcinoma of the pancreas (Table 5.2). This is the diagnosis of exclusion in the setting of a focal or infiltrative pancreatic mass characterized by decreased signal on T1-weighted images, decreased enhancement, and proximal ductal obstruction. Rarely, focal chronic pancreatitis may have an identical appearance, and if the history suggests this diagnosis biopsy is indicated for definitive diagnosis.

However, solid lesions will occasionally have features that suggest a diagnosis other than adenocarcinoma. Two findings in particular indicate an alternate diagnosis: the absence of proximal ductal dilatation and the presence of early enhancement, a feature strongly associated with pancreatic endocrine tumors.

Once a solid pancreatic lesion is diagnosed, it is the radiologist's job to clearly describe the extent of the lesion. It is necessary to define the lesion's size, anatomic boundaries, and the presence or absence of invasion of adjacent structures, particularly the peripancreatic vessels. If malignancy is suspected, a careful search for lymphadenopathy or metastases should follow. These details allow one to predict if the patient is a candidate for surgical resection and are essential in counseling the patient regarding prognosis.

Pancreatic ductal adenocarcinoma is the most common pancreatic malignancy and is the fourth most common cause of cancer death in the United States. It is often diagnosed late in the course of the disease and has a 5-year survival rate of less than 5%. In the 15% to 20% of patients with a potentially resectable tumor, 5-year survival rates improve to 15% to 20% among those who undergo a successful pancreaticoduodenectomy. Pancreatic carcinoma primarily affects the elderly, with

Table 5.2 SOLID LESIONS OF THE PANCREAS: DIFFERENTIAL DIAGNOSIS

LESION	DUCTAL OBSTRUCTION	DEFINING FEATURES
Pancreatic adenocarcinoma	Almost always present	Infiltrative mass Abrupt narrowing of duct "Double duct sign" predictive of malignancy Decreased enhancement Proclivity for vascular invasion May occur with hepatic, mesenteric, or nodal metastases
Mass-like chronic pancreatitis	May be present	Smooth, stenotic duct penetrating mass, "duct penetrating sign," may differentiate from adenocarcinoma
Endocrine neoplasm	Rare in small tumors May be present in large tumors	Well defined Often show avid enhancement on early post-contrast images Heterogeneous enhancement and signal, necrosis when large Calcification may be present in large tumors. If functional, clinical symptoms reflect cell of origin.
Acinar cell carcinoma	Rare	Well circumscribed Large at diagnosis Partially or completely exophytic Heterogeneous; cystic components may predominate when very large
Solid pseudopapillary tumor	Absent	Young women are usually affected. Well circumscribed Large at diagnosis Hemorrhagic debris with high signal on T1-weighted images Cystic components often predominate.
Pancreatic lymphoma	May cause mild dilatation	Well circumscribed or infiltrative May infiltrate mesentery, surround arteries If secondary, often associated with lymphadenopathy below the renal veins (unlike adenocarcinoma)
Accessory spleen	Absent	Pancreatic tail location Follows signal and enhancement characteristics of spleen
Lipoma	Rare	Follows fat signal on all sequences
Metastases	Rare	Solitary, multifocal, or diffuse Often with rim enhancement Melanoma: often high signal on T1-weighted images Renal cell CA (clear cell): may show loss of signal on opposed-phase images

80% of cases occurring in individuals between the ages of 60 and 80. It is slightly more common in African Americans and individuals of Ashkenazi Jewish descent. Cigarette smoking is believed to double the risk of pancreatic cancer. Chronic pancreatitis and diabetes are associated with an increased risk of pancreatic cancer, but a causal role in the development of the tumor has not been established.

The poor prognosis of pancreatic adenocarcinoma is in part due to its tendency to remain clinically silent until the tumor has invaded adjacent structures; this is illustrated by the fact that in fortunate individuals in whom cancer is discovered at a very early stage (less than 1 cm), 5-year survival is 100%.[20] Unfortunately, screening tests have not proven beneficial in cancer detection. Serum antigens (e.g., CEA, CA19-9) are useful in measuring response to treatment but are insufficiently sensitive and specific in establishing the diagnosis of pancreatic adenocarcinoma. Pain is the most common first symptom, and when there is pain the cancer is usually beyond cure. Obstructive jaundice may occur if the lesion is in the pancreatic head involving and obstructing the CBD. Weight loss, anorexia, and weakness indicate advanced disease (Table 5.3).

Pancreatic adenocarcinoma occurs throughout the pancreas, with 60% of cases arising in the head, 15% in the body, and 5% in the tail, and 20% showing diffuse involvement. The cancer is usually a moderately to poorly differentiated adenocarcinoma with a deeply infiltrative growth pattern and a proclivity for perineural, lymphatic, and vascular invasion. The cancer elicits a desmoplastic response; consequently, dense fibrosis accompanies the invasive cancer.[21]

The fibrotic and infiltrative nature of the cancer accounts for many of its imaging characteristics. The tumor and associated fibrosis efface the pancreatic acini; as a consequence, the tumor appears as a region of low signal intensity on non-contrast-enhanced T1-weighted images, against a background of the relatively high signal intensity of the normal pancreatic tissue. As fibrosis restricts tumor vascularity, the tumor shows decreased enhancement on early post-gadolinium-contrast-enhanced

images when compared to normal parenchyma (Fig. 5.17). The appearance on interstitial-phase images is variable, but desmoplastic content may cause gradual delayed enhancement. Tumor signal intensity on T2-weighted images is strongly affected by necrosis, inflammation, and hemorrhage and is therefore variable; consequently, T2-weighted images are poorly suited for detection or assessment of tumor extent.

As pancreatic adenocarcinoma arises in the ductal epithelium, it invariably causes abrupt narrowing of the main pancreatic duct with upstream dilatation, best appreciated on MRCP images. Pancreatic head cancers may also cause stenosis and proximal (upstream) dilatation of the common bile duct, leading to the "double duct" sign, a finding strongly associated with malignancy. Glandular tissue distal to an obstructing cancer (closer to the tail) will often be affected by chronic inflammation, leading to progressive fibrosis and atrophy; in such cases, it is difficult to assess tumor extent on non-contrast-enhanced T1-weighted images. However, on immediate post-contrast-enhanced images the tumor will show decreased enhancement compared to the adjacent chronically inflamed tissue.

The CT literature has shown that greater than 10% of pancreatic adenocarcinomas have density and enhancement characteristics indistinguishable from that of adjacent normal pancreatic tissue. Such cancers may be appreciated only by an interrupted pancreatic duct, distal parenchymal atrophy, or glandular contour abnormality. As MRI provides superior contrast resolution and acquires a greater variety of imaging data, it has been shown to be more useful in the detection of these small cancers, particularly the lesions that do not deform the contour of the pancreas.[22]

A focal pancreatic mass causing ductal dilatation and having characteristic signal and enhancement features will, in most cases, be pancreatic adenocarcinoma. Chronic pancreatitis, however, may cause a focal mass-like lesion with similar imaging characteristics. Effacement of the fine lobular architecture of the pancreas may support the diagnosis of adenocarcinoma. The presence of a well-defined demarcation between normal and abnormal tissue on early post-contrast-enhanced T1-weighted images favors the diagnosis of adenocarcinoma, but it is recognized that some tumors appear as poorly marginated lesions. Differentiation is particularly difficult in cases where adenocarcinoma causes pancreatitis or develops in the setting of chronic pancreatitis. However, invasion of peripancreatic vessels, the presence of lymphadenopathy, or visualization of hepatic metastases indicates pancreatic cancer.

Resection of pancreatic adenocarcinoma leads to a modest decrease in mortality, as 5-year survival rates improve from 5% to 15% to 20% among patients who undergo a successful pancreaticoduodenectomy. Therefore, once the diagnosis of adenocarcinoma is strongly suspected or established, the role of the imaging study is to determine resectability (Table 5.4). A pancreatic cancer is characterized as resectable if there is no evidence of involvement of the SMA or celiac axis, preserved patency of the superior mesenteric–portal venous confluence, and no evidence of distant metastatic disease (i.e., T3 [or less] M0) (Fig. 5.17); although patients with regional nodal metastases have a poorer long-term prognosis, the presence of

Table 5.3 TNM STAGING OF PANCREATIC CANCER

Primary Tumor
  Tx: Primary tumor cannot be assessed
  T0: No evidence of primary tumor
  Tis: Carcinoma *in situ*
  T1: Tumor limited to the pancreas, 2 cm or less in greatest dimension
  T2: Tumor limited to the pancreas, more than 2 cm in greatest dimension
  T3: Tumor extends beyond the pancreas but without involvement of the celiac axis or the superior mesenteric artery
  T4: Tumor involves the celiac axis or the superior mesenteric artery
Regional Lymph Nodes
  Nx: Regional lymph nodes cannot be assessed
  N0: No regional lymph node metastasis
  N1: Regional lymph node metastasis
Distant Metastasis
  M0: No distant metastasis
  M1: Distant metastasis

Adapted with permission from American Joint Committee on Cancer. *AJCC Cancer Staging Manual*, 7th ed. Springer, 2010.

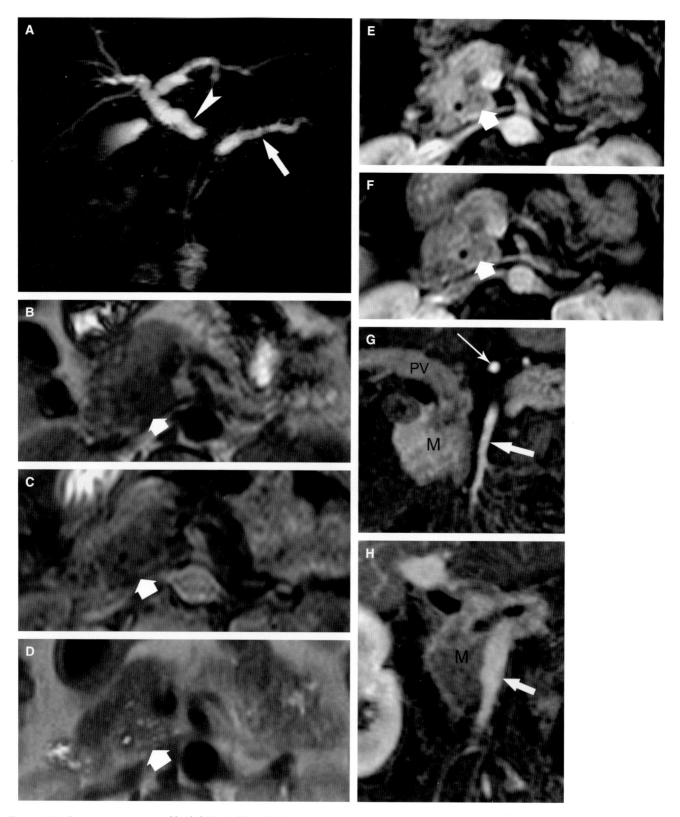

Figure 5.17 *Pancreatic cancer, resectable.* (**A**) Thick-slab MRCP image reveals abrupt stenosis of both the CBD (*arrowhead*) and main pancreatic duct (*arrow*), with proximal dilatation. Axial T1-weighted gradient-echo images without (**B**) and with (**C**) fat saturation show a 2-cm mass (*arrow*) in the head of the pancreas. The mass displays lower signal intensity than the adjacent normal pancreatic parenchyma. (**D**) Axial T2-weighted single shot FSE/TSE image at the same level shows the mass (*arrow*) to have slightly increased signal compared to normal pancreatic parenchyma; however, the mass is less conspicuous compared to its appearance on the T1-weighted image. (**E**) Following the administration of intravenous gadolinium-based contrast material, the mass (*arrow*) appears as a region of decreased enhancement on the axial T1-weighted fat-saturated pancreatic parenchymal-phase image. (**F**) The mass (*arrow*) is markedly less conspicuous during the portal venous phase of imaging. (**G**) On the coronal T1-weighted fat-saturated contrast-enhanced MRA image, the SMA (*arrow*) and the celiac axis (*skinny arrow*) are completely surrounded by fat and are free of disease. *M*, mass. *PV*, portal vein. (**H**) Coronal T1-weighted fat-saturated contrast-enhanced MRV image shows the mass (*M*) to focally abut the SMV (*arrow*). This finding does not preclude resection.

enlarged regional nodes does not preclude resection. Recently, a subset of T4 tumors has been classified as "borderline resectable" if the tumor has any of the following characteristics: (1) abutment of the SMA or celiac axis is no more than 180 degrees; (2) limited abutment/encasement of the common or proper hepatic artery, typically at the gastroduodenal artery origin, allowing segmental reconstruction of the hepatic artery; and (3) short segment occlusion of the SMV or portal vein with sufficient flow above and below the occlusion to allow interposition grafting (Fig. 5.18).[23] These patients may benefit from resection following preoperative systemic chemotherapy and local radiation therapy.

At MRI, arterial involvement is appreciated as intermediate-intensity tissue infiltrating and effacing the fat plane surrounding peripancreatic vessels, usually the SMA (Fig. 5.19). This is best appreciated on non–fat-suppressed T1-weighted or post-gadolinium-contrast-enhanced fat-suppressed images. Arterial patency is best depicted on immediate post-contrast-enhanced MRA images. Venous narrowing or occlusion is best seen on portal venous-phase enhanced MRA images.

Regional nodal metastases are suspected when lymph nodes measure more than 10 mm in short axis in the axial plane. Regional lymph nodes for tumors in the head and neck of the pancreas include lymph nodes along the CBD, common hepatic artery, portal vein, posterior and anterior pancreaticoduodenal arcades, the SMV, and the right lateral wall of the SMA. For cancers of the body and tail, regional lymph nodes include lymph nodes along the common hepatic artery, celiac axis, splenic artery, and splenic hilum.[24] Lymph nodes are best seen as foci of low/intermediate signal intensity against a background of high-signal-intensity fat on T1-weighted images, or high signal intensity against a background of low signal on T2-weighted or post-contrast-enhanced fat-suppressed images.

Liver metastases may be round or irregular in shape. They display low signal intensity on T1-weighted and mildly increased signal intensity on T2-weighted images compared to the adjacent normal hepatic parenchyma. The increase in

Table 5.4 CRITERIA FOR PANCREATIC CANCER RESECTABILITY

Resectable:
    No evidence of involvement of the celiac axis or SMA (T3 or less)
    No distant metastases (M0)
Borderline Resectable:
    T4 lesions with:
        ≤180° tumor abutment of the SMA or celiac axis
        Short segment abutment or encasement of the common hepatic artery
        Segmental venous occlusion allowing reconstruction (adequate SMV below and portal vein above region of tumor involvement)
    No distant metastases (M0)
Non-resectable:
    T4 lesions with vascular involvement that does not qualify as "borderline"
    Presence of distant metastases (M1)

signal intensity on T2-weighted images is much less than that of hemangiomas or hepatic cysts, due to the relatively low water content and hypovascular nature of adenocarcinoma metastases. On early post-contrast-enhanced images, metastases usually show irregular rim enhancement with decreased central enhancement; very small lesions may show homogeneous early enhancement. Small hypervascular subcapsular metastases are seen in more than 80% of patients with pancreatic cancer metastases and may be the sole manifestation of hepatic metastases in up to 20% of patients.[25]

Peritoneal metastases may be difficult to detect on preoperative imaging, but their presence, like liver metastases, will preclude surgery. Peritoneal metastases are best seen as foci of high signal on post-contrast-enhanced fat-suppressed T1-weighted images.

Pancreatic Endocrine Neoplasms. Commonly called "islet cell tumors," the preferred term for tumors of the pancreatic islet cells is pancreatic endocrine neoplasms. Endocrine neoplasms are rare and account for less than 2% of pancreatic neoplasms. Although most common in young to middle-aged adults, pancreatic endocrine neoplasms may occur throughout

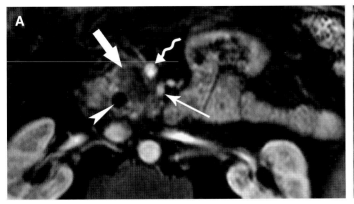
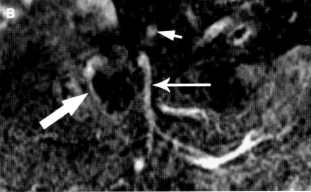

Figure 5.18 *Pancreatic cancer, borderline resectable.* (**A**) Axial T1-weighted fat-saturated post-gadolinium-contrast-enhanced gradient-echo image obtained during the parenchymal phase through the pancreatic head shows the 3-cm carcinoma (*arrow*) as a region of markedly decreased enhancement. Abnormal soft tissue abuts the SMA (*skinny arrow*), however, circumferential involvement is less than 180 degrees. The tumor also abuts the SMV (*squiggly arrow*) and the CBD (*arrowhead*). (**B**) Coronal reconstruction from a contrast-enhanced 3D gradient-echo sequence for shows the mass (*arrow*) to enhance peripherally, with decreased central enhancement secondary to necrosis. Focal enhancing soft tissue extends from the left side of the mass and abuts the SMA (*skinny arrow*) without encasement. The celiac axis (*short arrow*) is not involved by tumor.

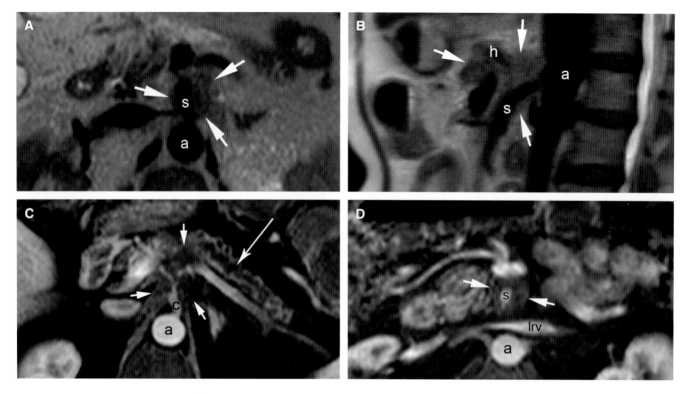

Figure 5.19 *Pancreatic cancer, nonresectable.* (**A**) Axial T2-weighted single-shot FSE/TSE image through the SMA origin from the aorta (*a*) shows abnormal intermediate-signal-intensity tumor (*short arrows*) surrounding the SMA (*s*), precluding resection. (**B**) Sagittal T2-weighted image through the SMA origin from the aorta (*a*) shows tumor (*short arrows*) surrounding both the SMA (*s*) and the proximal common hepatic artery (*h*). (**C**) Axial T1-weighted fat-saturated post-contrast-enhanced gradient-echo image obtained during the pancreatic parenchymal phase shows infiltrating tumor (*short arrows*) as tissue that enhances to a lesser degree than the pancreatic parenchyma. The tumor originates at the junction of the pancreatic body and tail and causes proximal ductal dilatation (*long arrow*) and parenchymal atrophy. Infiltrative tumor surrounds and narrows the celiac axis (*c*) and its branches, the proximal splenic and common hepatic arteries. *a*, aorta. (**D**) Axial image obtained inferior to image C shows infiltrating tumor (*short arrows*) surrounding the SMA (*s*). *a*, aorta. *lrv*, left renal vein.

life, with several reported cases in newborns. With the exception of gastrinoma, pancreatic endocrine neoplasms have a slightly higher incidence in females. Pancreatic endocrine neoplasms have an increased incidence in VHL disease and multiple endocrine neoplasia type 1 (MEN 1) but are more commonly not associated with a syndrome. Clinical features reflect the cell of origin. Functional pancreatic endocrine neoplasms tend to present when the lesion is still small, as unregulated hormone production heralds the presence of disease. Nonfunctional tumors usually present with symptoms related to mass effect or metastatic disease, and therefore tend to present when large. Insulinomas, the most common pancreatic endocrine neoplasm, are benign in 90% of cases. The remaining pancreatic endocrine neoplasms, both functional and nonfunctional, are malignant in 60% to 90% of cases.

The various types of pancreatic endocrine neoplasms share many MR imaging characteristics, and differences in appearance tend to be based on size rather than cell origin. Although classically described as well-defined lesions with relatively high signal intensity on T2-weighted images and avid enhancement on early contrast-enhanced images, these tumors have a broad spectrum of appearances. Tumor conspicuity is generally highest on unenhanced, fat-suppressed T1-weighted images, because of the high contrast between the low-signal-intensity tumor and the background high signal intensity of the normal pancreas. Endocrine tumors typically display increased signal intensity on T2-weighted images but may also be iso- or hypointense compared to the normal pancreas.

The classically described pattern of homogeneous intense enhancement on early post-contrast-enhanced images is most commonly seen in small pancreatic endocrine neoplasms. However, even small lesions may show variable degree and timing of enhancement, with some tumors best seen on venous-phase enhanced images and some tumors remaining inconspicuous as they have similar perfusion characteristics to the normal pancreas; consequently, it is necessary to closely evaluate unenhanced T1-weighted images and all phases of the dynamic contrast enhancement acquisition. Ring-like enhancement is another characteristic pattern and may be seen on early or delayed gadolinium-contrast-enhanced images.

As pancreatic endocrine neoplasms become larger, enhancement tends to be more variable and heterogeneous. The largest tumors, usually nonfunctional, may have necrotic areas, which lack enhancement and demonstrate high signal intensity on T2-weighted images. If the necrotic portion is sufficiently large, the tumor may resemble a pseudocyst or cystic neoplasm; the presence of a rim of solid enhancing tissue favors the diagnosis of a necrotic solid tumor. It is uncommon for endocrine tumors to cause ductal obstruction and dilatation, particularly when small; this feature, along with characteristic early enhancement, when present helps differentiate endocrine tumors from the far more common adenocarcinoma. Signs of malignancy include vascular invasion, invasion of adjacent organs, or metastases to peripancreatic lymph nodes or the liver. Signal and enhancement characteristics of hepatic metastases from pancreatic endocrine neoplasms tend to resemble those of the primary lesion.[26]

Characteristic clinical or imaging features of the various pancreatic endocrine tumors are discussed in the following paragraphs.

Insulinomas (beta-cell tumor) are the most common pancreatic endocrine neoplasm, accounting for 50% to 55% of islet cell tumors. Hypoglycemia, caused by unregulated insulin secretion, is the most common presenting symptom and is mild in all but 20% of cases. Insulinomas are usually benign (90%) and solitary (90%). Tumors are usually discovered when small (less than 2 cm) and may be found anywhere in the pancreas. Histologically, the lesions look like giant islets. Diagnosis of malignancy is based on the detection of local invasion or distant metastases, as the primary malignant lesion may show little evidence of anaplasia. At MR imaging, insulinomas are commonly detected when small and show homogeneous low signal on non-contrast-enhanced T1-weighted images, homogeneous high signal on T2-weighted images, and uniform intense enhancement on early contrast-enhanced images (Fig. 5.20).

Gastrinomas are the second most common pancreatic endocrine neoplasm, accounting for approximately 30% of islet cell tumors. They are sporadic in approximately 70% of patients and seen in MEN 1 in the remaining 30%. When associated with MEN 1, gastrinomas are often multiple; sporadic gastrinomas are usually solitary. Approximately 65% of patients are male. Hypersecretion of gastrin leads to Zollinger-Ellison syndrome, whose features include abdominal pain, diarrhea, nausea/vomiting, gastrointestinal bleeding caused by duodenal ulcers, and weight loss. The histologic appearance of gastrinomas is similar to that of insulinomas. Unlike insulinomas, gastrinomas have a strong predilection for occurring within the "gastrinoma triangle," bounded by the junction of the cystic duct and CBD superiorly, the junction of the second and third portions of the duodenum inferiorly, and the junction of the neck and body of the pancreas medially. The MR appearance is similar to that of insulinomas, as gastrinomas are usually detected when small (mean size less than 4 cm). Unlike insulinomas, gastrinomas may arise in the duodenal wall (40% to 50%), and affected patients may have duodenitis or duodenal ulcers. Because more than 60% of gastrinomas are malignant, they are more likely to show locally aggressive features or metastases than insulinomas.

Nonfunctioning islet cell tumors are the third most common pancreatic endocrine neoplasm, accounting for approximately 15% to 25% of islet cell tumors. Because nonfunctioning islet cell tumors do not produce a clinically significant amount of hormones, the patient's symptoms are usually related to the tumor's mass effect or the presence of metastatic disease. Consequently, they are much larger at diagnosis (6 to 10 cm) than functioning tumors, are malignant in more than 80% of cases, and commonly present with evidence of locally advanced or metastatic disease. At MR imaging, these large tumors often

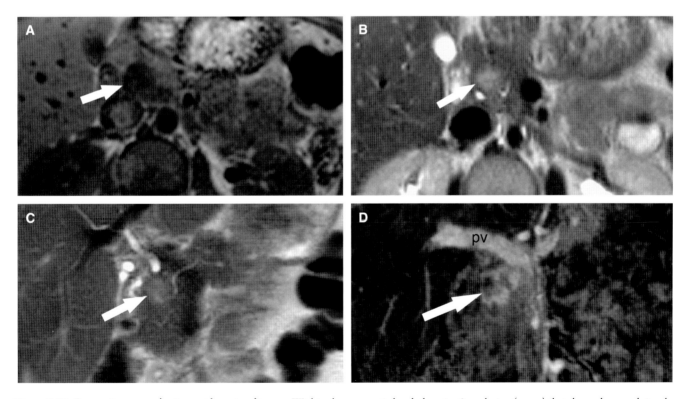

Figure 5.20 *Pancreatic neuroendocrine neoplasm, insulinoma.* Within the pancreatic head, there is a 2-cm lesion (*arrow*) that shows decreased signal intensity compared to normal parenchyma on the axial T1-weighted gradient-echo image (**A**) and mildly increased signal intensity on the axial (**B**) and coronal (**C**) T2-weighted image single-shot FSE/TSE. (**D**) On the coronal T1-weighted fat-suppressed image from a gadolinium-contrast-enhanced MRA sequence acquired during the late-arterial phase, the lesion (*arrow*) shows avid early enhancement. *pv,* portal vein.

show cystic degeneration, foci of necrosis, and markedly heterogeneous enhancement (Fig. 5.21). Calcification, if present, will appear as a signal void on all sequences and is better appreciated at CT; when visualized, this finding differentiates an endocrine neoplasm from the far more common adenocarcinoma.

Rare pancreatic endocrine neoplasms, including glucagonomas, VIPomas, and somatostatinomas, are usually malignant (60% to 80%) and tend to present late in the course of disease because of their uncommon and often nonspecific signs and symptoms.

Glucagonomas (alpha-cell tumors) occur most frequently in peri- and postmenopausal women. High plasma glucagon

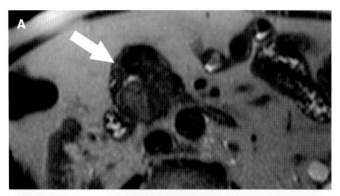

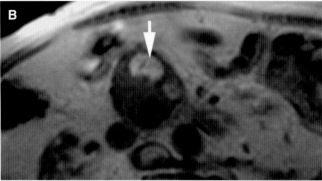

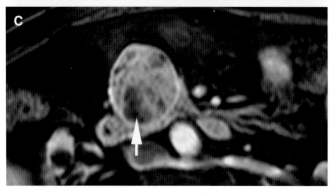

Figure 5.21 *Pancreatic endocrine neoplasm, nonfunctioning.* (**A**) Axial T2-weighted single-shot FSE/TSE image through a 4-cm pancreatic head mass shows a predominantly solid lesion (*arrow*) with heterogeneous signal intensity. (**B**) Axial T1-weighted gradient-echo image obtained at the same level reveals regions of hemorrhagic necrosis as foci with high signal intensity (*short arrow*). (**C**) Axial T1-weighted fat-suppressed post-contrast-enhanced gradient-echo image shows heterogeneous enhancement, with regions of absent enhancement (*short arrow*), representing necrosis. Of note, this large mass did not cause ductal obstruction.

levels lead to mild diabetes mellitus. A characteristic skin rash, necrolytic migratory erythema, is seen in tissues exposed to friction or pressure. Other symptoms include anemia and venous thromboembolism. The tumor is most frequently found in the pancreatic tail but may also arise in the body or head and may rarely arise in the stomach or duodenum.

VIPomas secrete vasoactive intestinal polypeptide (VIP), which causes watery diarrhea that persists despite fasting and leads to electrolyte abnormalities such as hypokalemia and achlorhydria. Ninety percent arise in the pancreas; the remainder are found in paraganglionic tissues, the adrenal glands, the colon, the bronchi, or the liver.

Somatostatinomas (delta-cell tumors) secrete somatostatin, which inhibits the secretion of many hormones, including insulin, glucagon, gastrin, cholecystokinin (CCK), and VIP, among others. Symptoms include diabetes mellitus, diarrhea and steatorrhea with weight loss, cholelithiasis, and hypochlorhydria. These tumors occur with equal frequency in the pancreas and duodenum and rarely arise in other locations such as the liver, kidneys, and lungs.

Primary pancreatic carcinoid tumors, which secrete serotonin, are exceedingly rare, as more than 95% arise in the gastrointestinal tract. When present, most pancreatic carcinoids occur in the tail. Calcification occurs far more frequently in carcinoid tumors than in other endocrine neoplasms.

Pancreatic acinar cell carcinomas account for only 1% of pancreatic exocrine tumors. Acinar cell carcinomas occur in the fifth to seventh decades and are more common in men. Symptoms are most commonly related to local mass effect and include abdominal pain, nausea/vomiting, and weight loss. As tumors are often large at diagnosis, a palpable abdominal mass may be present; however, jaundice is rare. At histology, the tumor shows prominent acinar differentiation; cells contain prominent zymogen granules, reflecting the high production of exocrine enzymes, including trypsin and lipase. The resultant lipasemia leads to the characteristic syndrome of subcutaneous fat necrosis, occurring in 15% of patients. Circulating exocrine pancreatic enzymes may also cause polyarthritis and lytic osseous lesions in the distal extremities. Tumors are evenly distributed throughout the pancreas. Acinar cell carcinomas are aggressive neoplasms, with a median survival of 19 months from diagnosis, but have a better prognosis than adenocarcinomas.

At MR imaging, acinar cell tumors are well marginated and, in most cases, partially or completely exophytic. Tumors are large at diagnosis, averaging 7 to 10 cm. Smaller tumors (less than 5 cm) are homogeneous and solid, with mildly increased signal on T2-weighted images and decreased signal on T1-weighted images compared to normal parenchyma. Larger tumors have cystic or necrotic components, with the largest lesions (more than 10 cm) having cystic areas constituting more than 75% of the tumor. In such lesions, the presence of a significant solid enhancing component differentiates the tumor from a pseudocyst or cystic pancreatic neoplasm; however, nonfunctioning endocrine neoplasms and solid pseudopapillary tumors may have an similar appearance. Like adenocarcinoma, acinar cell carcinoma typically enhances less than adjacent normal parenchyma; however, well-defined margins, large size, cystic components, and absence of pancreatic ductal dilatation differentiate this tumor from the far more common adenocarcinoma.[27]

Solid Pseudopapillary Tumor. The most characteristic feature of the rare solid pseudopapillary tumor is its demographic: 90% of affected patients are female, with a mean age of 24 to 30 years. Some case series show a predilection for African American or Asian women. These tumors account for 1% to 2% of pancreatic exocrine neoplasms. The tumors are often asymptomatic and painless and do not present until palpable or large enough to compress adjacent viscera. As a result, the lesions are relatively large when diagnosed, with a mean diameter of more than 9 cm. Solid pseudopapillary tumors have no specific predilection for any portion of the pancreas and may occur anywhere within the gland. Histologic evaluation reveals a well-circumscribed mass with cells that grow as solid sheets or papillary projections. As in other large pancreatic tumors, cystic and necrotic components may predominate; however, the presence of hemorrhagic debris is characteristic. Ductal obstruction is usually not present.

The tumors are rarely malignant (15%); they tend to displace the surrounding structures rather than invade them, and surgical resection usually leads to cure.

At non-contrast-enhanced MR imaging the tumors usually display heterogeneous signal intensity on both T1- and T2-weighted images, reflecting the complex nature of the lesions. Regions of high signal on T1-weighted images are present in more than 70% of lesions and reflect the presence of blood products; hemorrhagic degeneration may also demonstrate a fluid–fluid level due to an hematocrit effect. The solid and cystic nature of the tumor leads to markedly heterogeneous signal on T2-weighted images, with cystic portions occasionally having decreased signal if old blood products are present. In most cases, a low-signal fibrous capsule surrounds the tumor. Peripheral calcification is rare and better seen with CT. The most commonly described pattern of contrast enhancement is early peripheral heterogeneous enhancement with heterogeneous fill-in of the lesion on portal venous and delayed images. The tumor enhances less than normal pancreatic parenchyma on all phases (Fig. 5.22).[28]

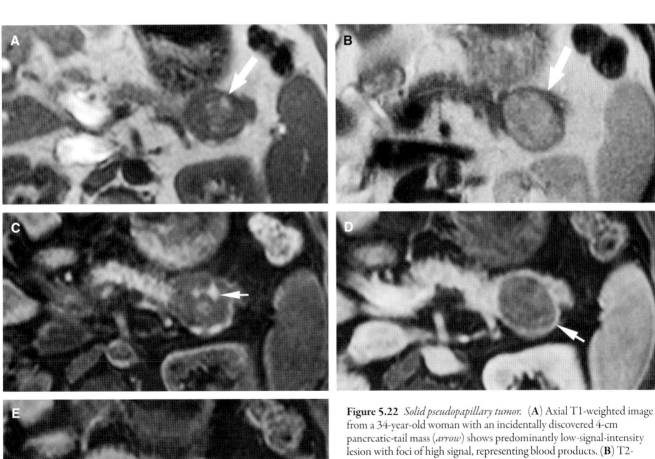

Figure 5.22 *Solid pseudopapillary tumor.* (**A**) Axial T1-weighted image from a 34-year-old woman with an incidentally discovered 4-cm pancreatic-tail mass (*arrow*) shows predominantly low-signal-intensity lesion with foci of high signal, representing blood products. (**B**) T2-weighted image through the lesion (*arrow*) shows a low-signal fibrous capsule and heterogeneously increased signal centrally. (**C**) Axial T1-weighted fat-suppressed pre-contrast-enhanced image again shows foci of high signal (*short arrow*) within the lesion, representing hemorrhage. (**D**) Axial T1-weighted fat-suppressed post-contrast-enhanced image obtained in the parenchymal phase shows heterogeneous peripheral, capsular enhancement (*short arrow*). The tumor enhances less than normal parenchyma. (**E**) Axial T1 weighted delayed post-contrast-enhanced image shows avid enhancement of the fibrous capsule (*short arrow*). Resected specimen confirmed a solid pseudopapillary tumor.

As solid pseudopapillary tumor is a mixed solid and cystic lesion, its spectrum of appearance can be similar to that of large nonfunctioning neuroendocrine neoplasms and acinar cell carcinomas. However, a partially solid lesion with foci of relatively high signal intensity on T1-weighted images in a young woman suggests the diagnosis.

Primary pancreatic lymphoma is a rare manifestation of non-Hodgkin's B-cell lymphoma. Although the gland is secondarily involved in more than 30% of patients with non-Hodgkin's lymphoma, fewer than 2% of extranodal non-Hodgkin's lymphomas arise in the pancreas. Incidence is slightly higher (5%) in patients with human immunodeficiency virus (HIV) because the gastrointestinal tract is the most common site of extranodal AIDS-related non-Hodgkin's lymphoma. Diagnostic criteria for primary pancreatic lymphoma include a mass predominantly within the pancreas, lymphadenopathy confined to the peripancreatic lymph nodes, no involvement of the liver or spleen, no mediastinal nodal involvement on chest radiography, no palpable superficial lymphadenopathy, and a normal leukocyte count.

Two different morphologic patterns of involvement are seen in primary pancreatic lymphoma. The more common tumoral type appears as a well-circumscribed mass within the pancreas; the less common diffuse infiltrating type appears as an infiltrating tumor through the gland parenchyma. In both cases, the tumor displays homogeneous decreased signal intensity compared to the gland on T1-weighted images and heterogeneous increased signal intensity compared to the gland on T2-weighted images. After administration of gadolinium-based contrast material the tumor will enhance to a lesser extent than normal pancreatic parenchyma. Pancreatic lymphoma can cause mild ductal dilatation and may involve the fat surrounding the celiac axis and superior mesenteric artery.

Differentiation between primary pancreatic lymphoma and secondary invasion is of little clinical importance. However, differentiation between lymphoma and adenocarcinoma is essential, as adenocarcinoma has a far worse prognosis and may require surgical staging or a Whipple procedure for treatment, whereas lymphoma is generally managed without surgery. At MR imaging, both malignancies have similar signal and enhancement characteristics; both may cause ductal dilatation and/or involve the peripancreatic vessels. However, ductal dilatation is less common and less marked in pancreatic lymphoma; also, lymphadenopathy below the level of the renal veins, often seen in secondary pancreatic lymphoma, is uncommon in adenocarcinoma.[29]

Intrapancreatic Accessory Spleen Accessory spleens are found in greater than 10% of the population; 16% of these are near or within the pancreatic tail. An accessory spleen will have MRI signal and enhancement characteristics identical to the native spleen (Fig. 5.23). Consequently, it will show relatively decreased signal compared to the pancreatic parenchyma on T1-weighted images, mildly increased signal on T2-weighted images, and avid enhancement on arterial-phase

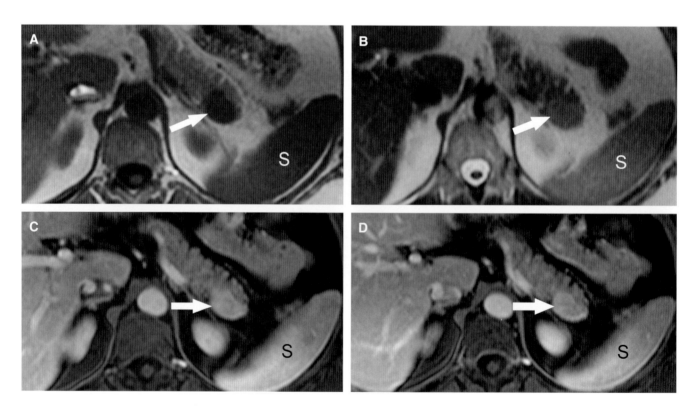

Figure 5.23 *Intrapancreatic accessory spleen.* The accessory spleen appears as a focal mass (*arrow*) within the pancreatic tail with signal characteristics that are identical to those of the native spleen (*S*) on both axial T1-weighted gradient-echo (**A**) and axial T2-weighted single-shot FSE/TSE (**B**) images. Contrast-enhanced fat-saturated gradient-echo images show that the enhancement characteristics of the accessory spleen (*arrow*) are identical to those of the native spleen (*S*) on both pancreatic parenchymal-phase (**C**) and portal venous-phase images (**D**).

enhanced images. An islet cell tumor has similar imaging features; however, signal and enhancement characteristics of an islet cell tumor do not follow splenic imaging characteristics to the same degree. Thus, considering the entity of an intrapancreatic accessory spleen when characterizing a solid pancreatic tail lesion is important and may consequently spare the patient an invasive diagnostic procedure or unnecessary distal pancreatectomy. Suspected ectopic splenic tissue may be confirmed with nuclear scintigraphy using technetium-99m-sulfur colloid or heat-damaged red blood cells. Alternatively, MR imaging following the administration of reticuloendothelial system-specific contrast media, such as superparamagnetic iron oxide particles that are taken up by such tissue, will show loss of signal within splenic tissue on T2-weighted images.[30]

Pancreatic lipomas are uncommon and are usually an incidental finding. These benign tumors are well circumscribed and composed almost entirely of fat, with a few scattered vessels or septa. Diagnosis is straightforward, as the mass will be iso-intense to peripancreatic fat on all imaging sequences; the diagnosis is established if the lesion shows loss of signal on fat-suppressed T1-weighted images. In the rare event that a pancreatic lipoma becomes sufficiently large to cause ductal obstruction or compression of the peripancreatic vessels, the lesion must be surgically removed; otherwise, these benign tumors can be managed conservatively.[31]

Focal fatty infiltration of the pancreas is a benign process that is associated with aging, obesity, diabetes mellitus, chronic pancreatitis, and steroids, among other causes. Lipid is confined to the interstitium of the pancreas and does not affect the exocrine or endocrine parenchymal cells. At first glance, this process may have a concerning appearance by imaging, as it may be mass-like in appearance and show decreased signal intensity compared to normal pancreatic parenchyma on fat-saturated T1-weighted images, mimicking the appearance of adenocarcinoma. However, focal fatty infiltration can be effectively diagnosed on chemical-shift imaging: on in-phase images, the lesion will be iso-intense or mildly hyperintense to normal parenchyma; on opposed-phase images, the lesion will show significant loss of signal and appear hypointense compared to normal parenchyma. Unlike a lipoma, the degree of signal loss will be greater on opposed-phase images than on fat-saturated images. Focal fatty infiltration has been reported throughout the pancreas but is most commonly seen in the posterior head and uncinate process because of the differences in fat content between the dorsal and ventral pancreas. Focal fatty infiltration is not border-deforming and is not associated with ductal obstruction or pancreatic atrophy.[32]

Metastases to the pancreas are rare and usually seen in the setting of advanced disease. Pancreatic metastases are most

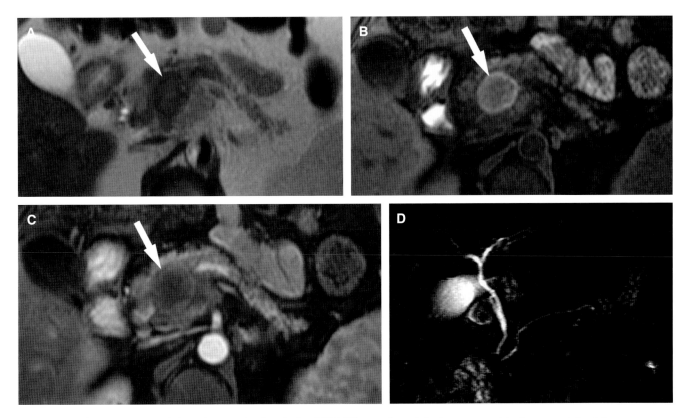

Figure 5.24 *Melanoma metastasis.* (**A**) Axial T2-weighted single-shot FSE/TSE image through the 3-cm metastasis in the pancreatic head demonstrates a solid mass (*arrow*) with decreased signal intensity compared to that of the normal pancreatic parenchyma. (**B**) Axial T1-weighted fat-saturated non-contrast-enhanced gradient-echo image at the same level shows the mass (*arrow*) displaying markedly increased inherent signal due to the presence of melanin. (**C**) After the administration of gadolinium-based contrast material the mass (*arrow*) shows mild peripheral enhancement and decreased central enhancement likely secondary to central necrosis. (**D**) Thick-slab MRCP image shows that this mass did not cause ductal obstruction despite its large size.

commonly caused by malignancies that spread hematogenously: renal cell carcinoma, breast cancer, colon cancer, bronchogenic carcinoma, and melanoma.

Three patterns of metastases are recognized: solitary, multifocal, or diffuse. In general, pancreatic metastases show decreased signal on T1-weighted and heterogeneous or increased signal on T2-weighted images compared to normal parenchyma. Metastases commonly show rim enhancement; even the most hypovascular metastases tend to enhance more than primary adenocarcinoma. Metastases may obstruct the pancreatic duct but are less prone to cause obstruction or duct dilatation than primary adenocarcinoma. Metastases are also less likely to encase the peripancreatic arteries than primary adenocarcinoma.

Some imaging features of pancreatic metastases may suggest a particular primary cancer. Melanoma metastases may show increased signal on T1-weighted images due to the presence of melanin or intratumoral hemorrhage (Fig. 5.24). Renal cell carcinomas tend to show avid and homogeneous enhancement, particularly when small; the clear cell subtype may show loss of signal on opposed-phase GRE imaging due to the presence of intracellular lipid.

Box 5.6 ESSENTIALS TO REMEMBER

- If a solid pancreatic lesion is identified, the diagnosis of exclusion is primary pancreatic carcinoma.

- Characteristic features of pancreatic adenocarcinoma are: (1) solid mass showing decreased signal on T1-weighted images, often with ill-defined margins; (2) proximal (upstream) ductal dilatation; (3) decreased gadolinium contrast enhancement compared to normal parenchyma; and (4) a propensity to infiltrate peripancreatic tissues, particularly the tissue surrounding the celiac axis and SMA.

- If pancreatic adenocarcinoma is suspected, it is the radiologist's job to carefully describe the local extent of the lesion, with particular attention to tumor involvement of peripancreatic vessels, as involvement of the celiac axis and SMA and the presence of metastatic spread disqualify the patient for tumor resection.

- The liver is the most common site of metastasis from pancreatic adenocarcinoma. Metastases display relatively low signal on T1-weighted images and mildly increased signal on T2-weighted images compared to the normal liver. Irregular rim contrast enhancement with central hypoenhancement is the most common feature of metastases, but very small lesions may show homogeneous early enhancement.

- The peritoneum is the second most common site of metastases from pancreatic cancer.

- Two imaging features usually indicate that a solid pancreatic lesion does not represent primary adenocarcinoma: (1) absence of proximal (upstream) ductal dilatation and (2) presence of early contrast enhancement.

- Functional pancreatic endocrine neoplasms generally present clinically when they are small due to unregulated hormone production. Nonfunctional tumors present when large, either from symptoms related to mass effect or from the presence of metastatic disease.

- The various pancreatic endocrine neoplasms have similar appearances at MR imaging; differences in appearance are based on size at presentation rather than cell of origin.

- Classically, a small pancreatic endocrine neoplasm shows homogeneous early enhancement and decreased signal on T1-weighted and mildly increased signal on T2-weighted images, and is not associated with ductal obstruction. As endocrine neoplasms enlarge, signal characteristics and enhancement become heterogeneous, with the largest tumors having central necrosis.

- The most characteristic feature of a solid pseudopapillary tumor is its demographic profile: 90% of affected patients are female; mean age at diagnosis is 24 to 30 years.

- Pancreatic lymphoma is rare, and secondary involvement is far more common than primary pancreatic lymphoma. Because lymphoma commonly appears as a mass, differentiation from adenocarcinoma is essential as a Whipple procedure is not indicated with lymphoma. Features favoring lymphoma include the absence of ductal dilatation and the presence of lymphadenopathy below the level of the renal veins.

- When evaluating a solid mass in the peripheral lateral aspect of the pancreatic tail, remember to consider an intrapancreatic accessory spleen, which will have signal and enhancement characteristics following those of the normal spleen.

- Focal fatty infiltration of the pancreas can mimic adenocarcinoma as fatty infiltration may appear as a focal lesion with decreased signal on fat-suppressed T1-weighted images. The diagnosis of focal fat can be made if the lesion is not border-deforming, is not associated with ductal dilatation, and shows loss of signal on opposed-phase gradient-echo images.

- Metastases in the pancreas from tumors elsewhere are rare and are usually seen in the setting of advanced disease. The metastases are caused by malignancies that spread hematogenously and include renal cell carcinoma, breast cancer, colon cancer, bronchogenic carcinoma, and melanoma.

REFERENCES

1. Yu J, Turner MA, Fulcher AS, et al. Congenital anomalies and normal variants of the pancreaticobiliary tract and the pancreas in adults: Part 2, pancreatic duct and pancreas. *AJR Am J Roentgenol.* 2006;187: 1544–1553.
2. Fields TM, Michel SJ, Butler CL, et al. Abdominal manifestations of cystic fibrosis in older children and adults. *AJR Am J Roentgenol.* 2006;187:1199–1203.
3. Queiroz-Andrade M, Blasbalg R, Ortega CD, et al. MR imaging findings of iron overload. *Radiographics.* 2009;29:1575–1589.
4. Leung RS, Biswas SV, Duncan M, et al. Imaging features of von Hippel-Lindau disease. *Radiographics.* 2008;28:65–79.
5. Marcos HB, Libutti SK, Alexander HR, et al. Neuroendocrine tumors of the pancreas in von Hippel-Lindau disease: spectrum of appearances at CT and MR imaging with histopathologic comparison. *Radiology.* 2002;225:751–758.
6. Heras-Castano G, Castro-Senosiain B, Fontalba A, et al. Hereditary pancreatitis: clinical features and inheritance characteristics of the R122C mutation in the cationic trypsinogen gene (PRSS1) in six Spanish families. *JOP.* 2009;10(3):249–255.
7. Balci NC, Bieneman BK, Bilgin M, et al. Magnetic resonance imaging in pancreatitis. *Top Magn Reson Imaging.* 2009;20:5–30.
8. Aghdassi A, Mayerle J, Kraft M, et al. Diagnosis and treatment of pancreatic pseudocysts in chronic pancreatitis. *Pancreas.* 2008;36: 105–112.
9. Martin DR, Karabulut N, Yang M, et al. High signal peripancreatic fat on fat-suppressed spoiled gradient echo imaging in acute pancreatitis: preliminary evaluation of the prognostic significance. *J Magn Reson Imaging.* 2003;18:49–58.
10. Miller FH, Keppke AL, Wadhwa A, et al. MRI of pancreatitis and its complications: part 2, chronic pancreatitis. *AJR Am J Roentgenol.* 2004;183:1645–1652.
11. Blasbalg R, Baroni RH, Costa DN, et al. MRI features of groove pancreatitis. *AJR Am J Roentgenol.* 2007;189:73–80.
12. Sahani DV, Kalva PS, Maher MM, et al. Autoimmune pancreatitis: imaging features. *Radiology.* 2004;233:345–352.
13. Kalb B, Sarmiento JM, Kooby DA, et al. MR imaging of cystic lesions of the pancreas. *Radiographics.* 2009;29:1749–1765.
14. Le Borgne J, de Calan L, Partensky FS. Cystadenomas and cystadenocarcinomas of the pancreas: a multi-institutional retrospective study of 398 cases. *Ann Surg.* 1999;230:152–161.
15. Tanaka M, Chari S, Adsay V, et al. International consensus guidelines for management of intraductal papillary mucinous neoplasms and mucinous cystic neoplasms of the pancreas. *Pancreatology.* 2006;6: 17–32.
16. Capitanich P, Iovaldi ML, Medrano M, et al. Lymphoepithelial cysts of the pancreas: case report and review of the literature. *J Gastrointest Surg.* 2004;8:342–345.
17. Handrich SJ, Hough DM, Fletcher JG, et al. The natural history of the incidentally discovered small simple pancreatic cyst: Long-term follow-up and clinical implications. *AJR Am J Roentgenol.* 2005;184:20–23.
18. Sahani DV, Saokar A, Hahn PF, et al. Pancreatic cysts 3 cm or smaller: How aggressive should treatment be? *Radiology.* 2006;238(3): 912–919.
19. Goh BKP. Letter to the editor: Pancreatic cysts 3 cm or smaller. *Radiology.* 2007;243(2):607.
20. Ariyama J, Suyama M, Satoh K, et al. Imaging of small pancreatic ductal adenocarcinoma. *Pancreas.* 1998;16:396–401.
21. Kumar V, Abbas AK, Fausto N, et al. *Robbins and Cotran Pathologic Basis of Disease,* 8th ed. Philadelphia: Saunders, 2009.
22. Vachiranubhap B, Kim YH, Balci NC, et al. Magnetic resonance imaging of adenocarcinoma of the pancreas. *Top Magn Reson Imaging.* 2009;20:3–9.
23. Varadhachary GR, Tamm EP, Abbruzzese JL, et al. Borderline resectable pancreatic cancer: definitions, management, and role of preoperative therapy. *Ann Surg Oncol.* 2006;13(8):1035–1046.
24. Greene FL, et al. *AJCC Cancer Staging Manual,* 7th ed. Springer-Verlag, 2010.
25. Danet IM, Semelka RC, Negase LL, et al. Liver metastases from pancreatic adenocarcinoma: MR imaging characteristics. *J Magn Reson Imaging.* 2003;18:181–188.
26. Herwick S, Miller FH, Keppke AL. MRI of islet cell tumors of the pancreas. *AJR Am J Roentgenol.* 2006;187:W472–W480.
27. Tatli S, Mortele KJ, Levy AD, et al. CT and MRI features of pure acinar cell carcinoma of the pancreas in adults. *AJR Am J Roentgenol.* 2005;184:511–519.
28. Cantisani V, Mortele KJ, Levy AD, et al. MR imaging features of solid pseudopapillary tumor of the pancreas in adult and pediatric patients. *AJR Am J Roentgenol.* 2003;181:395–401.
29. Merkle EM, Bender GN, Brambs HJ. Imaging findings of pancreatic lymphoma: differential aspects. *AJR Am J Roentgenol.* 2000;174: 681–675.
30. Boraschi P, Donati F, Volpi A, et al. Intrapancreatic accessory spleen: Diagnosis with RES-specific contrast-enhanced MRI. *AJR Am J Roentgenol.* 2005;184:1712–1713.
31. Katz DS, Nardi PM, Hines J, et al. Lipomas of the pancreas. *AJR Am J Roentgenol.* 1998;170:1485–1487.
32. Isserow JA, Siegelman ES, Mammone J. Focal fatty infiltration of the pancreas: MR characterization with chemical shift imaging. *AJR Am J Roentgenol.* 1999;163:1263.

6.

URINARY TRACT MR IMAGING

Tereza Poghosyan, MD

MR TECHNIQUES FOR THE URINARY TRACT

MR imaging has become one of the essential modalities for evaluating the urinary tract by providing exquisite and unique soft tissue contrast and allowing accurate assessment of a wide range of pathology. Existing and emerging applications include renal mass characterization, evaluation of the collecting systems and bladder, staging of malignancies, depiction of anomalies of the urinary system, MR angiography, and it has been used for guidance of percutaneous tumor ablation and post-procedural follow-up. Functional MR nephrourography is a developing technique combining structural and functional data within a single examination.

Multi-coil array body surface coils are used to increase the signal-to-noise ratio (SNR) and obtain high-resolution images. The standard protocols for renal imaging in most institutions currently include the following sequences:

1. Breath-hold T2-weighted localizer sequence that provides images in coronal, sagittal, and axial planes. This sequence allows a preliminary evaluation of anatomy and may reveal gross findings that require modification of the routine protocol.

2. Multislice or single-shot fast/turbo spin-echo (FSE/TSE) T2-weighted pulse sequence with or without breath-holding techniques is usually obtained in the axial or coronal plane. Non-breath-hold T2-weighted FSE/TSE pulse sequences are used with fat suppression and respiratory triggering for improved signal-to-noise ratio. T2-weighted imaging is most helpful in characterizing renal cysts. Simple cysts demonstrate high signal intensity, whereas complicated or complex cysts and partially cystic neoplasms demonstrate heterogeneous signal. Renal cell carcinoma (RCC), angiomyolipoma (AML), hematoma, and focal pyelonephritis can also demonstrate heterogeneous signal. Blood products within a hemorrhagic cyst and internal hemorrhage within AML

or RCC appear as low-signal areas on T2-weighted images. Heavily T2-weighted sequences with TE of more than 160 ms may also be added for improved discrimination between solid and cystic renal lesions.

3. Dual-echo gradient-echo (GRE) for in-phase and opposed-phase imaging is obtained to detect macroscopic or microscopic fat within renal masses. The gradient-echo images are acquired with specific TE values such that the signals from fat and water are either in phase or out of phase with one another. In general, at 1.5T, in-phase images are obtained with TE of approximately 4.4 ms and out-of-phase images are obtained with TE of about 2.2 ms. Loss of signal on opposed-phase images occurs when fat and water signal are present in the same voxel, signifying the presence of intracellular (microscopic) fat. Clear cell RCCs, adenomas, and renal AMLs with minimal fat can contain intracellular lipid. Opposed-phase imaging is also helpful for detecting macroscopic, focal fat within renal AMLs by demonstrating chemical-shift (India ink) artifact at the fat–water (soft tissue) interfaces. However, T1-weighted images with chemically selective fat saturation should be included in the renal protocol to reliably characterize a macroscopic fat-containing renal mass.

4. T1-weighted sequence with fat saturation can be obtained with either spin-echo or GRE technique. Spin-echo sequences were the standard of T1-weighted imaging in the past, but these have long acquisition times and images can therefore usually not be obtained within a breath hold. Fast T1-weighted imaging using GRE sequences is now the widely accepted alternative. The most commonly used GRE technique is the multislice gradient pulse sequence, which can provide full coverage of the kidneys in one 18- to 23-second breath hold.[1] 3D T1-weighted GRE imaging has advantages over 2D GRE imaging by providing thin sections, no interslice gaps, higher SNR, and comparable image contrast in a breath-hold time frame.[1]

Axial T1-weighted images with fat suppression are routinely obtained and may be supplemented with coronal images. Most of the solid renal masses demonstrate signal intensity that is slightly lower than that of the renal cortex. Simple cysts demonstrate low signal intensity. Hemorrhagic cysts, as well as renal AML and RCC with internal hemorrhage, demonstrate high signal intensity due to the presence of blood products. Cysts with high protein content, macroscopic fat-containing AMLs, and melanin-containing lesions (metastases) also demonstrate T1 shortening with resulting high signal intensity.

5. Dynamic post-contrast-enhanced imaging of the kidneys is the essential part of the examination. It allows characterization of enhancement pattern of the solid masses and detection of small solid renal lesions or small solid components within complex cystic lesions. Following acquisition of T1-weighted, fat-suppressed axial images intravenous (IV) gadolinium-containing contrast material is administered and post-contrast-enhanced images are obtained typically in the arterial, venous, nephrographic, and delayed excretory phases. The timing of post-contrast-enhanced image acquisition is critical for both lesion detection and characterization; therefore, bolus tracking or a test bolus can be used to determine the optimal timing of the gadolinium bolus injection and acquisition of the image data.

Subtraction imaging is often performed to detect subtle enhancement of small solid components within a cystic mass or at the margins of a renal mass previously treated with percutaneous ablation, indicating residual or recurrent tumor. This technique is based on subtraction of the unenhanced data set from each of the dynamic contrast-enhanced data sets. The acquisition of the pre- and post-contrast 3D GRE images is performed with the same parameters, including the field of view, resolution and slice thickness. The resulting subtracted images demonstrate only the areas of enhancement within normal or pathologic tissues and within the vessels.

6. MR urography (MRU) is a technique for evaluating the renal collecting systems, ureters, and bladder. It is based on two types of imaging: T2-weighted and excretory post-gadolinium contrast-enhanced T1-weighted imaging with fat suppression.

The intrinsic high signal of urine on T2-weighted images and intermediate signal of the urothelium allows detection of foci of low signal, or signal voids, caused by small lesions or stones within the urinary tract. Administration of furosemide results in distention of the urinary system and has been shown to be helpful for identifying these abnormalities.[2] The most commonly used T2-weighted sequences are relatively motion-insensitive half-Fourier acquisition single-shot FSE/TSE and breath-hold balanced steady-state free precession (SSFP). The advantage of T2-weighted image acquisition is that the urinary tract is depicted without the use of gadolinium-based contrast agents and the technique is therefore independent from the renal function.

3D GRE T1-weighted fat-suppressed post-gadolinium-contrast-enhanced images are another mainstay of MR urography. The early post-contrast-enhanced images allow detection of enhancing urothelial lesions against the background of low-signal-intensity urine before the excretion of contrast material. The delayed post-contrast-enhanced images in the excretory phase make the signal voids, showing as "filling defects", apparent, similar to CT urography.

Maximum-intensity-projection (MIP) reconstructions can be obtained with both T2-weighted and contrast-enhanced T1-weighted images to display the urinary tract anatomy and morphology in a 3D rotating manner.

Newer applications include the following:

1. Functional MR nephrourography is a novel technique that has the capacity to measure the glomerular filtration rate (GFR) by using rapid "snapshots" of the kidney at different time points following administration of gadolinium-based contrast agent,

---

Box 6.1 ESSENTIALS TO REMEMBER

- Dynamic post-gadolinium-contrast-enhanced T1-weighted sequences are essential for detecting and characterizing renal masses as cysts or as solid neoplasms. Detection of subtle lesion enhancement is improved by obtaining subtraction images.

- The presence of enhancement within a renal mass after intravenous administration of gadolinium-based contrast agents is the most reliable finding to differentiate solid renal tumors from benign cysts.

- Fat-suppression sequences are essential for demonstrating macroscopic fat, which characterizes angiomyolipomas.

- MR urography using heavily T2-weighted images and delayed post-gadolinium-contrast-enhanced excretory-phase coronal T1-weighted GRE images provides evaluation of the urinary collecting system, renal pelvises, ureters, and bladder. T2-weighted images may be used alone to evaluate the uroepithelium in patients with severe renal failure without the use of contrast agents or radiation. Maximum-intensity-projection reconstructions display the urinary system morphology in 3D images that can be rotated to demonstrate spatial relationships.

using mathematical modeling of tracer kinetics to determine the renal blood flow (RBF) and GFR similar to renal scintigraphy.

2. Diffusion-weighted imaging (DWI) of the abdomen has recently become feasible with new technologic advances in MRI techniques, including echoplanar imaging and parallel imaging, high-performance gradients, phased-array multichannel surface coils, and clinical use of higher magnetic field strengths. Potential applications of DWI in renal and urinary tract evaluation include differentiation of benign from malignant processes, characterization of tumors, detection of tumor recurrence, and assessment of diffuse renal parenchymal disease.

DWI is typically performed with at least two b values (degree of diffusion weighting) and interpreted in conjunction with the Apparent Diffusion Coefficient (ADP) map. The signal intensity of most simple renal cysts drops significantly on images obtained at a b value of 500 sec/mm^2 and is lost completely on images obtained at b values of 1,000 to 1,500 sec/mm^2.[2,3] In most benign processes, the signal intensity

at DWI decays with increasing b value. In contrast, slower signal-intensity decay or even signal-intensity enhancement with increasing b value may indicate malignancy or viable hypercellular tissue.[3]

ANATOMY

The normal kidney demonstrates relatively high signal intensity on T2-weighted images compared to the liver and other upper abdominal organs but is close in signal to the spleen. Normal corticomedullary differentiation appears as brighter-signal medulla and lower-signal cortex on T2-weighted images (Fig. 6.1A). On T1-weighted images this relationship is reversed, with the cortex demonstrating higher signal intensity and the medulla demonstrating lower signal intensity, similar to skeletal muscle (Fig. 6.1B).

After administration of gadolinium-based contrast material the renal cortex enhances first (corticomedullary phase) followed by enhancement of the medulla (nephrographic phase) and excretion of contrast from the renal collecting systems and pelvises into

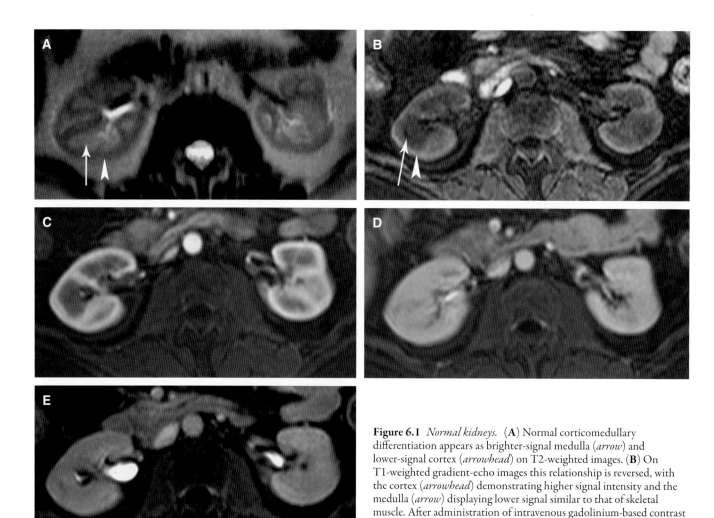

Figure 6.1 *Normal kidneys.* (**A**) Normal corticomedullary differentiation appears as brighter-signal medulla (*arrow*) and lower-signal cortex (*arrowhead*) on T2-weighted images. (**B**) On T1-weighted gradient-echo images this relationship is reversed, with the cortex (*arrowhead*) demonstrating higher signal intensity and the medulla (*arrow*) displaying lower signal similar to that of skeletal muscle. After administration of intravenous gadolinium-based contrast material the renal cortex enhances first (corticomedullary phase) (**C**) followed by enhancement of the medulla (nephrographic phase) (**D**) and excretion of contrast material into the renal collecting systems (**E**).

the ureters and into the bladder (Fig. 6.1C, D, E). The ureters have the same signal characteristics on T1- and T2-weighted images as skeletal muscle, demonstrating relative low to intermediate signal intensity. The four layers of the bladder wall—mucosa, submucosa, muscularis, and serosa—are not usually seen as separate layers. The normal bladder wall demonstrates homogeneous low to intermediate signal intensity on T1-weighted images and low signal intensity on T2-weighted images due to the dominant detrusor muscle. The bladder mucosa and submucosa enhance early following contrast material administration and the detrusor muscle enhances in the delayed phase.

The female urethra has a characteristic target-like appearance on T2-weighted images in the axial plane orientation with four concentric rings corresponding to mucosa, submucosa, smooth muscle, and striated muscle layers. The four segments of the male urethra (prostatic, membranous, bulbous, and penile) are evaluated in all three planes due to its complex anatomic course. The male urethra appears as a high-signal-intensity tubular structure with a low-signal-intensity rim on T2-weighted images.

CONGENITAL ANOMALIES

MRI allows comprehensive evaluation of renal anomalies of position and rotation. MR urography not only provides anatomic information about the location and relationship of the kidneys, the course and insertion of the ureters, and the degree of hydronephrosis, but also provides details of the vascular anatomy for surgical planning and allows differentiation of congenital hydronephrosis (obstruction vs. vesicoureteral reflux) and assessment of relative renal function without using ionizing radiation. It is increasingly used in the pediatric population, including neonates and infants.[4,5]

Renal agenesis is incompatible with life if bilateral. Unilateral renal agenesis is uncommon but accounts for 5% of all renal anomalies. It is usually asymptomatic and associated with abnormal shape of the unilateral adrenal gland. The solitary kidney undergoes compensatory hypertrophy. Renal agenesis is often associated with Mullerian duct fusion anomalies and other genital anomalies, more frequently in females (Fig. 6.2)

Duplication anomalies can be unilateral or bilateral and can involve the renal pelvis and ureters. The ureters can have orthotopic or ectopic insertion into the bladder, sometimes associated with ureterocele in ectopy.

Fusion anomalies include horseshoe kidney (Fig. 6.3), cross-fused ectopia (Fig. 6.4), and pelvic pancake kidney. The kidneys are joined with separate insertion of the ureters on each side of the bladder. Fusion anomalies are often associated with vesicoureteral reflux, obstruction, and stone disease.

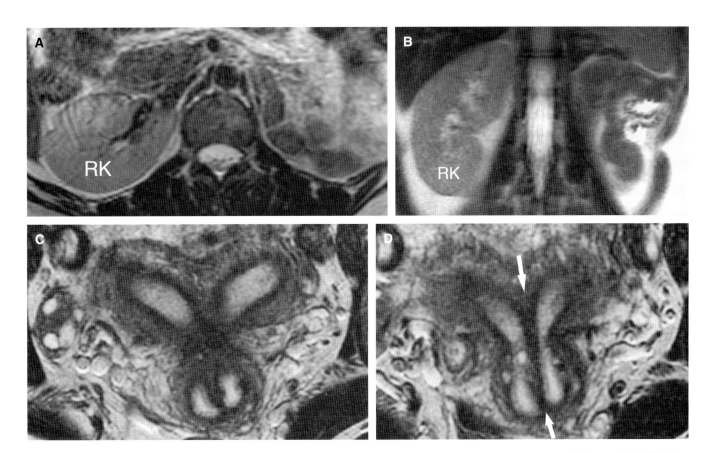

Figure 6.2 *Left renal agenesis.* Axial (**A**) and coronal (**B**) T2-weighted single-shot FSE/TSE images demonstrate congenital absence of the left kidney with compensatory hypertrophy of the right kidney (*RK*). This anomaly is associated with a Müllerian duct fusion anomaly of the uterus. (**C, D**) Axial T2-weighted images demonstrate bicornuate bicollis uterus with the muscular septum extending into the level of the uterine cervix (*arrows* in image D).

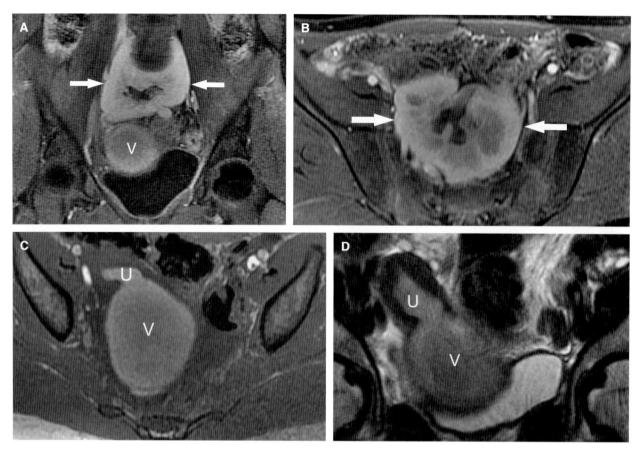

Figure 6.3 *Presacral fused kidney with associated unicornuate uterus and hematometrocolpos.* Coronal (**A**) and axial (**B**) post-contrast-enhanced T1-weighted gradient-echo images with fat saturation demonstrate a low-lying fused kidney (between *arrows*) with normal enhancement of the renal parenchyma. The vagina (*V*) distended with blood is partially visualized. Axial T1-weighted (**C**) and coronal T2-weighted (**D**) images demonstrate a single right-sided uterine horn (*U*) with marked distention of the vaginal (*V*) lumen by blood products, characterized by the relatively high signal intensity on T1-weighted and intermediate signal on T2-weighted images. Findings indicate unicornuate uterus, hematocolpos, and hematometra.

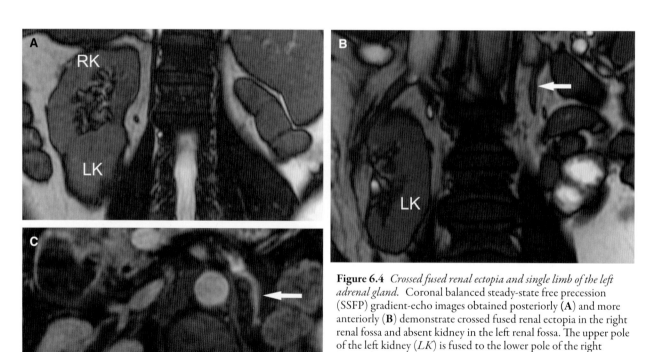

Figure 6.4 *Crossed fused renal ectopia and single limb of the left adrenal gland.* Coronal balanced steady-state free precession (SSFP) gradient-echo images obtained posteriorly (**A**) and more anteriorly (**B**) demonstrate crossed fused renal ectopia in the right renal fossa and absent kidney in the left renal fossa. The upper pole of the left kidney (*LK*) is fused to the lower pole of the right kidney (*RK*). The left adrenal gland (*arrow* in image B) is present in the normal location but has only a single limb. (**C**) Axial post-gadolinium-contrast-enhanced fat-suppressed T1-weighted image shows single limb of the malformed left adrenal gland (*arrow*) and normal appearance of the right kidney.

Malrotation results from a shift of the normal axis of the kidney and is usually asymptomatic. Renal ectopia is abnormal location of the kidney outside the renal fossa. It is the result of failed or incomplete ascent of the kidney from its site of origin in the true pelvis during embryonic development. Thoracic renal ectopia is extremely rare.

Multicystic dysplastic kidney (MDCK) is a form of renal dysplasia resulting from ureteral and pelviureteral atresia and abnormal renal development, and presents as a cluster of cysts of various sizes replacing the normal kidney. The natural history of MDCK is gradual involution of the nonfunctional kidney with an increase in size of the affected kidney in a small percentage of cases. Bilateral MDCK is incompatible with life. Ureteropelvic junction obstruction and vesicoureteral reflux are the most common associated congenital abnormalities of the contralateral kidney.

Sonography is the preferred initial study in newborns and infants with MDCK. MR urography can be used to characterize the complex cystic lesion replacing the involved kidney as well as to evaluate the contralateral kidney for ureteropelvic junction obstruction or vesicoureteral reflux. Limitations of the MRI technique in newborns and infants include need for sedation, availability, and cost.

SOLID RENAL MASSES

Renal cell carcinoma (RCC) is the most common solid renal mass, representing up to 90% of all renal malignancies. Its incidence has significantly increased over the past decade, in part due to increased use of cross-sectional imaging and subsequent early detection of asymptomatic small tumors. Up to 30% to 40% of tumors are currently discovered incidentally.[6] MRI has an important role in the diagnosis, staging, and treatment planning of RCC, as well as differentiating its subtypes and therefore estimating the disease prognosis. The 2004 World Health Organization classification of RCC includes clear cell, papillary, chromophobe, medullary, and collecting duct carcinoma.

Clear cell RCC is the most common type (70%) and typically presents as a solitary heterogeneous enhancing solid renal mass. It usually displays high or intermediate signal intensity on T2-weighted images (Fig 6.5A), low or intermediate signal intensity on T1-weighted images (Fig. 6.5B), and avid enhancement (Fig. 6.5C, D). Central areas of decreased or absent enhancement can be present caused by necrosis, cystic components, or hemorrhage. The lesion can demonstrate a

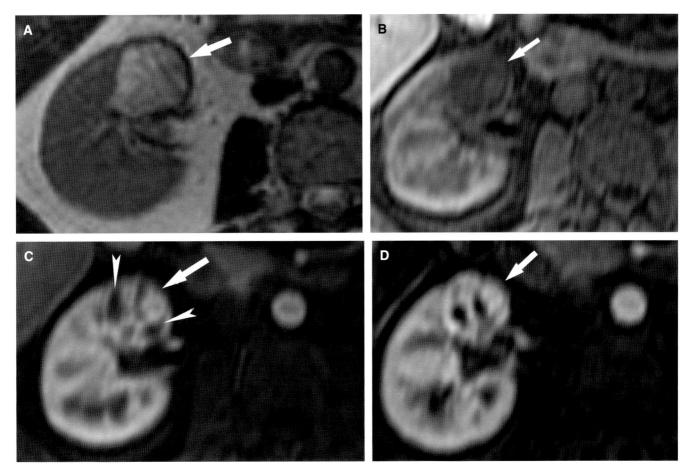

Figure 6.5 *Renal cell carcinoma, clear cell type.* (**A**) Axial T2-weighted image demonstrates a well-circumscribed ball-shaped mass (*arrow*) arising from the anterior aspect of the right kidney. (**B**) Unenhanced axial T1-weighted image with fat saturation shows low signal intensity within the mass (*arrow*). (**C**) Axial T1-weighted fat-suppressed post-gadolinium-contrast-enhanced image in corticomedullary phase demonstrates avid heterogeneous enhancement of the mass (*arrow*) with some areas of non-enhancement (*arrowheads*) representing necrosis or cystic degeneration. (**D**) Subtraction image confirms avid enhancement of the typical clear cell renal carcinoma (*arrow*).

decrease in signal on out-of-phase imaging due to the presence of microscopic intracellular fat. The pattern of avid enhancement is a distinctive feature of clear cell RCC, allowing its differentiation from non-clear cell subtypes. Up to 10% to 15% of clear cell RCCs can have calcifications (sometimes ossifications), which are usually not detectable with MRI.

Multilocular clear cell RCCs are predominantly cystic tumors, usually presenting as Bosniak category III cysts with enhancing, sometimes thick septations. This topic is discussed in greater detail in the "Renal cysts, cystic masses, and cystic disease" section. Papillary RCC represents up to 10% to 15% of all RCCs. Type 1 (pale cytoplasm, small cell) and type 2 (eosinophilic cytoplasm,

large cell) subtypes have been described. Type 1 is usually of lower stage and grade at the time of diagnosis. As opposed to the clear cell subtype, this lesion usually demonstrates low signal intensity on T2-weighted images (Fig. 6.6A), intermediate or high signal intensity on T1-weighted images (Fig. 6.6B), and a lesser degree of enhancement than clear cell RCC. The dynamic post-gadolinium-contrast-enhanced images also show gradual delayed enhancement, unlike the clear cell variety (Fig. 6.6C,D,E). The mass is commonly homogeneous but can be heterogeneous if hemorrhage and/or necrosis are present. The main differential diagnosis is lipid-poor AML, and biopsy is often required to establish the diagnosis.

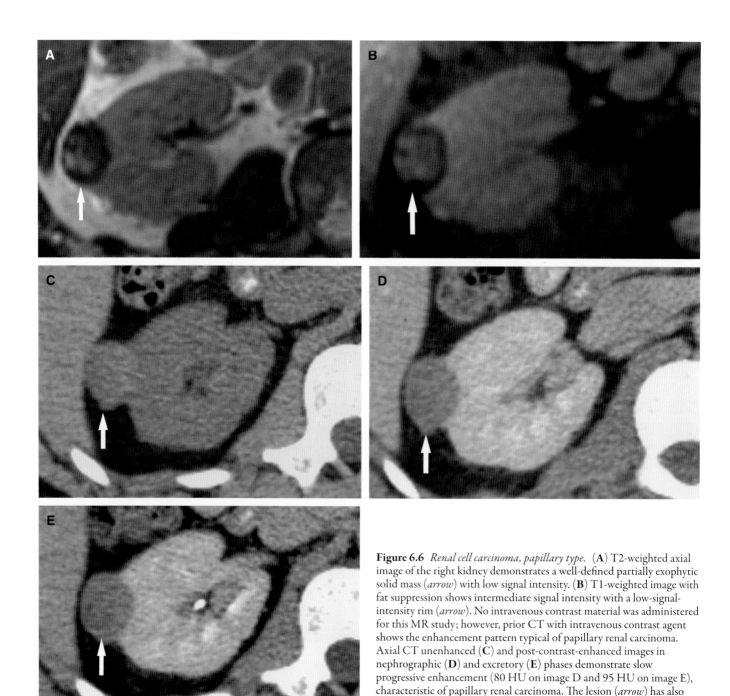

Figure 6.6 *Renal cell carcinoma, papillary type.* (**A**) T2-weighted axial image of the right kidney demonstrates a well-defined partially exophytic solid mass (*arrow*) with low signal intensity. (**B**) T1-weighted image with fat suppression shows intermediate signal intensity with a low-signal-intensity rim (*arrow*). No intravenous contrast material was administered for this MR study; however, prior CT with intravenous contrast agent shows the enhancement pattern typical of papillary renal carcinoma. Axial CT unenhanced (**C**) and post-contrast-enhanced images in nephrographic (**D**) and excretory (**E**) phases demonstrate slow progressive enhancement (80 HU on image D and 95 HU on image E), characteristic of papillary renal carcinoma. The lesion (*arrow*) has also relatively high attenuation pre-contrast enhancement (65 HU on image C), another characteristic of the papillary variety of renal cancer.

Table 6.1 TNM STAGING OF RENAL CELL CARCINOMA

STAGE		FINDINGS
T stage		**Size and location of the tumor**
TX		The primary tumor cannot be assessed (information not available)
T0		No evidence of primary tumor
T1		Tumor confined to kidney, <7 cm in largest diameter
	T1a	Tumor <4 cm in largest diameter, confined to kidney
	T1b	Tumor is 4–7 cm in largest diameter, confined to kidney
T2		Tumor confined to kidney, >7 cm in largest diameter
	T2a	Tumor is 7–10 cm in largest diameter, confined to kidney
	T2b	Tumor is >10 cm in largest diameter, confined to kidney
T3		Tumor has grown into major veins or perinephric tissue. Tumor does not involve the ipsilateral adrenal gland and does not extend beyond Gerota's fascia.
	T3a	Tumor involves the renal vein, or has spread to perinephric fat. Tumor does not extend beyond Gerota's fascia.
	T3b	Tumor involves the inferior vena cava below the diaphragm
	T3c	Tumor involves the inferior vena cava above the diaphragm
T4		Tumor has spread beyond Gerota's fascia and may involve the ipsilateral adrenal gland
N stage		**Involvement of lymph nodes**
NX		Regional lymph nodes cannot be assessed (information not available)
N0		No spread to regional lymph nodes
N1		Tumor has spread to regional lymph nodes
M stage		**Distant metastases**
MX		Presence of distant metastasis cannot be assessed (information not available)
M0		No metastatic disease
M1		Distant metastases are present (distant lymph nodes, lung, bones, brain, etc.)

STAGE GROUPING		5-year Survival
Stage I	T1, N0, M0	81%
Stage II	T2, N0, M0	74%
Stage III	T3, N0, M0 *or* T1 to T3, N1, M0	53%
Stage IV	T4, Any N, M0 *or* Any T, any N, M1	8%

Adapted with permission from American Joint Committee on Cancer. *AJCC Cancer Staging Manual*, 7th ed. Springer, 2010.

Chromophobe RCC accounts for less than 5% of RCCs. It had similarities with benign oncocytomas in histologic and sometimes imaging appearance.[6] It usually presents as a homogeneous tumor with less post-contrast enhancement than clear cell RCC. In general, if the solid renal mass enhances to a lesser degree compared to the renal cortex, it is likely to represent a non-clear cell subtype of RCC (papillary or chromophobe).[7] On T2-weighted images chromophobe RCC can show low signal intensity, similar to papillary RCC.

Medullary RCC is a rare subtype occurring almost exclusively in patients with sickle cell trait. The patients are usually young, with the typical age range between 10 and 40 years (mean age, 22 years). The male-to-female ratio is 2:1. Medullary RCC usually presents as a large infiltrative heterogeneous mass and is often metastatic at the time of diagnosis, with a poor prognosis.

Staging and treatment of RCC. The current standard of treatment of RCC is surgical, given the resistance of the tumor to most traditional oncologic treatments, including radiation therapy, chemotherapy, and hormonal therapy. Radical and partial nephrectomy are the mainstays of treatment, with the image-guided minimally invasive percutaneous tumor ablation procedures rapidly becoming an accepted alternative in poor surgical candidates with low-stage RCC.[8]

MRI allows accurate staging and preoperative assessment of RCC. Important criteria for staging include size of the tumor, extension into the perinephric fat or Gerota's fascia, involvement of the ipsilateral adrenal gland, invasion of the renal vein and inferior vena cava (IVC), lymphadenopathy, and distant metastases (Table 6.1).[9]

Tumor size. Tumors confined to the kidney and smaller than 4 cm (stage T1a) are generally treated with partial nephrectomy. In some cases partial nephrectomy can be performed on patients with larger tumors (less than 7 cm, stage T1b) if the location of the tumor permits and adequate surgical margins can be obtained.

Local invasion. MRI is accurate in detecting perinephric fat invasion and extension of the tumor into the adrenal gland (stage T3a) as a result of superior soft tissue contrast resolution. Invasion of the tumor beyond Gerota's fascia and into the adjacent organs (stage T4) is well demonstrated on MRI.

Venous invasion. Tumor thrombus in the renal vein and IVC is seen on T1- and T2-weighted images as a soft tissue mass filling the lumen of the vessel. Enhancement of the intraluminal mass following intravenous contrast media administration is diagnostic of a tumor thrombus (Figs. 6.7 and 6.8). There is often associated bland thrombus without enhancement showing relatively high signal intensity on T1-weighted images and intermediate signal intensity on T2-weighted images, with absence of expected flow void. Extent of the tumor thrombus beyond the renal vein (stage T3b), into the intrahepatic IVC (T3b) and into the right atrium (T3c), dictates a different surgical approach.

Lymphadenopathy. The presence of retroperitoneal lymphadenopathy is an important prognostic factor and can be readily assessed. Curative lymphadenectomy is not possible in

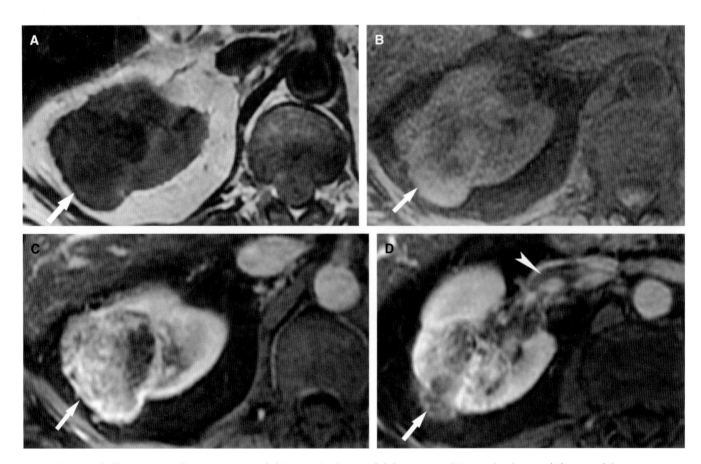

Figure 6.7 *Renal cell carcinoma with venous invasion.* (**A**) T2-weighted image, (**B**) fat-suppressed T1-weighted image, (**C**) post-gadolinium-contrast-enhanced arterial-phase, and (**D**) nephrographic-phase images demonstrate a large heterogeneously enhancing partially exophytic mass (*arrow*) in the upper pole of the right kidney with extension into the right renal vein (*arrowhead* in image D). Tumor thrombus in the renal vein or inferior vena cava is an important finding, impacting on the surgical approach for nephrectomy.

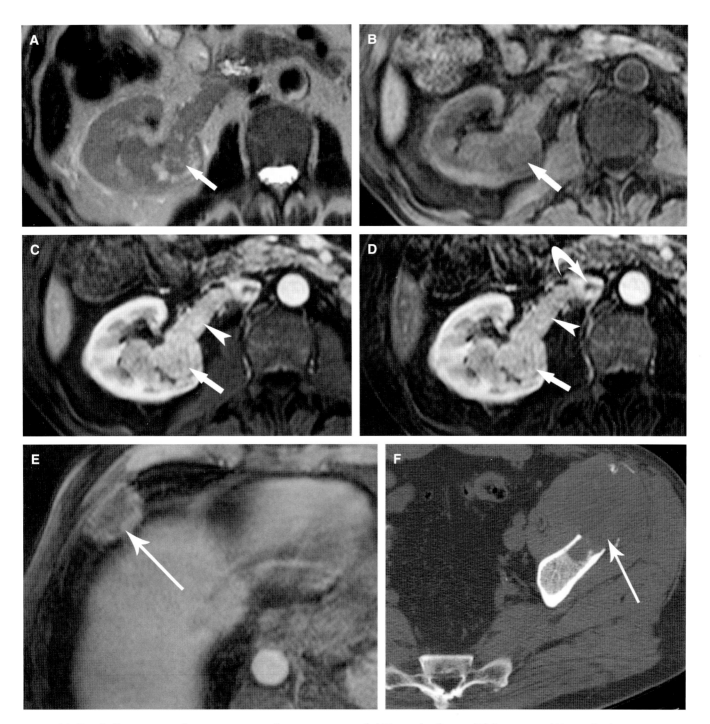

Figure 6.8 *Renal cell carcinoma with venous invasion and osseous metastases.* (**A**) T2-weighted image, (**B**) fat-suppressed T1-weighted pre-contrast image, (**C**) post-gadolinium-contrast-enhanced image, and (**D**) subtraction image demonstrate a heterogeneously enhancing solid right renal mass (*arrows*) representing a renal carcinoma extending into the renal vein (*arrowhead* in images C and D) and inferior vena cava (*curved arrow* in image D). (**E**) Axial fat-suppressed T1-weighted post-contrast-enhanced image of the right lung base demonstrates a pleural-based right middle lobe metastasis (*arrow*). (**F**) Axial CT image of the pelvis displayed with bone algorithm shows a lytic left iliac bone metastasis (*arrow*). Lung and bone are common sites of metastatic disease from renal cell carcinoma.

most cases, but lymph node dissection is performed to determine lymph node involvement and accurate staging.

Distant metastatic disease. Pulmonary, osseous, hepatic, pancreatic, and other metastases can be detected on MRI examination for a renal mass (Fig. 6.8F).

Angiomyolipoma (AML) is a benign renal hamartoma containing varying amounts of vascular, smooth muscle, and fat components. It is a rare solid renal tumor with incidence of approximately 0.3% to 3%.[10] About 20% of AMLs occur in patients with tuberous sclerosis and 80% occur sporadically. In 80% of patients with tuberous sclerosis, AMLs are present. In tuberous sclerosis the tumors are usually multiple, bilateral, and large, often replacing the kidney.

Patients with AMLs are usually asymptomatic but can present clinically with a palpable mass, flank pain, hematuria, or retroperitoneal hemorrhage when tumors are large. The characteristic absence of elastic tissue in the tumor vessels predisposes to aneurysm formation and spontaneous hemorrhage, which can be life-threatening. Tumors larger than 4 cm have an increased risk of hemorrhage and can be treated with selective embolization, nephron-sparing surgery, or nephrectomy. The asymptomatic small tumors can be managed conservatively.

Although renal AML is a benign tumor, it can invade the renal vein and extend into the IVC in rare cases. Very rarely it can be found in the regional lymph nodes.

Diagnosis of AML with MR imaging technique is based on detection of macroscopic fat components within the complex tumor. Adipose tissue is detected with fat-suppression technique, and its presence is virtually diagnostic of AML (Fig. 6.9). If the tumor is predominantly fatty it can be sometimes difficult to detect the lesion in the background of same-signal-intensity retroperitoneal fat. In these cases identification of tumor capsule and scant soft tissue components can be helpful (Fig. 6.10).

A few case reports of RCC containing macroscopic fat have been described, but for all practical purposes a macroscopic fat-containing lesion should be considered an AML if no aggressive features or calcifications are present.[11]

A small percentage of AMLs (approximately 5%) have a minimal amount of intralesional fat; these represent a

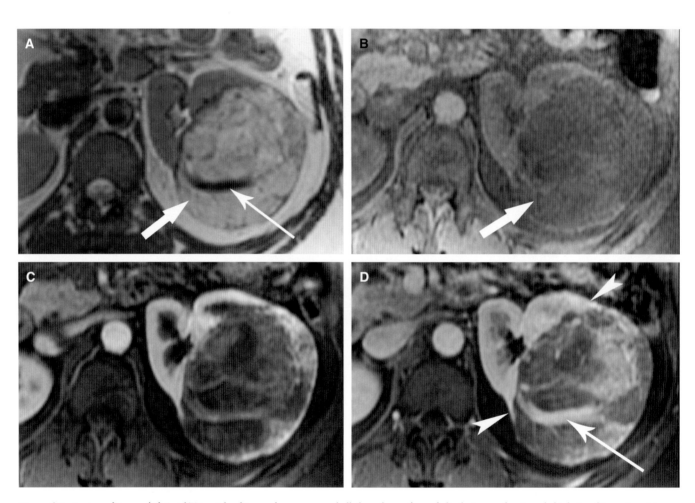

Figure 6.9 *Angiomyolipoma.* (**A**) Axial T2-weighted image demonstrates a ball-shaped mass (*arrow*) displaying predominantly high signal intensity arising from the left kidney. (**B**) Fat-suppressed axial T1-weighted image demonstrates decrease of signal within the renal mass (*arrow*) similar to that of subcutaneous and retroperitoneal fat signal, indicating the presence of macroscopic fat. Post-gadolinium-contrast-enhanced images in corticomedullary (**C**) and nephrographic (**D**) phases demonstrate heterogeneous enhancement of the mass. There is a prominent vessel (*skinny arrow*) traversing the highly vascularized angiomyolipoma, presenting as a linear signal void on T2-weighted images (**A**) and showing prominent enhancement on post-contrast-enhanced images (**C**, **D**). Note the claw sign (*arrowheads*), indicating renal origin of the fatty mass as opposed to an adrenal fatty mass (myelolipoma).

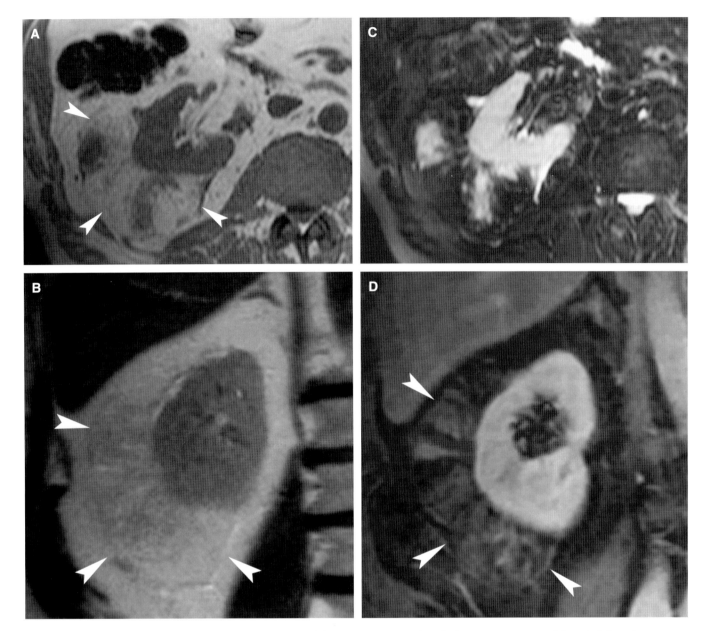

Figure 6.10 *Primarily extrarenal angiomyolipoma.* (**A**) Axial and (**B**) coronal T2-weighted single shot FSE/TSE images of the right kidney demonstrate a fat-containing exophytic lesion arising from the right kidney. The lesion is inconspicuous due to the similarity of signal to the adjacent retroperitoneal fat, but the borders of the mass and non-fatty components can be seen at close inspection (*arrowheads*). (**C**) Axial and (**D**) coronal post-gadolinium contrast-enhanced fat-suppressed T1-weighted gardient-echo images show enhancement of the non-fatty smooth muscle and vascular components (*arrowheads*).

diagnostic challenge.[12] These benign tumors cannot be reliably differentiated from RCC on MRI or any other available imaging modality and require biopsy or excision to establish the diagnosis. Opposed-phase imaging can detect microscopic intracellular lipid within the AML with minimal fat; however, a subset of clear cell RCC is also known to contain intracellular fat and demonstrates the same characteristics. Opposed-phase gradient-echo imaging can be useful in the characterization of AML by demonstrating chemical-shift artifact at the fat-soft tissue boundaries within the mass only if macroscopic fat is present.

Leiomyoma is a rare benign tumor of the kidney found in approximately 5% of autopsy specimens.[13] It is composed of smooth muscle cells and usually arises from the renal capsule. It is considered a hamartomatous lesion similar to AML. In fact, AML also contains a variable amount of smooth muscle cells, and both lesions possibly represent components of a continuum along with renal lipoma. Leiomyoma most commonly presents as an exophytic or partially exophytic well-circumscribed rounded enhancing solid renal mass. Abundance of fibrous stroma results in low signal intensity on T2-weighted images and gradual delayed enhancement (Fig. 6.11).

Oncocytoma is a benign renal tumor that accounts for 5% of all cortical renal masses.[13] It presents as a well-defined rounded "ball-type" renal mass with relatively homogeneous

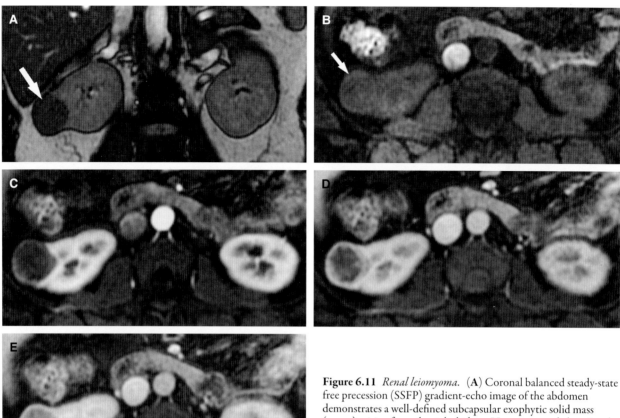

Figure 6.11 *Renal leiomyoma.* (**A**) Coronal balanced steady-state free precession (SSFP) gradient-echo image of the abdomen demonstrates a well-defined subcapsular exophytic solid mass (*arrow*) arising from the right kidney. Homogeneously low signal of the mass is due to abundance of fibrous stroma. (**B**) The mass (*arrow*) shows intermediate signal on T1-weighted fat-suppressed gradient-echo image. (**C, D, E**) Dynamic post-gadolinium-contrast-enhanced T1-weighted fat-suppressed gradient-echo images demonstrate slow progressive enhancement of the mass.

enhancement. The classical feature of oncocytoma is its central scar, which can be seen on all the cross-sectional modalities. It is present in a small percentage of cases and is not specific for oncocytoma, as it can be also seen in RCC, most commonly in the chromophobe type. Another classic feature of oncocytoma is a "spoke-wheel" appearance of its vasculature, which can be seen on MR angiography but is also nonspecific. Since no definitive diagnosis of oncocytoma can be made on imaging, biopsy and resection remain the most appropriate management options. Oncocytoma also has similarity at pathology to the chromophobe type of RCC, which mandates its resection. If a definitive diagnosis of oncocytoma is made on the basis of cytology, histology, or immunohistochemistry, a watchful-waiting therapeutic approach can be used.

Hereditary renal cancer syndromes are a group of familial diseases characterized by the development of multiple bilateral renal masses. It is estimated that approximately 4% of renal cancers are familial. The most common and best-known syndrome is *von Hippel-Lindau* (VHL) disease. Others include tuberous sclerosis, hereditary papillary RCC, Birt-Hogg-Dube, hereditary leiomyoma RCC, and familial oncocytoma. Medullary carcinoma is also included into this group because

it develops in patients with specific genetic makeup, namely sickle cell trait. The hereditary renal cancer syndromes usually develop at a younger age than sporadic renal cancers and affect males and females at similar frequency. Bilateral sporadic tumors can occur as well (Fig. 6.12).

VHL is an autosomal dominant disease caused by mutation of the tumor suppressor gene that results in development of multiple neoplasms, including hemangioblastomas of the central nervous system, retinal angiomas, endolymphatic sac tumors, pancreatic cysts and neoplasms, pheochromocytoma, and so forth. Renal manifestations include multiple bilateral synchronous and metachronous cysts and the clear cell type of RCC (Fig. 6.13). Approximately 28% to 45% of individuals with the VHL gene mutation develop RCC during their lifetime,[14] and approximately 60% to 70% develop renal cysts.[15] Because of the recurrent and progressive nature of disease, a nephron-sparing approach (partial nephrectomy, enucleation, radiofrequency ablation, and cryotherapy) is the preferred treatment in VHL patients, with close observation used as an alternative in carefully selected patients with multiple small tumors.

Hereditary papillary RCC is an autosomal dominant disease with multiple type 1 papillary renal cell tumors.

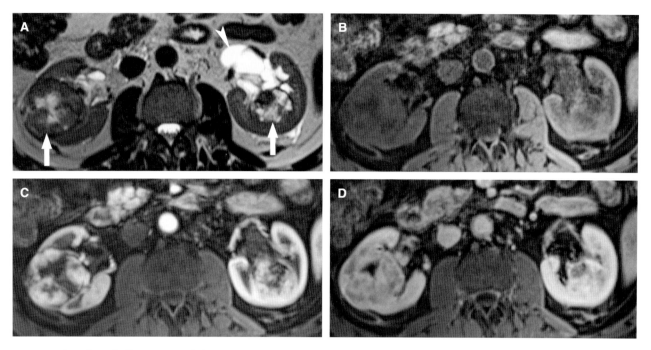

Figure 6.12 *Bilateral renal cell carcinomas.* (**A**) Axial T2-weighted FSE/TSE image demonstrates bilateral heterogeneous ball-shaped renal masses with central areas of high signal intensity (*arrows*). The left kidney has an extrarenal pelvis (*arrowhead*). Axial fat-suppressed T1-weighted pre-contrast gradient-echo image (**B**) and post-gadolinium-contrast arterial-phase (**C**) and nephrographic-phase (**D**) images demonstrate heterogeneous enhancement of both masses, consistent with clear cell renal cell carcinomas, proven at biopsy.

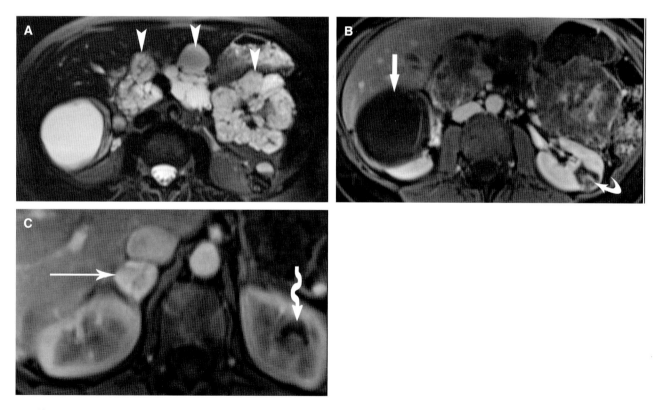

Figure 6.13 *von Hippel-Lindau disease.* Axial T2-weighted (**A**) and post-contrast-enhanced fat-saturated T1-weighted images obtained in a 35-year-old woman with von Hippel-Lindau disease demonstrate multiple serous cystadenomas (*arrowheads* in image A) of the pancreas. Arising from the left kidney is a heterogeneous round intrarenal mass (*curved arrow* in image B) resulting in mild contour deformity, representing a clear cell renal carcinoma. Arising from the right kidney is a Bosniak category III cystic lesion (*straight arrow* in image B) with an enhancing septation in the upper pole. (**C**) Fat-suppressed axial T1-weighted post-contrast-enhanced image at a different level demonstrates a second enhancing solid renal cell carcinoma (*squiggly arrow*) in the upper pole of the left kidney and an enhancing right adrenal pheochromocytoma (*skinny arrow*). The patient also has vertebral metastases from metastatic breast cancer shown with heterogeneous slightly increased signal intensity in the vertebral body.

The masses display the same imaging characteristics as the sporadic papillary type of RCC. Associated cysts are not common. No extrarenal manifestations have been described.

Hereditary leiomyoma RCC is an autosomal dominant disorder associated with cutaneous and uterine leiomyomas and type 2 papillary RCC.

Birt-Hogg-Dube syndrome is an autosomal dominant disease characterized by fibrofolliculomas of the face and trunk, pulmonary cysts, and renal tumors. The renal neoplasms are most commonly the chromophobe type of RCC and oncocytomas, but clear cell and papillary RCC can also occur.

Familial renal oncocytoma is a rare condition with probable overlap with Birt-Hogg-Dube syndrome.

Tuberous sclerosis is a genetic disorder with an autosomal dominant inheritance pattern and multiorgan involvement. Systemic manifestations include facial cutaneous angiofibromas, retinal hamartomas, cortical tubers, subependymal tubers, subependymal giant cell astrocytoma, cardiac rhabdomyoma, lymphangiomyomatosis, and so forth. The most common renal manifestations include AMLs and cysts, as previously discussed, with RCC occurring in 1% to 2% of patients.[15] Differentiation of AMLs with minimal fat from RCC requires tissue diagnosis.

Renal lymphoma. Kidneys are a common site of extranodal lymphomatous involvement of the genitourinary system, occurring in approximately 3% to 8% of patients with lymphoma. Primary renal lymphoma isolated to the kidneys, however, is very rare, being seen in less than 1% of extranodal disease cases.[16] There are several described patterns of renal involvement: multiple circumscribed bilateral renal masses (60%), solitary renal mass, diffusely infiltrative unilateral or bilateral tumor resulting in nephromegaly, direct extension from retroperitoneal lymphadenopathy, perinephric disease, and renal sinus involvement.

MRI is comparable to contrast-enhanced CT in the evaluation of renal and perirenal lymphoma, but it is superior in demonstrating bone marrow involvement.[16] The MR appearance of untreated lymphoma is similar to that of most malignant renal lesions, showing lower signal intensity on T1-weighted images relative to the normal renal cortex and slightly lower or equal signal intensity on T2-weighted images. The post-gadolinium-contrast enhancement is usually less than in the adjacent renal parenchyma, with some lesions demonstrating gradual delayed enhancement.[16] Perinephric soft tissue raises a strong suspicion of lymphoma. Peripelvic and periureteric lymphoma presents as unilateral or bilateral thickening of the renal pelvic and ureteral walls with enhancement.[17]

Renal metastases. Kidneys are a common site of hematogenous metastases due to their abundant blood supply. The most common primary malignancy to metastasize to the kidney is lung cancer, followed by breast cancer, gastric cancer, and melanoma, based on autopsy series.[16] Renal metastases are usually multiple and bilateral, with a nonspecific and variable appearance on MRI (Fig. 6.14). The diagnosis is usually suspected in the presence of widespread metastatic disease. The differential diagnosis includes renal lymphoma, hereditary renal cancer syndromes, acute multifocal pyelonephritis, renal abscesses, septic emboli to the kidneys, and infarcts.

Transitional cell carcinoma (TCC) accounts for approximately 10% of upper urinary tract neoplasms, and about 5% of TCC cases arise in the upper tracts. The lesions can be multicentric and bilateral, synchronous and metachronous. Approximately 2% to 4% of patients with bladder cancer develop TCC of the upper tracts, and 40% of patients with upper tract TCC develop bladder cancer.[18] TCC of the renal pelvis and calices typically has an infiltrative growth pattern and invades the renal parenchyma without significant change in the shape of the kidney in early stages. Direct invasion and lymphatic spread are typical, with hematogenous metastases occurring less frequently. Invasion of the renal vein can rarely be seen. Patients commonly present with microscopic or macroscopic hematuria as well as flank pain and renal colic due to

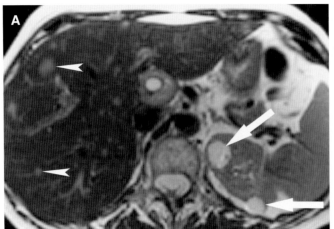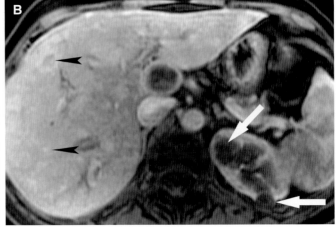

Figure 6.14 *Metastases to the kidneys.* MR images of 55-year-old woman with metastatic meningeal hemangiopericytoma. (**A**) Axial T2-weighted single-shot FSE/TSE image demonstrates two round high-signal intensity lesions (*arrows*) in the upper pole of the left kidney. Innumerable high-signal intensity liver metastases (*arrowheads*) of varying size are also evident. (**B**) Post-gadolinium contrast-enhanced T1-weighted fat-gradient-echo image at the same level shows the irregular borders and mild enhancement of the metastases (*arrows*). The liver metastases (*arrowheads*) also enhance.

obstruction in some cases. The TNM system is commonly used for staging of the upper-tract TCC.

The workup for urothelial neoplasms includes urinalysis with urine cytology, cystoscopy, and imaging of the upper urinary tract, most commonly with CT urography (CTU). MR urography can also be used to evaluate all the anatomic components of the urinary tract, similar to CTU. The heavily T2-weighted pulse sequences allow detection, localization, and characterization of urothelial neoplasms in case iodinated or gadolinium-based contrast material cannot be administered.

TCC presents as a low- to intermediate-signal-intensity signal void within the high-signal-intensity fluid-filled collecting system, pelvis, or ureter on T2-weighted images. It has a similar signal intensity to renal parenchyma on T1- and T2-weighted images; therefore, IV contrast material administration is required to determine renal parenchymal involvement. The degree of enhancement is less than that of the adjacent renal tissue due to relative tumor hypovascularity.[19] Dynamic post-contrast enhanced images performed in the corticomedullary, nephrographic, and delayed phases provide the necessary staging information (Table 6.2) about tumor location and extent and invasion of the adjacent structures or, rarely, the renal vein and IVC. The excretory images can be obtained after intravenous furosemide administration, which results in better distention of the renal collecting systems and the ureters, making the signal voids more conspicuous. Maximum-intensity projections of the urinary tract are usually obtained from both T2-weighted images and post-contrast-enhanced T1-weighted images with fat saturation and display the urinary tract in a 3D rotating manner, resembling conventional x-ray urography and demonstrating the filling defects in their entirety.

TCC of the ureter demonstrates intermediate signal intensity similar to that of the muscle on T1-weighted images and slightly high signal intensity on T2-weighted images. Small tumors are sometimes difficult to differentiate from calculi. Stones are usually better defined and have low signal intensity on both T1- and T2-weighted images. Enhancement of the tumor is crucial for differentiation from other potential causes of obstruction, such as stones and blood clots in patients with hematuria. Periureteric fat stranding can be seen with transureteric tumor extension.

RENAL CYSTS, CYSTIC MASSES, AND CYSTIC DISEASE

Bosniak Classification System. Any discussion of renal cystic lesions starts with the Bosniak classification system, which provides guidelines for the evaluation and management of these lesions, widely accepted by radiologists and urologists. Although the classification system is based on CT features of the cystic lesions, it can be applied to MRI most of the time. Nevertheless, MRI can reveal additional characteristics that can change the lesion's classification and potentially affect its management in some cases.[20]

Table 6.2 TNM STAGING OF TRANSITIONAL CELL CARCINOMA OF THE UPPER URINARY TRACT

STAGE	FINDINGS
T stage	**Size and location of the tumor**
TX	The primary tumor cannot be assessed (information not available)
T0	No evidence of primary tumor
Ta	Papillary non-invasive carcinoma
Tis	Carcinoma in situ
T1	Tumor invades subepithelial connective tissue
T2	Tumor invades the muscularis
T3	Tumor invades beyond muscularis into peripelvic fat or the renal parenchyma (for renal pelvis only)
T3	Tumor invades beyond muscularis into periureteric fat (for ureter only)
T4	Tumor invades adjacent organs, or through the kidney into the perinephric fat
N stage	**Involvement of regional lymph nodes**
NX	Regional lymph nodes cannot be assessed (information not available)
N0	No spread to regional lymph nodes
N1	Metastasis in a single lymph node, 2 cm or less in greatest dimension
N2	Metastasis in a single lymph node, >2 cm but <5 cm in greatest dimension, or in multiple lymph nodes not >5 cm in greatest dimension
N3	Metastasis in a lymph node, >5 cm in greatest dimension
M stage	**Distant metastases**
MX	Presence of distant metastasis cannot be assessed (information not available)
M0	No metastatic disease
M1	Distant metastases are present

STAGE GROUPING

Stage 0a	Ta, N0, M0
Stage 0is	Tis, N0, M0
Stage I	T1, N0, M0
Stage II	T2, N0, M0
Stage III	T3, N0, M0
Stage IV	T4, N0, M0 or Any T, N1, M0 or Any T, N2, M0 or Any T, N2, M0 or Any T, N3, M0 or Any T, any N, M1

Adapted with permission from American Joint Committee on Cancer. *AJCC Cancer Staging Manual*, 7th ed. Springer, 2010.

Box 6.2 ESSENTIALS TO REMEMBER

- MR has assumed an increasing role in the diagnosis, staging, and treatment planning of RCC, which is by far the most common renal malignancy. The morphology of RCC varies and includes: (1) a solitary avidly but heterogeneously enhancing solid mass, the most common appearance and characteristic of clear cell carcinoma; (2) a multicystic mass with enhancing, usually thick septations and nodular wall; fluid content is usually proteinaceous or hemorrhagic, demonstrating high signal intensity on T1-weighted images; (3) a homogeneous solid mass with low-grade enhancement is typical of chromophobe RCC or of benign oncocytoma, which is indistinguishable from malignancy by imaging; and (4) a heterogeneous infiltrative mass, which is characteristic of medullary RCC.

- Loss of signal intensity in solid portions of clear cell RCC may be observed on opposed-phase images. Signal loss is caused by the presence of cytoplasmic fat within tumor cells.

- Necrosis is common in RCC and is seen on MR as foci of low signal intensity on T1-weighted images, with moderate to high signal intensity in the same foci on T2-weighted images.

- Intratumoral hemorrhage is also common but is variable in appearance on MR, depending on the degradation stage of blood products.

- Invasion of the renal vein or IVC by RCC appears as a soft tissue mass within the vessels, usually displaying intermediate low signal intensity on T1-weighted images and intermediate high signal intensity on T2-weighted images. Intravascular flow is absent. Tumor thrombus shows enhancement, while bland thrombus does not.

- The MR appearance of AML reflects the constituents of the tumor: fat, smooth muscle, and blood vessels. Diagnosis on MR is made most reliably by comparing images with and without selective fat suppression to diagnose the presence of macroscopic (bulk) fat within the tumor.

- Transitional cell carcinoma of the urothelium is often multifocal. TCC of the renal pelvis is often infiltrative, iso-intense to the renal medulla, and difficult to detect on T1-weighted images. On T2-weighted images the low signal intensity of the tumor appears as a low signal intensity mass within high-signal-intensity urine. Low-grade enhancement of the tumor differentiates TCC from nonenhancing blood clots. Subtraction images may be necessary to confirm tumor enhancement.

- Renal lymphoma appears as: (1) multiple, or occasionally solitary, homogenous masses with low-level enhancement; (2) infiltrative masses showing a lesser degree of enhancement than the renal parenchyma; or (3) extension of a retroperitoneal mass into the kidney.

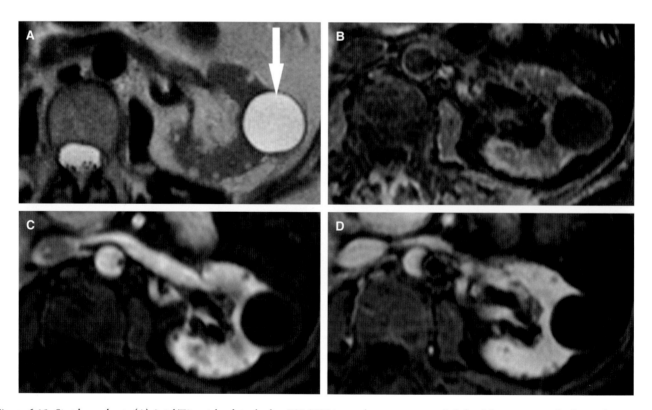

Figure 6.15 *Simple renal cyst.* (**A**) Axial T2-weighted single-shot FSE/TSE image demonstrates a well-defined, homogeneous, high-signal-intensity, round, partially exophytic left renal lesion (*arrow*) without internal septations or wall thickening. (**B**) Fat-suppressed axial T1-weighted gradient-echo image shows homogeneous low signal intensity within the lesion. The wall is uniformly thin. Axial T1-weighted fat-suppressed post-gadolinium-contrast enhanced images in corticomedullary (**C**) and nephrographic (**D**) phases demonstrate no enhancement. Findings are indicative of a benign simple renal cyst (Bosniak category I). Additional tiny cortical renal cysts are also evident.

Category I lesions are simple cysts with water-density content and no septations or mural calcifications. Renal cysts occur with increased frequency in older individuals and are more common in men than women. Renal cysts show high signal intensity on T2-weighted images, low signal intensity on T2-weighted images, and no enhancement following contrast material administration (Fig. 6.15). Heavily T2-weighted sequences allow both detection and characterization of very small cysts as they result in an increase in signal intensity of the lesion with increased T2 weighting.

Category II lesions are benign cysts with a hairline-thin septation and no measurable enhancement. These cysts can contain fine wall calcifications that are often not seen on MRI. Another group of minimally complex cysts included in category II is hemorrhagic and proteinaceous cysts measuring less than 3 cm in diameter. These cysts demonstrate high signal on T1-weighted images, intermediate or low signal intensity on T2-weighted images, and no post-gadolinium-contrast enhancement. These lesions are equivalent to hyperdense cysts on CT.

Category IIF ("F" for follow-up) was introduced later and includes cysts with multiple but thin septations, thicker mural calcifications, and no measurable enhancement. In addition, completely intrarenal hemorrhagic and proteinaceous cysts measuring more than 3 cm in diameter are included in this category. Most of these lesions are benign, yet they require follow-up imaging for confirmation.

Category III cysts are truly indeterminate lesions; approximately 60% represent cystic RCC. These lesions have thicker walls and septa with measurable enhancement. MRI may have added value in differentiating category IIF and III lesions by demonstrating septal enhancement in cases of equivocal enhancement on CT.[21]

Category IV cystic lesions clearly demonstrate malignant features, with thick irregular walls, enhancing septations, and mural nodularity or solid components.

Simple Renal Cyst. The most common cystic lesion of the kidney is simple cyst. It is common in the elderly and can be seen in about 50% of people older than 50 years of age. The cysts can be a few millimeters in size or may grow up to 10 cm or more. Solitary cysts can be seen, although multiple and bilateral cysts are more frequent. Histologically these cysts are lined by flattened cuboidal epithelium and contain clear fluid, which is the basis of their MRI appearance. The cysts demonstrate uniform high signal on T2-weighted images and low signal on T1-weighted images, similar to cerebrospinal fluid. There is a smooth hairline-thin wall with no enhancement (Fig. 6.15).

Parapelvic simple renal cysts arising from the renal parenchyma and extending into the renal sinus should be differentiated from peripelvic cysts. The latter are thought to have a lymphatic origin and are extraparenchymal. Both are located in the renal sinus; however, the peripelvic cysts usually present as multiple and bilateral clusters of cysts filling the renal sinuses and do not contain contrast material on the excretory phase, allowing their distinction from hydronephrosis.[22]

The vast majority of simple cysts are asymptomatic and do not require treatment; however, cyst aspiration, usually with

injection of a sclerosing agent, can be performed if large cysts result in hydronephrosis or cause pain.

Complicated cysts are simple cysts that are hemorrhagic or infected. These are usually classified as Bosniak category II cysts. Hemorrhagic cysts usually demonstrate high signal intensity on T1-weighted images and low signal on T2-weighted images, which indicates the presence of blood products. Sometimes simple cysts demonstrate high signal intensity on T1-weighted images related to high protein content of the cystic fluid.

Cystic nephroma is a multiloculated cystic neoplasm of the kidney, usually with a central location. Pediatric and adult cystic nephromas are now considered entirely different tumors. Pediatric cystic nephroma was previously classified as a tumor in the spectrum of cystic partially differentiated nephroblastoma, but now these two tumors are believed to represent a single entity. It usually occurs in boys less than 2 years of age. Adult cystic nephroma is considered a neoplasm in the same spectrum with mixed epithelial and stromal tumor and occurs in adult women. Adult cystic nephroma is characterized by thin fibrous septa, whereas mixed epithelial and stromal tumor contains thick and dense septa and ovarian-like stroma.[23]

On MRI both adult and pediatric cystic nephromas appear as a well-defined encapsulated multiloculated cystic renal lesion of variable size, with individual loculi measuring up to 4 cm.[24] They are usually centrally located and may herniate into the renal pelvis. The capsule and septa demonstrate low signal intensity on T1- and T2-weighted images due to the presence of fibrotic tissue and usually enhance following administration of IV contrast material. The intensity of fluid signal on T1- and T2-weighted images may vary based on the presence of hemorrhage or high protein content (Fig. 6.16).

Cystic nephroma presents as a Bosniak category III lesion and cannot be reliably differentiated from cystic RCC or other cystic renal tumors; therefore it requires nephron-sparing surgery or nephrectomy.

Cystic Renal Cell Carcinoma. RCC can present as a complex cystic mass either because of areas of central necrosis or due to its multilocular cystic nature. Rarely RCC can arise adjacent to a simple cyst. The multilocular variety of clear cell RCC on pathology contains clusters of clear cells in the septa of the complex cystic mass. This tumor can be seen in adults aged 26 to 71 years (mean age 51) and has a 3:1 male-to-female predominance. On imaging it usually presents as a Bosniak category III or, less commonly, category IIF lesion. MRI demonstrates the multilocular cystic nature of the renal mass, a fibrous capsule, and irregular thickening and enhancement of the walls and septa.[6]

Localized cystic disease of the kidney should be considered in the differential diagnosis of a multilocular cystic renal mass. It presents as a cluster of simple renal cysts of variable sizes separated by thin bands of normal renal parenchyma. It is a non-hereditary rare lesion that is usually asymptomatic. The condition commonly affects one kidney; however, simple renal cysts are often present in the contralateral kidney as well. The cyst aggregates can replace variable volumes of the kidney and sometimes the entire kidney, but the renal

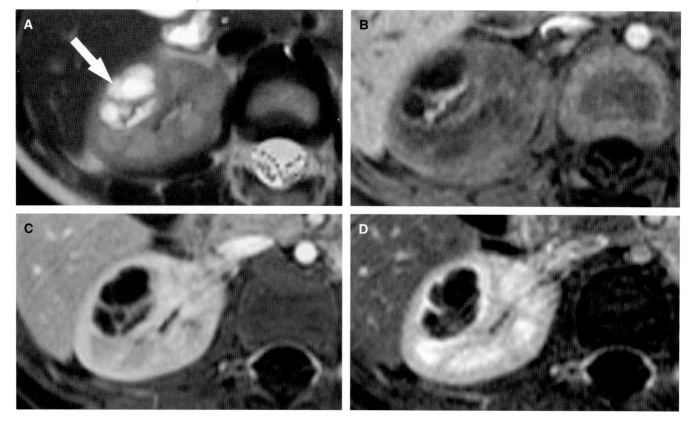

Figure 6.16 *Cystic nephroma.* MR images of a 4-year-old boy. Axial T2-weighted (**A**) and T1-weighted fat-suppressed (**B**) images demonstrate a multiseptated intraparenchymal renal cystic lesion (*arrow* in image A), consistent with Bosniak category III cyst. Axial T1-weighted fat-suppressed post-gadolinium-contrast-enhanced images in nephrographic phase (**C**) with corresponding subtraction image (**D**) demonstrate enhancement of the septa. Lesion was confirmed to be a cystic nephroma.

function is usually preserved, in contradistinction to multicystic dysplastic kidney. Absence of defined capsule and lobulated contour is another useful feature differentiating localized cystic disease of the kidney from ball-shaped cystic renal masses (e.g., cystic RCC, cystic nephroma). No mural or septal nodularity is present. Splaying of the intrarenal vessels around the cysts within the cluster could also aid in differential diagnosis if present.[25]

MRI features of localized cystic disease are similar to those seen on CT. It presents as an aggregate of simple cysts separated by normal enhancing renal parenchyma. Differentiation of the bands of intervening parenchyma may be difficult at times from true septations, so evaluation in the coronal and sagittal planes is important.[26] After administration of gadolinium-based contrast material the insinuating renal parenchyma should enhance similar to the rest of the kidney. Isolated simple renal cysts are usually present in the ipsilateral and contralateral kidney.

Autosomal recessive polycystic disease (ARPKD), also known as infantile polycystic renal disease, is a rare condition (1 in 50,000) associated with generalized dilatation of the collecting tubules with formation of innumerable microcysts. A varying degree of hepatic fibrosis is always present and is inversely related to renal involvement. The imaging diagnosis is usually based on the ultrasound appearance of the kidneys with bilateral symmetrical enlargement, increased echogenicity, and preservation of the reniform shape. MRI is

rarely necessary and shows bilateral smooth enlargement of the kidneys occupying most of the abdomen.

Autosomal dominant polycystic renal disease (ADPKD), also known as adult polycystic renal disease, is more common than ARPKD (1 in 400 to 1,000) and usually manifests in the third or fourth decades. Pathologically both the glomeruli and collecting tubules are involved, with resulting formation of innumerable bilateral renal cysts and marked enlargement of the kidneys. Cysts can also be seen in the liver and pancreas and have been described in the spleen, thyroid, parathyroid, pituitary, pineal gland, seminal vesicles, epididymis, testes, ovaries, endometrium, and breast (Figs. 6.17 and 6.18).

Sonography is routinely used for screening and diagnosis of ADPKD, with CT and MRI reserved for problem cases. MRI is more sensitive and specific for evaluation of small renal cysts and also provides the opportunity to detect and characterize extrarenal manifestations of disease. In addition, complications of ADPKD, such as cyst hemorrhage and infection, as well as RCC development can be evaluated. MRI is the best imaging modality for assessing the renal size and progression of disease. It is used as the standard to monitor renal volume changes in response to medication treatment in clinical trials.

Various numbers of bilateral cysts can be seen early in the disease. Polycystic kidneys have a characteristic appearance on MRI in the late phase and usually present as markedly enlarged

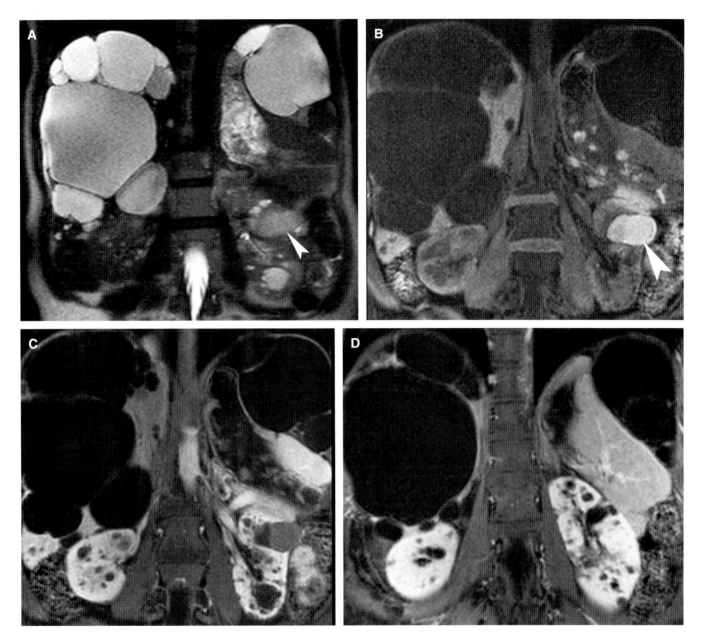

Figure 6.17 *Autosomal dominant polycystic disease with large liver cysts.* (**A**) Coronal T2-weighted single shot FSE/TSE and (**B**) T1-weighted gradient-echo image with fat saturation show innumerable large cysts replacing the liver and innumerable small simple renal cysts in both kidneys. A hemorrhagic cyst (*arrowheads*) in the left kidney shows high signal intensity on fat-suppressed T1-weighted and intermediate signal on T2-weighted images. Some of the cysts demonstrate lower signal on T2-weighted images due to their protein content. (**C, D**) Post-gadolinium-contrast-enhanced coronal T1-weighted fat-suppressed images make the smaller cysts more conspicuous because they remain low in signal without enhancement against the background of brightly enhancing renal parenchyma.

kidneys containing innumerable cysts of various sizes and no detectable normal parenchyma. Internal hemorrhage is often present in many of the cysts, manifesting as high signal intensity on T1-weighted fat-suppressed images and low signal intensity on T2-weighted images (Fig. 6.19). The reniform shape of the kidneys is usually preserved and the kidneys occupy most of the upper abdominal cavity, displacing adjacent viscera. The risk of RCC development in ADPKD is thought to be increased,[27] so evaluation of post-gadolinium-contrast enhancement of the lesions is very important for the detection of solid masses.

Acquired renal cystic disease (ACDK) is a condition associated with the development of multiple bilateral simple cysts in individuals without a history of hereditary cystic disease. It occurs in end-stage renal disease and uremia and most commonly is discovered inadvertently on cross-sectional imaging in patients on dialysis. Rarely it antedates the clinical recognition of renal failure, and radiologists can aid in establishing this diagnosis. Although acquired cystic disease is not a consequence of dialysis, the incidence and the number and size of the cysts correlate with the number of years the patient had been on dialysis because it prolongs patient's life, allowing

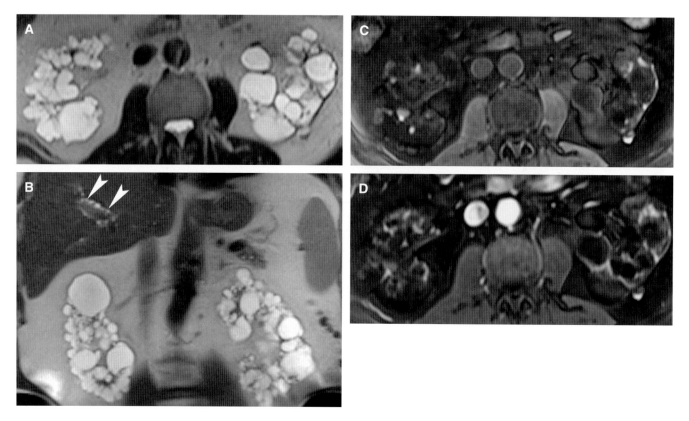

Figure 6.18 *Autosomal dominant polycystic disease with Caroli's disease.* Axial (**A**) and coronal (**B**) T2-weighted single shot FSE/TSE images demonstrate innumerable cysts of various sizes obscuring the intervening renal parenchyma of both kidneys. Small cysts (*arrowheads*) along the portal vein are due to coexisting Caroli's disease. (**C**) Some of the renal cysts demonstrate high signal intensity on axial pre-contrast-enhanced T1-weighted fat-suppressed image, indicative of internal hemorrhage. (**D**) Post-gadolinium-contrast-enhanced T1-weighted fat-suppressed image demonstrates enhancement of the renal parenchyma that is compressed by the multitude of cysts. No solid masses are seen.

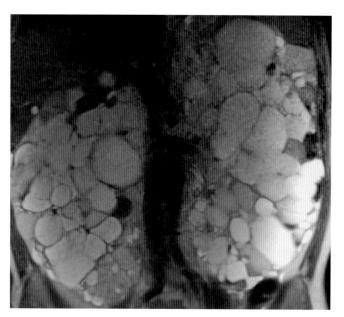

Figure 6.19 *Autosomal dominant polycystic disease, advanced.* Coronal T2-weighted image demonstrates innumerable renal cysts of various sizes in massively enlarged kidneys. The majority of the cysts demonstrate high signal intensity, consistent with their simple fluid nature. Some of the cysts show low signal intensity due to internal hemorrhage.

more time for cysts to develop. It is a progressive disease but can be reversible after successful renal transplantation. The disease is usually asymptomatic, but occasional manifestations include retroperitoneal hemorrhage, hematuria, flank pain, renal colic, cyst infection or hemorrhage, erythrocytosis, or distant metastatic disease from RCC.

The MRI appearance of the acquired cystic disease is similar to that of ADPKD, with the most important difference being the renal size. In acquired cystic disease the kidneys are normal or small in size due to underlying end-stage renal disease. The intervening parenchyma with discernible corticomedullary differentiation can be seen in ACDK as opposed to ADPKD. Another helpful distinguishing feature is the presence of cysts only in the kidneys in ACDK, while cysts can be seen in the liver, pancreas, and other organs in ADPKD. Otherwise, the appearance of the cysts can be similar, with many of them containing hemorrhage. The cysts are usually small (up to 1 cm) but can reach 2 to 4 cm in size.

CT is the modality of choice in detecting complications of ACDK, including hemorrhage and cyst infection, with MRI used in problem cases. It has a role in the detection and characterization of solid renal neoplasms in ACDK, since there is 40-fold increase in the incidence of RCC in patients with this disease compared to the general population (Fig. 6.20). Renal cancers develop in 2% to 7% of patients with ACDK.[28] The tumors are commonly multicentric and bilateral in this

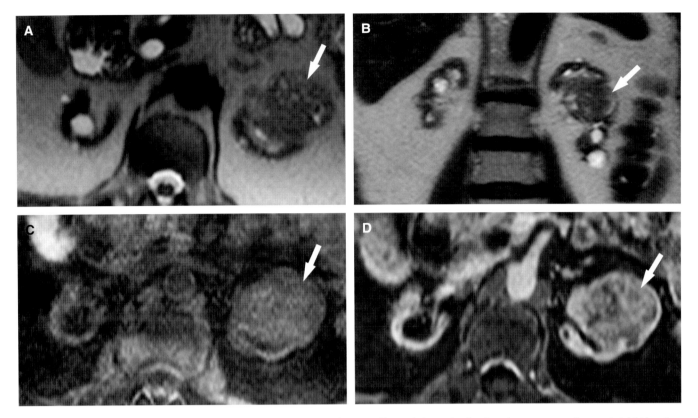

Figure 6.20 *Cystic uremic disease.* A 69-year-old patient with a 12-year history of hemodialysis who developed cystic uremic disease. Axial (**A**) and coronal (**B**) T2-weighted single shot FSE/TSE images demonstrate the small kidneys of end-stage renal disease. Cystic uremic disease is characterized by development of numerous small cysts in the end-stage kidneys of patients on long-term hemodialysis. Patients are at increased risk of developing renal carcinoma. MR reveals a heterogeneous exophytic solid mass (*arrows*) arising from the left kidney. Pre-contrast (**C**) and post-contrast (**D**) axial T1-weighted fat-suppressed images show enhancement of the mass (*arrow*), proven by nephrectomy to represent chromophobe renal cell carcinoma.

patient population and are predominantly of the papillary subtype. Assessment of lesion enhancement is crucial for detection of RCC and can be performed with CT and MRI. However, gadolinium-based contrast agent administration should be used with caution in patients with renal failure. The American College of Radiology recommends that gadolinium-based contrast agents not be administered in patients with a GFR of less than 30 mL/min due to the high risk of gadolinium-induced nephrogenic systemic fibrosis (NSF). A standard dose of 0.1 mmol/kg or less of the contrast material

is recommended to minimize the risk of NSF.[29] The risk of nephrotoxicity from the iodinated contrast agents used in CT is higher than the risk of NSF from gadolinium-based contrast agents, so it is generally not recommended to switch patients to contrast-enhanced CT just to avoid NSF.[29] Diffusion-weighted MR imaging can serve as an alternative to contrast-enhanced sequences. ADC values of simple and complicated cysts are usually higher than those of solid lesions.[30]

Lithium nephropathy has been described to present with innumerable parenchymal microcysts (Fig. 6.21).

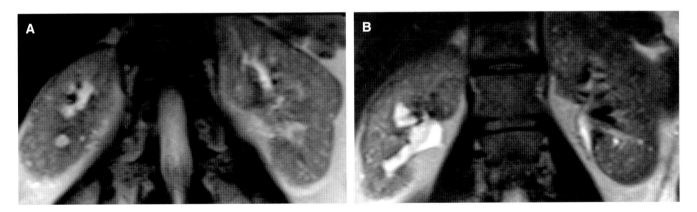

Figure 6.21 *Lithium nephropathy.* (**A, B**) Coronal T2-weighted images demonstrate innumerable minute cortical cysts measuring 1 to 2 mm. No cysts are present in the medulla.

Box 6.3 ESSENTIALS TO REMEMBER

- Simple cysts of the kidneys have a thin wall that does not enhance. The cysts contain serous fluid that shows low signal intensity on T1-weighted images and high signal intensity on T2-weighted images.

- Renal cysts complicated by infection or hemorrhage contain proteinaceous or hemorrhagic fluid characterized by intermediate to high signal intensity on T1-weighted images and intermediate to low signal intensity on T2-weighted images.

- Cystic renal tumors, including cystic RCC, cystic nephroma, and cystic metastases, are diagnosed by the presence of enhancement of solid tissue nodules, septations, or thickened walls. Contained fluid shows variable signal intensity.

- MR demonstrates the same morphology of the various forms of renal cystic disease as does CT and ultrasound. Cysts with internal hemorrhage, debris, or proteinaceous material are more specifically characterized by MR.

INFECTION

Pyelonephritis has a similar imaging appearance on CT and MRI, presenting with "striated nephrogram," alternating radial bands of normal and decreased enhancement extending from the renal sinus to the periphery of the renal cortex. Focal pyelonephritis involves only a portion of the renal parenchyma, which shows decreased enhancement. The differential diagnosis of focal pyelonephritis includes renal infarct. CT, however, has the advantage of demonstrating renal stone disease, often associated with pyelonephritis, to a better extent.

Renal abscess can result from ascending urinary tract infection and pyelonephritis (corticomedullary abscess). It can also be caused by hematogenous infection (cortical abscess). Renal abscess can perforate the capsule and extend into the perirenal space, thus forming a perirenal abscess. Risk factors include recurrent urinary tract infections, urinary tract anomalies, stone disease, recent instrumentation, vesicoureteral reflux, and diabetes mellitus. Renal abscess appears on MRI as a rim-enhancing thick-walled fluid collection within the renal parenchyma. Gradient-echo images can show small pockets of gas within the abscess, resulting in blooming artifact. Other features may include perinephric fat stranding, fluid, and thickening of Gerota's fascia.

Xanthogranulomatous pyelonephritis (XGP) is a chronic longstanding infection of the kidney associated with granulomatous inflammation extending beyond the kidney into the perirenal fat, Gerota's fascia, and retroperitoneum. Histologically the granulomatous tissue contains a large number of lipid-laden foamy macrophages (i.e., xanthoma cells). XGP is associated with renal calculus in approximately 75% of cases, and half of them are staghorn in shape. Diffuse and focal forms of XGP are described. MRI has no advantage over CT for characterizing XGP because it has a nonspecific appearance on MRI and can mimic other inflammatory and neoplastic lesions.

OBSTRUCTION

MR urography is similar to CT urography in terms of allowing the evaluation of urinary tract obstruction caused by stone disease, urothelial neoplasms, and other causes; however, it is inferior to CT in detecting stones due to their poor visualization (Fig. 6.22). T2-weighted images, excretory-phase T1-weighted images, post-contrast-enhanced imaging with fat saturation, and MIP reconstructions are used to evaluate obstructive uropathy.

TRAUMA

CT scanning is the preferred and widely used modality for evaluating traumatic injuries of the urinary system. MRI can be used as an alternative and allows evaluation of renal parenchymal, urinary tract, and vascular injuries. The disadvantage of MRI in the setting of trauma is the long scanning time, availability, cost, and limited patient access during the scan.

BLADDER

Bladder cancer is the most common neoplasm of the urinary system. 90% of all bladder cancers are TCC, with squamous cell carcinoma and adenocarcinoma accounting for approximately 9% and other rare tumors for less than 1%. Bladder cancer can present with superficial (70% to 80%) and invasive forms. The superficial form has a high rate of recurrence when treated and can progress into the invasive form at the time of recurrence.[31] Transmural invasion into the perivesical fat can be seen with the invasive form and carries a poor prognosis. The prostate, vagina, uterus, and pelvic wall can be involved with advanced TCC. Regional metastases occur into the pelvic lymph nodes, and distant hematogenous metastases can be seen in lung, liver, and bone. The TNM staging system is currently preferred.

Cystoscopy and deep biopsy involving all four layers of the bladder wall are usually performed for initial staging of the tumor (Table 6.3). CT and MRI are used as adjuncts for tumor staging and have comparable accuracy. Evaluation of the entire urinary tract (upper and lower) is indicated to evaluate for multicentric disease and for treatment planning.

Assessment of the bladder wall requires distention of the bladder. The tumor can be seen as a polypoid or nodular mass,

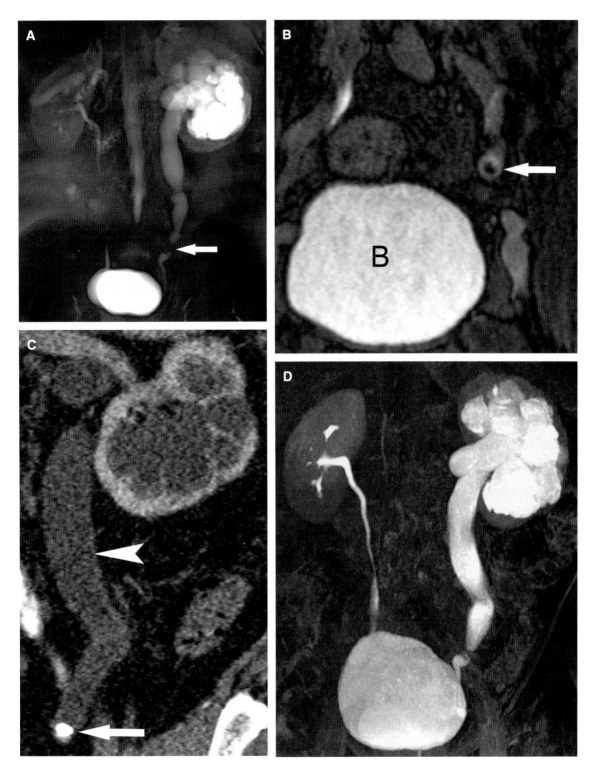

Figure 6.22 *Chronic hydronephrois, MR urogram.* (**A**) Coronal T2-weighted thick-slab MR urogram (acquired with the same thick slab single-shot FSE/TSE pulse sequence technique typically used for MRCP) shows marked left hydronephrosis and hydroureter with a low-signal intensity "filling defect" (*arrow*) in the distal third of the left ureter. The degree of dilatation of the collecting system and ureter indicates chronic obstruction. (**B**) Detailed view of the distal ureter and bladder (*B*) on a 5-minute-delayed post-gadolinium contrast-enhanced coronal T1-weighted fat-suppressed image demonstrates a focal signal void (*arrow*) in the distal left ureter. (**C**) Early post-contrast-enhanced coronal image from a CT urogram in the same patient shows the high-attenuation calculus (*arrow*) in the distal portion of the markedly dilated left ureter (*arrowhead*). (**D**) Maximum-intensity-projection (MIP) image of the urinary tract in excretory phase generated from a 3D T1-weighted gradient-echo sequence provides the complete picture of left hydronephrosis, hydroureter, and calculus in the distal left ureter. The right ureter is normal.

Table 6.3 TNM STAGING OF UROTHELIAL CARCINOMA OF THE URINARY BLADDER

STAGE		FINDINGS
T stage		**Size and location of the tumor**
TX		The primary tumor cannot be assessed (information not available)
T0		No evidence of primary tumor
Ta		Non-invasive papillary carcinoma
Tis		Carcinoma in situ: "flat tumor"
T1		Tumor invades subepithelial connective tissue
T2		Tumor invades the muscularis
	pT2a	Tumor invades superficial muscle (inner half)
	pT2b	Tumor invades deep muscle (outer half)
T3		Tumor invades perivesical tissue
	pT3a	Microscopically
	pT3b	Macroscopically (extravesical mass)
T4		Tumor invades any of the following: prostate, uterus, vagina, pelvic wall, abdominal wall. Includes prostatic stromal invasion directly from bladder cancer. Subepithelial invasion of prostatic urethra will not constitute T4 status.
	T4a	Tumor invades prostate, uterus, vagina
	T4b	Tumor invades pelvic wall, abdominal wall
N stage		**Involvement of regional lymph nodes**
NX		Regional lymph nodes cannot be assessed (information not available)
N0		No spread to regional lymph nodes
N1		Single node metastasis in primary drainage regions
N2		Multiple node metastases in primary drainage regions
N3		Common iliac node involvement
M stage		**Distant metastases**
MX		Presence of distant metastasis cannot be assessed (information not available)
M0		No metastatic disease
M1		Distant metastases are present

STAGE GROUPING

Stage 0a	Ta, N0, M0
Stage 0is	Tis, N0, M0
Stage I	T1, N0, M0
Stage II	T2a, N0, M0 or T2b, N0, M0
Stage III	T3a, N0, M0 or T3b, N0, M0 or T4a, N0, M0
Stage IV	T4b, N0, M0 or Any T, N1, M0 or Any T, N2, M0 or Any T, N2, M0 or Any T, N3, M0 or Any T, any N, M1

Adapted with permission from American Joint Committee on Cancer. *AJCC Cancer Staging Manual*, 7th ed. Springer, 2010.

or focal thickening (Fig. 6.23). With advanced disease diffuse irregular bladder wall thickening can be seen. The high inherent soft tissue contrast on MRI shows distinctly the bladder wall layers and allows evaluation of the depth of tumor invasion. The tumor demonstrates intermediate signal intensity on T2-weighted images, whereas the normal detrusor muscle shows low signal intensity, permitting assessment of bladder wall invasion. Both T1- and T2-weighted images show the tumor as an intermediate-signal-intensity lesion and can depict transmural extension of the tumor into the perivesical fat, which displays intrinsic high signal on both sequences (Fig. 6.24). T1- and T2-weighted imaging are also used to evaluate adjacent organ invasion, lymph node metastases, and bone metastases. Dynamic post-gadolinium-contrast-enhanced imaging shows early enhancement of the tumor and simultaneous enhancement of the metastatic pelvic lymph nodes. The early and avid enhancement of the tumor helps differentiate it from fibrosis, edema, and post-biopsy changes.

Squamous cell carcinoma (SCC) is the second most common bladder cancer and is much more frequent in countries where schistosomiasis is endemic. In the United States the risk factors for SCC of the bladder are chronic irritation from indwelling bladder catheters, bladder calculi, and chronic infection. Smoking, cyclophosphamide use, and intravesical administration of bacillus Calmette-Guérin have also been implicated in the development of SCC of the bladder.

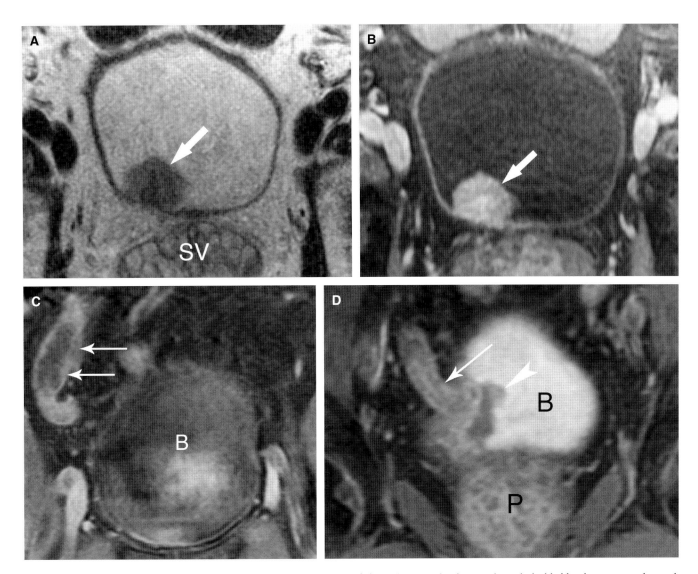

Figure 6.23 *Multifocal transitional cell carcinoma of the bladder and ureter.* (**A**) Axial T2-weighted image through the bladder shows an intraluminal polypoid mass (*arrow*). The fluid-filled seminal vesicles (*SV*) are high in signal intensity. (**B**) Post-gadolinium-contrast-enhanced axial fat-suppressed T1-weighted image shows enhancement of the mass (*arrow*), confirming tumor. (**C**) Coronal post-contrast-enhanced fat-suppressed T1-weighted image shows nodularity and wall thickening (*arrows*) of the enhancing wall of the distal right ureter. This T1-weighted urogram with intravenous contrast material reveals tissue enhancement against a background of low-signal urine. *B*, bladder. (**D**) Another coronal image from the T1-weighted post-contrast-enhanced urogram shows extension of wall thickening (*arrow*) of the distal right ureter and a mass (*arrowhead*) protruding into the bladder (*B*) through the ureteral orifice. Findings were confirmed as multifocal transitional cell carcinoma of the right ureter and bladder. The patient had undergone a prior left nephrectomy for transitional cell carcinoma. *P*, prostate.

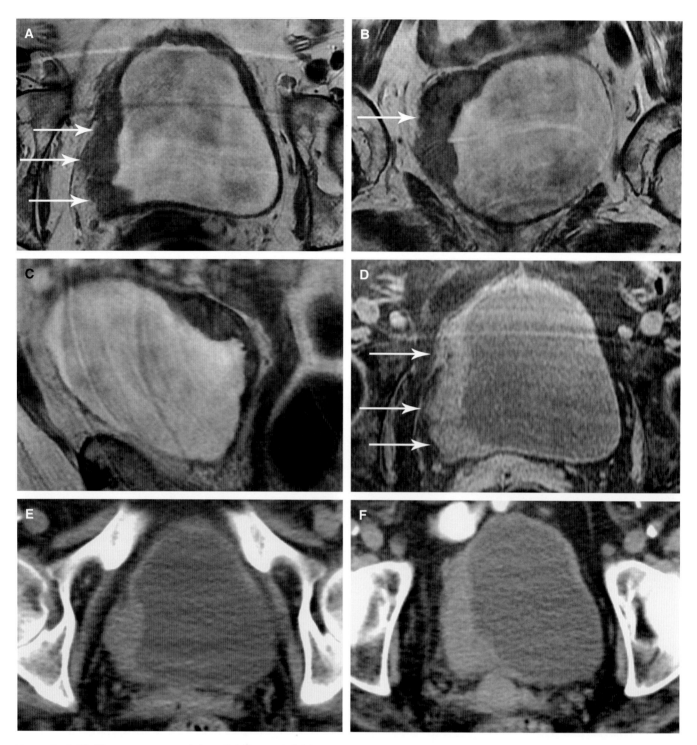

Figure 6.24 *Bladder cancer, stage III.* (**A**) Axial, (**B**) coronal, (**C**) sagittal T2-weighted FSE/TSE, and (**D**) axial fat-suppressed T1-weighted gadient-echo images of the urinary bladder demonstrate irregular thickening of the right and posterior wall of the bladder caused by transitional cell carcinoma. The indistinct border between the bladder wall and perivesical fat indicates transmural extension (*arrows* in images A, B, and D) of the tumor (TNM stage T3). (**E, F**) CT images of the same patient for comparison. Note the more distinct depiction of perivesical fat infiltration on MR images compared to the CT images.

The imaging findings are nonspecific. The tumors are usually high grade and invasive at initial presentation and can appear as a mass or as diffuse or focal bladder wall thickening. SCC commonly occurs in the region of the trigone and lateral bladder wall, and it can occur in bladder diverticulum.[32]

Adenocarcinoma is the third type of bladder cancer that commonly arises in a urachal remnant or in case of bladder exstrophy. Secondary metastatic adenocarcinoma is more common than primary and occurs as a result of direct invasion from adjacent organs (colon, prostate, rectum). Hematogenous and lymphogenous metastatic adenocarcinomas from breast, stomach, or lung are less frequent. Urachal adenocarcinoma has a characteristic location in the dome of the bladder and typically has a large extravesical component. Tumors have a complex solid and cystic appearance on MRI, and T2-weighted imaging shows high-signal-intensity components, consistent with collections of mucin within the tumor.[32]

TCC and SCC can also occur in the urachal remnant but are less common (20%).

Other malignant bladder tumors are rare and represent less than 1% of all bladder cancers. These include small cell or neuroendocrine tumor, leiomyosarcoma, and rhabdomyosarcoma. Carcinoid and paraganglioma are less likely to be malignant (Fig 6.25).

Leiomyoma is the most common benign mesenchymal bladder tumor and represents approximately 0.43% of all bladder tumors. It is usually asymptomatic but can manifest with urinary frequency, hesitancy, dribbling, hematuria, pressure from mass effect, and urinary obstruction if large. Leiomyoma comprises smooth muscle cells and arises from the submucosal layer of the bladder wall. The growth can be submucosal (7%), intravesical (63%), and extravesical (30%). The imaging features of bladder leiomyoma are similar to those of the uterus on ultrasound, CT, and MRI, with the latter offering the best

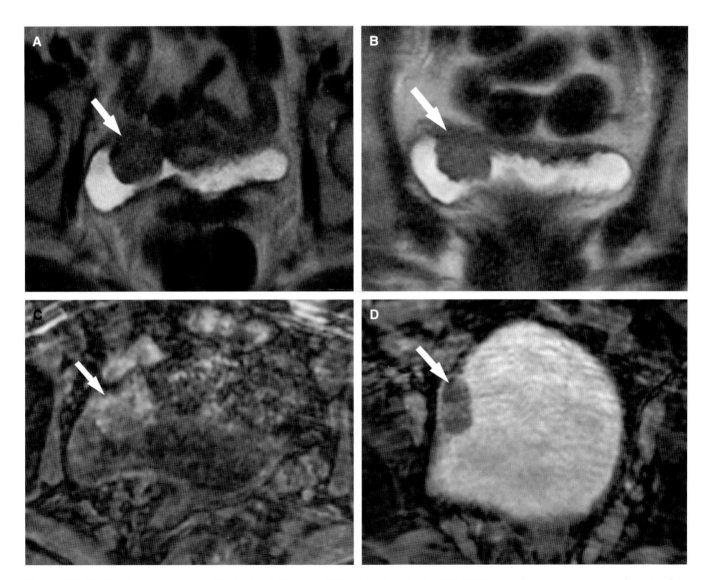

Figure 6.25 *Bladder pheochromocytoma.* (**A**) Axial and (**B**) coronal T2-weighted single-shot FSE/TSE images demonstrate an intermediate-signal-intensity polypoid mass (*arrows*) in the anterior-right lateral wall of the bladder protruding into the lumen. (**C**) Pre-contrast and (**D**) post-gadolinium-contrast-enhanced T1-weighted fat-suppressed images demonstrate 200% enhancement of the mass (*arrows*) by signal intensity measurement. Bladder pheochromocytomas are typically well-marginated submucosal masses, displaying low signal on T1-weighted and moderately high signal on T2-weighted images, and showing moderate to avid contrast enhancement.

soft tissue contrast. Leiomyomas display intermediate signal intensity on T1-weighted imaging and low signal intensity on T2-weighted images with homogeneous contrast enhancement. If areas of cystic degeneration are present, they demonstrate high signal intensity on T2-weighted images and do not enhance.

Paraganglioma of the bladder is a rare tumor arising from the chromaffin cells of the sympathetic chain in the muscular layer. It is also known as pheochromocytoma of the bladder. The symptoms of functioning paraganglioma are rather peculiar and are caused by catecholamine release during micturition, precipitating a "micturition attack" with severe headache, palpitations, hypertension, anxiety, sweating, and tremor.

Bladder paraganglioma appears as a well-marginated, sometimes lobulated submucosal mass displaying low signal intensity on T1-weighted images and moderately high signal intensity on T2-weighted images.[32] Post-contrast-enhanced images usually demonstrate avid enhancement (Fig 6.25). Central areas of necrosis and hemorrhage as well as peripheral calcifications can give the tumor a heterogeneous appearance.

Neurofibroma is a rare benign tumor of the bladder that can be isolated or associated with neurofibromatosis type 1. Tumors can be localized, diffuse, or plexiform, with the plexiform neurofibroma having the most characteristic appearance of a "bag of worms" or "knots" on a cord, representing thickened nerve and its branches. The tumors markedly thicken the bladder wall and can lead to ureteral obstruction and hydronephrosis. Involvement of the adjacent pelvic organs can occur.

On MRI the tumor presents with marked nodular thickening of the bladder wall, usually in the region of the trigone, where the nerve plexuses enter the bladder. T1-weighted imaging shows the tumor with low signal intensity, although the signal is slightly higher than that of skeletal muscle. T2-weighted imaging shows a characteristic target sign: low-signal-intensity fibrosis surrounded by high-signal-intensity myxoid stroma.[32] Enhancement of myxoid stroma is seen after contrast material administration. Extension of nodular masses through the neural foramina into the spinal canal is highly suggestive of plexiform neurofibroma.

Inflammatory pseudotumor, also known as pseudo-sarcomatoid fibromyxoid tumor, is a non-neoplastic proliferation of myofibroblastic spindle cells and inflammatory cells with myxoid components. It can mimic malignancy clinically, on cystoscopy and imaging, and therefore histologic diagnosis is essential.[33]

Inflammatory pseudotumor appears as an exophytic or polypoid, sometimes ulcerated bladder mass. Intramural cystic and solid variants have been described as well. The region of the trigone is usually spared. Large lesions may extend through the bladder wall into the adjacent structures, mimicking invasive bladder cancers. A heterogeneous appearance with a central hyperintense component with peripheral low signal intensity is seen on T2-weighted images. Peripheral enhancement is seen after contrast material administration, with less enhancement seen centrally.

Endometriosis. 11% to 8% of women with endometriosis have bladder involvement. It can occur from direct implantation of endometrial tissue or after pelvic surgery. Cyclic hematuria is the most specific symptom; however, this occurs in only 20% of cases. Other clinical manifestations of bladder endometriosis include cyclic pain, urgency, and dysuria. Patients may be asymptomatic as well.

The vesicouterine pouch is the most common site of bladder endometriosis. The lesions can extend through the bladder wall, forming a polypoid intraluminal mass. Focal areas of endometriosis can also be seen over the serosal surface of the bladder.

MRI provides excellent contrast resolution and tissue characterization compared to ultrasound and CT and is therefore the preferred modality for detection, localization, and characterization of bladder endometriosis. High-signal-intensity foci within the lesions on T1-weighted images with and without fat suppression caused by blood products from recurrent hemorrhage are characteristic of endometriosis. These foci can occur in areas of fibrosis, which demonstrate low signal intensity on T1- and T2-weighted images. Sometimes moderately high signal intensity can be seen within the lesions on T2-weighted imaging.[34] These images also delineate the bladder wall layers and allow for assessment of the depth of bladder wall invasion. Post-contrast-enhanced images demonstrate enhancement of the lesions homogeneously or in the periphery.

Lymphoma. There are three types of bladder involvement with lymphoma: (1) primary, isolated to the bladder; (2) secondary, with the primary involvement of the lymph nodes, spleen, and bone marrow; and (3) manifestation of systemic lymphoma. Secondary lymphoma of the bladder is the most common type and occurs in 10% to 25% of patients with lymphoma and leukemia.[34] On imaging and cystoscopy multiple masses are present, usually in the bladder dome and lateral walls, that mimic urothelial neoplasm.

Metastatic Disease. Direct invasion from adjacent pelvic organs is the most common type of metastatic process involving the bladder. The prostate and rectum are the most common sites of malignancies spreading to the bladder in men (Fig. 6.26). Cervical and uterine cancers commonly invade the bladder in women. Hematogenous and lymphatic metastatic lesions usually occur with widespread disease.

URETHRA

Urethral diverticulum occurs predominantly in women and represents an outpouching of the urethra formed from a distended Skene gland with subsequent rupture into the lumen. It usually occurs in the posterolateral wall of the middle third of the urethra. Axial T2-weighted images best demonstrate the characteristic crescent-shaped, sometimes septated fluid-filled lesion "hugging" the target-shaped urethra (Fig 6.27). Bilateral diverticula can also occur. Heterogeneous signal is sometimes seen within the diverticulum if superimposed infection or inflammation is present.[34]

Primary Urethral Tumors. The vast majority of urethral tumors are malignant, with SCC being the most common

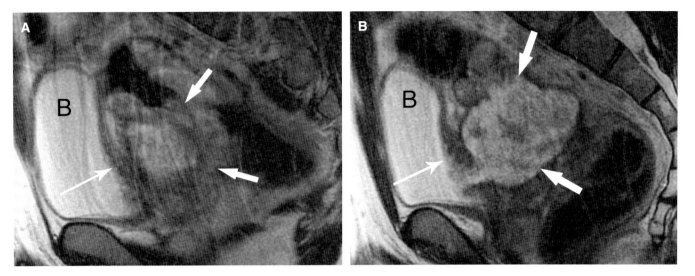

Figure 6.26 *Local invasion of the bladder by rectosigmoid carcinoma.* (**A, B**) Consecutive sagittal T2-weighted FSE/TSE images demonstrate an irregular heterogeneous circumferential (*fat arrows*) rectosigmoid mass displaying predominantly high signal intensity and invading (*skinny arrows*) the posterior wall of the urinary bladder (*B*).

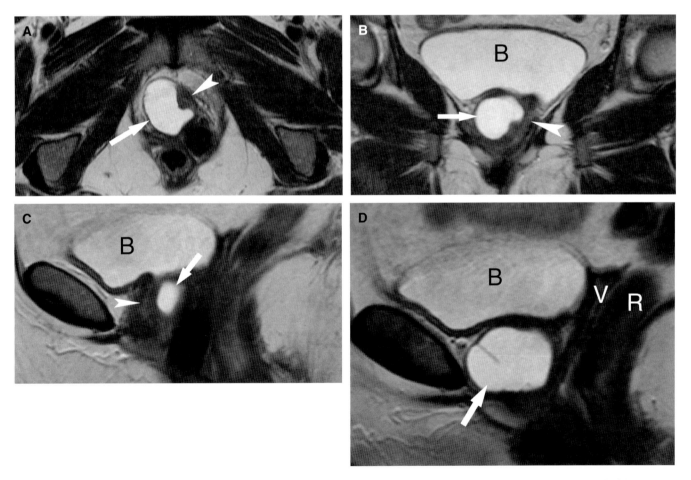

Figure 6.27 *Urethral diverticulum.* Axial (**A**), sagittal (**B**), and coronal (**C, D**) T2-weighted FSE/TSE images of the pelvis at the level of the pubic symphysis demonstrate a crescent-shaped fluid-filled diverticulum (*arrows*) "hugging" the right side of and displacing the female urethra (*arrowheads*). Coronal image D was obtained to the right of image C and shows the full size of the diverticulum (*arrow*). The uterus is surgically absent. *B*, bladder. *V*, vagina. *R*, rectum.

- Urothelial cancer is commonly multicentric, with synchronous tumors in the bladder, ureter, and renal pelvis. Patients with a history of urothelial cancer may develop tumors anywhere in the urothelium later in the course of disease. Bladder cancers are multicentric within the bladder in up to 40% of cases.

- On T1-weighted images tumors of the bladder wall display intermediate signal intensity; the lesions are well outlined by low-signal-intensity urine. Invasion of tumor through the bladder appears as intermediate tumor signal extending into high-signal-intensity perivesical fat.

- T2-weighted images show bladder tumors as intermediate signal intensity lesions, contrasting with the low signal intensity of the bladder wall and the high signal intensity of urine.

- Dynamic T1-weighted post-gadolinium-contrast-enhanced sequences show tumor of the bladder enhancing to a greater extent than the normal bladder wall. Recurrent or residual tumor also enhances to a greater degree than fibrosis that forms following resection.

- Involved lymph nodes show early enhancement similar to that of the primary tumor. Lymph nodes containing tumor metastases may not be enlarged.

- Tumors in the midline of the lower abdominal wall between the bladder and the umbilicus are very likely to be adenocarcinomas arising from the urachus or a urachal remnant.

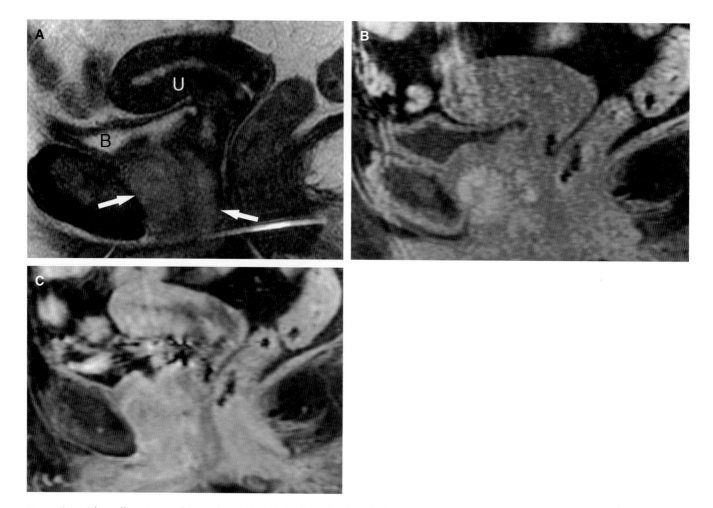

Figure 6.28 *Clear cell carcinoma of the urethra.* (**A**) Sagittal T2-weighted single-shot FSE/TSE image demonstrates an infiltrative mass (*arrows*) involving the entire female urethra and extending into the periurethral soft tissues, the vagina, and the base of the bladder (*B*). (**B**) Sagittal pre-contrast and (**C**) post-gadolinium-contrast-enhanced T1-weighted fat-suppressed gradient-echo images demonstrate avid enhancement of the mass, proven to be clear cell carcinoma of the urethra. *U*, uterus.

malignant tumor in both men and women. SCC is followed by TCC and adenocarcinoma in decreasing frequency. In men, SCC is more common in the penile, bulbous, and membranous portions of the male urethra, while TCC is more common in the prostatic portion.

MRI allows accurate local staging of the urethral cancer and treatment planning.[34] In men, the tumor usually displays low or intermediate low signal intensity on both T1- and T2-weighted images. Sometimes higher signal intensity can be seen on T2-weighted images. In women, the tumors usually demonstrate low signal intensity on T1-weighted images and moderately high signal intensity on T2-weighted images. Post-contrast-enhanced images show mild enhancement (Fig. 6.28). Invasion of adjacent organs is common.

Secondary Uretral Tumors. Direct invasion of the urethra by neoplasms from adjacent organs is common. Cervical, vaginal, ureteral, renal and bladder cancers can invade the urethra in female patients, while cancers of the prostate, bladder, testes, kidney, and ureter can lead to local spread with involvement of the male urethra.

REFERENCES

1. Zhang R, Pedrosa I, Rofsky NM. MR techniques for renal imaging. *Radiol Clin North Am.* 2003;41:877–907.
2. Kawashima A, Glockner JF, King BF. CT urography and MR urography. *Radiol Clin North Am.* 2003;41:945–961.
3. Jeon JY, Kim SH, Lee HJ, Sim JS. Atypical low-signal-intensity renal parenchyma: causes and patterns. *Radiographics.* 2002;22:833–846.
4. Riccabona M. Pediatric MRU: its potential and its role in the diagnostic work-up of upper urinary tract dilation in infants and children. *World J Urol.* 2004;22:79–87.
5. Grattan-Smith JD, Jones RA. MR Urography in children. *Pediatr Radiol.* 2006;36:1119–1132.
6. Prasad SR, Humphrey PA, Catena JR, et al. Common and uncommon histologic subtypes of renal cell carcinoma: imaging spectrum with pathologic correlation *Radiographics.* 2006;26:1795–1806.
7. Virkra R, Ng CS, Tamboli P, et al. Papillary renal cell carcinoma: radiologic-pathologic correlation and spectrum of disease. *Radiographics.* 2009;29:741–754.
8. Sheth S, Scatarige JC, Horton KM, et al. Current concepts in the diagnosis and management of renal cell carcinoma: role of multidetector CT and three-dimensional CT. *Radiographics.* 2001;21:S237–S254.
9. American Joint Committee on Cancer. Kidney. In: *AJCC Cancer Staging Manual*, 7th ed. New York: Springer, 2010:479–486.
10. Rakowski SK, Winterkorn EB, Paul E, et al. Renal manifestations of tuberous sclerosis complex: incidence, prognosis, and predictive factors. *Kidney Int.* 2006;70:1777–1782.
11. Prando A, Prando D, Prando P. Renal cell carcinoma: unusual imaging manifestations. *Radiographics.* 2006;26:233–244.
12. Dyer R, DiSantis DJ, McClennan BL. Simplified imaging approach for evaluation of the solid renal mass in adults. *Radiology.* 2008; 247:331–343.
13. Wagner BJ, Wong-You-Cheong JJ, Davis CJ Jr. Adult renal hamartomas. *Radiographics.* 1997;17:155–169.
14. Choyke PL, Glenn GM, Zbar B, Linehan WM. Hereditary renal cancers. *Radiology.* 2003;226:33–46.
15. Choyke PL. Imaging of hereditary renal cancer. *Radiol Clin North Am.* 2003;41:1037–1051.
16. Sheth S, Ali S, Fishman E. Imaging of renal lymphoma: patterns of disease with pathologic correlation. *Radiographics.* 2006;26: 1151–1168.
17. Pedrosa I, Sun MR, Spencer M, et al. MR imaging of renal masses: correlation with findings at surgery and pathologic analysis. *Radiographics.* 2008;28:985–1003.
18. Vikram R, Sandler CM, Ng CS. Imaging and staging of transitional cell carcinoma: part 2, upper urinary tract. *AJR Am J Roentgenol.* 2009;192:1488–1493.
19. Brown RFJ, Meehan CP, Colville J, et al. Transitional cell carcinoma of the upper urinary tract: spectrum of imaging findings. *Radiographics.* 2005;25:1609–1627.
20. Israel GM, Hindman N, Bosniak MA. Evaluation of cystic renal masses: comparison of CT and MR imaging by using the Bosniak classification system. *Radiology.* 2004;231:365–371.
21. Israel GM, Bosniak MA. How I do it: evaluation of renal masses. *Radiology.* 2005;236:441–450.
22. Rha SE, Byun JY, Jung SE, et al. The renal sinus: pathologic spectrum and multimodality imaging approach. *Radiographics.* 2004;24: S117–S131.
23. Takahashi N, Kawashima A, Lewin M, et al. Invited commentary. *Radiographics.* 2008;28:1225–1226.
24. Silver IMF, Boag AH, Soboleski DA. Multilocular cystic renal tumor: cystic nephroma. *Radiographics.* 2008;28:1221–1225.
25. Slywotzzky CM, Bosniak MA. Localized cystic disease of the kidney. *AJR Am J Roentgenol.* 2001;176:843–849.
26. Israel GM, Bosniak MA. Pitfalls in renal mass evaluation and how to avoid them. *Radiographics.* 2008;28:1325–1338.
27. Bonsib SM. Renal cystic disease and renal neoplasms: a mini-review. *Clin J Am Soc Nephrol.* 2009;4:1998–2007.
28. Choyke PL. Acquired cystic kidney disease. *Eur Radiol.* 2000; 10:1716–1721.
29. Prince MR, Zhang HL, Prowda JC, et al. Nephrogenic systemic fibrosis and its impact on abdominal imaging. *Radiographics.* 2009;29:1565–1574.
30. Saremi F, Knoll AN, Bendavid OJ, et al. Characterization of genitourinary lesions with diffusion-weighted imaging. *Radiographics.* 2009;29:1295–1317.
31. Vikram R, Sandler CM, Ng CS. Imaging and staging of transitional cell carcinoma: part 1, lower urinary tract. *AJR Am J Roentgenol.* 2009;192:1481–1487.
32. Wong-You-Cheong JJ, Woodward PJ, Manning MA, Sesterham IA. Neoplasms of the urinary bladder: radiologic-pathologic correlation. *Radiographics.* 2006;26:553–580.
33. Wong-You-Cheong JJ, Woodward PJ, Manning MA, Davis CJ. Inflammatory and nonneoplastic bladder masses: radiologic-pathologic correlation. *Radiographics.* 2006;26:1847–1868.
34. Ryu J, Kim B. MR imaging of the male and female urethra. *Radiographics.* 2001;21:1169–1185.

7.

ADRENAL AND RETROPERITONEAL MR IMAGING

Matthew J. Bassignani, MD

ADRENAL GLANDS

MR TECHNIQUE

Adrenal MRI should encompass the entirety of both adrenal glands on all sequences (Fig. 7.1). Our protocol begins with a T2-weighted fast localizer using half-Fourier acquisition single-shot fast/turbo spin-echo (single-shot FSE/TSE) scan in axial, coronal and sagittal planes, in-phase and opposed-phase gradient-echo (GRE) T1-weighted images (preferably using a dual-echo technique) for chemical-shift imaging, T1-weighted GRE sequences without and with frequency-selective fat saturation, dedicated multislice T2-weighted FSE/TSE imaging (as necessary), and a dynamic contrast-enhanced T1-weighted 3D GRE sequence with fat saturation following intravenous administration of a gadolinium contrast agent. Each sequence is performed during a single breath hold. This protocol may be tailored (with removal or modification of some sequences) to answer a specific question if prior imaging or clinical presentation has already narrowed the differential diagnosis.[1,2] Visualization of the adrenal glands is facilitated when there is sufficient retroperitoneal fat surrounding the adrenal gland. Adrenal visualization can be limited in patients with little suprarenal fat. The adrenal glands are iso- to hypointense to normal liver on T1- and T2-weighted images.

With gradient-echo imaging, chemical-shift artifact results in a decrease of signal intensity at the interfaces between (water-containing) soft tissues and fat, giving the so-called "India ink" appearance. This dropout of signal can be seen at the interface of the retroperitoneal fat and normal adrenal gland limbs (Fig. 7.1F). When a lesion displays high signal intensity on the pre-gadolinium contrast-enhanced images, it is helpful to generate subtraction images using an algorithm that subtracts, on a pixel-by-pixel basis, the signal of the pre-contrast images from that of the post-contrast images. Using this technique, lesions that do not enhance but display relatively high signal intensity on the pre-contrast-enhanced images, such as a hemorrhagic cyst, will appear black because the signal intensity values of the pixels on the pre- and post-contrast images are equal, resulting in no signal when subtracted. On the other hand, high-signal-intensity lesions

that truly enhance on post-gadolinium-contrast-enhanced images, such as cystic renal cell carcinoma containing protein-aceous fluid, will show increased intensity on subtraction images as the signal intensity values of the pixels on the post-contrast-enhanced images are greater than those of the pixels of the pre-enhanced images.

ANATOMY

The adrenal glands are paired retroperitoneal structures that sit in the right and left suprarenal space enclosed by Gerota's fascia along with the kidneys and surrounded by perirenal fat. A thin transverse fibrous lamella separates the kidneys from the adrenal glands within the perirenal space.[3,4] These endocrine glands weigh approximately 6 grams in adults and typically have an upside-down "y" or "v" configuration, with the medial and lateral limbs of the gland separated slightly by intervening perirenal fat. The normal adult glands measure 2 to 4 cm in length and 2 to 6 mm in thickness. Medial and lateral limbs join centrally to the adrenal body. The limbs should not measure more than 10 mm in thickness.[1,5] The right gland is typically closely applied to the posterior surface of the sub-diaphragmatic inferior vena cava. The left gland is more variable in position: it usually sits atop the left kidney or is closely applied to the left diaphragmatic crus. In the setting of renal agenesis or nephrectomy, the ipsilateral adrenal gland may assume a configuration other than a "v" or "y" shape. The adrenal gland may appear flattened with the two limbs closely apposed in the so-called "lying down adrenal" configuration. This is a normal variant and should not be considered pathologic. The adrenal gland is supplied by arterial branches of the inferior phrenic artery, the renal arteries, and the adrenal artery, which arises directly from the aorta. Venous drainage occurs on the left by a long left adrenal vein to the inferior phrenic vein that ultimately empties into the left renal vein. The right adrenal vein is quite short and enters directly into the posterior aspect of the inferior vena cava. Multiple accessory adrenal veins follow the arterial branches.[3]

The *microscopic anatomy* of the adrenal gland consists of an outer adrenal cortex derived from mesoderm, which makes up 90% of the gland's weight. The central adrenal medulla, which

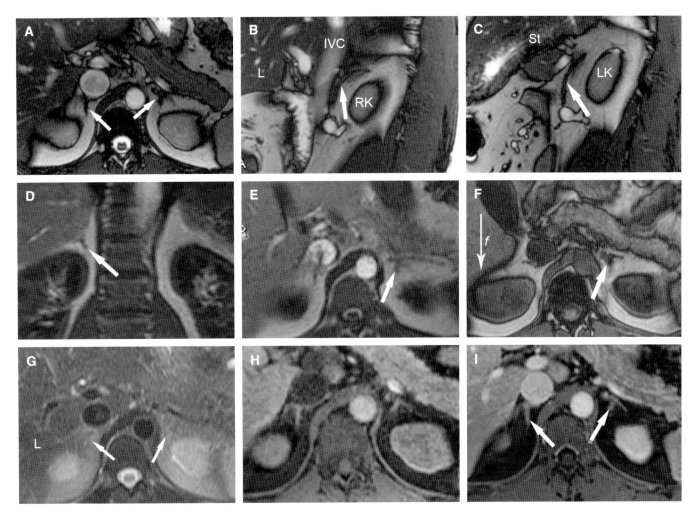

Figure 7.1 *Normal adrenal gland.* (**A**) Balanced steady-state free precession (SSFP) gradient-echo sequence in axial plane shows the normal adrenal glands (*arrows*) as upside-down "v" and "y" configurations. (**B**) Sagittal SSFP image of the right adrenal gland (*arrow*) shows that the gland is tightly applied to the posterior surface of the inferior vena cava (*IVC*), anterior and superior to the upper pole of the right kidney (*RK*) and posterior to the liver (*L*). (**C**) Sagittal SSFP image acquired adjacent to **B** shows an adrenal limb (*arrow*) extending inferior from the left adrenal body along the anterior superior left kidney (*LK*), posterior to the stomach (*St*). (**D**) Coronal T2-weighted single-shot FSE/TSE image shows only the right adrenal body and limbs (*arrow*), while the left gland is out of plane. (**E**) Axial T1-weighted gradient dual-echo sequence obtained in phase (TE ~4.6 msec) and (**F**) opposed-phase (TE ~2.3 msec). Note that on the opposed-phase sequence, all fat-soft tissue interfaces demonstrate signal drop-out (*skinny arrow, f*). This artifact can also be seen at the normal left adrenal gland (*arrows*). (**G**) Axial T2-weighted FSE/TSE image with fat saturation shows the adrenal glands (*arrows*) poorly because their signal is near iso-intense to that of both liver (*L*) and surrounding fat. Axial T1-weighted dynamic 3D gradient-echo images without (**H**) and with (**I**) gadolinium contrast enhancement. On the non-enhanced study, the higher-signal-intensity adrenal glands are conspicuous as the signal of the surrounding fat is suppressed by fat saturation. The adrenal glands enhance homogeneously following intravenous gadolinium contrast material injection.

accounts for 10% of the gland's weight, is derived from ectodermal neural crest cells that have migrated to this location as a part of the parasympathetic nervous system. The cortex cannot be differentiated from the medulla on MRI. Microscopic zonal anatomy within the cortex depicts three layers with three distinct cell types that produce three separate endocrine steroid hormones. From outer to inner, the cell layers are the zona glomerulosa, the zona fasciculata, and the zona reticularis (Fig. 7.2). The zonal anatomy cannot be discerned on MRI, but it is functionally important to know that these layers exist. Many remember the function of these cells by using the mnemonic, "the deeper you go, the sweeter it gets." Thus, the outer cell layer (zona glomerulosa) produces mineralocorticoids (e.g., aldosterone), which are responsible

for salt metabolism; the middle cell layer (zona fasciculata) produces glucocorticoids (the most important being cortisol), which regulate glucose metabolism; and the inner cell layer (zona reticularis) produces sex hormones (estrogens and androgens). The adrenal medulla is made up of neural crest tissue that produces the adrenergic substances known as catecholamines, primarily epinephrine.[6]

ADRENAL PATHOLOGY

Adrenal adenoma is a common entity that is encountered in up to 9% of autopsy series, with an increased prevalence in older patients. These adrenal masses are at least 1 cm in diameter and are conspicuous as a focal nodule (composed of bland

Adrenal Cortex

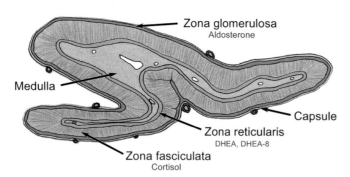

Figure 7.2 *Zonal anatomy of the adrenal cortex.* Line drawing shows normal zonal anatomy of the adrenal gland. (Thanks to Laurie Persson of the University of Virginia Radiology Department Graphics and Design Illustration Lab.)

adrenal cortical cells) within the otherwise normal-appearing adrenal gland. With increased use of imaging, adrenal adenomas are detected in up to 5% of CT scans performed for a reason other than assessment of the adrenal glands. These incidentally discovered adrenal masses are thus termed "adrenal incidentalomas."

The vast majority of adrenal incidentalomas represent nonfunctioning adrenal adenomas, but there is a differential diagnosis to consider. Chief considerations are the size of the incidentally discovered mass, and whether the patient has a known extra-adrenal malignancy. In the setting of no known primary malignancy, a small adrenal mass (less than 3 cm) is highly likely to be a benign adrenal adenoma. Two thirds of small adrenal incidentalomas are benign in the absence of a primary malignancy. In a patient with a known primary malignancy, there is a 50% chance that an incidentally discovered adrenal mass is metastatic. Thus, when a mass is found in the adrenal gland in a patient with a primary malignancy, further evaluation is required to determine its true nature so as to appropriately stage the patient's primary malignancy. The size of an adrenal mass is important in differentiating between benign and malignant disease. Most adrenal adenomas are small (less than 3 cm), while lesions greater than 6 cm are almost uniformly malignant, representing metastatic disease or primary adrenal cortical carcinoma.

Adrenal adenomas detected at imaging are nonfunctioning in 94% of cases, with 6% representing functioning adrenal adenomas producing cortisol (5%) or aldosterone or sex hormones (1%). The adrenal steroid hormones are synthesized by the adrenal cortex using a cholesterol precursor. It is this cholesterol substrate that gives adrenal adenomas their characteristic lipid signature that imparts low attenuation on CT and a decrease in MR signal on opposed-phase chemical-shift imaging compared to in-phase images. Importantly, up to 30% of adrenal adenomas lack sufficient intracytoplasmic lipid to be characterized on chemical-shift MRI or unenhanced CT (so-called *lipid-poor adrenal adenomas*). These lipid-poor adenomas must be characterized in some other manner (e.g., showing rapid washout of iodinated contrast material on CT).

With non-contrast-enhanced CT scan up to 70% to 80% of adrenal adenomas can be adequately characterized based on the presence of lipid within the lesions. Most of the remaining lipid-poor adenomas can be characterized based on the rate at which iodinated contrast material washes out of the lesion from the enhanced to the delayed contrast-enhanced images on the CT scan. With MRI, characterization of lipid-rich adenomas is performed with non-contrast-enhanced images (Fig. 7.3). No reliable washout criteria for diagnosing lipid-poor adrenal adenomas using gadolinium contrast agents have been currently defined. Adrenal adenomas appear on MR as small, well-defined round or oval lesions with homogeneous signal intensity on T1- and T2-weighted images. Heterogeneous signal intensity on T1- or T2-weighted images is associated with an increased risk of malignancy. Heterogeneous enhancement on post-gadolinium contrast-enhanced images is common in both benign and malignant adrenal lesions. Most (70% to 80%) of adrenal adenomas contain sufficient lipid to be detected with chemical-shift MRI. Chemical-shift imaging with T1-weighted gradient-echo imaging is used to detect the lipid component of adrenal adenomas by demonstrating a drop in signal within the adenoma on opposed-phase images compared with in-phase images.[3] Using this technique, we take advantage of the chemical-shift artifact that occurs when the opposed signals from the intracytoplasmic fat (from cholesterol) and the water containing soft tissue are in the same image voxel, as is commonly found in adrenal adenomas. Chemical-shift imaging makes use of the different resonant frequencies of the protons associated with fat versus those associated with water, as discussed in Chapters 1 and 2. On in-phase images, the signals from lipid and soft tissue will summate, giving a higher signal, whereas on opposed-phase images, the signals from lipid and soft tissue will negate one another, leading to a decrease in signal. With window width and window center settings identical between the in-phase and opposed-phase sets of images, the reader visually compares the two sequences, and if the adrenal mass gets darker on opposed-phase images, the mass is said to contain sufficient lipid to diagnose an adrenal adenoma, with sensitivity and specificity ranging from 81% to 100% and 94% to 100%, respectively, using this qualitative measurement. Loss of signal intensity in the adenoma parallels the loss of signal intensity in normal marrow of the adjacent vertebral body. A signal-intensity drop of greater than 20% on matched dual-phase chemical-shift gradient-echo images is considered diagnostic of benign adrenal adenoma. Heterogeneous loss of signal intensity on opposed-phase images is a common finding (~14% of cases) associated with benign adrenal adenomas. The portion of the adrenal gland that is not involved by the adenoma will follow the same signal as displayed by the contralateral normal adrenal gland on T1- and T2-weighted images. The glands, including the adenoma, will enhance following gadolinium contrast administration.

Most adenomas can be diagnosed using qualitative visual comparison of the lesion between in-phase and opposed-phase images so long as the values for window width and window center are kept the same. If there is not a clear drop in signal on opposed-phase sequences, a signal intensity index may be calculated using the spleen as an internal control. To diagnose an

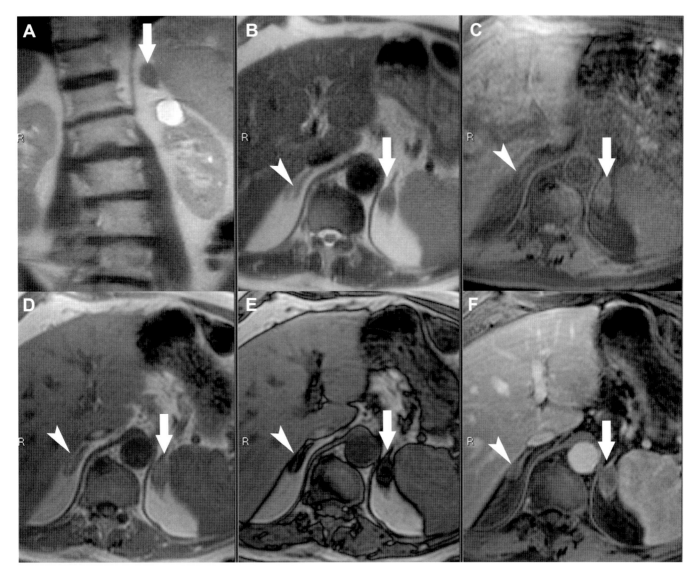

Figure 7.3 *Lipid-containing adrenal adenoma.* Patient with melanoma. (**A**) Coronal T2-weighted single-shot FSE/TSE image shows a lesion in the left adrenal gland that at first glance may be interpreted as a metastasis from the melanoma (*arrow*). (**B**) Axial T2-weighted single-shot FSE/TSE image shows the same lesion (*arrow*) with similar signal intensity to the normal right adrenal gland (*arrowhead*). (**C**) Axial T1-weighted gradient-echo image with fat saturation shows no signal decrease of the mass (*arrow*), indicating it is not a fat-containing lesion. Note that the left adrenal mass and the normal right adrenal gland (*arrowhead*) have the same signal intensity. (**D**) Axial T1-weighted in-phase gradient-echo image shows the same lesion (*arrow*) with similar signal intensity to the normal right adrenal gland (*arrowhead*). (**E**) Axial T1-weighted opposed-phase gradient-echo image shows a substantial decrease in signal compared with the in-phase image, indicating that the lesion (*arrow*) contains intracytoplasmic lipid, consistent with a lipid-containing adrenal adenoma. The functioning right adrenal gland (*arrowhead*) also shows a normal signal drop. (**F**) Post-gadolinium contrast-enhanced axial T1-weighted image with fat saturation shows enhancement of the right adrenal gland (*arrowhead*) and left adrenal gland, including the mass (*arrow*).

adrenal adenoma, the mass must drop in signal by approximately 25% on the opposed-phase image to diagnose the presence of lipid within the adenoma, with a sensitivity and specificity of 100% and 82%- respectively. The formula for the adrenal–spleen signal intensity index is {[(adrenal signal intensity on opposed-phase imaging /spleen signal intensity on opposed-phase imaging)/(adrenal signal intensity on in-phase imaging/spleen signal intensity on in-phase imaging)] – 1} × 100%.

The differential diagnosis for adrenal incidentaloma depends on many factors, including the patient's age, clinical presentation, history of prior malignancy, and size of the adrenal mass. The primary concern is whether the adrenal mass in question represents a benign (nonfunctioning or otherwise) adrenal adenoma versus a metastatic focus or a primary adrenal cortical carcinoma. When an adrenal mass does not show a signal drop on opposed-phase images, it is important to state that the lesion does not meet the criteria for a lipid-rich adrenal adenoma. The differential diagnosis then includes adrenal adenoma (lipid-poor), metastatic disease, pheochromocytoma, primary adrenal carcinoma, adrenal cyst or pseudo-cyst, adrenal hemorrhage, adrenal hyperplasia, myelolipoma, and rare entities such as infection, ganglioneuroma, neurofibroma, and teratoma.[4]

Conn's syndrome of hypertension and hypokalemia is caused by a hyperfunctioning aldosterone-secreting adrenal

Box 7.1 ESSENTIALS TO REMEMBER

Important caveats to diagnose lipid-rich adenomas include:

- The adrenal mass should display relatively homogeneous signal intensity on all sequences.

- The signal drop-out should be uniform throughout the mass. Heterogeneous lesions may show foci of decreased signal intensity on opposed-phase images and other areas that do not decrease in signal. These cannot be definitively diagnosed as adrenal adenomas.

- Signal intensities may vary artifactually between in-phase and opposed-phase images if separate pulse sequences are used to acquire the images instead of a single dual-echo sequence that acquires both in- and opposed-phase images together by varying the echo time. Also, images from independent pulse sequences may not match exactly with respect to their slice positions, resulting in errors when comparing.

adenoma, an *aldosteronoma*. Imaging plays a major role in the assessment of these patients and typically reveals a characteristic adrenal adenoma. Adrenal vein sampling is performed to demonstrate excessive levels of aldosterone ipsilateral to the adrenal adenoma, confirming that it is a functioning aldosteronoma. Adrenalectomy is curative.

The 2003 National Institutes of Health state-of-the-science conference proceedings regarding adrenal adenomas suggested that in the absence of clinical findings for hyperfunctioning adrenal adenoma or pheochromocytoma, a follow-up imaging examination be performed between 3 and 12 months to assess for interval growth.[1] Slight growth can be seen in some adenomas and myelolipomas, but substantial growth would indicate the need for biopsy or surgical removal owing to the increased risk of malignancy. The laboratory workup for subclinical Cushing's syndrome (i.e., subclinical hypercortisolism) and pheochromocytoma includes a dexamethasone suppression test and an assay for plasma free metanephrines, respectively.

Adrenal metastases are the most common malignant lesions to involve the adrenal glands. Adrenal metastases are found in up to 27% of autopsies in patients with extra-adrenal malignancies. The presence of an adrenal metastasis usually indicates advanced disease, with limited treatment options and shortened survival. Metastatic spread to the adrenal glands is facilitated by the rich vascular network that supplies the adrenal glands. Primary tumors that have a propensity for adrenal involvement include lung, breast, renal, melanoma, and gastrointestinal tract tumors.

Most adrenal metastases are carcinomas that result in enlargement of the gland to a mean of 2 cm. Isolated adrenal metastasis is an uncommon finding and there are usually other sites of metastatic disease in addition to the adrenal gland. Symptomatic adrenal metastases causing pain or hormonal disturbance are unusual, although a small percentage of patients with bilateral adrenal metastases will present with adrenal insufficiency (Addison's disease).

All entities in the differential diagnosis must be considered when an adrenal mass is found at MRI (Fig. 7.4). Size and shape should be noted. Benign entities are usually small and well defined with homogeneous signal intensity. In-phase and opposed-phase gradient-echo images are reviewed to determine if there is drop in signal on opposed-phase images compared with the in-phase images, which would confirm that the lesion is a lipid-rich adrenal adenoma. Heterogeneous signal intensity excludes definitive characterization of the lesion as a benign adenoma. Increased signal on T1-weighted images suggests areas of hemorrhage; proteinaceous debris,

Box 7.2 ESSENTIALS TO REMEMBER

- Most small (<3 cm) adrenal masses are benign, nonfunctioning adrenal adenomas. Benign adenomas are homogeneous, round, and well defined.

- Patients with primary adrenal malignancy have a 50% chance that the mass is a metastatic focus rather than a benign adrenal adenoma.

- Most benign adrenal adenomas can be characterized by the presence of intracellular fat due to accumulation of cholesterol, a precursor to hormone production.

- In-phase and out-of-phase MR gradient-echo imaging demonstrates the presence of intracytoplasmic lipid by showing a decrease in signal intensity on the opposed-phase images compared to the in-phase images.

- Failure to demonstrate an MR signal drop-out does not mean the lesion is a metastasis; it just means that such lesions cannot be definitively diagnosed as a lipid-rich benign adrenal adenoma

- Additional evaluation of an adrenal adenoma diagnosed by imaging may include biochemical tests to exclude subclinical hypercortisolism and pheochromocytoma plus follow-up imaging to confirm size stability.

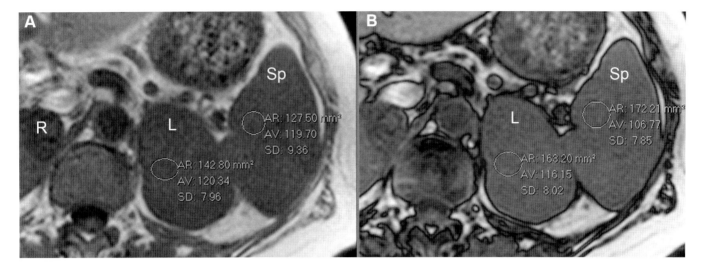

Figure 7.4 *Adrenal metastases.* Patient with history of melanoma has bilateral adrenal masses on MR. (**A**) Axial T1-weighted in-phase gradient-echo image shows right (*R*) and left (*L*) adrenal masses. A region of interest is drawn within the left adrenal mass and in the spleen (*Sp*). The average signal intensity (*AV*) for the left adrenal mass and for the spleen is 120. (**B**) Axial T1-weighted opposed-phase image shows regions of interest drawn in the left adrenal mass (*L*) and the spleen (*Sp*). If one visually compares the left adrenal masses between the in-phase and opposed-phase images, no significant decrease in signal can be appreciated. The average signal intensity (*AV*) for the adrenal lesion is 116 and for the spleen is 107. Signal intensity index was calculated to 8%, with criteria requiring a 25% decrease in signal; therefore, this left adrenal lesion is not consistent with a benign adrenal adenoma. This patient went on to have percutaneous left adrenal biopsy, which showed malignant melanoma at cytology. *AR*, area. *SD*, standard deviation.

which can be seen in metastasis; melanin, as seen in melanoma metastases; or macroscopic fat representing adipose tissue of a myelolipoma. The presence of macroscopic fat is excluded if the areas of increased T1-signal intensity fail to show a decrease in signal on fat-suppressed T1-weighted images. Increased signal intensity on T2-weighted images is a common but not specific finding in adrenal metastases. Contrast enhancement is likely to be homogenous in small (less than 2 cm) metastases, while larger ones may show heterogeneous enhancement with areas of necrosis or hemorrhage. Enhancement may be strong, as seen with melanoma metastases; patchy, as may be seen with hemorrhagic metastases; or absent in extensively necrotic metastases.

Importantly, the study should be compared to available prior imaging examinations to determine if the adrenal lesion is new. In the setting of a primary malignancy, a new adrenal lesion should be considered as a metastatic focus (Fig. 7.5). Biopsy may be needed to appropriately stage the patient's primary malignancy prior to definitive treatment. Growth of the lesion within 6 months is usually an indication of malignancy. Since solitary adrenal metastases are rare, a search for additional metastatic foci should be performed of all structures visualized on the MRI.

MR findings alone cannot definitely determine whether a mass in the adrenal gland is metastasis. However, in the setting of a primary extra-adrenal malignancy, a new adrenal lesion must be considered a metastatic focus until proven otherwise. Adrenal biopsy is safe, with a complication rate of 0% to 3%. Biopsy can be performed after appropriate evaluation to exclude pheochromocytoma. Biopsy of a pheochromocytoma may precipitate a hypertensive crisis. A positive diagnosis is definitive as to the nature of an adrenal mass. A negative biopsy showing no malignancy but not yielding a definite diagnosis may be due to sampling error. Negative biopsy rates range from 4% to 17%. When clinical suspicion of metastatic disease is high, an initial negative biopsy should be repeated.

Myelolipoma is one of the few adrenal lesions with a pathognomonic appearance on MR and CT. These are well-circumscribed benign adrenal lesions that consist of mature adipose tissue and hematopoietic (myeloid) elements in varying proportions, mimicking the appearance of bone marrow on microscopic examination.[5] An autopsy series found the prevalence of myelolipoma to be between 0.08% and 0.2%. These lesions are benign neoplasms that arise within the adrenal gland. They have no malignant potential and are hormonally inactive, although some are associated with adrenal cortical dysfunction. Non-hemorrhagic myelolipomas were reported to have a mean size of 10.4 cm in one series from the Armed Forces Institute of Pathology, but this size seems greater than is encountered in routine clinical practice.[7] Most tumors are

---

Box 7.3 **ESSENTIALS TO REMEMBER**

- In patients with a known extra-adrenal primary malignancy, an adrenal mass is likely to be metastatic in 50% of cases

- Once pheochromocytoma is excluded biochemically, biopsy may be required for definitive diagnosis and staging.

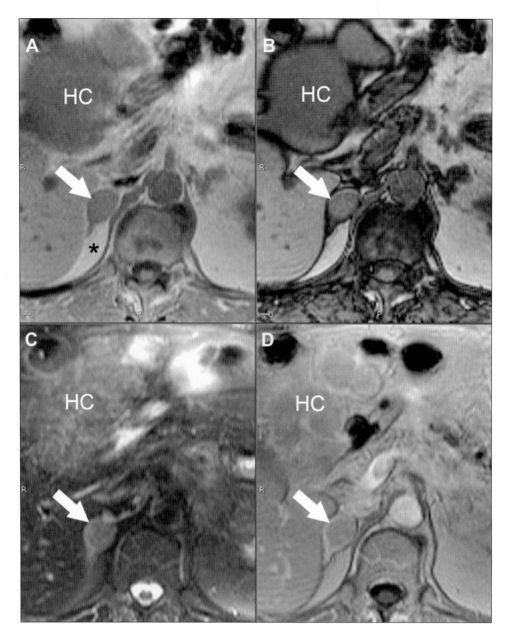

Figure 7.5 *Adrenal metastasis.* MR shows a right adrenal gland mass in a patient with hepatocellular carcinoma (*HC*). (**A**) Axial T1-weighted in-phase gradient-echo image shows a 2-cm right adrenal mass (*arrow*). The lesion is not high in signal like the background retroperitoneal fat (*), and thus the adrenal mass is not a myelolipoma. (**B**) Axial T1-weighted opposed-phase gradient-echo image shows no significant decrease in signal compared with the in-phase image; thus, the lesion (*arrow*) is not consistent with a lipid-rich adrenal adenoma. (**C**) Axial T2-weighted image with fat saturation shows the right adrenal lesion (*arrow*) displaying homogeneous high signal. (**D**) Axial T1-weighted gradient-echo image following gadolinium shows the lesion (*arrow*) to enhance homogeneously.

unilateral. Myelolipomas occur with equal frequency in men and women and are rare in patients younger than 30. Myelolipomas are almost always detected incidentally and are asymptomatic unless complicated by hemorrhage. Follow-up imaging may show interval growth.

MR imaging accurately detects macroscopic fat within an adrenal mass by use of T1- or T2-weighted fat-suppressed techniques (Fig. 7.6). A well-circumscribed focal mass originating within the adrenal substance with high signal on T1-weighted images with a drop in signal intensity on fat-saturated images confirms the diagnosis of myelolipoma. Myelolipomas contain varying amounts of mature fat and soft tissue hematopoietic elements. Some are made up entirely of

fat, while most contain soft tissue elements interspersed within the fat, giving the tumor a heterogeneous appearance. The soft tissue elements demonstrate intermediate signal intensity on T2-weighted images and will enhance following gadolinium contrast material administration. The appearance of interspersed soft tissue foci should not raise concern. It is the presence of macroscopic fat in any amount within the adrenal lesion that confirms the diagnosis of myelolipoma. When a myelolipoma contains no demonstrable fat, it is impossible to make a definitive diagnosis using MRI. One should not be confused when a fat-containing myelolipoma does not show a significant drop in signal on opposed-phase gradient-echo images. Since myelolipomas are predominantly made up of

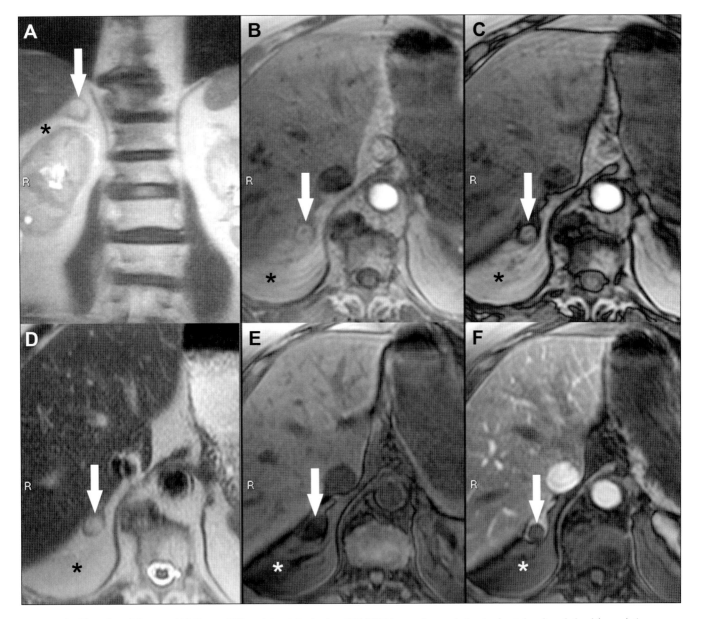

Figure 7.6 *Adrenal myelolipoma.* (**A**) Coronal T2-weighted single-shot FSE/TSE image shows a lesion in the right adrenal gland (*arrow*) that follows the same signal intensity as that of the surrounding retroperitoneal fat (*) on all sequences. Axial T1-weighted in-phase (**B**) and opposed-phase (**C**) gradient-echo images show no substantial decrease in signal. Thus, this lesion (*arrow*) is not a lipid-rich adrenal adenoma. (**D**) Axial T2-weighted single-shot FSE/TSE image shows that the right adrenal lesion (*arrow*) has signal intensity equal to that of fat. (**E**) Pre-gadolinium contrast-enhanced axial T1-weighted image with fat saturation applied shows the signal of the lesion (*arrow*) is decreased, similar to that of the surrounding retroperitoneal fat (*), indicating that the lesion predominantly consists of macroscopic (adipose) fat. (**F**) Post-gadolinium-contrast-enhanced axial T1-weighted image with fat saturation shows that the adrenal gland enhances but the central fat-containing myelolipoma (*arrow*) does not enhance because there are few soft tissue hematopoietic elements in the lesion.

adipose cells, there is little or no intracellular water or soft tissue component to cause significant loss in signal on opposed-phase images. 20% of myelolipomas contain calcification, but this is unlikely to be appreciated on MRI due to MRI's insensitivity to calcification detection.

To be certain that a lesion is an adrenal myelolipoma and not a retroperitoneal liposarcoma, the lesion must be seen to arise from the substance of the adrenal gland. A fatty neoplasm outside of the adrenal gland may represent a retroperitoneal lipoma or liposarcoma. A fatty lesion invading the adrenal is likely a liposarcoma. Assessment of sagittal and coronal images

in addition to axial images is particularly helpful for determining the origin of the lesion and its relationship with the adrenal gland. When the radiologist is uncertain whether the lesion is arising from or is adjacent to the adrenal gland, a differential diagnosis must be rendered and biopsy is needed for definitive diagnosis. The *differential diagnosis* includes exophytic angiomyolipoma from the adjacent kidney, retroperitoneal lipomas, and retroperitoneal liposarcoma.

Myelolipomas with internal hemorrhage will have a more complex appearance, making a definitive diagnosis more challenging. If characteristic signal of hemorrhage is detected

Box 7.4 **ESSENTIALS TO REMEMBER**

- Myelolipomas are well-circumscribed fat-containing masses with varying proportions of soft tissue hematopoietic elements and mature fat that arise within the adrenal gland.

- MR or CT demonstration of macroscopic fat (adipose tissue) within the adrenal lesion is pathognomonic of myelolipomas.

- Myelolipomas are benign masses with no malignant potential. They are "leave-alone" lesions in the absence of hemorrhagic complications.

superimposed upon a fatty adrenal lesion, a short-term follow-up examination (e.g., 3 months) will allow time for hemorrhage to resolve and reveal the underlying true fat signal of the adrenal mass.

Myelolipomas are benign, with no malignant potential. Recommendations are to "leave it alone," with no further imaging workup required. Pain from hemorrhagic myelolipomas should remit once the hemorrhage resolves. Recurrent hemorrhage may be an indication for surgical removal.[8]

Adrenal cysts are rare lesions. True cysts have a wall lined by cells, while ***pseudocysts*** do not. Most simple cysts are unilocular, fluid-containing structures with thin walls (Fig. 7.7). The spectrum of adrenal cysts can include large, heterogeneous masses with lobular contours, thick walls, and calcifications that can mimic the appearance of adrenal cortical carcinoma.[6] The origin of adrenal cystic lesions is varied, with most pseudo-cysts arising from prior traumatic hemorrhage. Rare true adrenal cysts have an endothelial or epithelial lining. Some are the result of hydatid disease. In a review of 41 cystic adrenal lesions from the Mayo Clinic, 78% were pseudo-cysts, 20% were endothelial cysts, and 2% were epithelial cysts. No parasitic cysts were reported.[7] In the Mayo review, most cystic adrenal lesions were symptomatic. Symptoms included pain, gastrointestinal distress, or a palpable mass. 17% of lesions were discovered incidentally. The mean age of patients was 50 years, with a nearly equal number of male and female patients. All cysts were unilateral, with mean cyst size of 9.3 cm.

Simple adrenal cysts arise within the adrenal gland and follow the signal of simple fluid on all sequences (signal similar to that of cerebrospinal fluid on T1- and T2-weighted images). They do not show central enhancement following gadolinium contrast material administration. A peripheral rim of enhancement is often detected, representing normal adrenal tissue compressed by the cyst capsule. Complex cystic lesions may show septa within the cyst that enhance. Hemorrhagic cysts and pseudo-cysts show MR features of hemorrhage with high signal on T1-weighted images, low signal intensity on T2-weighted images, and lack of enhancement following gadolinium contrast material administration (Fig. 7.8). Pseudo-cysts can show markedly heterogeneous signal and areas of enhancement or calcification (Fig. 7.9). Benign heterogeneous cysts overlap in appearance with cystic degeneration or necrosis seen in adrenal carcinomas or pheochromocytoma.

Pheochromocytomas and primary adrenal carcinomas may appear as predominantly cystic masses due to marked hemorrhage or degeneration. No specific imaging findings are known to separate a complicated benign adrenal cyst from a cystic pheochromocytoma or a cystic primary adrenal cortical carcinoma. Necrotic metastases may also appear cystic, but these lesions usually have a variable amount of enhancing soft tissue detectable within the lesion. Still, the Mayo review

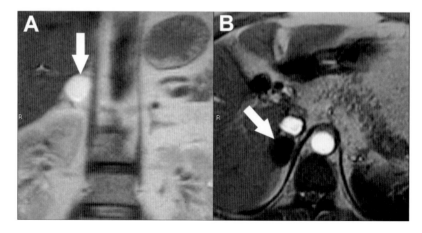

Figure 7.7 *Simple adrenal cyst.* (**A**) Coronal T2-weighted single-shot FSE/TSE image shows a lesion (*arrow*) in the right adrenal gland displaying high signal intensity, slightly higher than that of the retroperitoneal fat (*). (**B**) Axial T1-weighted gradient-echo image shows the lesion (*arrow*) is dark and is set off by the high-signal retroperitoneal fat. The lesion is not fat-containing, but rather displays the signal intensity of simple fluid on all sequences. The lesion did not enhance following intravenous admninstration of gadolinium-based contrast material (image not shown) confirming that the lesion was a simple cyst.

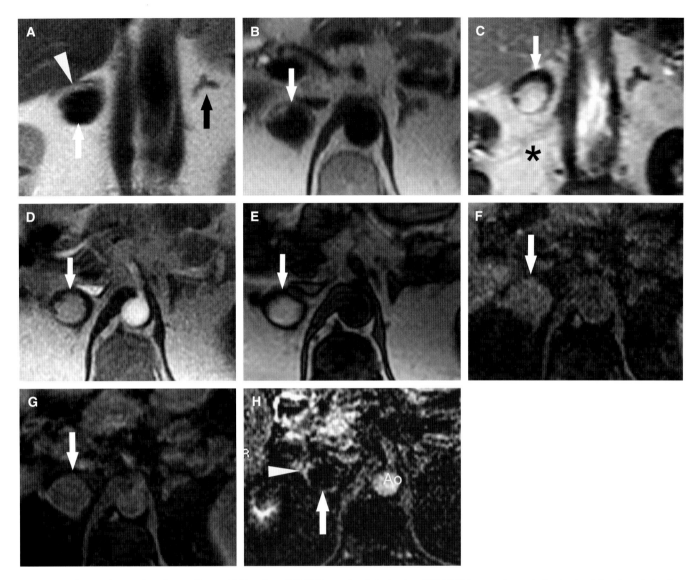

Figure 7.8 *Hemorrhagic adrenal cyst.* Coronal (**A**) and axial (**B**) T2-weighted single-shot FSE/TSE images show a lesion in the right adrenal gland (*white arrows*) with low, though not that of simple fluid, signal intensity. One adrenal limb is discernable (*arrowhead*). The left adrenal gland (*black arrow*) is normal. (**C**) Coronal T1-weighted gradient-echo image shows the right adrenal lesion (*arrow*) displaying high signal intensity similar to that of retroperitoneal fat (*). Axial T1-weighted in-phase (**D**) and (**E**) opposed-phase (**E**) gradient-echo images show no substantial decrease in signal within the lesion (*arrow*), indicating that this lesion is not a lipid-rich adrenal adenoma. (**F**) Pre-gadolinium contrast-enhanced axial T1-weighted image with fat saturation shows the lesion (*arrow*) with intermediate high signal. The signal does not saturate to black, indicating that the lesion does not contain macroscopic fat. (**G**) Post-gadolinium-contrast-enhanced axial T1-weighted image with fat saturation shows the lesion (*arrow*) with approximately the same signal intensity as that on the pre-contrast image (**F**), so subtle enhancement is difficult to detect. Therefore, post-processing was performed to create a subtraction image (**H**). Signal intensity on the post-contrast-enhanced image is mathematically subtracted from the pre-contrast-enhanced image. Areas that show true enhancement are high in signal on subtraction images. In this case the aorta (*Ao*) and the visible limb of the right adrenal gland (*arrowhead*) show enhancement. The non-enhancing adrenal lesion (*arrow*) is dark. The findings indicate a hemorrhagic adrenal cyst.

found two pheochromocytomas and two primary adrenal carcinomas that had imaging features of simple cysts but that were found to have neoplastic cells in the cyst wall at microscopic inspection. The differential diagnosis includes adrenal hemorrhage, cystic pheochromocytoma, necrotic primary adrenal carcinoma, and metastatic focus.

Simple adrenal cysts have no malignant potential and are hormonally inactive. All reported cystic pheochromocytomas were symptomatic, and one of the two cystic adrenal carcinomas was hormonally active. As with other adrenal lesions discovered incidentally, it is recommended to perform biochemical tests to exclude adrenal cortical dysfunction and pheochromocytoma. Follow-up imaging in 3 to 12 months is also recommended to ensure stability. Adrenal cortical hormonal hyperactivity or interval growth is an indication for surgical removal. The surgical literature suggests resection when the etiology of the lesion is uncertain, the lesion is larger than 5 cm, symptoms are present, and there is hormonal imbalance. Simple adrenal cysts less than 4 cm in size may be followed with imaging to confirm stability.

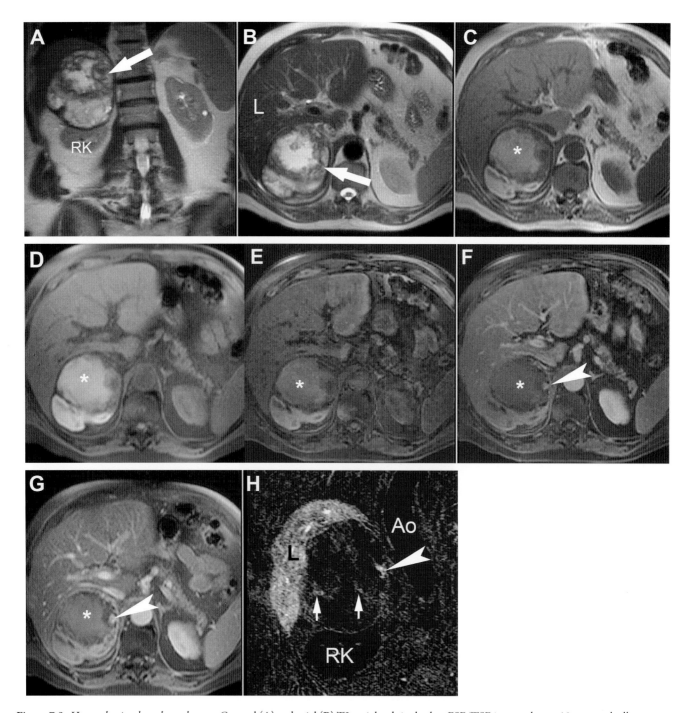

Figure 7.9 *Hemorrhagic adrenal pseudo-cyst.* Coronal (**A**) and axial (**B**) T2-weighted single-shot FSE/TSE images show a 10-cm, markedly heterogeneous lesion (*arrows*) in the right adrenal gland, displacing the right kidney (*RK*) inferiorly. The axial image shows mass effect on the liver (*L*). Axial T1-weighted images without (**C**) and with fat suppression (**D**) show that the high-signal areas (*) within the adrenal mass do not decrease in signal and therefore do not represent macroscopic fat. Pre-gadolinium, (**E**), early post-gadolinium-enhanced (**F**), and late post-gadolinium-enhanced (**G**) axial T1-weighted gradient-echo images with fat saturation show nodular enhancement (*arrowhead*) within the mass. The large central high-signal component (*) shows no significant enhancement. (**H**) A coronal subtraction image shows very little enhancement within most of the mass. However, nodular enhancement (*arrowhead*) and areas of linear enhancement (*short arrows*) are identified within the lesion. Because of its large size and enhancing components, adrenal cortical carcinoma was suspected. At surgery the lesion was proven to be an adrenal hemorrhagic pseudocyst, with no tumor identified. We can speculate that the enhancing areas were normal residual adrenal gland or organizing granulation tissue. *L*, liver. *RK*, right kidney. *Ao*, aorta.

Adrenal hematoma can result from traumatic and nontraumatic causes. Trauma is most common and the adrenal hematoma is often found in association with other abdominal parenchymal injuries found at the time of imaging workup for the trauma. Nontraumatic causes in adults are related to physiologic stressors (pregnancy, major surgery, burns, sepsis), bleeding diatheses and coagulopathy, hemorrhage occurring in preexisting adrenal neoplasms, and idiopathic. Posttraumatic adrenal hematoma is found in 2% of patients who undergo CT scanning for a traumatic event.[7]

Box 7.5 **ESSENTIALS TO REMEMBER**

- Simple adrenal cysts less than 4 cm in size can be observed. Microscopic deposits of tumor will be impossible to detect on imaging.

- Complex cysts and pseudocysts have varied etiologies, from benign post-hemorrhagic to cystic pheochromocytoma to malignant cystic adrenal carcinoma and cystic degeneration of metastatic disease. Imaging findings are not specific.

- Surgical literature recommends resection of non-simple cysts, simple cysts larger than 4 cm in size, and simple cysts that are symptomatic.

Adrenal MR is not indicated in the setting of acute trauma. A review of trauma-caused acute adrenal hematomas showed the lesions to be round or oval, well-defined masses averaging 2.8 cm and most often (77%) involving the right gland. Adrenal injuries are found with increasing frequency as the severity of the patient's other injuries increases. In non-trauma cases, most adrenal hematomas are detected incidentally since most patients are asymptomatic. Symptoms and signs associated with adrenal hemorrhage include abdominal pain, hypotension and anemia.

MR may be performed to further evaluate an adrenal mass that is suspected to represent hematoma (Fig. 7.10). Signal intensities of the hematoma vary depending on the age of the clot and show a predictable pattern of evolution to complete resolution with time.[8] In the early phase of the hematoma, there may be periadrenal soft tissue stranding seen as linear high signal around the adrenal gland on T2-weighted images. This stranding will enhance. The stranding in the perirenal space may make localization of the process to the adrenal gland problematic. Deviation of structures away from the adrenal hematoma is a good indication that the process arises in the adrenal gland. In the subacute phase, periadrenal edema resolves and signal intensity changes indicating methemoglobin become apparent. Over time, clot retraction becomes evident. The adrenal mass continues to decrease in size and often resolves completely. However, some hemorrhagic adrenal lesions will go on to form an adrenal pseudocyst. The signal intensities of post-hemorrhagic pseudocysts are quite variable. Calcifications in the pseudocyst may result in magnetic susceptibility artifact, further complicating the MR picture. Some pseudocysts show areas of enhancement from granulation tissue or capillary ingrowth into fibrotic tissue.[9]

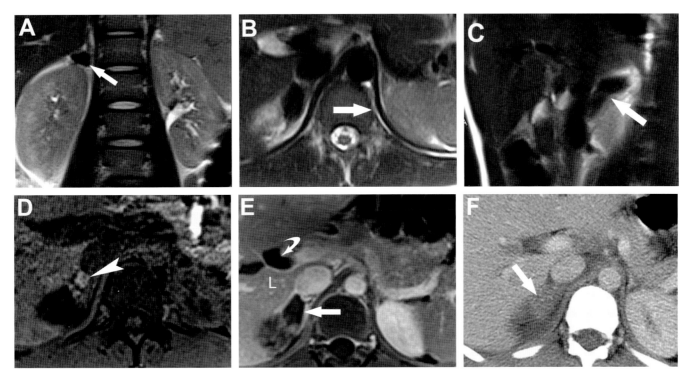

Figure 7.10 *Acute traumatic adrenal hemorrhage.* Coronal (**A**), axial (**B**), and sagittal (**C**) T2-weighted single-shot FSE/TSE images show a lesion in the right adrenal gland (*arrows*) with markedly low signal intensity consistent with intracellular methemoglobin, indicating previous adrenal hemorrhage. (**D**) Axial T1-weighted image with fat saturation shows the right adrenal hematoma to be heterogeneous, with foci of high signal (*arrowhead*) representing extracellular methemoglobin. (**E**) Post-gadolinium-contrast-enhanced axial T1-weighted gradient-echo image with fat saturation shows no enhancement within the adrenal hematoma (*arrow*). A low-signal laceration (*curved arrow*) is seen in the liver (*L*) on this same image. (**F**) Corresponding axial CT scan performed 1 day prior to the MR shows the adrenal hematoma (*arrow*).

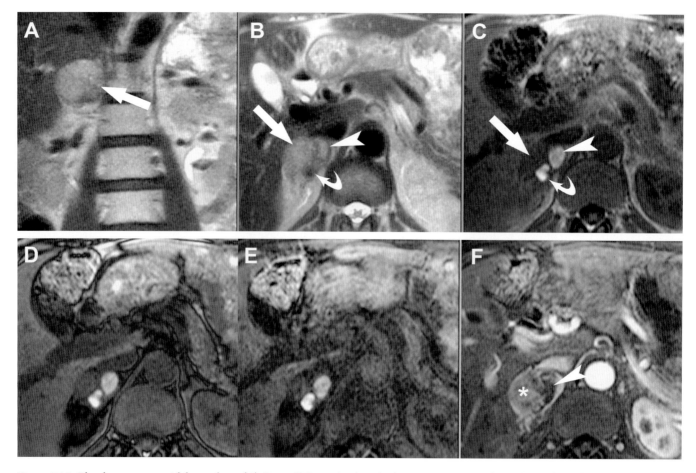

Figure 7.11 *Pheochromocytoma with hemorrhage.* (**A**) Coronal T2-weighted single-shot FSE/TSE image shows a lesion (*arrow*) displaying moderate signal intensity in the right adrenal gland. (**B**) Axial T2-weighted image obtained with same technique shows the same lesion (*arrow*) with a high-signal-intensity focus anteromedially (*arrowhead*) and a low-intensity focus posteromedially (*curved arrow*). (**C**) Axial T1-weighted in-phase gradient-echo image shows that the right adrenal lesion is now low in signal intensity (*arrow*) while the focal areas medially, one bright (*arrowhead*) and one dark (*curved arrow*) on the T2-weighted image, now both display high signal intensity. (**D**) Axial T1-weighted opposed-phase image shows these focal abnormalities do not decrease in signal compared with the in-phase images (i.e., they are not lipid-rich adrenal adenomas). (**E**) Pre-gadolinium-contrast enhanced axial T1-weighted gradient-echo image with fat saturation shows no change in the low-signal portion of the lesion or the focal high-signal areas medially. The absence of signal loss on fat-suppressed images indicates the absence of fat. (**F**) Early post-enhanced axial T1-weighted image with fat saturation obtained at a slightly different level within the lesion shows the large adrenal lesion (*) to enhance significantly while the anteromedial lesion (*arrowhead*) does not.

When dealing with an adrenal mass that has characteristics suggestive of adrenal hematoma it is important not to overlook an enhancing component that may indicate an underlying adrenal neoplasm that has undergone hemorrhage. Adrenal cortical carcinoma, pheochromocytoma, adrenal myelolipoma, adrenal adenoma, and metastases from bronchogenic carcinoma and melanoma may all undergo hemorrhage (Fig. 7.11). Most acute hemorrhagic lesions do not show areas of enhancement. If an adrenal hemorrhagic lesion does show areas of enhancement, close follow-up to ensure resolution should be performed. If the lesion does not completely resolve, adrenal biopsy or surgical resection should be considered.

It is important to be certain that the hemorrhagic mass is arising within the adrenal gland and not from some another structure, such as a ruptured hemorrhagic renal cyst or a renal angiomyolipoma. Hemorrhage within a retroperitoneal sarcoma adjacent to the adrenal gland may present with similar imaging findings. If the origin of the retroperitoneal hematoma is not certain, follow-up imaging is indicated to follow clot evolution or confirm resolution. With follow-up imaging, as the hematoma resolves, the organ from which it originated may become more apparent. The differential diagnosis includes adrenal hematoma, hematoma in a primary adrenal tumor, hematoma from metastatic disease, and juxta-adrenal hematoma (e.g., renal tumor, retroperitoneal sarcoma).

With an adrenal mass that has all the characteristics of adrenal hematoma (i.e., signal intensity features consistent with the various stages of blood breakdown and showing no enhancement following gadolinium contrast enhancement), follow-up imaging may be unnecessary. If adrenal hematoma is bilateral, adrenal insufficiency (Addisonian crisis) may occur if greater than 90% of the adrenal glands are destroyed. Addisonian crisis is life-threatening, requiring hospitalization of the patient and administration of adrenal hormone replacement therapy. When the cause of the adrenal hematoma is unclear, follow-up imaging is indicated to confirm resolution and/or reveal an underlying tumor as the origin.

Box 7.6 ESSENTIALS TO REMEMBER

- Adrenal hematoma is found in 2% of abdominal trauma CTs. Additional parenchymal injuries are usually present.

- Nontraumatic causes of adrenal hematoma include physiologic stress, coagulopathy and bleeding diatheses, and hemorrhage in an underlying adrenal neoplasm. Some cases are idiopathic.

- Because of the characteristic features of hematoma on MR the modality can be effectively used to clarify whether an adrenal mass is caused by hematoma or is a true neoplasm.

- Most adrenal hematomas will resolve with time, although some will form chronic adrenal pseudocysts.

Adrenal carcinoma is a very rare malignancy of the adrenal cortex (incidence of 1 to 2 per 1,000,000 persons). The tumors are often difficult to differentiate from normal adrenal cortical tissue by microscopic inspection alone. The biological behavior of the tumor must be taken into account to determine its true nature and the prognosis for the patient. A large tumor that shows adrenal cortical cells on pathologic examination and demonstrates invasion of the adrenal vein or inferior vena cava will be classified as an adrenal cortical carcinoma primarily based on its biological behavior. The corollary is that a tumor showing adrenal cortical cells on microscopic inspection that is small, round, and well circumscribed will be categorized as an adrenal cortical neoplasm, requiring clinical and imaging follow-up to determine its true nature.

Adrenal cortical carcinomas show a bimodal distribution, with one peak in childhood and another in the fourth to fifth decade. The mean age of diagnosis is 40 to 70 years. Women are affected 1.5 times more commonly than men. Symptoms are related to excessive adrenal cortical hormone production (60% of patients) or to pain from mass effect. Excess hormone secretion most often results in Cushing's syndrome. Other adrenal cortical hormones cause hypertension, virilization in females, or feminization in males. Most tumors are large (7 to 17 cm).

Size and tumor behavior are important indictors of the nature of the adrenal mass (Fig. 7.12). Adrenal lesions larger than 6 cm in size are likely adrenal carcinoma and are considered for surgical removal. Adrenal cortical carcinomas are aggressive tumors that invade adjacent structures, including the adrenal vein, the inferior vena cava, and adjacent retroperitoneal structures. Signal characteristics on MR are not particularly specific. Most tumors are iso-intense to liver on T1-weighted images and show heterogeneous, intermediate signal intensity on T2-weighted images. Variable enhancement is seen on post-gadolinium contrast-enchanced imaging. Large tumors appear heterogeneous because of hemorrhage or outgrowth of their blood supply, leading to necrosis.

It is important to note that although they are rare, primary adrenal carcinomas can present as entirely cystic lesions. Further, they can also contain enough lipid to show signal drop on opposed-phase T1-weighted gradient-echo images. Size and behavior trump other imaging characteristics. Other large retroperitoneal masses, such as exophytic renal carcinomas and retroperitoneal sarcomas, should be considered in the differential diagnosis. Assessment of the tumor in the sagittal and coronal orientation is important in determining the tumor's origin. Look for vascular invasion into the adrenal and renal veins and the inferior vena cava. Evidence of adjacent organ and bone invasion should be carefully evaluated.

The differential diagnosis includes retroperitoneal sarcoma, adrenal hemorrhage, retroperitoneal lymphadenopathy or lymphoma, pheochromocytoma, metastasis, and chronic organizing adrenal pseudocyst.

There are case reports of adrenal carcinoma being found in the walls of otherwise simple adrenal cysts. The tumor deposits were not identifiable on imaging. There are also case reports of adrenal carcinomas containing sufficient lipid to be detected on CT and MR, mimicking lipid-rich adrenal adenomas.

For any chance for cure, surgical resection of the large adrenal mass is undertaken. Pheochromocytoma should be excluded prior to surgery. The mean survival for patients with primary adrenal carcinoma is 2 years for those who undergo complete surgical resection. With resection of the

Box 7.7 ESSENTIALS TO REMEMBER

- Size matters with adrenal tumors. Those larger than 6 cm in size should be considered as possible primary adrenal carcinoma.

- Recommendation is for surgical removal of adrenal tumors of 6 cm or larger.

- Size and aggressive behavior are paramount in making the diagnosis.

- Signal characteristics and enhancement are quite variable, and both lipid- and fluid-containing lesions should not dissuade the radiologist from making the diagnosis of primary adrenal carcinoma when the tumor is large or displays aggressive behavior.

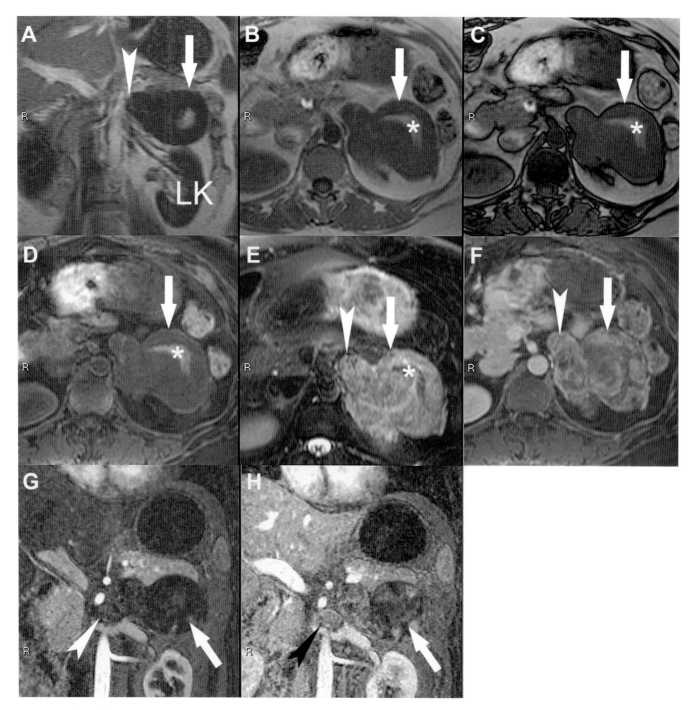

Figure 7.12 *Adrenal carcinoma.* (**A**) Coronal T1-weighted gradient-echo image shows a large low-signal intensity left adrenal mass (*arrow*) displacing the left kidney (*LK*) inferiorly. Tumor extending towards the midline (*arrowhead*) represents tumor invasion into the left renal vein. (**B**) Axial T1-weighted in-phase image shows the left adrenal lesion (*arrow*) with central high signal (*) representing hematoma. (**C**) Axial T1-weighted opposed-phase image shows no decrease in lesion signal (*arrow*) when compared with the in-phase images, indicating that the lesion does not contain intracellular lipid. The central high signal (*) area representing hematoma does not change. (**D**) Axial T1-weighted image with fat saturation shows no signal change in the lesion (*arrow*) or in the area (*) with high signal intensity, indicating absence of adipose tissue. (**E**) Axial T2-weighted FSE/TSE image with fat saturation shows the lesion (*arrow*) with markedly increased signal. The area (*) of the lesion that was bright on the T1-weighted image is now dark on the T2-weighted image, consistent with hematoma. Note the tumor shows extension towards midline (*arrowhead*) as it invades the left renal vein. (**F**) Axial post-gadolinium-enhanced axial T1-weighted image with fat saturation shows heterogeneous enhancement of the tumor (*arrow*) and the tumor thrombus in the left renal vein (*arrowhead*). Early (**G**) and late (**H**) post-gadolinium-contrast-enhanced images in the coronal plane using 3D T1-weighted gradient-echo imaging with fat saturation shows the tumor (*arrows*) and the tumor thrombus (*white arrowhead*) in the left renal vein. Note enhancement of the tumor thrombus (*black arrowhead*) on the delayed contrast-enhanced image.

primary tumor, signs and symptoms related to the excessive production of adrenal cortical hormones should also abate. Patients with incomplete tumor resection have a much shorter survival.

Adrenal hyperplasia is enlargement of one or both of the adrenal glands while maintaining the normal adreniform shape. Hyperplasia can be diffuse, involving the entire gland or both glands uniformly, or can present as one or more discernible nodules. Multinodular adenomatous hyperplasia is uncommon.[10] Adrenal hyperplasia occurs almost always in response to excess levels of adrenocorticotropic hormone (ACTH) derived from either a pituitary adenoma (Cushing's disease) or an ACTH-producing tumor. ACTH stimulates the adrenal glands to become hyperplastic and to produce excess levels of cortisol, leading to Cushing's syndrome.[11]

In Cushing's syndrome, hypercortisolism results in hypertension, centripetal obesity, poor wound healing, impaired immune responses, osteoporosis, mood changes, and a myriad of other signs and symptoms. Some patients present with diffuse adrenal enlargement on imaging studies as the first indication of hormonal imbalance. Non-ACTH-dependent cases of hypercortisolism result from hyperfunctioning adrenal adenoma or adrenal carcinoma.

Hyperplasia appears as a diffusely enlarged adrenal gland that maintains its overall adrenal shape (Fig. 7.13). It may be unilateral or bilateral. The signal intensity of the adrenal glands will be normal on T1- and T2-weighted images. If there is a high lipid content within the enlarged adrenal gland, opposed-phase imaging will show visibly decreased signal compared with in-phase T1-weighted images.[12]

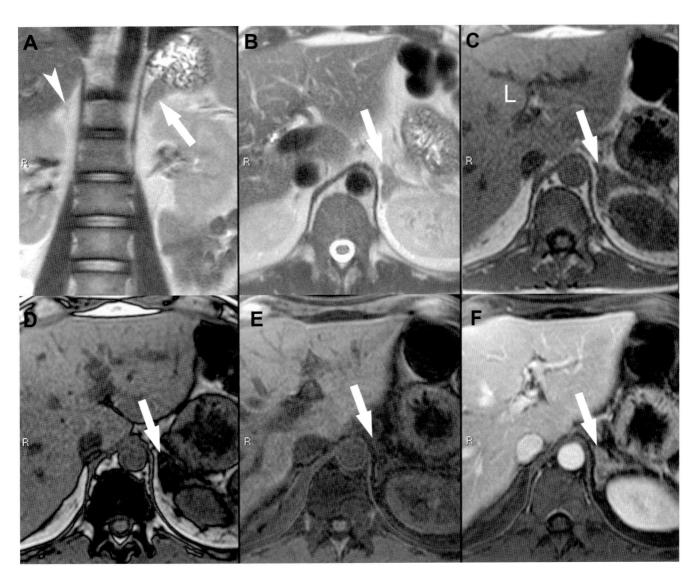

Figure 7.13 *Adrenal hyperplasia.* (**A**) Coronal and (**B**) T2-weighted single-shot FSE/TSE images show a lesion displaying intermediate signal in the left adrenal gland (*arrow*) having the same signal as that of the normal right adrenal gland (*arrowhead*). The images show the enlarged left adrenal gland (*arrow*) that otherwise maintains its normal shape. (**C**) Axial T1-weighted in-phase gradient-echo image shows that the right adrenal lesion (*arrow*) is iso-intense to liver (*L*). (**D**) Axial T1-weighted opposed-phase image shows decrease in signal, indicating a high intracellular lipid content within the enlarged left adrenal gland (*arrow*). The finding is consistent with functioning adrenal tissue and adenomatous hyperplasia. (**E**) Pre-gadolinium contrast-enhanced axial T1-weighted gradient-echo image with fat saturation shows that the adrenal gland is less conspicuous due to loss of signal from surrounding fat. (**F**) Post-gadolinium-enhanced axial T1-weighted image with fat saturation shows normal enhancement in the enlarged left adrenal gland (*arrow*).

Hyperplasia is uniform enlargement with no focal mass seen. If a focal adrenal mass is seen, this mass should be assessed as any other adrenal mass would be assessed. This includes imaging to characterize the lesion and an endocrine workup as recommended by the National Institutes of Health consensus statement on adrenal incidentalomas.[1] The *differential diagnosis* includes nonfunctioning adrenal adenoma, adrenal metastasis, adrenal carcinoma, pheochromocytoma, and adrenal pseudo-cyst.

Macronodular adrenal hyperplasia is a variant of hyperplasia found in the minority of cases with hypercortisolism not related to the ACTH pathway. The nodules within the adrenal gland are multiple and generally less than 3 cm in size.

Treatment of Cushing's disease is directed at resection of the pituitary adenoma, with return of adrenal function to normal once the ACTH overstimulation is removed. Functioning adrenal adenomas require localization with imaging since surgical removal is indicated to return the patient to hormonal balance. Once an adrenal mass is localized, adrenal vein sampling is performed to ensure the identified nodule is responsible for the hormone excess. Surgical removal of the hyperfunctioning adrenal nodule will restore hormonal balance. In the setting of bilateral adrenal hyperplasia in the absence of a ACTH-producing pituitary tumor, medical therapy is directed at blocking formation of cortisol.

Pheochromocytoma is a neoplasm of the adrenal medulla derived from the chromaffin cells of neural crest origin, a component of the sympathetic nervous system. Pheochromocytomas produce an excess of the catecholamines epinephrine and norepinephrine. Catecholamine-producing tumors of the sympathetic nervous system outside of the adrenal gland are defined as paragangliomas. Pheochromocytoma is found most commonly in the fourth to fifth decades, with an equal frequency in men and women.

The "rule of 10s" has traditionally been used to list important epidemiology factors: 10% are bilateral, 10% are extra-adrenal paragangliomas, 10% are familial, and 10% are malignant. However, new genetic information on pheochromocytoma has made the rule of 10s much less cogent: up to 30% of pheochromocytomas have now been associated with genetic defects. The malignancy rate depends on the presence of a specific genetic defect in a tumor-suppressor gene.

Overproduction of catecholamines results in sustained or paroxysmal hypertension or hypertensive crisis associated with diaphoresis, palpitations, and headaches. It is important to note that some pheochromocytomas will be subclinical. Nonetheless, during tumor manipulation at biopsy, with induction of general anesthesia, or a host of other stimuli, the unsuspected pheochromocytoma may put out large quantities of catecholamines, resulting in a hypertensive crisis and its attendant morbidity.

Pheochromocytomas have a "classic" appearance in 65% of cases, appearing as an adrenal mass showing iso-intense signal on T1-weighted images, high signal described as "light bulb" bright on T2-weighted images, and intense enhancement following gadolinium contrast material administration (Fig. 7.14). Hemorrhage and necrosis result in variable signal intensity on T1- and T2-weighted images and less-than-intense enhancement following gadolinium administration (see Fig. 7.11). Cystic pheochromocytomas have been reported (Fig. 7.15).

Pheochromocytoma must be considered in the differential diagnosis of any adrenal mass. With clinical suspicion of pheochromocytoma, the adrenal glands should be evaluated first, since 90% of pheochromocytomas are found within one of the adrenal glands. If the adrenal glands are entirely normal, the examination should include imaging of the abdomen and pelvis, including the organ of Zuckerkandl at the level of the inferior mesenteric artery, and the bladder. Close attention to the paraspinal regions is necessary to detect extra-adrenal paragangliomas, since 98% of these tumors are found along these regions in the abdomen. In the setting of strong clinical evidence of pheochromocytoma, even a small adrenal nodule may represent the pheochromocytoma. Also, keep in mind that 10% are bilateral, so don't get trapped into "satisfaction of search" when one adrenal mass is found.

Biochemical testing is not 100% sensitive for the detection of pheochromocytomas. This should be kept in mind when imaging is consistent with pheochromocytoma but the patient is asymptomatic. MR imaging is 90% to 100% sensitive for the detection of pheochromocytoma but has limited specificity (as low as 50%). Radionuclide imaging with metaiodobenzylguanidine (MIBG) may be indicated in equivocal cases. MIBG is a precursor in the synthesis of norepinephrine taken up in the catecholamine-producing tissue. Specificity of MIBG imaging approaches 100%. Anesthesia or tumor manipulation may cause a paroxysm of hypertension. Preprocedure adrenergic blocking is therefore recommended.

Box 7.8 ESSENTIALS TO REMEMBER

- Cushing's syndrome is a clinical diagnosis.

- Adrenal hyperplasia presents as bilaterally or asymmetrically enlarged adrenal glands that maintain their adreniform shape.

- Most cases are related to ACTH-secreting pituitary adenoma (Cushing's disease).

- Treatment of Cushing's syndrome varies: surgical removal for the pituitary adenoma that causes Cushing's disease, and adrenalectomy for an autonomously functioning adrenal adenoma.

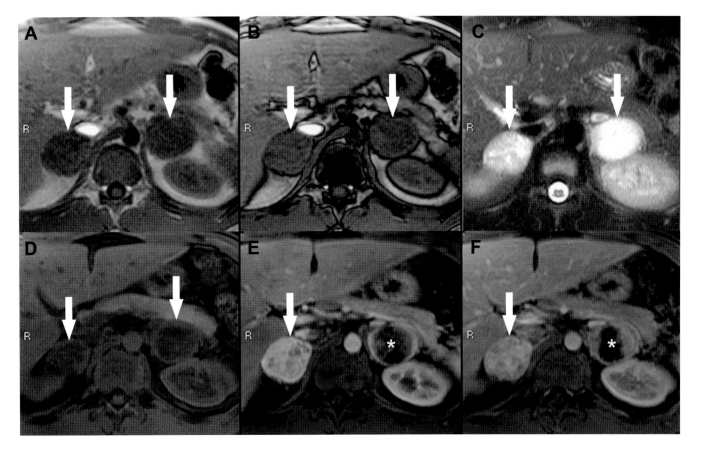

Figure 7.14 *Bilateral pheochromocytomas.* 17-year-old boy with von Hippel-Lindau disease and hypertension. (**A**) Axial T1-weighted in-phase image shows bilateral low-signal-intensity adrenal masses (*arrows*). (**B**) Axial T1-weighted opposed-phase image shows no decrease in signal in either of the adrenal masses (*arrows*) and, therefore, there is no evidence of significant intracytoplasmic lipid. Thus, these are not lipid-rich adrenal adenomas. (**C**) Axial T2-weighted single-shot FSE/TSE image with fat saturation shows intensely high signal in both adrenal masses (*arrows*). (**D**) Pre-gadolinium contrast-enhanced axial T1-weighted image with fat saturation applied shows bilateral low-signal intensity adrenal masses (*arrows*). Immediate (**E**) and late (**F**) post-gadolinium-enhanced axial T1-weighted images with fat saturation show intense enhancement in the right adrenal mass (*arrow*), but the left adrenal mass enhances poorly centrally (*) because of central necrosis.

Lymphoma. It is extremely rare for primary lymphoma to involve the adrenal gland. Primary adrenal lymphoma is a B-cell-origin lymphoma that diffusely infiltrates the gland.[13] Primary adrenal lymphoma affects men twice as often as women at a mean age of 65 years. It is much more common for a retroperitoneal non-Hodgkin's lymphoma to invade the adrenal gland.

Replacement of the adrenal glands by lymphoma may present as adrenal insufficiency. Patients may manifest classic symptoms of lymphoma, including fever of unknown origin, soaking night sweats, weight loss, unexplained pruritus, or alcohol-induced pain at the sites of disease. Generalized lymphadenopathy may be present on physical examination.

Box 7.9 ESSENTIALS TO REMEMBER

- Pheochromocytoma is a neoplasm of the catecholamine-producing adrenal medulla.

- The classic clinical triad is that of headaches, palpitations, and diaphoresis in a patient with hypertension.

- Classic imaging features of the lesion on MR images found in 65% of patients are iso-intense signal on T1-weighted images, high signal on T2-weighted images, and intense enhancement following intravenous administration of gadolinium contrast material.

- Non-classic imaging features of pheochromocytoma include findings of hemorrhage, necrosis, and weak contrast enhancement.

- Prior to surgical removal or biopsy of adrenal masses that may be pheochromocytomas, the patient should undergo adrenergic blockage to prevent a hypertensive crisis.

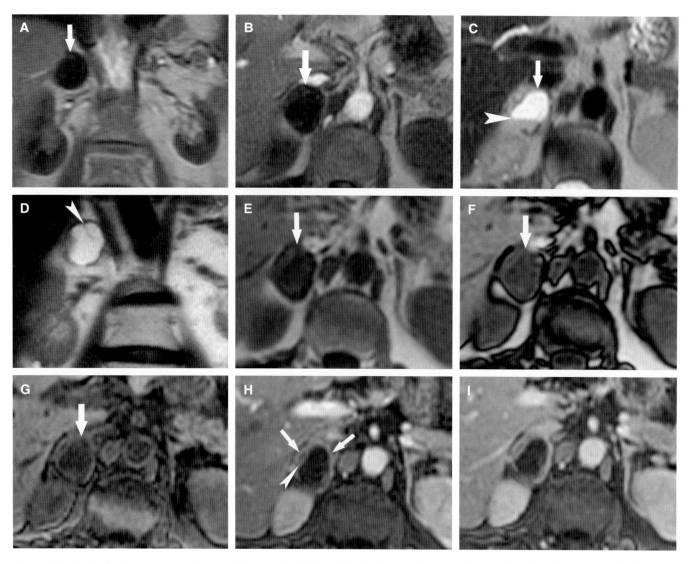

Figure 7.15 *Cystic pheochromocytoma.* Coronal (**A**) and axial (**B**) T1-weighted gradient-echo images show a right adrenal lesion (*arrow*) displaying low in signal intensity, similar to fluid. (**C**) Axial and (**D**) coronal T2-weighted single-shot FSE/TSE image shows high signal intensity of simple fluid in the right adrenal gland (*arrow*). A fluid–fluid level (*arrowhead*) is seen in **C** representing layering debris within the cystic lesion. Coronal image shows a low-signal septum (*arrowhead*) in the cyst. Axial T1-weighted in-phase (**E**) and opposed-phase (**F**) gradient-echo images show no substantial decrease in signal in the cyst (*arrow*). Pre-gadolinium (**G**) and early post-gadolinium-contrast-enhanced (**H**) axial T1-weighted gradient-cho with fat saturation show enhancement of the adrenal limbs (*arrows*) and the septum (*arrowhead* in image H) but not the remainder of the lesion, confirming cyst fluid. (**I**) Late post-gadolinium-contrast-enhanced image shows no additional enhancing elements.

Bilateral adrenal masses are the most commonly reported presentation (80% of cases) in primary adrenal lymphoma. The affected adrenal glands will be enlarged and diffusely infiltrated (Fig. 7.16). They are lower in signal on T1-weighted images and higher in signal on T2-weighted images, compared with the signal of the normal gland. Lymphoma does not cause a drop in signal on opposed-phase sequences because they contain no fat. Enhancement is variable but usually heterogeneous.[14] MRI and CT are equally accurate in the detection of lymph nodes and tumor infiltration into parenchymal organs. Retroperitoneal lymphadenopathy appears as a mass that is separate from the adrenal gland, either with mass effect upon the gland or with invasion of the adrenal gland. The differential diagnosis includes tumor extension from another retroperitoneal neoplasm, retroperitoneal

hemorrhage, adrenal infection (granulomatous), adrenal hyperplasia, and sequelae of pancreatitis. Benign lymphadenopathy from inflammatory disease diminishes over time as the inciting inflammatory process resolves. Follow-up imaging confirms resolution.

Biopsy of an adrenal mass thought to represent lymphoma is as safe as most other percutaneous image-guided abdominal biopsies. Once pheochromocytoma is excluded, fine-needle aspiration may be performed for flow cytometry to aid in the diagnosis of a population of monomorphic lymphocytes. Core biopsy may be required when cytologic sampling is inadequate or when there is need for immunohistochemical stains to determine the definitive type of tumor. Lymphadenopathy in other locations may be found with diffuse metastatic disease or widespread non-Hodgkin's lymphoma.

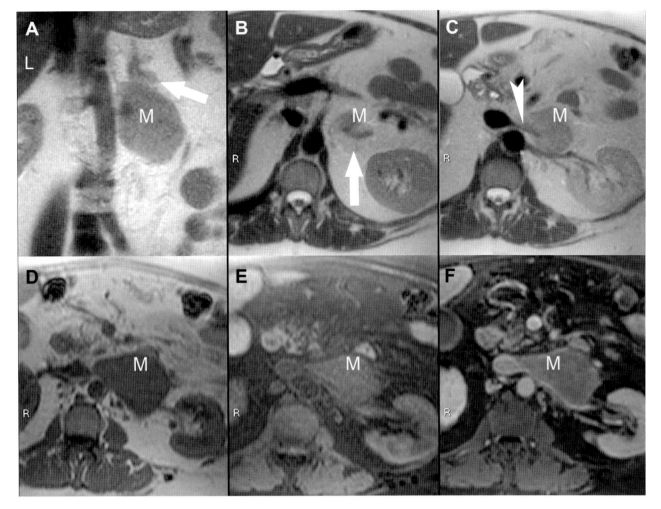

Figure 7.16 *Lymphoma invading the adrenal gland.* (**A**) Coronal and (**B, C**) axial T2-weighted single-shot images shows a left retroperitoneal mass (*M*) to be slightly higher in signal than the liver (*L*). The mass is invading the undersurface of the left adrenal gland (*arrow*). Axial image shows the mass (*M*) invading the left adrenal gland (*arrow*). On axial image A obtained at a more caudal level than B the bulk of the mass (*M*) is seen arising in the left retroperitoneum and engulfing the left renal vessels (*arrowhead*). (**D**) Axial T1-weighted in-phase gradient-echo image at a more caudal level than image C shows that the lesion (*M*) displays low signal intensity and has no fat in it. (**E**) Axial T1-weighted image with fat saturation shows that the mass (*M*) is relatively homogeneous and without macroscopic fat content. (**F**) Post-gadolinium-contrast-enhanced axial T1-weighted image with fat saturation shows minimal enhancement of the mass (*M*). A homogeneous mass with minimal enhancement is typical of lymphoma.

RETROPERITONEUM

Most primary retroperitoneal malignant tumors are tumors of the sarcoma line (liposarcoma, fibrosarcoma, angiosarcoma). These tumors are rare, with approximately 1,400 cases diagnosed in the United States in 2007. Most patients present with an abdominal mass or with abdominal pain as their chief complaint. Many tumors are clinically silent. When diagnosed, the tumors are often quite large (more than 10 cm). About 11% of cases will already have metastatic disease when first discovered.

Box 7.10 **ESSENTIALS TO REMEMBER**

- Primary adrenal lymphoma is extremely rare.

- Primary adrenal lymphoma is most commonly bilateral.

- Much more common is contiguous spread of non-Hodgkin's lymphoma from the peri-aortic region to the adrenal gland.

- Lymphadenopathy in other areas may be an important clue to the diagnosis of lymphoma involving the adrenal gland when an enlarged adrenal gland is found at imaging.

- Fine-needle aspiration biopsy with flow cytometry is safe and efficacious for the diagnosis of adrenal lymphoma.

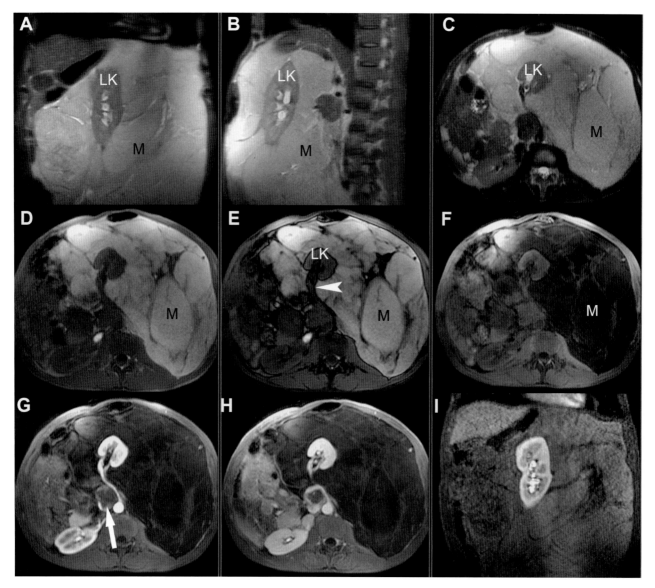

Figure 7.17 *Retroperitoneal liposarcoma.* Coronal (**A**), sagittal (**B**), and axial (**C**) T2-weighted single-shot FSE/TSE images show the left kidney (*LK*) displaced anteriorly and surrounded by a very large retroperitoneal high-signal intensity mass (*M*). (**D**) Axial T1-weighted in-phase gradient-echo image shows that the large mass (*M*) displays high signal intensity . (**E**) Axial opposed-phase image shows no decrease in signal compared with the in-phase image, indicating that the mass (*M*) does not have significant intracytoplasmic lipid. It is clear that the mass is retroperitoneal because it is deviating the retroperitoneal structures, including the left kidney (*LK*), anteriorly. The left kidney's vascular pedicle is stretched (*arrowhead*). (**F**) Pre-enhanced axial T1-weighted image with fat saturation shows that the high-signal intensity mass (*M*) decreases significantly in signal intensity, confirming that this mass consists of adipose tissue. (**G**) Early post-gadolinium-contrast-enhanced axial T1-weighted image with fat saturation shows enhancement of the arterial structures and both kidneys. The left renal artery is deviated around a right para-aortic nodal mass (*arrow*), indicative of metastatic spread of a malignant tumor. Findings are most indicative of retroperitoneal liposarcoma. (**H**) Late contrast-enhanced axial T1-weighted image with fat saturation shows no significant enhancement within the fatty mass. Central low-signal necrosis is evident in the right para-aortic lymph node. (**I**) Late contrast-enhanced coronal T1-weighted image with fat saturation shows the mass enveloping the left kidney as excreted contrast material is filling its collecting system.

Box 7.11 ESSENTIALS TO REMEMBER

- Retroperitoneal sarcoma is a rare tumor but is the most common primary soft tissue malignancy of the retroperitoneum.

- Tumors are usually larger than 10 cm at diagnosis.

- Tumors with aggressive histology have a 33-month median survival.

- Surgery performed by a qualified sarcoma surgeon is diagnostic and is the therapeutic option of choice. Pre-operative biopsy is often not performed because the variable histolology of many large sarcomas may result in sampling error.

The mean age of diagnosis is 50 years, with men slightly more often affected than women. Liposarcoma and leiomyosarcoma are the most common. Median survival is 33 months in high-grade aggressive tumors and 149 months in low-grade sarcomas. Complete resection of retroperitoneal sarcomas is often limited by the proximity of vital structures to the large tumor. Local tumor recurrence is common due to incomplete resection.[15]

The approach to the diagnosis of a retroperitoneal tumor is first to exclude the adrenal, kidney, pancreas, and gastrointestinal tract as the origin of the tumor. A primary retroperitoneal sarcoma is then the next most likely diagnosis (Fig. 7.17). Some tumors are more easily diagnosed by the presence of fat components, as seen with liposarcoma. Often the tumor is a nonspecific retroperitoneal mass. If the mass appears to arise from a vascular structure, angiosarcoma is highly likely.

Invasion of or close proximity to vital structures is important for determining the feasibility of complete surgical resection. With surveillance imaging following definitive surgical therapy, a change in the tumor characteristics, such as absence of fat in a liposarcoma, may indicate dedifferentiation of the tumor into a more primitive and more aggressive type. The *differential diagnosis* includes retroperitoneal lymphoma, retroperitoneal hemorrhage, retroperitoneal fibrosis, neurogenic mass, vascular aneurysm, pancreatic tumor or pancreatitis, metastatic disease, gastrointestinal stromal tumor, and retroperitoneal cyst or lymphangioma.

Definitive treatment of sarcoma includes *en bloc* tumor resection for both staging and treatment. Biopsy is sometimes not performed since sarcoma resection will be done by a qualified sarcoma surgeon who will be following appropriate staging and containment procedures during the surgery. Prognosis is linked to the success of complete tumor resection. An aggressive surgical approach is favored.

REFERENCES

1. Grumbach MM, Biller BM, Braunstein GD, et al. Management of the clinically inapparent adrenal mass ("incidentaloma"). *Ann Intern Med.* 2003; 138:424–429.
2. Erickson LA, Lloyd RV, Hartman R, Thompson G. Cystic adrenal neoplasms. *Cancer.* 2004;101:1537–1544.
3. Boland GW, Blake MA, Hahn PF, Mayo-Smith WW. Incidental adrenal lesions: principles, techniques, and algorithms for imaging characterization. *Radiology.* 2008;249:756–775.
4. Gross MD, Korobkin M, Bou Assaly W, et al. Contemporary imaging of incidentally discovered adrenal masses. *Nature Rev Urol.* 2009;6:363–373.
5. Olobatuyi FA, Maclennan GT. Myelolipoma. *J Urol.* 2006;176:1188.
6. Nigawara T, Sakihara S, Kageyama K, et al. Endothelial cyst of the adrenal gland associated with adrenocortical adenoma: preoperative images simulate carcinoma. *Intern Med.* 2009; 48:235–240.
7. Rana AI, Kenney PJ, Lockhart ME, et al. Adrenal gland hematomas in trauma patients. *Radiology.* 2004;230:669–675.
8. Kawashima A, Sandler CM, Ernst RD, et al. Imaging of nontraumatic hemorrhage of the adrenal gland. *Radiographics.* 1999;19:949–963.
9. Ishigami K, Stolpen AH, Sato Y, et al. Adrenal adenoma with organizing hematoma: diagnostic dilemma at MRI. *Magn Reson Imaging.* 2004;22:1157–1159.
10. Doppman JL, Miller DL, Dwyer AJ, et al. Macronodular adrenal hyperplasia in Cushing disease. *Radiology.* 1988;166:347–352.
11. Robbins SL, Kumar V, Cotran RS. *Robbins and Cotran Pathologic Basis of Disease,* 8th ed. Philadelphia: Saunders/Elsevier, 2010:1450.
12. Elsayes KM, Mukundan G, Narra VR, et al. Adrenal masses: MR imaging features with pathologic correlation. *Radiographics.* 2004;24:S73–86.
13. Zhang LJ, Yang GF, Shen W, Qi J. Imaging of primary adrenal lymphoma: case report and literature review. *Acta Radiol.* 2006;47:993–997.
14. Lee FT, Jr, Thornbury JR, Grist TM, Kelcz F. MR imaging of adrenal lymphoma. *Abdom Imaging.* 1993;18:95–96.
15. Hueman MT, Herman JM, Ahuja N. Management of retroperitoneal sarcomas. *Surg Clin North Am.* 2008;88:583–597.

8.

GASTROINTESTINAL TRACT, PERITONEAL CAVITY, AND SPLEEN MR IMAGING

William E. Brant, MD, FACR and Drew L. Lambert, MD

GASTROINTESTINAL TRACT

MR imaging of the gastrointestinal (GI) tract is fraught with difficulties. Besides the breathing motion that plagues abdominal MR imaging generally, bowel peristalsis is a significant obstacle. Adequate distention of the gut is required to fully evaluate the luminal gastrointestinal tract, a concern not isolated to MR. However, as MR imaging techniques have advanced, so has its ability to capture diagnostic images of the bowel. For imaging the bowel MR offers the advantages of superior tissue characterization, multiplanar imaging, and lack of use of ionizing radiation. Applications of MR imaging the GI tract include determining the presence and severity of inflammatory bowel disease; preoperative staging and post-treatment assessment of malignant neoplasms; detection of peritoneal abscesses and enteric fistulas; diagnosis of appendicitis, especially in pregnant women and children; and, increasingly, colorectal cancer screening. This chapter is devoted to MR imaging of the gastrointestinal tract, peritoneal cavity, and spleen.

MR TECHNIQUES

Basic sequences commonly used to image the bowel include breath-hold T2-weighted single-shot fast/turbo spin-echo (FSE/TSE) with half-Fourier acquisition and gadolinium contrast-enhanced fat-suppressed T1-weighted gradient-echo. Single-shot FSE/TSE imaging is sensitive to intraluminal fluid and is relatively resistant to susceptibility effects of intraluminal air. Rapid steady state free precession (SSFP) gradient-echo techniques in which the image contrast depends on both the T1 and T2 relaxation times provide single breath-hold sharp motion-free images of the fluid-filled bowel.

An important aspect of MR imaging of the GI tract is the use of enteric contrast agents. Enteric contrast material makes the lumen of the bowel apparent and provides luminal distention, features necessary for diagnostic characterization of the hollow viscera. Luminal distention can be achieved by using positive, negative, or biphasic enteric contrast materials.[1] Positive enteric contrast materials display high signal intensity on both T1- and T2-weighted sequences and include diluted gadolinium agent, high-fat-content milk, ferrous ammonium citrate, iron phytate, and manganese chloride. Negative contrast agents display low signal intensity on both T1- and T2-weighted MR sequences, and include barium sulfate and superparamagnetic iron oxide (ferumoxil oral suspension). Biphasic enteric contrast agents display low signal intensity on T1-weighted images and high signal intensity on T2-weighted images. Agents that cause low signal intensity on T1-weighted sequences allow for accurate assessment of enhancement of the bowel wall and mass lesions when additional intravenous gadolinium-based contrast agents is administrated. Biphasic enteric contrast materials are generally preferred for MR imaging of the GI tract. The prototypical biphasic agent is water. However, water is absorbed substantially in the jejunum, making it therefore an unsuitable contrast agent for use in the small bowel when administered orally. Water can be administered rectally to distend the colon. Other available biphasic contrast materials consist of a water solution mixed with substances such as methylcellulose, mannitol, sorbitol, and polyethylene glycol to make the solution hyperosmolar to decrease bowel absorption.

MR enterography and ***MR enteroclysis*** are two similar techniques for imaging the small bowel.[2] Both involve administration of a large volume of fluid to distend the small bowel. For MR enterography, 1,000 to 1,500 mL of an enteric contrast agent is ingested orally by the patient during the 45 to 60 minutes prior to the MR examination. For MR enteroclysis, a nasojejunal catheter with an occlusion balloon at the tip is placed through the nose to the proximal jejunum under fluoroscopic guidance. The enteric agent is then pumped into the small bowel at a set rate of 80 to 120 mL/min until the terminal ileum is reached, at which time the rate may be increased to 200 to 300 mL/min to induce reflex atony of the small bowel. The technique of MR enteroclysis produces greater bowel distention than MR enterography, but comes at the cost of additional radiation and discomfort to the patient. Enteroclysis requires a procedurally skilled radiologist for placement of the nasojejunal tube. For both MR enteroclysis and MR enterography, an antispasmodic agent (glucagon) is administered to limit bowel peristalsis. Patients are imaged in the prone or supine position. The prone position is less comfortable but facilitates separation of small bowel loops. With use of biphasic contrast agents axial- and coronal-plane T2-weighted single shot FSE/TSE sequences provide bright-lumen images. Intravenous gadolinium-based contrast material is administered to detect the hyperenhancement of active inflammation in the bowel wall and hyperenhancing neoplastic lesions (Fig. 8.1). Use of a fast 3D T1-weighted gradient-echo sequence obtained with fat saturation before and after intravenous contrast administration provides dark-lumen images that optimize demonstration of contrast enhancement. Gadolinium contrast agents are administered intravenously at a dosage of 0.1 mg/kg.

MR colonography offers a significant advantage over CT colonography for colorectal cancer screening by avoiding the use of ionizing radiation.[3] CT colonography is more commonly available, however, and its use is much better researched. The availability of 3.0T MR and fecal tagging is bringing MR colonography into clinical use both for colorectal cancer screening and for detection of other diseases of the colon.[4] MR colonography currently requires bowel preparation similar to that for CT colonography and optical colonoscopy. Colon distention is achieved by placing a soft-tipped rectal catheter in the rectum and use of an antispasmodic agent such as glucagon to minimize peristalsis. Patients are scanned in both supine and prone positions to optimize distention. Bright-lumen colonography is achieved by use of enema fluid with added gadolinium chelate (1:100) enema fluid, while air, water, or fat enemas are used for dark-lumen colonography. Bright-lumen colonography typically uses a 3D T1-weighted gradient-echo sequence with high-performance gradients and multi-coil array surface coils to allow single breath-hold acquisition. Dark-lumen colonography sequences are obtained as T1-weighted spoiled gradient echo sequences with fat suppression pre- and post-intravenous contrast enhancement. The low signal intensity of the lumen and the low signal intensity of the surrounding fat accentuates detection of contrast enhancement of the wall of the colon.

MR IMAGING OF THE ESOPHAGUS

MR is not generally used as a primary method of imaging the esophagus. Because the esophagus is a rapid-transit structure, optimal distention of the esophagus is not an attainable goal.

The esophagus is a muscular tube consisting of mucosa, submucosa, muscularis propria with inner circular and outer longitudinal muscle layers, and a loose connective tissue adventitia.

The surrounding loose connective tissue allows early spread of esophageal cancer into the fat of the mediastinum. The esophagus enters the abdomen through the esophageal hiatus anterior to the aorta. The esophagus courses to the left to join the stomach. The esophagus is usually collapsed, though a small amount of air in portions of the lumen is normal. Normal wall thickness is 3 mm. MR imaging of the esophagus is limited by cardiac motion and breathing. The normal esophagus follows the signal of muscle and displays intermediate signal intensity on T1- and T2-weighted images (Fig. 8.2). The mucosa-submucosa shows slight enhancement on fat-suppressed post-contrast-enhanced images.

Esophageal cancer treatment requires complete resection of the primary tumors and adjacent malignant lymph nodes. Imaging is used to provide accurate preoperative staging and to assess response to neoadjuvant chemotherapy. CT is the primary imaging modality for tumor staging. Squamous carcinoma and adenocarcinoma have similar appearance on MR. Tumor growth patterns are polypoid, ulcerating, infiltrating, and superficial spreading. Tumors appear as eccentric or circumferential wall thickening (Fig. 8.3). The esophagus is often dilated and filled with fluid and debris proximal to an obstructing lesion. Periesophageal fat stranding is often present. The presence of enlarged lymph nodes (more than 1 cm) or numerous (more than five) normal-size lymph nodes is evidence of metastatic spread. Tumor contact with the aorta exceeding 90 degrees is evidence of aortic invasion. Tumors are iso-intense to the wall of the esophagus on T1-weighted images and mildly hyperintense on T2-weighted images.

Esophageal leiomyomas are the most common benign submucosal tumors of the esophagus, occurring most frequently in the distal esophagus. The lesions vary in size (2 to 15 cm), may be solitary or multiple, and occasionally are pedunculated. They appear as smooth, well-defined, oval masses eccentrically within the wall of the esophagus. They are near iso-intense to the esophageal wall on T1- and T2-weighted images and enhance homogeneously to a greater extent than the esophageal wall.

Esophageal duplication cysts occur adjacent to the esophagus in the cervical region (20%), mid-esophagus (20%), and distal esophagus (60%). About half are lined with ectopic gastric mucosa. They appear as thin- or thick-walled spherical cystic masses. Signal intensity on T1-weighted images varies with the concentration of protein and mucin within the cyst. Most are high in signal intensity on T2-weighted images. The wall may enhance avidly if gastric mucosa is present, but the fluid does not.

Esophageal varices occur along the lower esophagus and extend into the stomach in association with portal venous hypertension or splenic vein thrombosis. Delayed fat-suppressed T1-weighted post-gadolinium contrast-enhanced gradient-echo images show an enhancing network of tubular structures within and adjacent to the esophageal wall. Spin-echo T1-weighted images show the lumen of the varices as signal voids (Fig. 8.4).

Esophagitis causes thickening of the wall of the esophagus with luminal narrowing and proximal esophageal dilatation

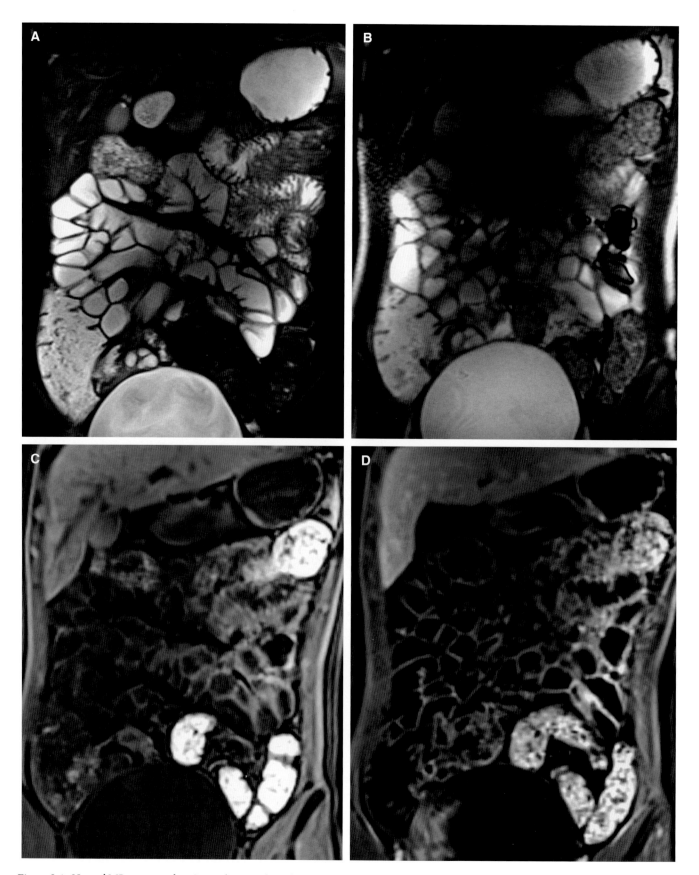

Figure 8.1 *Normal MR enterography.* Coronal images show the normal appearance of small bowel on standard sequences used for MR enterography. (**A**) T2-weighted single-shot FSE/TSE image with fat saturation shows bright enteric lumen. (**B**) steady state free precession (SSFP) gradient-echo image is used to assess adequacy of luminal distention. (**C**) Pre-contrast-enhanced T1-weighted gradient-echo image shows dark enteric lumen. (**D**) Post-gadolinium-contrast enhanced image at the same level shows dark enteric lumen with enhancement of the enteric wall. The large volume of contrast agent ingested orally commonly results in increased urine output and bladder filling.

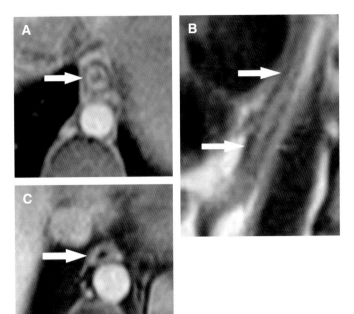

Figure 8.2 *Normal esophagus.* (**A**) Axial T2-weighted single-shot FSE/TSE image of the distal esophagus (*arrow*) shows the normal multilayer appearance with the low-signal-intensity muscular layer between the high-signal-intensity mucosa/submucosa and the high-signal-intensity serosa with surrounding tissues. Normal wall thickness from lumen to serosa is 3 mm. (**B**) Sagittal T2-weighted image of the distal esophagus (*arrows*) shows the normal multilayer appearance dominated by the low signal intensity of muscle in the wall. Images of the distal esophagus are degraded by cardiac motion. (**C**) Post-contrast-enhanced T1-weighted axial gradient-echo image with fat suppression shows enhancement of the wall of the esophagus (*arrow*).

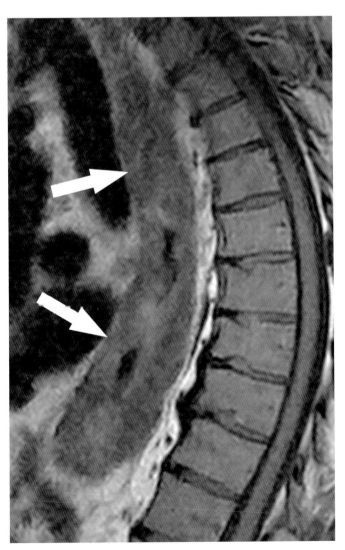

if fibrosis and strictures are present. Active inflammation is manifest by edema, ulceration, stranding in periesophageal fat, and marked wall enhancement after intravenous contrast material administration. Causes include gastroesophageal reflux, infection (*Candida albicans*, cytomegalovirus, herpes simplex virus), ingestion of corrosive agents, and radiation.

Achalasia refers to beak-like narrowing of the distal esophagus at the gastroesophageal junction associated with striking dilatation and tortuosity of the proximal esophagus, often containing retained fluid and debris. Primary achalasia results from an inability of the lower esophageal sphincter to relax in response to passage of food or liquids in the esophagus. Secondary achalasia occurs with Chagas disease and distal esophageal cancer. The underlying cause of achalasia is absence or destruction of the myenteric plexus innervating the lower esophageal sphincter. MR imaging may be used to detect neoplasm. MR of primary achalasia reveals the dilated esophagus with variable fluid and solid contents creating air–fluid levels. The esophageal wall is of uniform thickness without associated mass.

MR IMAGING OF THE STOMACH

MR of the stomach is performed most commonly to evaluate gastric malignancy and gastrointestinal stromal tumors (GISTs).

Figure 8.3 *Diffuse esophageal cancer.* Sagittal T1-weighted image reveals nodular poorly marginated circumferential thickening of the wall of the esophagus (*arrows*). This patient has diffuse esophageal cancer. Compare to Figure 8.1B. (Case courtesy of Dr. Sara Moshiri, Duke University and University of Virginia.)

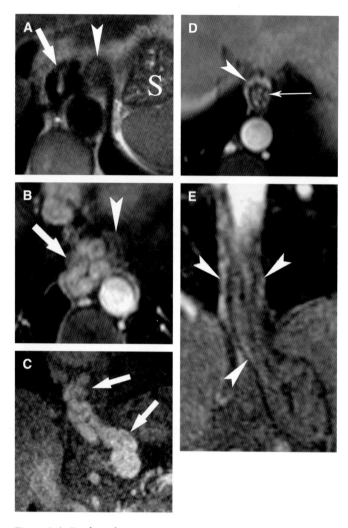

The appearance of the stomach varies with patient position, degree of distention, and size and shape of surrounding organs, and varies from one individual to another. Wall thickness is greatly affected by gastric distention, with normal thickening forming a pseudo-tumor near the gastroesophageal junction, a common finding in the nondistended stomach. The stomach, like the remainder of the abdominopelvic GI tract, has four distinct layers in its wall: mucosa, submucosa, muscularis propria, and serosa. The well-distended gastric wall is 2 to 3 mm thick in the body and 5 to 7 mm thick in the antrum. Rugal folds are normally prominent in the fundus and proximal gastric body but are usually absent in the antrum. T1-weighted images show the gastric wall with intermediate signal intensity.[5] T2-weighted images without fat suppression show the low-signal-intensity bowel wall sandwiched between the high-signal-intensity fluid-containing lumen and the high-signal-intensity periserosal fat. Normal gastric mucosa enhances uniformly and more avidly than the remainder of the GI tract. Avid mucosal enhancement is a diagnostic feature of ectopic gastric mucosa in duplication cysts and Meckel's diverticulum.

Gastric cancer is a deadly disease that is curable with surgical resection when detected early. Most tumors (95%) are adenocarcinomas, with the remainder being squamous cell carcinoma and tumors with rare cell types. The tumor grows in four morphologic patterns: polypoid masses within the gastric lumen, ulcerated masses, focal plaque-like lesions, and diffusely infiltrating tumor with diffuse wall and fold thickening and narrowing of the lumen (scirrhous carcinoma). T1-weighted images show the tumor as iso-intense to the gastric wall, manifest as a mass (Fig. 8.5) or polyp, or as wall thickening. On T2-weighted images the tumor is mildly hyperintense to the normal gastric wall. Dynamic post-contrast-enhanced MR shows heterogeneous tumor enhancement compared to avid uniform tumor enhancement of the normal gastric wall. Tumor detection is improved by obtaining a series of post-contrast-enhanced images that emphasize differential enhancement between tumor and normal wall on early and late images. Tumors of the diffusely infiltrating scirrhous type are more fibrotic and therefore lower in signal intensity on pre-contrast and show less enhancement on post-contrast enhanced sequences. Fat-suppressed

Figure 8.4 *Esophageal varices.* **Large varices:** (**A**) Axial T2-weighted image demonstrates varices (*arrow*) as tubular structures with internal signal void adjacent to the esophagus (*arrowhead*). *S*, stomach. (**B**) Axial T1-weighted post-gadolinium contrast-enhanced image demonstrates varices as a network of enhancing tubular structures (*arrow*) adjacent to the esophagus (*arrowhead*). (**C**) Coronal T1-weighted post-contrast-enhanced images show the varices (*arrows*) communicating with large portosystemic collateral vessels in the abdomen. **Small varices:** (**D**) T1-weighted post-contrast image of the distal esophagus shows a varix (*arrowhead*) looping around the esophagus, and a network of enhancing varices (*arrow*) in the wall of the esophagus. (**E**) Coronal T1-weighted post-contrast-enhanced image shows varices (*arrowheads*) coursing longitudinally in the wall of the esophagus.

Box 8.1 ESSENTIALS TO REMEMBER

- The normal wall of the esophagus does not exceed 3 mm in thickness.

- The wall of the esophagus displays intermediate signal intensity on T1- and T2-weighted images, and follows the signal intensity of smooth muscle.

- Esophageal cancer appears as eccentric wall thickening or a mass that is iso-intense to the esophageal wall on T1-weighted images and slightly hyperintense to the wall on T2-weighted images.

- Duplication cysts occur adjacent to the esophagus and are smooth, well defined, and cystic, with uniform walls and variable signal intensity of fluid content.

- Varices appear as tubular signal voids or as an enhancing vascular tangle in and around the distal esophagus.

- Active esophagitis appears as wall thickening with avid contrast enhancement and periesophageal edema.

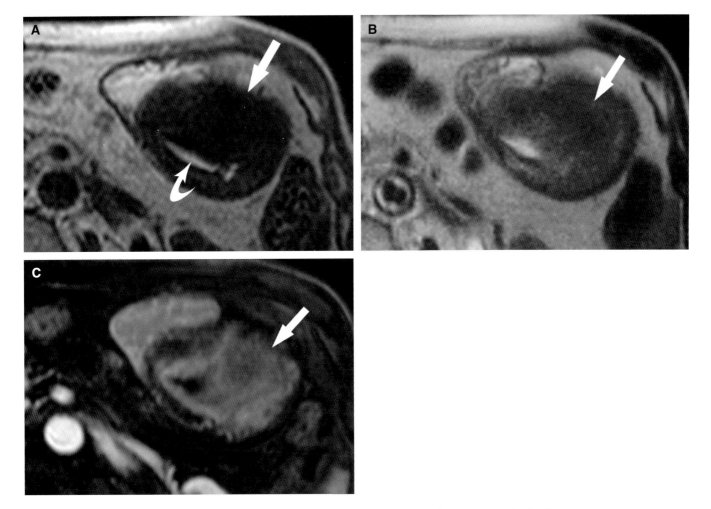

Figure 8.5 *Gastric cancer.* MR reveals a large gastric mass in a patient with a history of partial gastrectomy and Billroth II anastomosis presenting with weight loss and symptoms of gastric outlet obstruction. Axial plane T1-weighted gradient-echo (**A**) and T2-weighted single-shot FSE/TSE (**B**) images show a large gastric mass (*straight arrows*) eccentrically narrowing the lumen (*curved arrow* in image A). (**C**) Post-contrast T1-weighted gradient-echo image shows moderate contrast enhancement of the mass (*arrow*). Pathology at surgery revealed a well-differentiated adenocarcinoma arising from the stomach wall, likely within a rest of pancreatic tissue.

T1-weighted post-contrast images best reveal tumor extension into the perigastric fat. Nodal metastases enhance conspicuously. The liver must be carefully evaluated for metastatic disease.

Gastric GISTs may be benign or malignant.[6] Tumors presenting with symptoms are usually malignant. Histologic differentiation of benign (low grade) from malignant (high grade) tumors is difficult and is aided by the imaging findings.[7] The stomach is the most common site for GISTs. Arising from the gastric wall beneath the mucosa, the tumors are predominantly extraluminal. Benign lesions are generally small (4 to 5 cm average), uniform in signal intensity, and homogeneous in enhancement. Malignant tumors are larger (average more than 10 cm), are heterogeneous with areas of necrosis and hemorrhage, and show uneven enhancement. On T1-weighted MR images the solid components display intermediate low signal, with areas of necrosis and hemorrhage showing high signal intensity. On T2-weighted images malignant GISTs show increased heterogeneity, with irregular areas of high and

mixed signal intensity. Benign GISTs show moderate uniform enhancement (Fig. 8.6). Malignant GISTs enhance more avidly and irregularly. Irregular margins with adjacent fat, tumor extension to adjacent organs, and ulceration are evidence of malignancy. Dystrophic calcifications seen as foci of signal void are relatively common with both high-grade and low-grade tumors.

Gastric lymphoma consists almost entirely of B-cell non-Hodgkin's lymphoma. Primary GI lymphoma is most common in the stomach.[8] Chronic gastric infection with *Helicobacter pylori* predisposes to development of mucosa-associated lymphoid tissue (MALT) lymphomas. Lymphoma has four growth patterns demonstrated by imaging: solitary polypoid mass, bulky tumors with large ulcerated cavities, multiple submucosal nodules, and diffuse infiltration causing wall thickening. MR shows marked thickening of the gastric wall, often exceeding 3 cm. A characteristic appearance of lymphoma is a bulky tumor, often circumferential and associated with minimal narrowing of the gastric lumen. Gastric carcinomas much

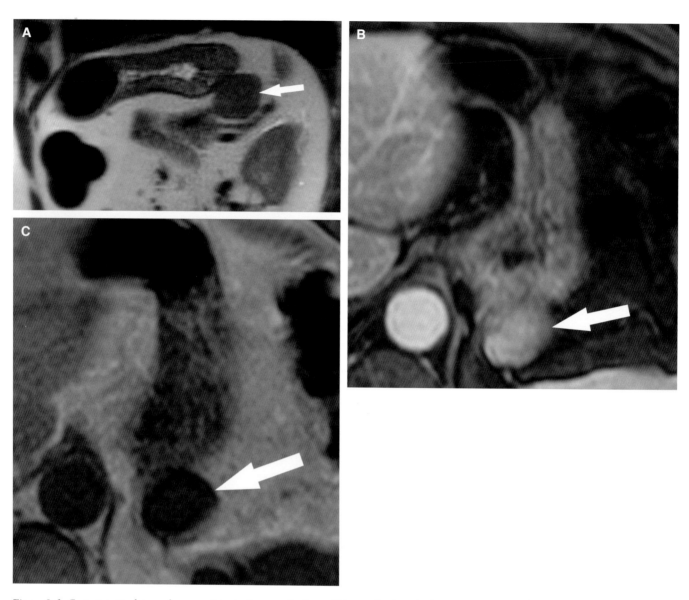

Figure 8.6 *Gastrointestinal stromal tumor arising in the stomach.* Sagittal T2-weighted single-shot FSE/TSE (**A**) and axial T1-weighted gradient-echo (**B**) images show a well-defined homogeneous mass (*arrows*) exophytic to the stomach. (**C**) Post-gadolinium-contrast enhanced axial T1-weighted image shows moderate uniform enhancement of the mass (*arrow*). Pathology confirmed a GIST of low risk for metastatic disease arising from the stomach.

more commonly show luminal narrowing. Transpyloric spread of tumor from stomach to duodenum is common (30%) and highly indicative of lymphoma. Signal intensity of lymphoma is intermediate on T1-weighted images, homogeneous in small tumors and heterogeneous in larger ones. Increasing signal heterogeneity correlates with tumors of higher aggressiveness and poorer prognosis.

Gastric volvulus may present as an acute abdominal emergency or with intermittent chronic symptoms.[9] Acute twisting of the stomach more than 180 degrees may result in ischemia, necrosis, perforation, shock, and death. Volvulus results from laxity of the stomach's attachments. Mesenteroaxial volvulus refers to rotation of the stomach about its short axis. Organoaxial volvulus describes rotation of the stomach about its long axis. With mesenteroaxial volvulus MR shows the stomach as "right side up" with the pylorus rotated from right

to left. With organoaxial volvulus the stomach is "upside down" with low position of the gastroesophageal junction and with the lesser curvature of the stomach lower than the greater curvature.

Gastric duplication cysts are uncommon but most frequently seen along the greater curvature of the stomach. Some calcify. About 15% communicate with the stomach. Like other GI duplication cysts they are well defined, with uniform wall thickness and variable signal intensity of the cyst contents (Fig. 8.7).[9]

MR IMAGING OF THE SMALL BOWEL

Indications for MR of the duodenum include staging of malignant tumors, characterization of benign tumors, duodenitis, pancreatitis, and trauma. Indications for MR imaging of the

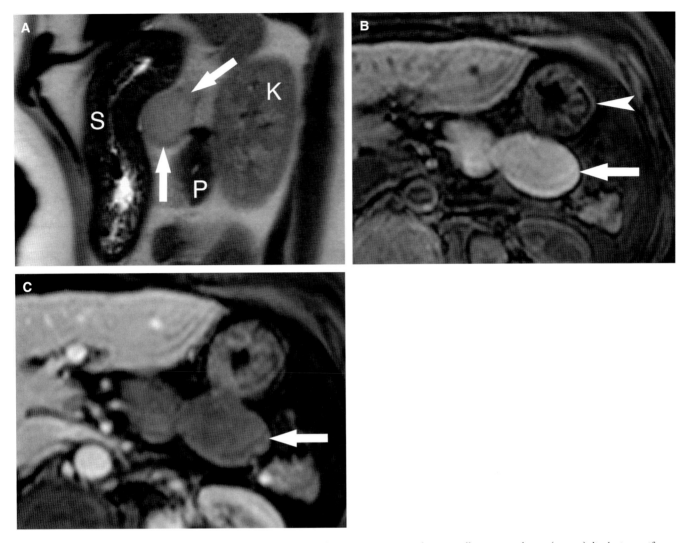

Figure 8.7 *Gastric duplication cyst.* (**A**) Sagittal T2-weighted single-shot FSE/TSE image shows a well-marginated mass (*arrows*) displaying uniform moderately high signal intensity between the stomach (*S*), left kidney (*K*), and pancreas (*P*). (**B**) Axial pre-contrast-enhanced T1-weighted gradient-echo image shows the mass (*arrow*) to be bilobed and demonstrating uniform high signal intensity. Sharp margination and close proximity to the stomach (*arrowhead*) are confirmed. (**C**) Axial T1-weighted post-gadolinium-contrast-enhanced image shows no enhancement of the mass (*arrow*). Fine-needle aspiration guided by endoscopic ultrasound yielded thick fluid containing gastric cells, consistent with gastric duplication cyst.

Box 8.2 ESSENTIALS TO REMEMBER

- When the stomach is only partially distended, the normal gastric folds appear prominent in the fundus; the resulting wall thickening may be striking, and a pseudo-tumor is often evident at the gastroesophageal junction. With full distention, the wall thickness is less than 3 to 4 mm in the body and fundus, and less than 5 to 7 mm in the antrum.

- Gastric cancers appear as luminal masses, ulcers within a mass, or focal or diffuse wall thickening. Scirrhous carcinoma stiffens the gastric wall and narrows the lumen.

- GISTs are usually large predominantly extraluminal smooth-walled tumors. The risk of malignancy increases with size, heterogeneity, and ulceration.

- Gastric lymphomas produce striking wall thickening and bulky masses that are relatively homogeneous, and characteristically cross the pylorus to involve the duodenum as well as the stomach.

mesenteric small bowel include Crohn's disease, bowel obstruction, and tumor staging.[2]

The duodenal bulb or "cap" is intraperitoneal and is the first portion of the duodenum adjacent to the pylorus. The second (descending) portion of the duodenum descends in the retroperitoneum adjacent to the head of the pancreas. It receives the common bile duct and pancreatic duct at the ampulla of Vater in its medial distal portion. The third or horizontal portion of the duodenum continues leftward in the retroperitoneum posterior to the uncinate process of the pancreas and the superior mesenteric blood vessels anterior to the inferior vena cava and aorta. The fourth (ascending) portion of the duodenum ascends just to the left of the aorta to the ligament of Treitz at the level of the L2 vertebra. The intestine turns abruptly ventrally at the duodenal–jejunal junction. Normal wall thickness of the distended duodenum is a uniform 3 mm.

The jejunum occupies the upper left abdomen while the ileum occupies the right lower abdomen. No discrete boundary separates the two portions of the mesenteric small bowel.

The jejunum has a wider lumen and more numerous folds, while the ileum has a narrower lumen and fewer folds. The mesenteric border of the bowel is concave and the antimesenteric border is convex. Wall thickness of the mesenteric small bowel normally does not exceed 3 to 4 mm.

The signal intensity of small bowel on MR images is similar to that of the stomach except that the submucosa/mucosa enhances only mildly.

Crohn's disease is the most common indication for MR imaging of the small bowel.[1,2,10,11] The disease starts typically at a young age and is characterized by numerous periods of high activity and many complications requiring repeated imaging. Traditional methods of imaging these patients includes fluoroscopy and CT, techniques that expose the patients to high lifetime doses of ionizing radiation. MR enterography is increasingly favored as an accurate imaging method to stage the disease, detect complications, and follow response to treatment without the use of ionizing radiation. Crohn's disease affects the small bowel in 80% of cases but

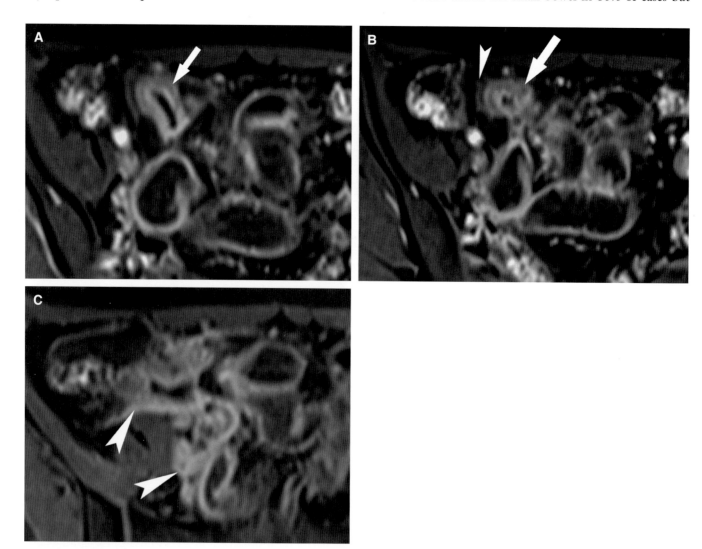

Figure 8.8 *Crohn's disease: wall thickening and mesenteric inflammation.* (**A**) Post-gadolinium contrast-enhanced T1-weighted gradient-echo black-lumen MR enterography image shows wall thickening and luminal narrowing of the terminal ileum (*arrow*). (**B**) Post-contrast-enhanced T1-weighted image shows a transverse view of the terminal ileum (*arrow*) illustrating circumferential narrowing, avid wall enhancement, and extension of inflammation into the adjacent mesenteric tissues (*arrowhead*), findings of active Crohn's disease. (**C**) Postcontrast enhanced image at a different level shows extensive extraluminal inflammation (*arrowheads*) characteristic of Crohn's disease.

may affect any portion of the GI tract, commonly at multiple sites. Bowel involvement is characteristically segmental, with healthy bowel segments interspersed between diseased bowel segments. Transmural inflammation leads to transmural ulceration, resulting in fistulas, sinus tracts, and abscesses. Chronic inflammation causes proliferation of fat both within the bowel wall and in the mesentery. MR, like CT, provides accurate assessment of the bowel wall, extraluminal complications, extent of disease, and disease activity. The earliest findings of Crohn's disease, superficial aphthous ulcers, mucosal nodularity, and erythema, are shown by endoscopy and high-quality barium contrast studies, but not by MR. MR findings of active disease are (Figs. 8.8 and 8.9): bowel wall thickening greater than 4 mm; intramural and mesenteric edema; mucosal hyperemia, manifested by increased visualization of blood

vessels and prominent contrast enhancement; transmural ulceration; fistulas; vascular engorgement; and enlarged, inflamed mesenteric lymph nodes showing hyperenhancement.[1,2,10,11] Small bowel folds may be uniformly and diffusely thickened ("picket fence pattern"), may be distorted or reduced in number, or may show the "cobblestone" pattern. Longitudinal and transverse mucosal ulceration separated by mounds and ridges of edema produces the cobblestone pattern, with knobs of high signal separated by ridges of low signal intensity. Transmural disease and wall thickening typically lead to irregular narrowing of the lumen. Caution must be taken to avoid misinterpretation of incomplete luminal distention for pathologic luminal narrowing. Ulceration is typically linear, appearing as transverse or longitudinal lines of high signal intensity on T2-weighted images, best seen when the bowel is

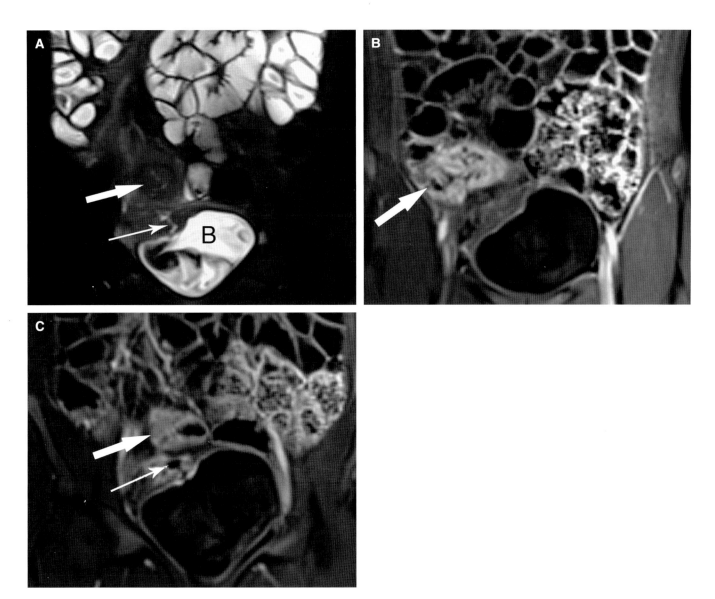

Figure 8.9 *Crohn's disease: enterovesical fistula.* (**A**) T2-weighted single-shot FSE/TSE image from MR enterography examination shows bright bowel lumen and a high-signal-intensity fistulous tract (*skinny arrow*) from a markedly thickened terminal ileum (*fat arrow*) to the bladder (*B*). (**B**) Post-gadolinium-contrast-enhanced T1-weighted gradient-echo image shows dark bowel lumen and marked inflammation and enhancement (*arrow*) in the right lower quadrant of the abdomen involving multiple loops of small bowel and adjacent mesentery, highly indicative of active Crohn's disease. (**C**) Post-contrast-enhanced T1-weighted image shows wall thickening and enhancement of the terminal ileum (*fat arrow*) as well as the low-signal-intensity fistulous tract to the bladder. A small abscess cavity (*skinny arrow*) is evident along the fistulous tract.

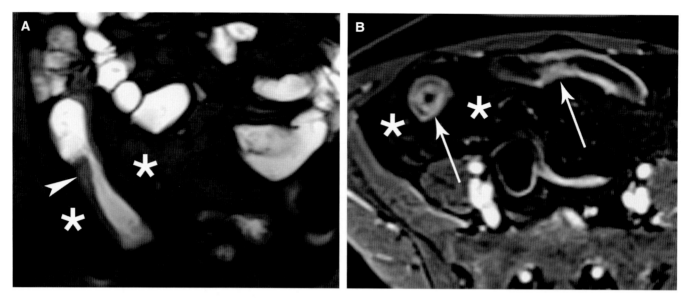

Figure 8.10 *Crohn's disease: fibrofatty proliferation.* (**A**) Coronal fat-suppressed T2-weighted image in a patient with chronic Crohn's disease shows asymmetric wall thickening and luminal narrowing (*arrowhead*) of a loop of distal ileum. The involved bowel loop is isolated and separated from adjacent bowel loops by fibrofatty proliferation (*) of the mesentery. This is a finding of longstanding Crohn's disease. (**B**) Axial T1-weighted fat-suppressed post-contrast-enhanced image shows isolation of bowel loops by fibrofatty proliferation (*), skip lesions (*arrows*), and asymmetric circumferential involvement of the bowel wall. Clinically and by imaging this patient has low-grade activity of chronic Crohn's disease.

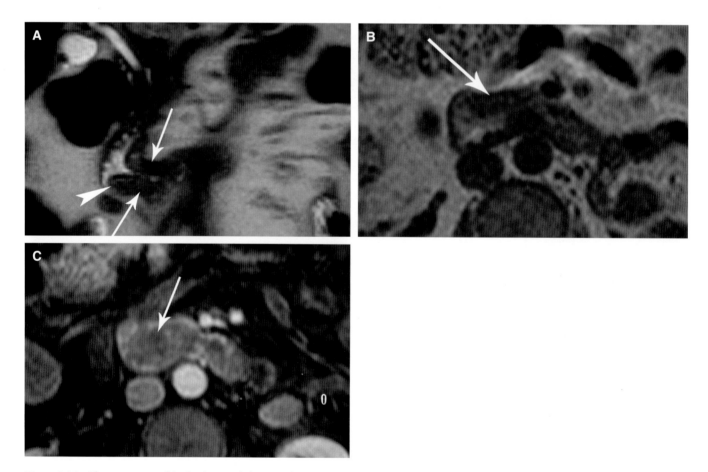

Figure 8.11 *Adenocarcinoma of the duodenum.* (**A**) Coronal T2-weighted single-shot FSE/TSE image reveals circumferential wall thickening (*arrows*) of the third portion of the duodenum. Note the shouldering (*arrowhead*) and abrupt narrowing of the lumen caused by the tumor. (**B**) Axial T1-weighted gradient-echo image shows nodularity of the wall and irregularity of the lumen resulting from the tumor (*arrow*). (**C**) Post-contrast fat-suppressed T1-weighted gradient-echo image shows mild tumor enhancement (*arrow*).

well distended. Edema of the bowel wall increases the wall signal intensity on T2-weighted images, best seen on fat-suppressed T2-weighted images. Increased-signal-intensity edema frequently extends into the mesenteric fat. Wall enhancement is best judged by comparing thickened, diseased bowel segments with thin-walled normal-appearing bowel segments. Stratified, layered enhancement of the bowel wall indicates active disease. Diffuse enhancement of thickened wall indicates transmural inflammation. Minimal enhancement indicates chronic disease with fibrosis.[1] Fat proliferation in the mesentery causing increased separation of bowel loops and fat infiltration of the thickened bowel wall are findings of chronic disease (Fig. 8.10). The "comb sign" is produced by a series of engorged vasa recta in mesenteric fat and is best seen on post-contrast-enhanced T1-weighted images as a series of parallel high-signal-intensity enhanced structures. Fistulas and sinus tracts appear as high-signal-intensity extraluminal tracts on T2-weighted images. Because of accompanying inflammation the tracts enhance prominently on post-contrast-enhanced images. Fistulas may extend between small bowel loops (enteroenteric), between small bowel and colon (enterocolic), between small bowel and skin (enterocutaneous), and between small bowel and the bladder (enterovesical) (Fig. 8.9). Sinuses are blind-ending tracts. Abscesses are localized collections of pus that may be found in the mesentery, between bowel loops, or anywhere in the peritoneal cavity or retroperitoneum. MR is sensitive for demonstrating abscesses, appearing as complex fluid collections. Colonic involvement is common and is reviewed further in the colon section.

Small bowel adenocarcinoma is a rare disease occurring most commonly in the duodenum (60% of tumors).[12] Tumors near the ampulla may cause jaundice. Tumors may obstruct the bowel or present with anemia from frequent bleeding. On MR adenocarcinomas (Fig. 8.11) appear as polypoid intraluminal masses, infiltrative wall thickening with luminal strictures, or focal wall thickening.[13] Lesions display intermediate to high signal on T2-weighted images and may blend in with luminal contents. Enhancement is usually heterogeneous and greater than the normal bowel wall, aiding in tumor detection. Staging includes assessment of extraluminal spread, lymphadenopathy, and liver metastases.

Small bowel lymphoma has findings similar to those of gastric lymphoma (Fig. 8.12): conspicuous concentric symmetric or asymmetric wall thickening, often striking for the

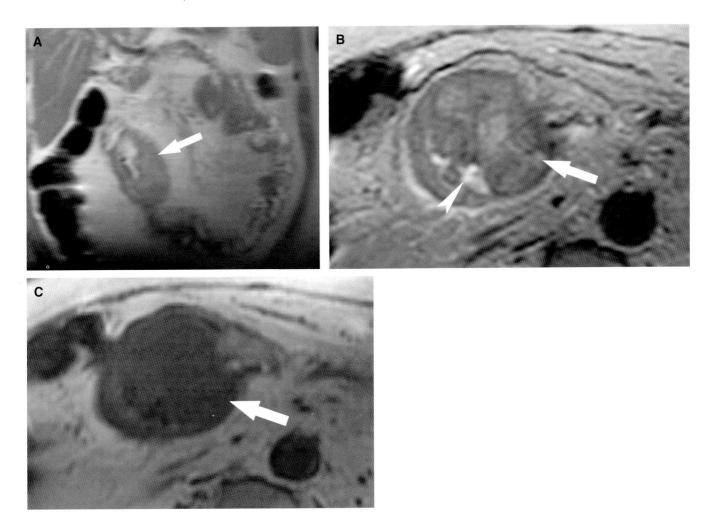

Figure 8.12 *Lymphoma involving the jejunum.* (**A**) Coronal T2-weighted single-shot FSE/TSE image demonstrates a bulky tumor (*arrow*) involving the distal jejunum. Despite the large size of the tumor there is no evidence of bowel obstruction. (**B**) Axial T2-weighted single-shot FSE/TSE image shows the tumor (*arrow*) with intermediate signal intensity asymmetrically narrowing the lumen (*arrowhead*). (**C**) T1-weighted axial gradient-echo image shows that the signal intensity of the tumor (*arrow*) is similar to that of muscle.

absence of significant luminal narrowing; effacement or thickening of small bowel folds; aneurysmal dilatation of the lumen; and uncommonly luminal strictures.[8,14] Additional findings include mesenteric fat stranding and lymphadenopathy in the mesentery and elsewhere.[12]

Carcinoid tumors of the jejunum and ileum frequently metastasize to mesenteric lymph nodes, producing excessive fibrous reaction in the mesentery. The mesenteric disease is often more prominent than the primary tumor. Mesenteric fibrosis causes kinking of the small bowel by scarring and retraction. The differential diagnosis includes sclerosing mesenteritis. The primary carcinoid tumor appears as a solitary, usually intraluminal, polyp or mass.[12] The most common location is the distal ileum. Carcinoid tumors of the duodenum (Fig. 8.13) account for only 2% of small bowel carcinoids and are associated with multiple endocrine neoplasia. Small tumors are easily overlooked, as signal intensity on MR imaging often parallels that of the normal bowel. Larger tumors are identified by heterogeneous enhancement (Fig. 8.14). The mesenteric reaction shows as low signal intensity on T1- and T2-weighted images with little to no enhancement reflecting fibrosis.

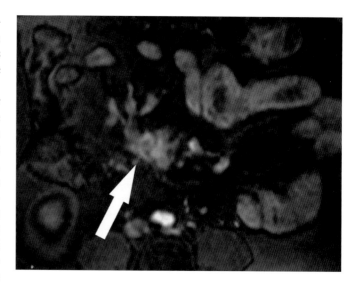

Figure 8.14 *Carcinoid tumor in the mesentery.* Axial fat-saturated T1-weighted post-gadolinium-contrast-enhanced gradient-echo image demonstrates a spiculated enhancing mass (*arrow*) in the small bowel mesentery in this patient with metastatic carcinoid tumor of the ileum.

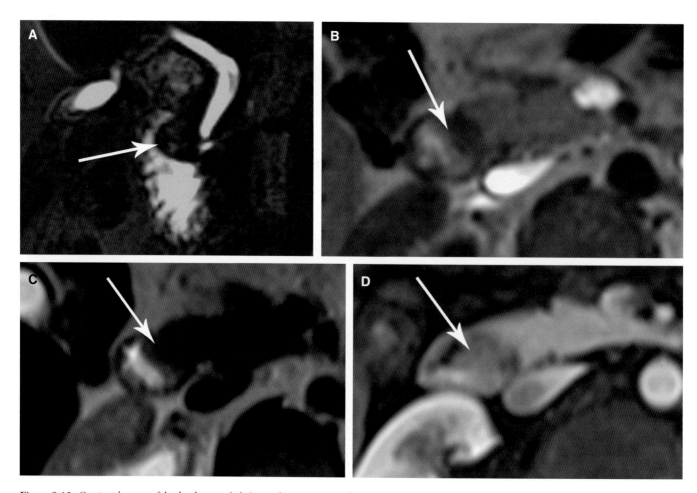

Figure 8.13 *Carcinoid tumor of the duodenum.* (**A**) Coronal source image of a 3D multislice FSE/TSE sequence for MRCP shows a well-defined tumor (*arrow*) bulging into the lumen of the descending duodenum near the ampulla. The common bile duct and pancreatic duct are unaffected by the presence of the tumor. (**B**) T1-weighted axial gradient-echo image shows the tumor (*arrow*) to display low signal intensity, similar to that of the muscular wall of the duodenum. (**C**) On T2-weighted axial single-shot FSE/TSE image the tumor (*arrow*) continues to follow the signal intensity of muscle and is low in signal intensity. (**D**) Early post-gadolinium-contrast-enhanced T1-weighted fat-suppressed image shows mild tumor enhancement (*arrow*).

Small bowel obstruction is usually diagnosed clinically, by conventional radiography, or by CT. However, MR is highly accurate in identifying bowel obstruction and its cause.[2] MR shows dilated fluid-filled small bowel loops to the point of obstruction. High intraluminal signal from fluid in the bowel loops on T2-weighted images improves conspicuity. T2-weighted images may show adhesions as high-signal-intensity bands coursing through the peritoneal cavity. As with CT, MR enteroclysis improves diagnostic accuracy.

Small bowel hematomas occur most commonly as a result of blunt trauma to the abdomen.[15] CT is the imaging method of choice but has the lowest sensitivity for injuries to the bowel and mesentery. MR may be indicated if the CT findings are equivocal, especially for injuries in the peripancreatic region. MR cholangiopancreatography (MRCP) accurately assesses the duodenum, pancreas, and bile and pancreatic ducts. The MR appearance of hematomas varies with age (see Table 2.2). Signal intensity is variably high on T1-weighted images and may be high or low on T2-weighted images (Fig. 8.15).

Mesenteric cysts are lymphangiomas or pseudo-cysts that lack an epithelial lining.[16] They arise in the mesentery of the small bowel, are of variable size, and are usually solitary. Most are unilocular with uniform thin walls and occasionally thin septations. MR most often shows cyst contents to have the signal intensity of simple fluid—that is, low signal intensity on T1-weighted images and high signal intensity on T2-weighted images. Prior hemorrhage or increased protein content causes increased signal on T1-weighted images. Septations are best visualized on T2-weighted images. Post-contrast enhanced images show no enhancement of cyst contents, with mild enhancement of the wall and septa.

Desmoid tumor, also called aggressive fibromatosis, is an infiltrative fibrous tumor of the mesentery, abdominal wall, and pelvis. The tumor is strongly associated with Gardner syndrome (familial adenomatous polyposis). The growth pattern is aggressive, with common recurrences after surgical resection. The lesions contain abundant fibrous tissue, resulting in low signal intensity on T1-weighted images and usually also on T2-weighted images. High signal on T2-weighted images correlates with more aggressive lesions showing more rapid growth.[17] Enhancement is variable and heterogeneous.

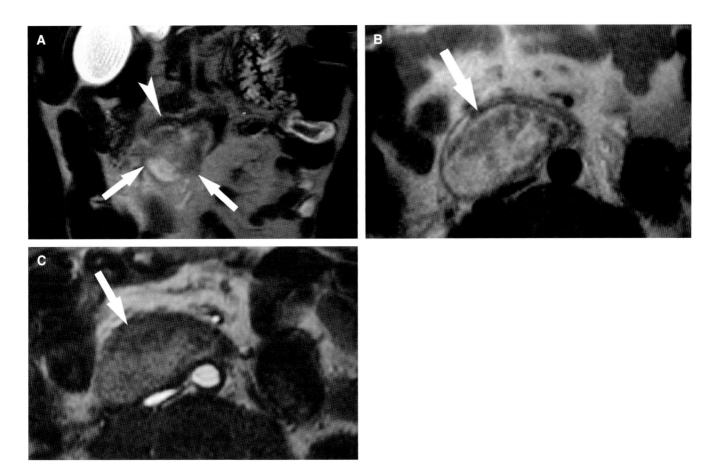

Figure 8.15 *Hematoma of the duodenum.* A patient presenting with gastric outlet obstruction was believed to have a neoplasm. MR revealed a hematoma in the wall of the third portion of the duodenum. (**A**) Coronal T2-weighted single-shot FSE/TSE image shows the hematoma (*arrows*) extending from the wall of the third duodenum (*arrowhead*). The mass shows foci of high and low signal intensity. (**B**) Axial T2-weighted image demonstrates sharp definition of the wall of the mass (*arrow*). (**C**) Axial T1-weighted gradient-echo image demonstrates intermediate low signal intensity of the mass (*arrow*). Post-gadolinium-contrast-enhanced MR sequences revealed no enhancement of the mass. Follow-up CT confirmed complete resolution of the hematoma.

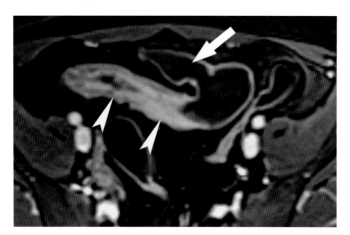

Figure 8.16 *Meckel's diverticulum: Crohn's disease.* Axial post-gadolinium contrast-enhanced T1-weighted fat-suppressed gradient-echo image from an MR enterography examination demonstrates a blind-ended sac (*arrow*) extending from a portion of the distal ileum. The ileum has a thickened wall (*arrowheads*) showing avid contrast enhancement, indicative of active Crohn's disease.

Meckel's diverticulum results from failure of involution of the omphalomesenteric duct that provided embryonic connection of the ileum to the yolk sac.[7] The "rule of 2's" describes their features: they occur in 2% of the population, are usually 2 inches (about 5 cm) in size, and occur within 2 feet (about 60 cm) of the ileocecal valve (Fig. 8.16).[9] Most contain heterotopic mucosa, either gastric or pancreatic. They may obstruct and become inflamed. MR reveals a saccular air- and fluid-containing mass attached as a blind sac to the ileum. Meckel's is a true diverticulum, containing all the normal layers of the bowel wall, and will therefore have the same MR signal characteristics as the ileum on non-contrast enhanced images. Marked enhancement of the mucosa on post-gadolinium-contrast enhanced images is strongly indicative of the presence of ectopic gastric mucosa.

MR IMAGING OF THE APPENDIX

While CT remains the modality of choice for the imaging diagnosis of acute appendicitis, concerns about radiation exposure have led to increased use of MR for diagnosis of patients with abdominal pain, especially pregnant women and children.[18–20] Ultrasound is highly beneficial in this clinical setting but is limited by operator dependence and inability to reliably provide reassuring demonstration of the normal appendix.

The normal appendix is a blind-ending tube less than 6 mm in diameter and averaging 10 cm in length.[20] The appendix arises from the medial aspect of the cecum, always on the same side as and approximately 3 cm inferior to the ileocecal valve. The normal appendix is often collapsed, or may be partially filled with fluid or air. The normal appendix shows low signal intensity on T1-weighted images, often blending in with other bowel loops. The normal appendix is best seen on T2-weighted images as a hypointense muscular tube with a high-intensity fluid center (Fig. 8.17). Though the origin of the appendix is reliably found by its relationship to the cecum and terminal ileum, the cecum itself is variable in location in the right lower quadrant, pelvis, or mid-abdomen, or even on the left side. In addition, the appendix wanders anterior, posterior, superior, or inferior to the cecum. The enlarging gravid uterus progressively displaces the appendix superiorly during pregnancy. Administration of oral and intravenous contrast agents improve visualization of the appendix. Because the effects of intravenous gadolinium agents on the unborn child are unknown, only oral enteric contrast agents are used in pregnant women. The normal appendix is reported to be visualized on MR in 90% of pregnant women and 83% to 89% of nonpregnant adults, but only 48% of children.[18–20]

Acute appendicitis is the most common cause of acute abdomen in adults and children and is the most common cause of abdominal pain requiring emergency surgery in

---

Box 8.3 **ESSENTIALS TO REMEMBER**

- Normal wall thickness of the distended small bowel does not exceed 4 mm.

- Active Crohn's disease shows bowel wall thickening greater than 4 mm and avid enhancement of the bowel wall.

- Skip lesions with normal small bowel segments intervening between diseased small bowel segments are characteristic of Crohn's disease.

- Full distention of the small bowel by intraluminal contrast agents is essential to avoid misdiagnosis of strictures and to visualize subtle findings such as ulceration.

- Fibrofatty proliferation of the mesentery, fatty infiltration of the bowel wall, and reduced contrast enhancement of the bowel wall are findings of chronic Crohn's disease.

- Fistulas and sinus tracts appear as high-signal-intensity streaks and bands on T2-weighted images. They are evident as enhancing curvilinear tracts on fat-suppressed post-contrast T1-weighted images.

- Adenocarcinoma of the small bowel appears as wall thickening, intraluminal mass, and luminal narrowing.

- Lymphoma of the small bowel shows marked wall thickening and mass, usually without significant luminal narrowing.

- Heterotopic gastric mucosa in a Meckel's diverticulum is identified by avid contrast enhancement.

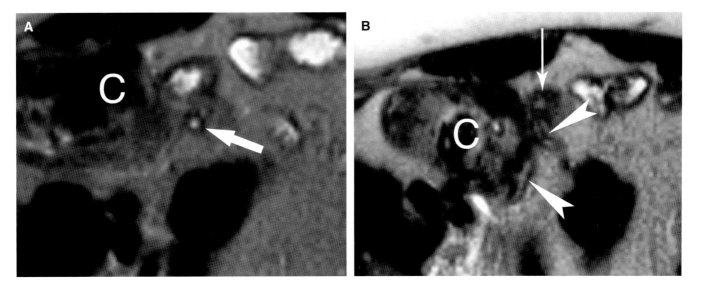

Figure 8.17 *Normal appendix.* With clinical suspicion of appendicitis, MR was performed on a 24-year-old pregnant woman at 10 weeks' gestational age. (**A**) Coronal T2-weighted single-shot FSE/TSE image shows a cross-sectional view of the appendix (*arrow*). The wall of the appendix displays low signal intensity and the nondilated lumen of the appendix is high in signal intensity. No findings of inflammation are present in the periappendiceal fat. The appendix measured a uniform normal 5 mm in diameter. *C*, cecum. (**B**) On axial T2-weighted single-shot FSE/TSE image parts of the appendix are seen to be coursing horizontal (*arrowheads*). As is usually the case, numerous images must be carefully examined to evaluate the twists and turns of the normal appendix. The appendix is identified by using the cecum (*C*) and terminal ileum (*arrow*) as anatomic landmarks. T2-weighted sequences usually provide the best demonstration of the appendix.

pregnant women.[19] Because the clinical presentation is commonly atypical and clinical diagnosis is inaccurate, many patients are sent for imaging diagnosis. If appendicitis is not present, imaging commonly provides an alternative diagnosis such as hemorrhagic ovarian cyst, Crohn's disease, ovarian torsion, or renal colic. MR diagnosis of acute appendicitis is based on demonstration of a fluid-filled appendix dilated to 7 mm in diameter or greater (Fig. 8.18).[20] Additional findings include periappendiceal edema and inflammation, best seen on fat-suppressed T2-weighted images as bright signal intensity in dark-signal-intensity fat. The wall of the appendix is thickened more than 3 mm. An appendicolith, which is a calcified nidus of inspissated feces, appears as a focal signal void on MR. Appendicoliths are more reliably seen on CT, however. Periappendiceal phlegmon appears as a heterogeneous, poorly marginated area of high signal intensity surrounding the distended appendix. Appendiceal rupture results in abscess, seen on MR as a discrete fluid collection adjacent to or surrounding the appendix. The entire appendix must be inspected, as acute appendicitis may be confined to the tip of the appendix.

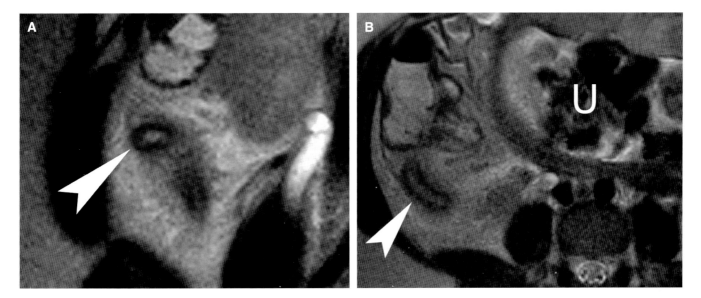

Figure 8.18 *Acute appendicitis.* MR was performed in 19-year-old pregnant woman at 22 weeks' gestational age. Coronal (**A**) and axial (**B**) T2-weighted single-shot FSE/TSE images demonstrate that the appendix (*arrowheads*) is dilated to 9 mm, has thickened walls, and there is inflammatory stranding into the periappendiceal fat. Surgery confirmed acute gangrenous appendicitis. *U*, the gravid uterus.

Box 8.4 ESSENTIALS TO REMEMBER

- The MR diagnosis of acute appendicitis is based on the depiction of an obstructed blind-ending bowel loop with thickened wall, adjacent inflammation, and a luminal diameter greater than 7 mm.

- MR is indicated for the diagnosis of acute appendicitis in pregnant women. No gadolinium contrast agent should be given.

- An appendix lumen diameter of greater than 15 mm should raise suspicion for the presence of an appendiceal mucocele or carcinoma.

- Although carcinoid tumor is the most common neoplasm of the appendix, it is commonly overlooked on imaging studies because of its small size. The appendix should be carefully examined on every image for the presence of focal wall thickening and small nodules.

Appendiceal mucocele refers to chronic dilatation of the appendix by mucus.[20] The appendix is chronically obstructed by a mucinous cystadenoma, mucinous cystadenocarcinoma, a mucous retention cyst, or a hyperplastic mucosal polyp. Continued secretion of mucus over time progressively dilates the appendix. Rupture of the mucocele seeds the abdominal cavity with mucin-producing cells that cause focal or diffuse pseudomyxoma peritonei. T2-weighted MR images show a dilated appendix filled with high-signal-intensity mucin. Dilatation of the appendix to a diameter greater than 15 mm suggests a possible mucocele. Wall thickening and periappendiceal inflammation tend to be minimal with a mucocele. The obstructing lesion is usually visualized and characterized as tumor, polyp, or cyst. Mucinous adenocarcinoma may show spread beyond the appendix.[21]

Appendiceal carcinoid tumor is the most common neoplasm of the appendix, accounting for 80% of all appendiceal tumors.[20] About one third of GI carcinoid tumors occur in the appendix. Most are discovered incidentally and are often overlooked on imaging studies. Carcinoid tumors are found in up to 25% of cases of acute appendicitis. Most tumors are small (1 to 2 cm). MR shows focal wall thickening and heterogeneous enhancement.

Appendiceal adenoma and adenocarcinoma are predominantly of the mucinous variety. While they are less common than appendiceal carcinoid tumors, they are more likely to be detected on imaging studies. Many are discovered as the causative lesion of an appendiceal mucocele or in association with acute appendicitis. MR shows an enhancing mass lesion. Spread through the appendiceal wall with soft tissue strands in the periappendiceal fat may be evident. Enlarged regional lymph nodes and liver metastases should be sought.

MR IMAGING OF THE COLON

MR of the colon is used for tumor staging, for assessment of inflammatory bowel disease, and, using MR colonography, for colorectal cancer screening.

The colon is 120 to 150 cm in length, consisting of the cecum with its attached appendix and terminal ileum, ascending colon, transverse colon, descending colon, sigmoid colon, and rectum. The ascending and descending colon are retroperitoneal in the anterior pararenal space. The transverse colon and sigmoid colon are intraperitoneal and suspended on a mesentery of variable length. The gastrocolic ligament is the mesentery of the transverse colon connecting the transverse colon to the lesser curvature of the stomach. When the gastrocolic ligament is long the mesentery of the sigmoid colon is short, and vice versa. This results in much individual variation in the length and position of these sections of the colon. The rectum is extraperitoneal and fixed in position. The colon wall consists of mucosa, submucosa, muscularis, and serosa. The muscularis has inner circular and outer longitudinal muscle layers. The large intestine is characterized by the taenia coli, three longitudinal bands of muscle that traverse the colon, shortening it to form haustra, the sacculations created by puckering of the bowel wall. The normal, distended colonic wall is less than 4 mm thick. High-resolution T2-weighted images demonstrate the mucosa and submucosa as a high-signal-intensity layer bordered by low-signal-intensity muscularis with outer high-signal-intensity serosa and pericolic fat.

Colorectal adenocarcinoma is the most common GI tract malignancy. Cancers occur most frequently in the rectum and sigmoid colon. Tumor morphology includes annular constricting ("apple core") lesions; polypoid masses, some with the frond-like appearance of villous carcinoma; and uncommonly infiltrating scirrhous tumors. Nearly all colorectal adenocarcinomas are believed to arise from preexisting adenomas. This is the primary rationale for colorectal cancer screening, with the goal of detecting high-grade adenomas or cancers at the small polypoid stage before they have had a chance to spread. Predisposing conditions include the polyposis syndromes and ulcerative colitis. Colon cancer spreads by direct invasion through the bowel wall, by spread into the lymphatic channels to regional lymph nodes, and hematogenously via the mesenteric veins to the liver and systemic circulation. Intraperitoneal spread occurs with tumors arising from the intraperitoneal segments of the colon. Complications include bowel obstruction, perforation, intussusception, abscess, and fistula formation.

Staging of rectal tumors for local spread with MR is increasingly being used (Figs. 8.19 and 8.20 and Table 8.1).[22,23] High accuracy for absence of local invasion has been reported (negative predictive value 93% to 100%).[22] The muscularis propria layer displays low signal intensity on T1- and T2-weighted

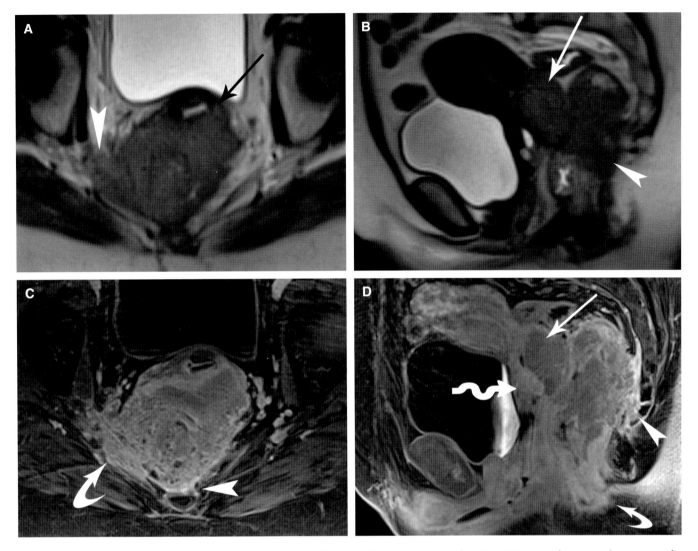

Figure 8.19 *MR staging of carcinoma of the rectum.* (**A**) Axial and (**B**) sagittal T2-weighted single-shot FSE/TSE images document a large tumor of the rectum with extension into perirectal fat (*arrowhead*) and tumor invasion of the cervix (*arrow*). On sagittal image B the bulky tumor is seen to extend posteriorly (*arrowhead*) and the cranial extent of tumor involves the cervix (*arrow*). (**C**) Early axial image from dynamic post-gadolinium-contrast-enhanced T1-weighted fat-suppressed gradient-echo sequence shows tumor extension to the distal sacrum (*arrowhead*) and invasion of the right piriformis muscle (*curved arrow*). (**D**) Sagittal image from the dynamic post-contrast-enhanced T1-weighted fat-suppressed series reveals tumor invasion of the perineum (*curved arrow*), tumor extension to the sacrum and coccyx (*arrowhead*), and tumor invasion of the cervix (*skinny arrow*) and upper vagina (*squiggly arrow*). Tumor stage by MR findings is T4b.

images and remains low in signal intensity following intravenous contrast administration. Interruption of the low-signal muscle layer by the tumor displaying increased signal intensity on T2-weighted images or by enhancing tumor on post-contrast enhanced T1-weighted images indicates tumor invasion of muscle (stage T2 disease). Tumor signal extending into perirectal fat on fat-suppressed T2-weighted images or fat-suppressed post-contrast enhanced T1-weighted images indicates tumor extension beyond the colon (stage T3 disease). Tumor invasion of the sacrum is evidenced by visualization of high-signal-intensity tumor invading the low-signal-intensity marrow on fat-suppressed T1- or T2-weighted images.

Tumor recurrences are most common at the operative site, in regional lymph nodes that drain the operative site, in the peritoneal cavity, and in the liver and distant organs. Recurrent tumors display low signal intensity on T1-weighted images and moderately high signal intensity on T2-weighted images. Post-contrast enhanced images show moderate enhancement. In the first year after therapy postoperative and post-radiation fibrosis may show as high signal intensity on T2-weighted images. After 1 year fibrosis usually shows as low signal intensity on both T1- and T2-weighted images. However, since colorectal cancers can produce significant amounts of fibrous tissue (desmoplastic reaction), foci of recurrent tumor may not always be easily detectable within the low-signal-intensity post-surgery/radiation fibrosis. Fibrosis may show enhancement for 1.5 to 2 years following therapy.

Colon lymphoma is uncommon except in patients with human immunodeficiency virus (HIV) or with chronic ulcerative colitis. The cecum and rectosigmoid colon are most

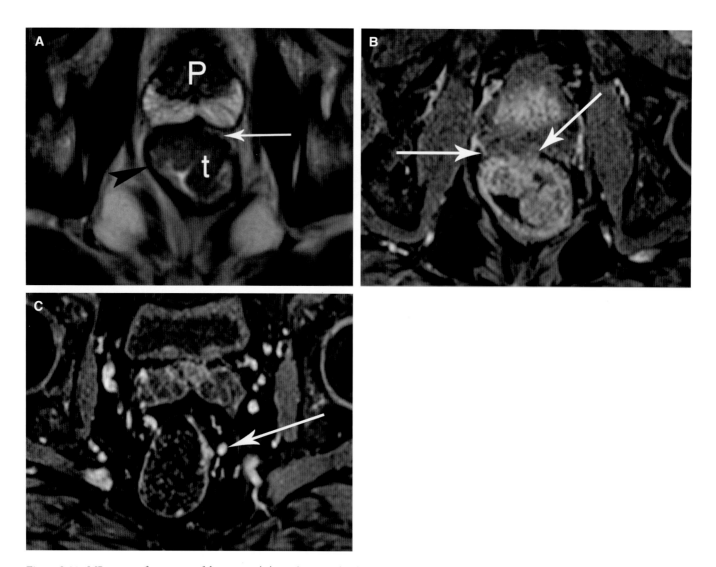

Figure 8.20 *MR staging of carcinoma of the rectum.* (**A**) Axial T2-weighted single-shot FSE/TSE image shows a lobulated tumor (*t*) within the lumen of the rectum. The normal low signal intensity of the muscular layer (*arrowhead*) is disrupted anteriorly (*arrow*), indicating tumor extension through the rectal wall. *P*, prostate. (**B**) Axial image from dynamic post-gadolinium-contrast-enhanced fat-suppressed T1-weighted gradient-echo sequence confirms enhancing tumor extension (*arrows*) through the rectal wall to the prostate. (**C**) Post-contrast-enhanced image at a higher level reveals a small but intensely enhancing lymph node (*arrow*) suspicious for tumor involvement.

often involved. Extracolonic disease may be widespread, with lymphadenopathy and splenic lesions. The findings in the colon are similar to those in the small bowel and stomach. MR shows wall thickening, bulky masses, or multiple nodules.[8]

Colon lipoma is a common benign neoplasm of the colon. The colon is the most common site for GI tract lipoma (65% to 75% of tumors).[24] The cecum and right colon are the most common locations. Most are solitary. Lipomas may serve as a lead point for intussusception. MR findings are diagnostic. The fat in lipomas shows high signal intensity on T1-weighted images and loss of signal on fat-suppressed T1-weighted images. Chemical-shift imaging shows the typical phase-cancellation artifact as a black rim at the fat–water interface on opposed-phase images.

Ulcerative colitis is an idiopathic chronic inflammatory disease limited to the large intestine.[4] The disease is characterized by superficial ulceration of the mucosa. It typically involves the rectum and spreads contiguously, without skip lesions, through the remainder of the colon. The rectosigmoid region is involved in 95% of cases, with pancolitis in 45% of cases. Involvement of the terminal ileum ("backwash ileitis") is rare (5%) and occurs only in the setting of pancolitis. Backwash ileitis is characterized by a patulous ileocecal valve in distinction from the typically narrowed ileocecal valve seen in Crohn's disease. Early-phase disease with superficial edema and hyperemia is not detected by MR. Active disease shows the following progressive changes: thickening of the colon wall due to mucosa and wall edema; wavy configuration of the inner wall due to ulceration; smooth contour of the outer wall; avid enhancement of the thickened wall with intravenous contrast administration (a crucial finding of active disease); loss of haustra, producing a tube-like colon; engorgement of the pericolic vasa recta, appearing as enhancing vascular structures adjacent to the colon; and the occasional presence of pericolic free fluid.

Table 8.1 TNM STAGING OF COLON AND
RECTAL CANCER

STAGE	FINDINGS
T stage	**Size and location of the tumor**
TX	Primary tumor cannot be assessed (information not available)
T0	No evidence of primary tumor
Tis	Carcinoma in situ (preinvasive)
T1	Tumor invades the submucosa
T2	Tumor invades the muscularis propria
T3	Tumor invades through the muscularis propria into immediately contiguous structures
T4a	Tumor penetrates to the surface of the visceral peritoneum
T4b	Tumor directly invades or is adherent to other organs or structures
N stage	**Involvement of regional lymph nodes**
NX	Regional lymph nodes cannot be assessed (information not available)
N0	No regional lymph node metastases
N1a	Metastasis in one regional lymph node
N1b	Metastasis in 2 or 3 regional lymph nodes
N1c	Tumor deposits in the subserosa, mesentery, or nonperitonealized pericolic or perirectal tissues without regional nodal metastasis
N2	Metastasis in 4 or more regional lymph nodes
N2a	Metastasis in 4–6 regional lymph nodes
N2b	Metastasis in 7 or more regional lymph nodes
M stage	**Distant metastases**
M0	No distant metastasis
M1	Distant metastasis
M1a	Metastasis confined to one organ or site
M1b	Metastases in more than one organ or site or in the peritoneum

Adapted with permission from American Joint Committee on Cancer. *AJCC Cancer Staging Manual*, 7th ed. Springer, 2010.

In distinction with Crohn's colitis, the outer wall of the colon remains smooth, and wall thickening is less prominent with ulcerative colitis. Chronic inactive ulcerative colitis shows loss of haustra, narrowing and rigid tube shape of the colon, smooth contours, and absence of contrast enhancement.

Crohn's colitis often represents extension of small bowel disease to involve the colon. However, in up to 35% of cases the colon is involved alone.[4] As in the small bowel, colon involvement is transmural and segmental. Involved colon segments commonly show various stages of activity. On MR active disease shows thickening of the colon wall, usually to a greater extent than is seen with ulcerative colitis; coalescent deep ulcers and mural edema, causing a wavy inner profile to the colon wall on T1- and T2-weighted images; hyperenhancement of the thickened wall, a key finding of active disease; loss of haustration; polypoid lesions and ulceration, producing a cobblestone pattern; engorgement of the pericolonic vasa recta similar to that in ulcerative colitis; fistulas and sinus tracts forming adjacent to the colon, especially in the perirectal region, a finding distinctive to Crohn's colitis; deep confluent ulcers that may be evident in the thickened colon wall; and narrowing and fibrosis of the lumen. Chronic inactive Crohn's colitis shows tubular shape and rigidity of the colon lumen, loss of haustra, fibrofatty pericolic proliferation with fatty infiltration of the colon wall, and absence of contrast enhancement.

Infectious colitis is most often caused by *Clostridium difficile* infection, occurring as a complication of use of broad-spectrum antibiotics. Pseudo-membranous colitis involves any or all of the colon, most commonly in a patchy distribution. Neutropenic enterocolitis (typhlitis) occurs in patients who become neutropenic, most often as a result of treatment for leukemia or lymphoma. Neutropenic colitis characteristically involves only the cecum and ascending colon. *Salmonella*, *Shigella*, and *Escherichia coli* are additional causes of infectious colitis. The MR findings do not differentiate between the various causes of infectious colitis. Typically the bowel wall is thickened and enhances markedly. Pericolic edema and fluid may also be present.

Diverticulitis is primarily a disease of older patients.[19] In Western populations 80% of people over age 80 have diverticula. MR findings (Fig. 8.21) include inflamed diverticulum; thickening of the bowel wall; segmental narrowing of the lumen; and inflammatory infiltration and edema of pericolonic fat. Complications include abscess, sinus tracts, and fistulas (most common to the bladder). Free perforation is rare. Inflammation is evident as high-signal-intensity wall thickening and pericolonic fat infiltration on fat-saturated T2-weighted images. Enhancement of inflamed tissue may be more evident on post-contrast-enhanced images.

PERITONEAL CAVITY

The peritoneal cavity is seldom the primary objective for MR imaging, yet it is present on every MR imaging study of the abdomen or pelvis. Diseases involving the peritoneum are frequently encountered and can be accurately characterized.

MR TECHNIQUES

The peritoneal cavity is imaged using pulse sequences for routine abdominal MR imaging. These generally include breath-held single-shot T2-weighted FSE/TSE images in axial, coronal, and sagittal planes and gradient-echo T1-weighted chemical-shift in-phase and out-of-phase images in the axial plane. A dynamic gadolinium-enhanced fat-suppressed 3D gradient-echo sequence is needed to assess for contrast enhancement, which occurs late with many peritoneal diseases.

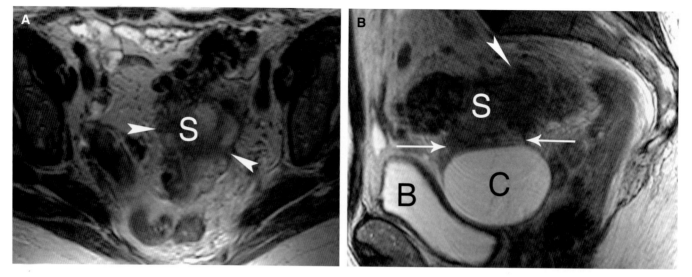

Figure 8.21 *Acute diverticulitis.* Axial (**A**) and sagittal (**B**) T2-weighted FSE/TSE images show a deformed and thick-walled sigmoid colon (*S*) with inflammatory changes extending into the pericolonic fat (*arrowheads*) and involving the bladder (*arrows* in image B). The patient has a large benign ovarian cyst (*C*). *B*, bladder.

ANATOMY

The peritoneal cavity is a complex sac with numerous recesses lined by mesothelium, a specialized type of epithelium. The continuous lining consists of parietal peritoneum, which lines the abdominal wall and covers the retroperitoneum, and the visceral peritoneum, which reflects over the abdominal organs and bowel. The small bowel mesentery extends diagonally across the posterior abdomen from the ligament of Treitz in the left upper quadrant to the cecum in the right lower quadrant. The visceral peritoneum extends from the small bowel mesentery to cover the entire small bowel. Similarly, the mesocolon extends from its attachments to cover the intraperitoneal portions of the colon. The parietal peritoneum defines the posterior aspect of the peritoneal

cavity, separating it from retroperitoneal structures. The greater omentum extends from the greater curvature of the stomach as a double layer of peritoneum enclosing fat and blood vessels, separating the abdominal viscera from the anterior abdominal wall. The greater omentum aids in the loculation of inflammatory processes and serves as fertile ground for implantation of metastases in the peritoneal cavity. The folds of the peritoneum and its extension over the abdominal organs form numerous recesses in which fluid, inflammatory processes, and neoplastic disease may extend. These include the right and left subphrenic spaces, the anterior and posterior subhepatic space (Morison's pouch), the gastrohepatic recess, the lesser peritoneal sac, the paracolic gutters, and the pelvic cul-de-sac. Diseases and fluid may also extend into the

---

Box 8.5 **ESSENTIALS TO REMEMBER**

- Most colon cancer occurs in the rectosigmoid region.

- MR demonstrates the wall of the colon on T2 weighted images with the low-signal-intensity muscularis propria sandwiched between high-signal-intensity submucosa and high-signal-intensity serosa/pericolic fat. Tumor invasion of the colon wall disrupts the low-signal muscle with the high signal intensity of tumor on T2-weighted images and T1-weighted contrast-enhanced images. Tumor extension through the colon wall shows tumor signal in the pericolic fat.

- Lipomas are definitively characterized by low signal intensity on fat-suppressed MR images.

- Active ulcerative colitis shows the colon with mild wall thickening and prominent contrast enhancement.

- Active Crohn's colitis shows marked wall thickening with prominent contrast enhancement.

- Extraluminal findings such as fistulas, sinus tracts, and abscesses differentiate Crohn's colitis from ulcerative colitis.

- Noncontiguous or skip lesions are seen in Crohn's colitis, whereas ulcerative colitis has continuous involvement.

- Backwash ileitis from ulcerative colitis is seen only with pancolitis and is characterized by a patulous ileocecal valve.

- All forms of active colitis show colonic wall thickening and wall enhancement.

numerous recesses formed by the loops of bowel. Study of the peritoneal recesses can be made on multiplanar MR images of the abdomen and pelvis in patients with copious serous ascites.

ABNORMALITIES

Intraperitoneal fluid may consist of transudative ascites, exudative ascites, or blood (hemoperitoneum).[16] Changes in MR signal intensities on various pulse sequences aid in determining the nature of intraperitoneal fluid. Transudative ascites is commonly associated with cirrhosis, hypoproteinemia, and congestive heart failure. Exudative ascites is associated with peritonitis, pancreatitis, bowel perforation, and malignant disease. Hemoperitoneum may result from trauma, surgery, or bleeding disorders. Simple transudates have signal characteristics of water, displaying low signal intensity on T1-weighted sequences, and high signal intensity on T2-weighted sequences (Fig. 8.22). Exudative ascites, having elevated protein content, shows as high signal intensity on T1-weighted sequences and variable high signal intensity on T2-weighted sequences (Fig. 8.23). The appearance of blood in the peritoneal cavity depends on its age and oxidative state. Acute hematoma (less than 48 hours) containing deoxyhemoglobin displays low signal intensity on both T1- and T2-weighted images. Subacute hematoma containing methemoglobin shows as high signal intensity on T1-weighted images. Intracellular methemoglobin shows as low signal intensity on T2-weighted images, while extracellular methemoglobin, found as red blood cells break down, is very high in signal intensity on T2-weighted images. Old hemorrhage containing hemosiderin shows very low

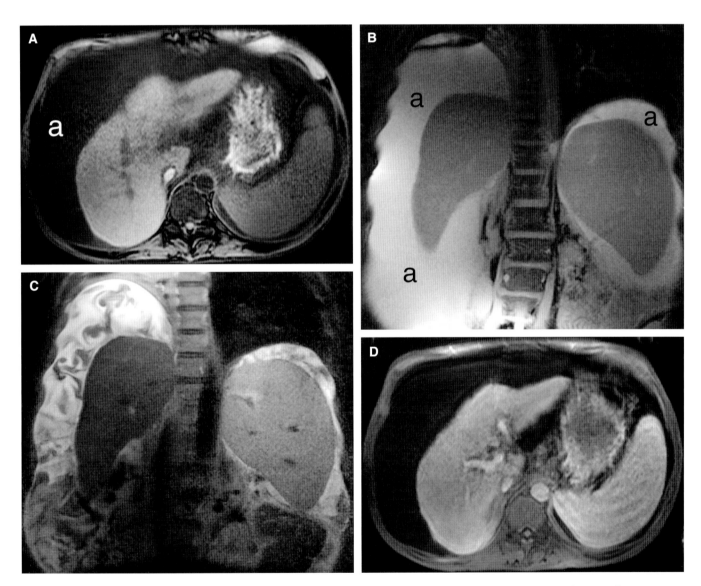

Figure 8.22 *Transudative free intraperitoneal fluid.* (**A**) In a patient with advanced cirrhosis, an axial T1-weighted gradient-echo image demonstrates a large volume of free intraperitoneal fluid (*a*), low in signal intensity, extending freely into peritoneal recesses. (**B**) Coronal SSFP gradient-echo image demonstrates uniform high signal intensity of the intraperitoneal fluid (*a*). (**C**) Coronal T2-weighted single-shot FSE/TSE image shows swirls of low signal intensity caused by fluid motion within the high-signal-intensity fluid (see Chapter 2 for further explanation about the fluid appearance with this pulse sequence). (**D**) Post-gadolinium-contrast-enhanced T1-weighted gradient-echo image shows uniform low signal intensity of the intraperitoneal fluid without enhancement of the peritoneal lining. Findings from the multiple MR sequences indicate that the fluid is transudative ascites.

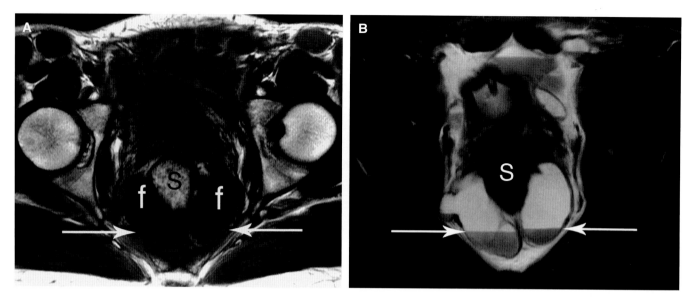

Figure 8.23 *Loculated exudative intraperitoneal fluid.* (**A**) Pockets of intraperitoneal fluid (*f*) extend to the pelvis and around the sigmoid colon (*S*) on this axial T1-weighted image. The fluid shows layering (*arrows*) with lower-signal-intensity fluid above dependent layering higher-signal-intensity fluid. Increased signal from fluid on T1-weighted images is indicative of increased protein concentration or blood in the fluid. The fluid causes mass effect on the sigmoid colon, providing evidence that the fluid is loculated. (**B**) Axial T2-weighted image at the same level shows the fluid layering (*arrows*), with high-signal-intensity fluid above and lower-signal-intensity fluid layering below. Summary of findings from the MR sequences indicates the fluid is exudative ascites or contains subacute hemorrhage with methemoglobin within red blood cells (intracellular methemoglobin). *S*, sigmoid colon. The patient has a Foley catheter in the bladder.

signal intensity on both T1- and T2-weighted images. Exudative ascites and hemoperitoneum are commonly associated with contrast enhancement of the peritoneal lining.

Fluid motion resulting from cardiac contractions, respiration, bowel peristalsis, arterial pulsations, and muscle activity can cause flow-related changes in signal intensity of fluid within the peritoneal cavity. Signal enhancement may be evident in ascites on T1-weighted gradient-echo images, causing transudative ascites to appear high instead of low in signal intensity. Similarly, fluid motion may show as swirls of low signal intensity within transudative ascites on single shot FSE/TSE T2-weighted images (Fig. 8.22).

Pneumoperitoneum may be a difficult diagnosis on MR. Often a careful assessment of the images is required to detect the signal void of air pockets in the non-dependent peritoneal recesses. Gradient-echo sequences are the most sensitive for depicting small volumes of air accentuated by susceptibility artifacts from rapidly dephasing magnetization.[16]

Pseudomyxoma peritonei ("jelly belly") refers to gelatinous ascites that occurs as a result of intraperitoneal spread of mucin-producing cells. It may caused by rupture of appendiceal mucocele, intraperitoneal spread of benign or mucinous cysts of the ovary, or mucinous adenocarcinoma of the colon or rectum. The thick deposits coat the peritoneal surfaces and scallop or indent the contours of involved abdominal organs. Post-contrast-enhanced MR imaging shows enhancement of thickened peritoneum.

Peritoneal metastatic disease most commonly occurs with peritoneal seeding by ovarian carcinoma, colon or gastric adenocarcinoma, or pancreatic carcinoma. Metastases are usually multiple, may be cystic or solid, large, small, or manifest only by focal peritoneal thickening. The lesions typically show low

to intermediate signal intensity on T1-weighted images and intermediate to high signal intensity on T2-weighted images (Fig. 8.24). Post-contrast enhanced fat-suppressed images show lesion enhancement, which increases conspicuity. All peritoneal surfaces must be carefully inspected to detect small lesions. Tumor implantation on the greater omentum produces "omental cake," seen as nodular thickening of the omentum displacing bowel away from the anterior abdominal wall.

Peritoneal mesothelioma is a rare, highly aggressive primary malignancy of the peritoneum typically associated with

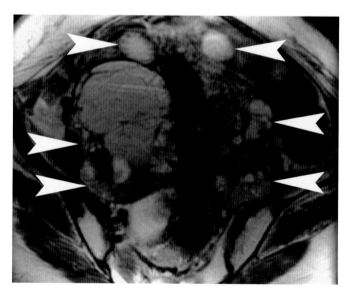

Figure 8.24 *Peritoneal metastatic disease.* Axial T2-weighted image shows widespread peritoneal implants (*arrowheads*) of ovarian carcinoma.

asbestos exposure.[25] The tumor may be a localized mass or may produce sheet-like or nodular thickening of the peritoneum. Tumor may also be cystic. The tumor appearance on MR overlaps with that of peritoneal metastatic disease.

Abscesses occur commonly in the abdomen and pelvis as a result of inflammatory disease (appendicitis, diverticulitis, pancreatitis, Crohn's disease), surgery (especially of the intestinal tract, pancreas, or biliary system), or trauma (infection of hematomas). Abscesses appear on MR as focal fluid collections that are usually round or oval and show mass effect by displacing adjacent structures (Fig. 8.25). Fluid within the abscess shows widely variable signal intensities depending upon its nature (containing pus, blood, cellular debris, bile, bowel contents, etc.). Abscesses may contain air, fluid layers, necrotic tissue, and foreign bodies. The primary MR finding that identifies a fluid collection as a potential abscess is rim enhacement of the collection after intavenous gadolinium contrast material administration. Fat suppression serves to highlight contrast enhancement. The diagnosis of an absecess is confirmed by fluid aspiration and drainage.

SPLEEN

The spleen is affected by a wide range of diseases that often overlap in appearance on imaging studies. MR imaging maximizes tissue characterization to improve the specificity of imaging diagnosis.

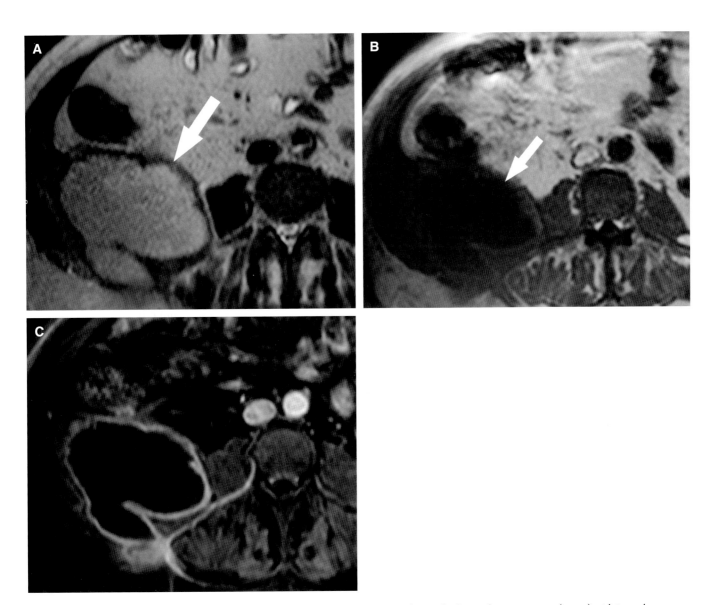

Figure 8.25 *Abdominal abscess.* (**A**) Axial T2-weighted single-shot FSE/TSE image shows a high-signal-intensity mass (*arrow*) with irregular low-signal-intensity rim. (**B**) Axial T1-weighted gradient-echo image at the same level shows the rim of the mass (*arrow*) to be of intermediate low signal intensity, while the contents are very low in signal intensity. (**C**) Post-gadolinium-contrast-enhanced T1-weighted image with fat saturation shows avid enhancement of the rim of the mass. Findings of the multiple MR sequences are highly suggestive of abscess. This abscess, confirmed by aspiration and drainage, occurred as a complication of perforation of the colon during colonoscopy.

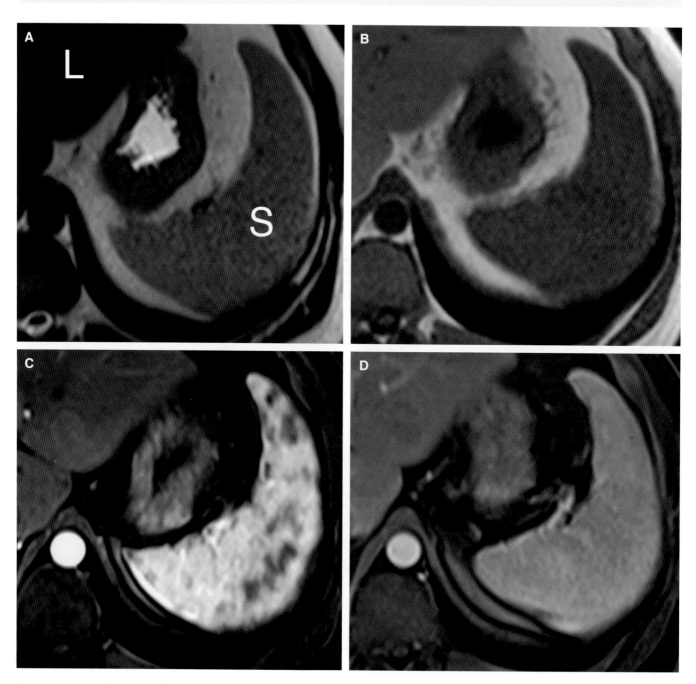

Figure 8.26 *Normal spleen.* Axial T2-weighted single-shot FSE/TSE (**A**) and T1-weighted (**B**) gradient-echo images demonstrate the normal spleen (*S*). Note the signal intensity of the spleen compared to that of the liver (*L*). (**C**) Early image from a dynamic post-gadolinium-contrast-enhanced T1-weighted fat-suppressed gradient-echo sequence shows the expected arcuate pattern of early splenic enhancement caused by slow flow of the contrast material through the red and white pulp. The spleen enhances maximally approximately 90 seconds sooner than the liver because 70% of the blood supply of the liver arrives via the portal vein, which fills with contrast material only after it perfuses the spleen and GI tract. (**D**) Mid-phase delayed image from the dynamic post-contrast-enhanced sequence shows uniform enhancement of the spleen and increasing enhancement of the liver compared to image C.

MR TECHNIQUES

MR imaging of the spleen uses standard pulse sequence techniques used for routine MR abdominal imaging. Breath-hold single-shot fast T2-weighted FSE/TSE sequences are obtained in the axial, coronal, and sagittal planes. Breath-hold T1-weighted chemical-shift in-phase and out-of-phase sequences are acquired in the axial plane. Dynamic pre- and post-contrast gadolinium-enhanced fat-saturated T1-weighted gradient-echo images are acquired to assess vascularity.

ANATOMY

The spleen is the body's largest lymphoid organ, occupying the left upper quadrant of the abdomen just below the diaphragm, posterior and lateral to the stomach. The spleen sequesters abnormal or aged red blood cells, white blood cells, and platelets, and serves as a reservoir for red blood cells. The diaphragmatic surface of the spleen is smooth and convex, conforming to the shape of the diaphragm. The visceral surface has concavities for the stomach, kidney, colon, and pancreas. Spleen size varies with age, nutrition, and hydration. The spleen is relatively large in children, reaching adult size by age 15. The average spleen dimensions in adults are 12 cm in length, 7 cm in width, and 3 to 4 cm in thickness. In older adults, the spleen progressively decreases in size with age. The splenic artery and vein course with the pancreas to the splenic hilum, where they divide into multiple branches. The splenic arteries are end arteries without anastomoses or collateral supply. As a result, occlusion of the splenic artery or its branches produces infarction of the spleen. On MR the spleen signal intensity is lower than that of hepatic parenchyma on T1-weighted images and higher than that of liver parenchyma on T2-weighted images (Fig. 8.26).[26]

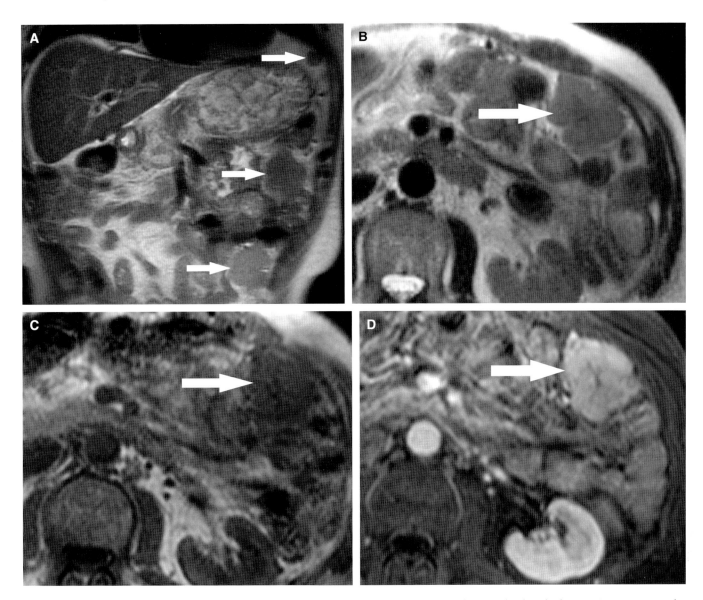

Figure 8.27 *Splenosis.* (**A**) In a patient with a history of splenectomy for traumatic injury, a coronal T2-weighted single-shot FSE/TSE image reveals several nodules (*arrows*) in the peritoneal cavity. Axial T2-weighted (**B**) and T1-weighted (**C**) images show the lobulated nodule (*arrows*) in the mid-left abdomen. (**D**) Post-contrast-enhanced T1-weighted fat-suppressed image shows avid enhancement of the nodule (*arrow*). A subsequent radionuclide sulfur colloid scan showed colloid uptake in each of the nodules, confirming the presence of reticuloendothelial cells in splenic tissue. Further confirmation of functioning splenic tissue was provided by a peripheral blood smear that showed the absence of Howell-Jolly bodies, indicating the presence of functioning splenic tissue.

Following intravenous contrast material injection, the enhancement pattern of the spleen reflects the normal rapid direct circulation of the white pulp, as well as the slow-flow, filtering circulation of the red pulp, which functions to clear aged and damaged blood cells. During the arterial phase contrast enhancement of the spleen appears as alternating bands of high and low density, the arciform or "tiger stripe" enhancement pattern. Delayed-contrast-enhanced images show homogeneous enhancement of the splenic parenchyma.

ABNORMALITIES

Splenomegaly is a frequent finding with many causes, most commonly including portal hypertension; portal or splenic vein thrombosis; myeloproliferative disorders; infection, including infectious mononucleosis, malaria, and AIDS; and infiltrative disorders such as Gaucher's disease.[26] The diagnosis of splenomegaly can be made by subjective assessment of spleen bulk. Any dimension that exceeds 14 cm is indicative of splenomegaly (see Fig. 8.29). Coronal images showing the spleen larger than the liver indicate splenomegaly.

Accessory spleens are detached nodules of normal splenic tissue found in 10% of the population. Most are located in close proximity to spleen, often near the splenic hilum (see Fig. 8.29). Signal intensity on MR imaging is identical to that of the spleen.

Splenosis occurs when splenic tissue implants in ectopic locations on peritoneal surfaces as a result of traumatic splenic rupture. The ectopic deposits may be found anywhere in the peritoneal cavity (Fig. 8.27). Occasionally they can be found

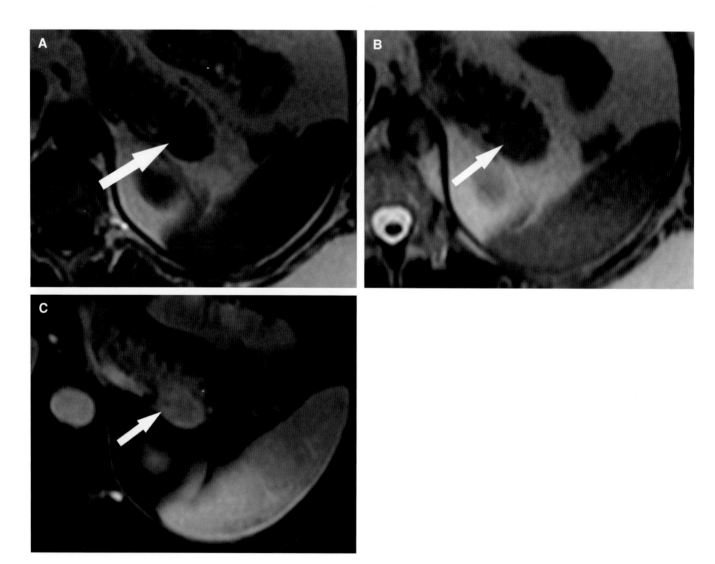

Figure 8.28 *Splenic rest in the pancreas.* (**A**) Axial T1-weighted gradient-echo image shows a well-defined nodule (*arrow*) in the tail of the pancreas showing signal intensity identical to that of the spleen. (**B**) T2-weighted single-shot FSE/TSE image also shows that the nodule (*arrow*) displays similar signal intensity as the spleen. (**C**) Images from dynamic gadolinium-contrast-enhanced T1-weighted fat-suppressed gradient-echo sequence show that the enhancement pattern of the nodule (*arrow*) is the same as that of the spleen. Surgical pathology confirmed a splenic rest in the pancreatic tail.

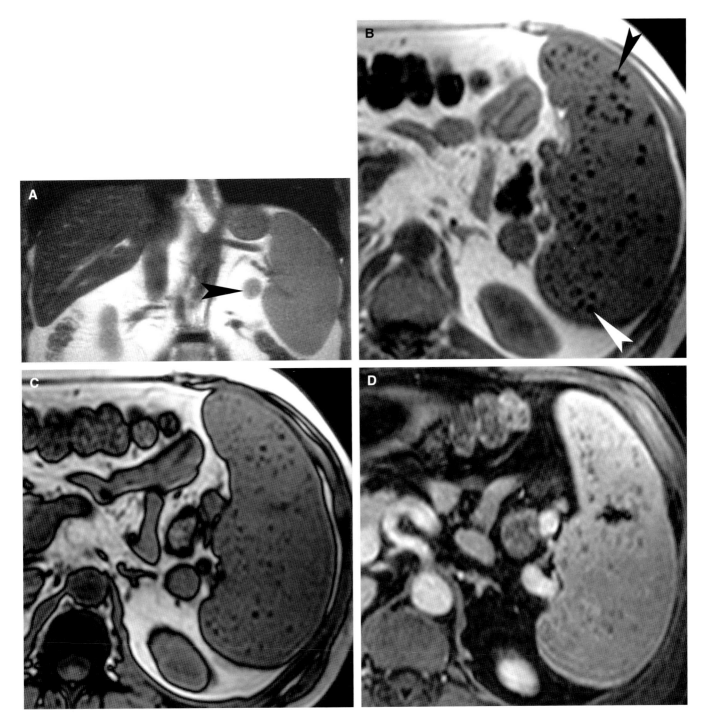

Figure 8.29 *Gamna-Gandy bodies.* (**A**) T2-weighted single-shot FSE/TSE coronal image in a patient with cirrhosis shows splenomegaly without focal splenic abnormalities. A hypertrophied splenule (*arrowhead*) is also present. T1-weighted in-phase (TE 4.6 ms) (**B**) and out-of-phase (TE 2.3 ms) (**C**) gradient-echo images show innumerable tiny foci (*arrowheads* in image B) of signal void throughout the spleen. These foci are deposits of hemosiderin resulting from tiny hemorrhages in the spleen caused by portal hypertension. Note that the hemosiderin-containing nodules cause susceptibility artifact, which is why they appear more prominent and larger on the in-phase gradient-echo image obtained with longer TE than the out-of-phase image obtained with shorter TE. (See Chapters 1 and 2 for further explanation of susceptibility.) (**D**) Post-gadolinium-contrast-enhanced T1-weighted image shows no enhancement of the lesions.

in the tail of the pancreas (Fig. 8.28). Fragments of spleen tissue regenerate and increase in size in the absence of the spleen. The splenules vary in size and shape. MR imaging shows the expected signal intensity of normal splenic tissue. Radionuclide scans using technetium sulfur colloid can be used to confirm functioning splenic tissue noninvasively.

Gamna-Gandy bodies, also called siderotic nodules, are tiny foci of hemorrhage that occur in the spleen as a result of portal hypertension. The microhemorrhages result in focal deposits of hemosiderin, seen best on MR as numerous tiny very-low-signal-intensity nodules on T1-weighted gradient-echo with relatively long TE (T2*-weighted images) (Fig. 8.29). Signal intensity is low because of the susceptibility artifact from hemosiderin. They do not enhance.

Genetic (primary, idiopathic) hemochromatosis is a disorder of excessive absorption of iron from the GI tract resulting in excessive iron deposition in the liver, pancreas, heart, joints, and skin. Excess iron is stored in the organ parenchyma, not in reticuloendothelial cells. Absence of involvement of the spleen is a diagnostic feature of primary hemochromatosis. ***Secondary (transfusional) hemochromatosis*** results from heavy iron stores that occur because of a large number of blood transfusions. Excessive iron from transfusions is stored in the reticuloendothelial system, and thus the spleen is involved. Iron is stored in Kupffer cells in both the liver and the spleen. Iron overload within abdominal organs results in substantially decreased signal on T2- and T2*-weighted images (Fig. 8.30). Mild forms of iron overload result in decreased organ signal intensity on gradient-echo and T2-weighted images, with T1-weighted spin-echo images being relatively unaffected. As iron deposition increases T1-weighted spin-echo images may also show decreased signal intensity in involved organs.

Spleen hemangioma is the most common primary neoplasm of the spleen, present in 14% of the population. Similar to liver hemangiomas the lesion consists of vascular channels of variable size lined by endothelium. On MR the lesions are

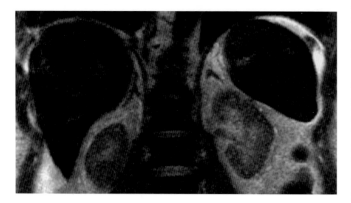

Figure 8.30 *Secondary hemochromatosis.* Coronal T2-weighted single-shot FSE/TSE image shows marked decrease in signal intensity of both the liver and spleen. Normal signal intensity of the liver and spleen is shown in Figure 8.26A. Signal loss results from excessive iron deposition in the reticuloendothelial cells of the liver and spleen resulting from a large number of blood transfusions that the patient received over several years.

typically hypointense to iso-intense on T1-weighted images and show high signal intensity relative to the spleen on T2-weighted images (Fig. 8.31). Three enhancement patterns have been described:

- Peripheral enhancement that progresses to complete uniform enhancement. This enhancement pattern is similar to that of liver hemangiomas but the delayed progressive peripheral nodular enhancement is less apparent.[27]

- Peripheral enhancement that progresses centrally but spares enhancement of a central low-signal-intensity scar.

- Immediate complete enhancement with persistence of enhancement on delayed contrast-enhanced images. This pattern is most common with small lesions.

Lesions are commonly multiple. A central scar resulting from focal chronic thrombosis shows as low signal intensity on T2-weighted images. Scars enhance minimally or not at all.

Spleen hamartoma is a benign mass of disorganized splenic tissue. Most are solitary and discovered as incidental findings. Lesions are well defined and spherical and closely follow the signal intensity of normal splenic tissue on MR. Post-contrast images most reliably demonstrate the lesions, which enhance early, heterogeneously, and diffusely. Enhancement frequently persists into the delayed phase (Fig. 8.32). The tumor may contain central foci, which do not enhance.[27]

Angiosarcoma, though rare, is the most common primary splenic malignancy. The tumor is aggressive, and metastasizes early and widely. Imaging appearance includes solitary mass, multiple splenic masses, or diffuse splenic enlargement with parenchymal replacement (Fig. 8.33). Coarse calcifications may be present, seen as signal voids on all MR sequences. The tumor is heterogeneous on T1-weighted images, with areas of high signal due to hemorrhage and low signal due to iron deposition. T2-weighted images are similar, with high signal intensity in necrotic areas and low signal intensity in foci of iron deposition. Post-contrast-enhanced images show marked hypervascularity with avid but very heterogeneous enhancement.[28]

Metastases to the spleen are frequent but often microscopic and are not detected by imaging. The most common metastases to be visualized arise from melanoma and lung, breast, ovary, and gastric carcinoma. Lesions are usually multiple but are occasionally solitary masses. Metastases are often iso-intense to spleen and may be overlooked on both T1- and T2-weighted images. Melanoma metastases contain melanin, which is paramagnetic, causing characteristic high signal intensity on T1-weighted images. Dynamic post-contrast-enhanced images significantly increase lesion conspicuity as the metastases enhance to a lesser or greater degree than the surrounding splenic parenchyma.

Lymphoma is the most common malignant tumor to involve the spleen. The morphology of splenic lymphoma includes diffuse splenomegaly, multiple masses of varying size,

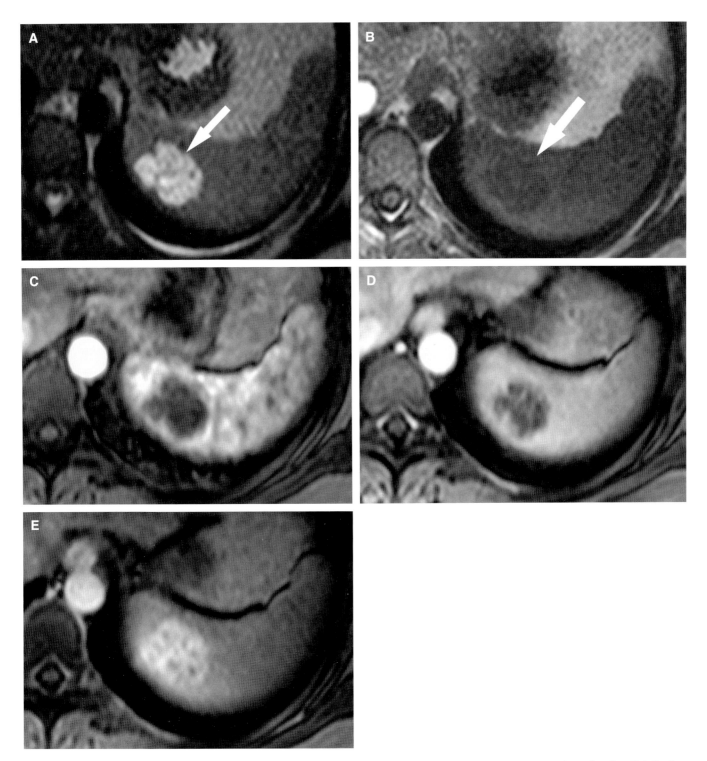

Figure 8.31 *Spleen Hemangioma.* (**A**) T2-weighted single-shot FSE/TSE axial image shows a high-signal-intensity mass (*arrow*) with well-defined nodular margins. (**B**) T1-weighted axial gradient-echo image shows that the lesion (*arrow*) displays slightly lower signal intensity than the spleen parenchyma. (**C**) Early image from dynamic post-contrast-enhanced T1-weighted fat-suppressed gradient-echo sequence shows early nodular peripheral enhancement. Note that the discontinuous peripheral nodular enhancement typical of liver hemangiomas is not evident. In distinction with the liver, early spleen enhancement is non-uniform. (**D**) Mid-phase post-contrast-enhanced image shows slow progressive enhancement of the lesion. The spleen is now uniformly enhanced. (**E**) Delayed post-contrast-enhanced image shows further progression of enhancement of the lesion.

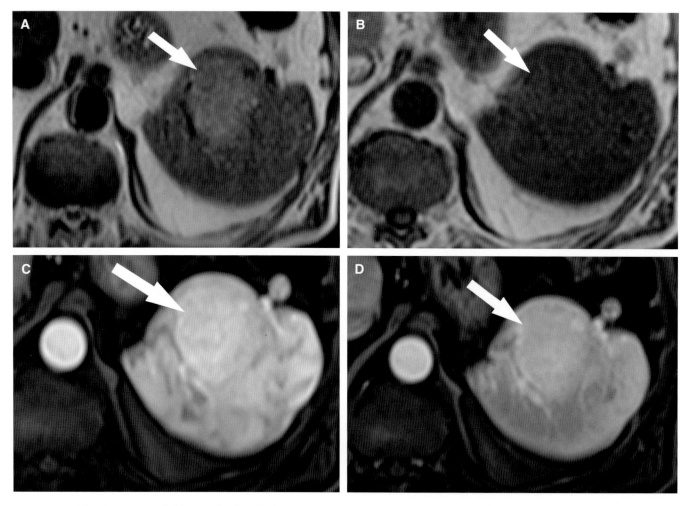

Figure 8.32 *Spleen hamartoma.* (**A**) T2-weighted single-shot FSE/TSE image shows a splenic mass (*arrow*) that is slightly higher in signal intensity than the splenic parenchyma. (**B**) Axial T1-weighted gradient-echo image at the same level shows that the mass (*arrow*) is entirely isointense to splenic parenchyma. (**C**) Early image from a dynamic post-contrast-enhanced T1-weighted gradient-echo sequence with fat suppression shows early intense enhancement of the mass (*arrow*). (**D**) Delayed post-contrast-enhanced image shows persisting enhancement (*arrow*). Because the patient had a history of malignancy elsewhere, fine-needle aspiration and core needle biopsies of the lesion were performed to exclude metastatic disease. The biopsies yielded only normal spleen cells, consistent with hamartoma. Two-year follow-up MR revealed no changes in the lesion.

miliary nodules resembling infection, a large solitary mass (Fig. 8.34), and contiguous invasion of the spleen from extrasplenic lymphomatous masses. On T1- and T2-weighted images lymphoma is commonly iso-intense to the splenic parenchyma. Low signal intensity is the most frequent finding to reveal the lesions. Dynamic post-contrast-enhanced images are the key to detection, as the lesions enhance less than splenic parenchyma on early acquisitions but become iso-intense on delayed images. Splenomegaly may be the only MR finding.

Splenic lymphangiomas are relatively rare benign tumors composed of small lymphatic channels showing cystic and fusiform dilatation of varying degrees.[28] Small lesions are asymptomatic and are discovered as incidental findings (Fig. 8.35). Large lesions may compress adjacent structures and cause pain, bleeding, or consumptive coagulopathy. The spleen may be one of the many organs involved by lymphangiomatosis. MR shows the lesions to be hypointense to

splenic parenchyma on T1-weighted images and hyperintense, with a multiloculated appearance, on T2-weighted images. Fibrous connective tissue septations enhance on late-phase post-contrast enhanced images.

Splenic infarction occurs most often in the setting of splenomegaly or trauma.[26] Embolus associated with endocarditis or valvular heart disease is an additional cause. While wedge-shaped is the classic description, the most diagnostic findings are extension of the lesion to the splenic capsule and lack of enhancement after contrast material administration (Fig. 8.36). T1-weighted images show variable signal depending upon the presence or absence of hemorrhage. T2-weighted images usually show high signal intensity. The lesions are commonly multiple.

Splenic cysts have a variety of etiologies. Most common is the post-traumatic cyst, which develops in intrasplenic areas of post-traumatic hemorrhage. Calcification showing signal void in the wall is common. Pancreatic pseudo-cysts track

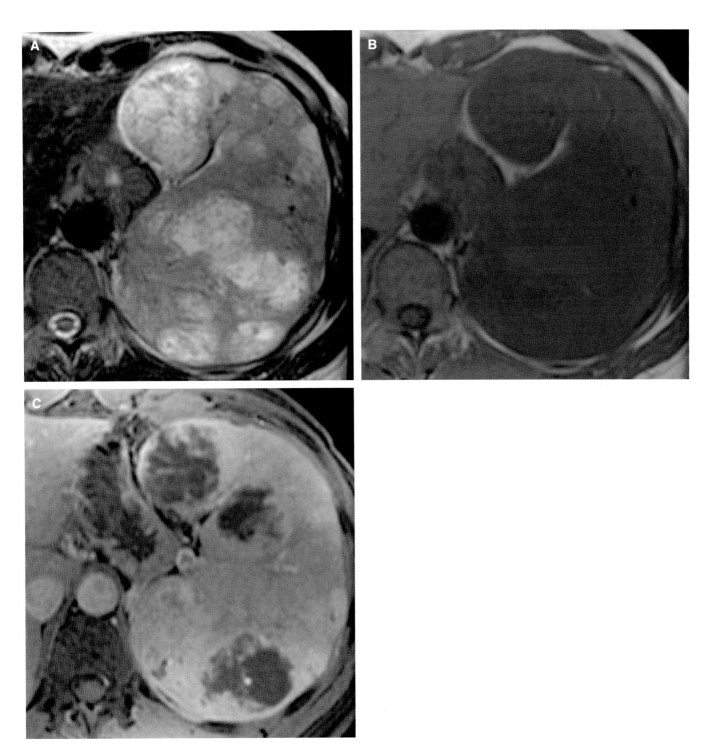

Figure 8.33 *Spleen angiosarcoma.* (**A**) Axial T2-weighted single-shot FSE/TSE image shows marked splenomegaly, with numerous nodules of variable signal intensity completely replacing the splenic parenchyma. (**B**) Axial T1-weighted gradient-echo image shows splenomegaly with only slight heterogeneity to the signal intensity of the splenic parenchyma. (**C**) Post-gadolinium contrast-enhanced T1-weighted image demonstrates intense, markedly heterogeneous contrast enhancement. Splenectomy confirmed angiosarcoma.

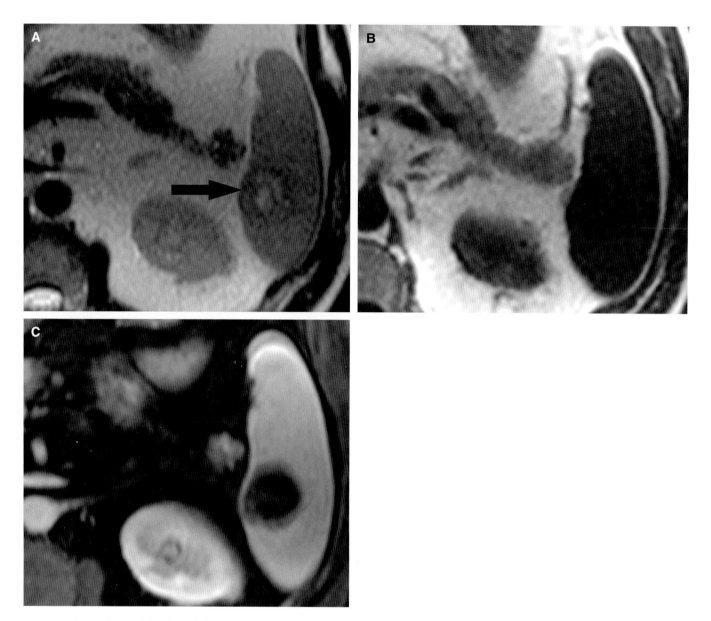

Figure 8.34 *Lymphoma of the spleen.* (**A**) Axial T2-weighted single-shot FSE/TSE image shows a mass (*arrow*) in the spleen displaying areas of high and intermediate signal intensity. The spleen is not enlarged. (**B**) Axial T1-weighted gradient-echo image at the same location fails to show the mass. (**C**) Dynamic post-gadolinium-contrast-enhanced T1-weighted image shows uniform enhancement of the spleen and lack of enhancement of the mass, which proved to be lymphoma.

along the splenic hilum to subcapsular locations in the spleen in association with acute pancreatitis. Congenital splenic cysts are epithelium-lined and appear simple. Abscesses usually occur from hematogenous spread of infection. The resulting fluid collection is complex and may contain air. Microabscesses usually occur in immune-compromised patients and are typically small (5 to 10 mm) and numerous. Spleen hydatid cysts generally occur only in the presence of hydatid disease else-

where in the lung or liver. Chronic hydatid cysts have ring-like calcifications. The cysts generally show with low signal intensity on T1-weighted images unless they contain acute hemorrhage, which increases the signal intensity. T2-weighted images show very high signal intensity. Post-contrast-enhanced images may show enhancement of the wall but not of the cyst contents. Diagnosis is made by correlation with clinical and associated imaging findings.[29]

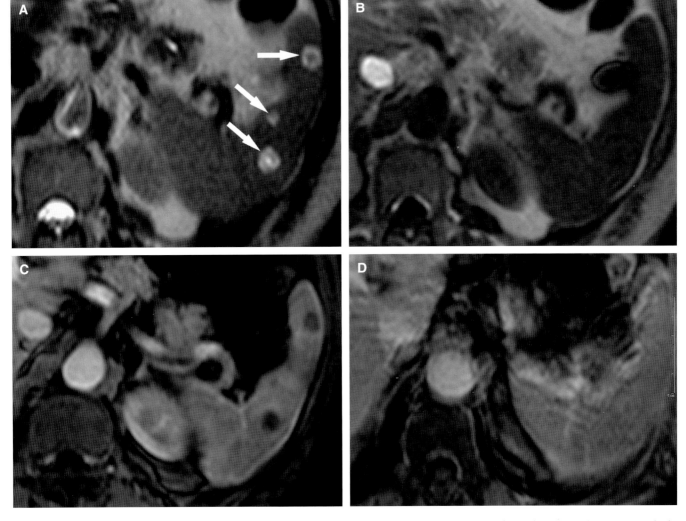

Figure 8.35 *Splenic lymphangioma.* (**A**) Axial T2-weighted single-shot FSE/TSE image shows three nodules (*arrows*) displaying heterogeneous high signal intensity. (**B**) The nodules are not evident on the T1-weighted gradient-echo image. (**C**) No enhancement is evident on early-phase image from dynamic post-gadolinium-contrast-enhanced T1-weighted fat-suppressed sequence. (**D**) On late-phase post-contrast-enhanced image the lesions are iso-enhancing with splenic parenchyma. Because of a history of colon cancer, the patient underwent splenectomy to exclude metastatic disease. Pathology revealed only lymphangioma.

Box 8.7 **ESSENTIALS TO REMEMBER**

- Many splenic lesions show common imaging characteristics. Lesions are differentiated by careful consideration of all MR findings and the clinical presentation.

- Intravenous gadolinium contrast material administration is essential to both detection and characterization of many splenic lesions.

- Splenomegaly is present when any splenic dimension exceeds 14 cm.

- Splenic infarctions are characterized as linear or triangular areas of low signal intensity on T2-weighted images extending to the splenic capsule and by lack of enhancement after contrast administration.

- While lymphoma is the most common malignancy involving the spleen, lesions may not be evident without administration of intravenous contrast material, and the only finding may be splenomegaly.

- Splenic cysts have many etiologies, determined by correlation with the clinical presentation and medical history.

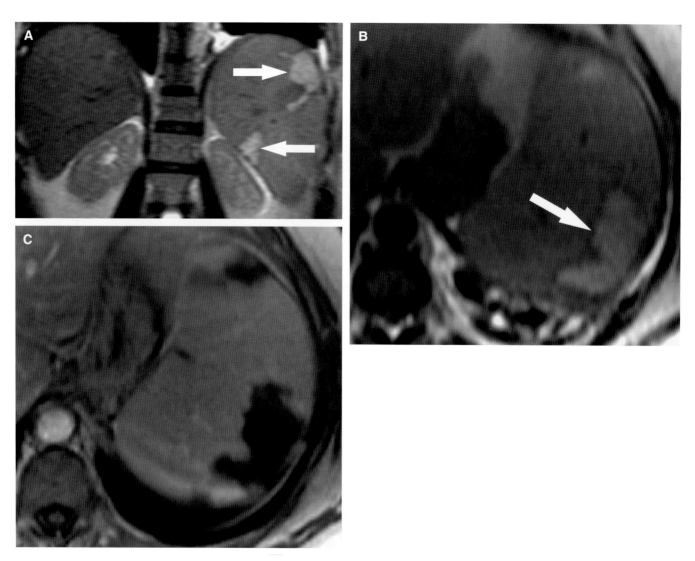

Figure 8.36 *Splenic infarctions.* (**A**) Coronal T2-weighted single-shot FSE/TSE image demonstrates two high-signal-intensity splenic lesions (*arrows*) abutting the capsule of the spleen. (**B**) Axial T2-weighted image shows the larger (*arrow*) of the two lesions, confirming extension of the lesion to the splenic capsule. (**C**) Image from dynamic post-contrast-enhanced T1-weighted gradient-echo sequence shows no enhancement of the lesions. The findings are consistent with splenic infarctions.

REFERENCES

1. Tolan DJM, Greenhalgh R, Zealley IA, et al. MR enterographic manifestations of small bowel Crohn disease. *Radiographics.* 2010;30:367–384.
2. Fidler JL, Guimaraes L, Einstein DM. MR imaging of the small bowel. *Radiographics.* 2009;29:1811–1825.
3. Thornton E, Morrin MM, Yee J. Current status of MR colography. *Radiographics.* 2010;30:201–218.
4. Rimola J, Rodriguez S, Garcia-Bosch O, et al. Role of 3.0-T MR colonography in evaluation of inflammatory bowel disease. *Radiographics.* 2009;29:701–719.
5. Martin DR, Danrad R, Hermann K, et al. Magnetic resonance imaging of the gastrointestinal tract. *Top Magn Reson Imaging.* 2005;16:77–98.
6. Sandrasegaran K, Rajesh A, Rydberg J, et al. Gastrointestinal stromal tumors: clinical, radiologic, and pathologic features. *AJR Am J Roentgenol.* 2005;184:803–811.
7. Levy AD, Remotti HE, Thompson WM, et al. Gastrointestinal stromal tumors: radiologic features with pathologic correlation. *Radiographics.* 2003;23:283–304.
8. Ghai S, Pattison J, Gahai S, et al. Primary gastrointestinal lymphoma: spectrum of imaging findings with pathologic correlation. *Radiographics.* 2007;27:1371–1388.
9. Lee NK, Kim SH, Jeon TY, et al. Complications of congenital and developmental abnormalities of the gastrointestinal tract in adolescents and adults: evaluation with multimodality imaging. *Radiographics.* 2010;30:1489–1507.
10. Leyendecker JR, Bloomfeld RS, DeSantis DJ, et al. MR enterography in the management of patients with Crohn disease. *Radiographics.* 2009;29:1827–1846.
11. Sinha R, Rajiah P, Murphy P, et al. Utility of high-resolution MR imaging in demonstrating transmural pathologic changes in Crohn disease. *Radiographics.* 2009;29:1847–1867.
12. Cronin CG, Lohan DG, DeLappe E, et al. Duodenal abnormalities at MR small-bowel follow-through. *AJR Am J Roentgenol.* 2008;191:1082–1092.
13. Van Weyenberg SJB, Meijerink MR, Jacobs MAJM, et al. MR enteroclysis in the diagnosis of small-bowel neoplasms. *Radiology.* 2010;254:765–773.
14. Lohan DG, Alhajeri AN, Cronin CG, et al. MR enterography of small-bowel lymphoma: potential for suggestion of histologic

subtype and the presence of underlying celiac disease. *AJR Am J Roentgenol.* 2008;190:287–293.

15. Tkacz JN, Anderson SA, Soto J. MR imaging in gastrointestinal emergencies. *Radiographics.* 2009;29:1767–1780.

16. Elsayes KM, Staveteig PT, Narra VR, et al. MRI of the peritoneum: spectrum of abnormalities. *AJR Am J Roentgenol.* 2006;186:1368–1379.

17. Azizi L, Balu M, Belkacem A, et al. MRI features of mesenteric desmoid tumors in familial adenomatous polyposis. *AJR Am J Roentgenol.* 2005;184:1128–1135.

18. Baldisserotto M, Valduga SG, Sotero Da Cunha CFJ. MR imaging evaluation of the normal appendix in children and adolescents. *Radiology.* 2008;249:278–284.

19. Heverhagen JT, Klose K. MR imaging for acute lower abdominal and pelvic pain. *Radiographics.* 2009;29:1781–1796.

20. Pedrosa I, Zeiku EA, Levine D, Rofsky NM. MR imaging of acute right lower quadrant pain in pregnant and nonpregnant patients. *Radiographics.* 2007;27:721–753.

21. Pickhardt PJ, Levy AD, Rohrmann CA, Jr, Kende AI. Primary neoplasms of the appendix: radiologic spectrum of disease with pathologic correlation. *Radiographics.* 2003;23:645–662.

22. Dresen RC, Kusters M, Daniels-Gooszen AW, et al. Absence of tumor invasion into pelvic structures in locally recurrent rectal cancer: prediction with preoperative MR imaging. *Radiology.* 2010;256:143–150.

23. Kim DJ, Kim JH, Lim JS, et al. Restaging of rectal cancer with MR imaging after concurrent chemotherapy and radiation therapy. *Radiographics.* 2010;30:503–516.

24. Thompson WM. Imaging and findings of lipomas of the gastrointestinal tract. *AJR Am J Roentgenol.* 2005;184:1163–1171.

25. Levy AD, Arnaiz J, Shaw JC, Sobin LH. Primary peritoneal tumors: imaging features with pathologic correlation. *Radiographics.* 2008;28:583–607.

26. Elsayes KM, Narra VR, Mukundan G, et al. MR imaging of the spleen: spectrum of abnormalities. *Radiographics.* 2005;25:967–982.

27. Ramani M, Reinhold C, Semelka RC, et al. Splenic hemangiomas and hamartomas: MR imaging characteristics of 28 lesions. *Radiology.* 1997;202:166–172.

28. Abbott RM, Levy AD, Aguilera NS, et al. Primary vascular neoplasms of the spleen: radiologic-pathologic correlation. *Radiographics.* 2004;24:1137–1163.

29. Urritia M, Mergo PJ, Ros LH, et al. Cystic lesions of the spleen: radiologic-pathologic correlation. *Radiographics.* 1996;16:107–129.

9.

GYNECOLOGIC MR IMAGING

Gia A. DeAngelis, MD

MR of the female pelvis affords superior soft tissue resolution and tissue characterization, multiplanar capacity, adequate field of view, and detection of vascularization. Its critical indications include detection and assessment of the extent of myometrial invasion and extrauterine extent of uterine and cervical malignancies, characterization of adnexal masses, and evaluation of congenital anomalies. Common indications for gynecologic MR are:

- Congenital anomalies: MR provides the gold standard for structural evaluation. It is particularly useful for assessing obstructed anomalies and vaginal agenesis in the prepubertal female patient.

- Endometrial cancer: MR provides high contrast between neoplasia and the myometrium and gives detailed information regarding pelvic lymph nodes. MR is used to identify reproductive-aged women with superficial myometrial invasion for fertility-sparing surgery. It is employed to select women for vaginal hysterectomy or intracavitary uterine brachytherapy and determine possible radiation therapy fields in patients who, for medical or surgical reasons, cannot undergo the standard surgical approach.

- Cervical cancer: MR provides high tissue contrast between the malignancy and the bladder base, the rectal wall, and the parametria and is well suited for detecting abnormal pelvic lymph nodes. This information is used for

selecting patients for surgical treatment or radiation therapy.

- Endometrial carcinoma - intrauterine mass: MR is used to determine the origin and extent of intrauterine masses and to differentiate benign leiomyomas from lesions that require further evaluation.

- Endometrial carcinoma - endometrium: MR depicts the endometrium in patients with pain or bleeding when ultrasound evaluation is nondiagnostic.

- Adenomyosis: MR can diagnose adenomyosis and differentiates leiomyomas from adenomyosis. Each condition requires different treatment.

- Adnexal masses: While ultrasonography characterizes the vast majority of adnexal masses, MR is of value in evaluating solid masses and in better detecting mural nodules in large cystic lesions. MR can well demonstrate whether a tumor is uterine or ovarian in origin, and may allow characterization of an adnexal mass as a pedunculated leiomyoma, fibroma, endometrioma, dermoid, or epithelial ovarian neoplasm.

- Leiomyomas: The superb contrast resolution of MR provides optimal assessment of leiomyomas before and after treatment with uterine artery embolization (UAE).

- Extrauterine malignancies and recurrent gynecologic cancer: MR provides diagnostic and staging information for treatment planning.

MR TECHNIQUES

MR provides excellent tissue characterization differentiating between water, fat, blood, proteinaceous or mucinous fluid, and vascularized tissue. High-resolution imaging and motion suppression is particularly needed for discerning alterations in the uterine zonal anatomy by cancer in case of invasion into the myometrium and involvement of the serosa, which have important implications for treatment. Spatial detail is critical in assessing for enhancing solid components and wall nodularity, indicative of cancer in adnexal masses. Methods for optimizing gynecologic MRI:

- *Antiperistaltic agents* can be used to suppress bowel motion artifact. Glucagon (0.75 to 1.0 mg) is effective when given intravenously (IV), intramuscularly (IM), or subcutaneously (SQ). It has an antiperistaltic effect for 30 minutes when injected IM or SQ and only a 10-minute effective period if given IV. If available, IV Buscopan (hyoscine butylbromide) can be used in 10-mg increments (10 to 40 mg total). Fasting for 4 to 6 hours can also help

suppress bowel motion. For pediatric patients, oral mebeverine 135 mg is an option.

- *Empty or near-empty bladder:* With a near-empty bladder, the uterus descends further in the pelvis and images are therefore less affected by artifacts from bowel motion. Ghosting artifact from a full bladder is also avoided when the bladder is empty. The anatomic plane between the uterus and the bladder is then also better delineated.

- *Vaginal gel:* The use of gel in the vagina separates the tissues and therefore allows for better delineation of the vagina and cervix (Fig. 9.1). The vaginal wall is thinner through distention, better differentiating the noncompliant tumor against the normal wall. The patient is given a 60-cc syringe filled with Surgilube and attached to a Foley catheter[1] and is asked to insert it into her vagina and inject it while laying on the MR table just prior to scanning.

- *High field strength and multichannel phased-array surface coils* increase the signal-to-noise ratio, allowing high-spatial-resolution imaging. Two coils are best employed if a

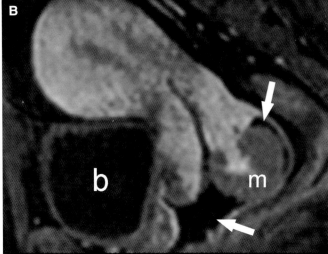

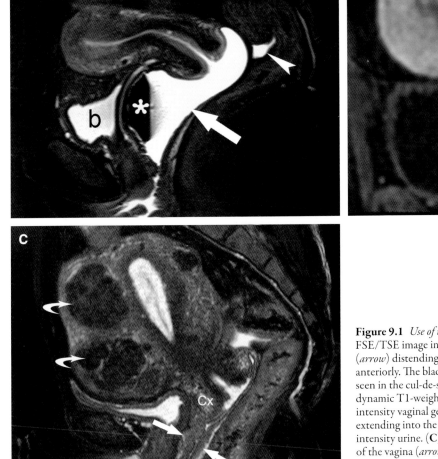

Figure 9.1 *Use of vaginal gel.* (**A**) Sagittal fat-suppressed T2-weighted FSE/TSE image in a normal patient shows high-signal-intensity gel (*arrow*) distending the vagina. A pocket of air (*asterisk*) is present anteriorly. The bladder (*b*) is partially filled. A small volume of fluid is seen in the cul-de-sac (*arrowhead*). (**B**) In a patient with cervical cancer a dynamic T1-weighted gradient-echo image shows the low-signal-intensity vaginal gel (*arrows*) surrounding an exophytic mass (*m*) extending into the vagina. The bladder (*b*) is filled with low-signal-intensity urine. (**C**) In another patient vaginal gel was not used. The wall of the vagina (*arrows*) shows irregular thickening, making it more difficult to determine involvement by tumor. This patient also has numerous leiomyomas (*curved arrows*). *Cx*, cervix.

sequence from the renal veins to the pelvis is included to detect adenopathy.

- *Endovaginal receiver coils*[2] are well tolerated and allow extremely high spatial detail, which is particularly valuable for assessing early cervical cancer. In-plane resolution approximates 0.4 mm. Any patient motion on the coil must be avoided, however. The coil can be supported with a rolled sheet or sandbag to avoid patient motion on the coil. The endovaginal coil may be combined with an external pelvic array coil.

- *Slice profile:* Thin slices through the uterus (e.g., 4 mm thickness using T2-weighted images and 1 to 2 mm using dynamic gadolinium contrast-enhanced T1-weighted imaging), small pixel size (0.7 to 1.0 mm), appropriate choice of frequency and phase-encoding directions, and use of flow compensation to reduce vascular artifact improve soft tissue detail.

- Saturation bands placed over the anterior abdominal wall decrease ghosting artifacts from the high-signal-intensity submucosal fat beneath the surface coil on non-fat-saturated sequences. Flow compensation or presaturation bands can reduce vascular artifact.

T1-weighted spin-echo imaging typically displays fat, blood, and other proteinaceous fluids with high signal intensity.

T2-weighted spin-echo images are the mainstay of diagnosis in pelvic gynecologic imaging, providing visualization of uterine zonal anatomy. On these images the higher signal intensity tumor is set off against the lower signal intensity stroma of the cervix and myometrium. Lymph nodes are well depicted on both T1- and T2-weighted images.

Fat saturation. Frequency-selective fat-saturation pulses on T2-weighted FSE/TSE imaging increase the dynamic range to improve delineation of the brighter cervical or

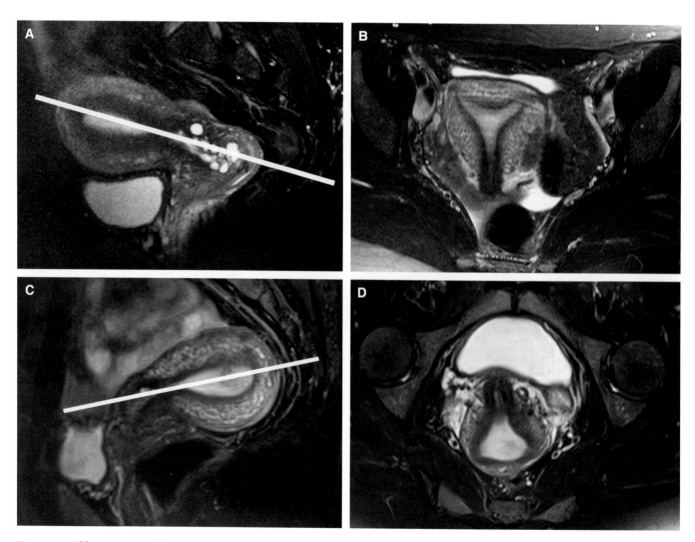

Figure 9.2 *Oblique projections through the uterine body.* (**A**) Sagittal T2-weighted FSE/TSE image shows anteflexed uterus. (**B**) Image of the same patient obtained in an oblique axial orientation taken through the long axis of the uterine body, indicated by the white line in image A. (**C**) Sagittal image of a different patient shows a retroflexed uterus. (**D**) Oblique axial view through the long axis of the uterus, indicated by the white line in image C, shows the contour of the uterus and the shape of the uterine cavity. Acquisition of oblique views paralleling the center of the uterine body is particularly important in assessing the uterus for congenital anomalies because it allows visualization of the external fundal contour.

endometrial carcinoma against the darker junctional zone and myometrium. Use of weaker fat suppression allows a windowing effect with good visualization of anatomic relationships. Fat saturation allows differentiation of macroscopic fat from hemorrhage and high-viscosity mucin, and typically detects macroscopic fat in dermoids. Opposed-phase gradient-echo (GRE) imaging may additionally detect components in dermoid tumors containing microscopic fat.

Specific anatomic planes for multiplanar imaging are selected to optimally define anatomic relationships. The sagittal projection provides the best evaluation of cervical or endometrial cancer invasion into the bladder or rectum. Image planes through the long and short axis of the uterine body (oblique axial and oblique coronal) (Fig. 9.2) best delineate the depth of myometrial invasion by endometrial cancer. In evaluating congenital abnormalities, the oblique coronal plane is helpful in differentiating a septate from a bicornuate uterus.

TISSUE CHARACTERIZATION

Tissue characterization can be done using a combination of T1- and T2-weighted and gadolinium-contrast-enhanced gradient-echo images with or without frequency-selective fat suppression (Fig. 9.3).

Mucins are high-molecular-weight glycosylated proteins that are characterized by their gel-like quality:

- Newly formed or low-viscosity mucin consists predominantly of water (98%) and glycoproteins (2%). It displays low signal on T1-weighted and high signal on T2-weighted images, similar to other fluids that consist predominantly of water.

- A chronically entrapped mucin collection inspissates over time, resulting in thicker mucus and increasing protein concentration. The increased protein shortens T1 relaxation time, causing the signal to change from low to

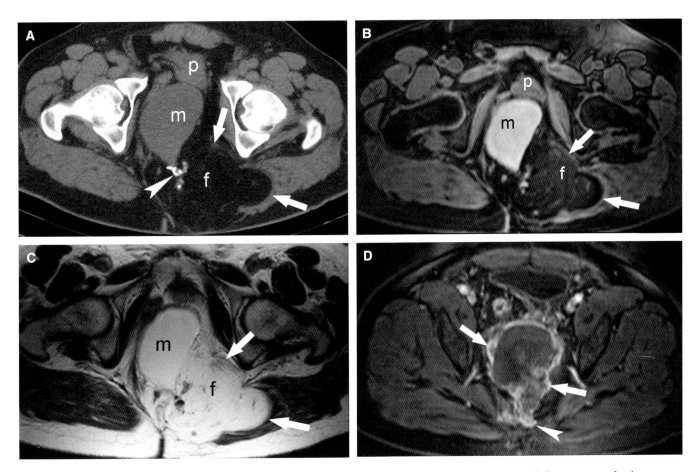

Figure 9.3 *Tissue characterization.* This patient had a known gluteal mass since childhood. New pressure symptoms led to suspicion of malignant degeneration. (**A**) Non-contrast-enhanced CT image demonstrates a complex pelvic mass with prominent fatty component (*f*, between *arrows*), a homogeneous soft tissue attenuation component (*m*), and a calcified osseous component (*arrowhead*). The prostate (*p*) is displaced far anteriorly. T1-weighted fat-suppressed gradient-echo (**B**) and T2-weighted FSE/TSE (**C**) images demonstrate that the non-fatty component of the mass (*m*) displays high signal intensity, suggestive of either mucin or hemorrhage. Histology revealed benign respiratory epithelium that secreted mucin. Note that the fatty component of the tumor (*arrows, f*) became low in signal on the fat-suppression sequence. *p*, prostate. (**D**) T1-weighted post-gadolinium-contrast-enhanced gradient-echo image obtained superior to the level of images B and C shows areas of enhancement (*arrows*) with infiltration of muscle posteriorly (*arrowhead*). Histology: adenocarcinoma of colonic type. The pluripotential cells of the sacrococcygeal teratoma can give rise to any type of malignancy.

higher signal intensity on T1-weighted images. On T2-weighted imaging inspissated mucus remains high in signal intensity until very high protein concentrations are reached, causing signal loss.

- In myxoid degeneration, mucin accumulates in the affected tissue, giving it a gel-like quality and also resulting in similar low signal on T1-weighted and high signal on T2-weighted images due to its high water content. However, since viable cells and vascularity are still present, contrast material administration results in a slow mesh-like enhancement, differentiating this from avascular cystic change.

Fat displays high signal intensity on T1-weighted images:

- Frequency-selective fat suppression suppresses the high signal of fat.

- On fat-suppressed T1-weighted images fat can be differentiated from hemorrhagic lesions, including endometrioma, hemorrhagic cyst, hematosalpinx, and ectopic pregnancy.

Blood. The appearance of *hemorrhage* on MRI depends on the age of the hematoma:

- An acute hemorrhagic collection or hemorrhage in a functional cyst displays initially intermediate signal intensity on T1-weighted and low signal on T2-weighted images. After approximately a week, hemoglobin is oxidized to methemoglobin, causing high signal on T1-weighted imaging. On T2-weighted imaging, methemoglobin may show low or high signal intensity depending on whether it is intracellular or extracellular, respectively. Subacute hemorrhagic lesions typically show high signal intensity on both T1- and T2-weighted images due to extracellular methemoglobin. Hemosiderin increases with the age of the hematoma and can lead to very low signal on T2-weighted images.

- A chronic pelvic hematoma may demonstrate a "concentric ring sign," best appreciated on T1-weighted images (Fig. 9.4). Over time, a low-signal thin outer rim develops due to ferritin within macrophages. This dark outer ring commonly does not extend around the entire circumference of the hemorrhage. A high-signal inner rim adjacent to the low-signal outer rim is caused by extracellular methemoglobin. Centrally, most of the hematoma displays low signal intensity due to the presence of still unoxidized hemoglobin.[3]

- T2-shading effect: The increasing concentration of hemosiderin in chronic hemorrhage layers dependently to result in a graded loss of signal intensity on T2-weighted images, called T2–shading. This feature helps differentiate endometriosis and other chronic blood-containing lesions from an acute hemorrhagic functional cyst. A chronic hematosalpinx can show a similar T2-shading effect.

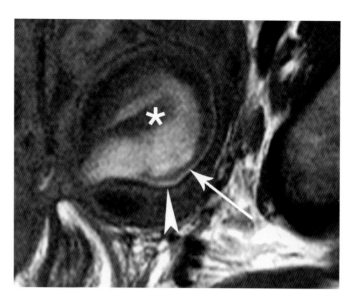

Figure 9.4 *Concentric ring sign.* A hemorrhagic tubo-ovarian abscess (*) shows a characteristic concentric ring sign. Axial T1-weighted image demonstrates a low-signal-intensity discontinuous peripheral ring (*arrowhead*), reflecting the presence of hemosiderin within macrophages. An adjacent high-signal-intensity inner ring (*arrow*) reflects the presence of extracellular methemoglobin. The heterogeneous central core of the hemorrhagic abscess reflects fluid and blood products in various stages of evolution. The concentric ring sign develops about 3 weeks after hemorrhage and is indicative of a chronic hemorrhage.

Fibrosis:

- Lesions composed of smooth muscle or extensive fibrosis include uterine leiomyomas and the ovarian fibroma-thecoma group tumors, respectively. They display low or low-intermediate signal on T2-weighted images because of low concentration of extracellular fluid and the T2-shortening effect of muscle and collagen.

Lymphadenopathy:

- A sequence covering the field from the renal veins to the pelvic brim can be included as part of a pelvic MR to assess for paraaortic lymphadenopathy in the staging examination for pelvic malignancies. Appropriate sequences include a fat saturated T2-weighted respiratory-gated sequence or a breath-held post-contrast enhanced fat saturated 3-dimensional (3D) gradient-echo sequence, the latter performed after the dynamic imaging in the pelvis.

INTRAVENOUS CONTRAST AGENTS

Use of intravenous gadolinium-containing contrast agents with fat-saturated T1-weighted sequences should be considered for most indications. Dynamically obtained contrast-enhanced sequences allow for differential enhancement of pathologic tissues. The image quality of a fat-saturated 3D GRE sequence is superior given the lack of motion and favorable slice profile of the 3D acquisition. Slices no greater than 1 to 2 mm in thickness allow for multiplanar reconstruction (MPR). Thickness may need to be increased to increase anatomic coverage or to prevent a parallel imaging artifact. Only cyclic or ionic linear gadolinium contrast agents are currently used at our institution.

Endometrial and cervical cancer. Dynamic contrast-enhanced sequences (every 30 seconds is adequate) are the standard in evaluating early-stage endometrial cancer. Dynamic post-contrast-enhanced sequences improve sensitivity and specificity over non-contrast T2-weighted images in determining the presence and depth of myometrial invasion. They show the critical but subtle differential enhancement between the tumor, junctional zone, and myometrium. At 50 to 120 seconds after contrast material injection the tumor enhances poorly in contrast to the strongly enhancing myometrium. The endometrium also enhances more than tumor, though not as much as the myometrium. The poorly defined junctional zone often seen in postmenopausal women is then made more apparent.[4] In addition, sensitivity of T2-weighted images is poor for myometrial invasion of adenomyosis, and dynamic contrast-enhanced sequences are essential. In cervical cancer, contrast enhancement has limited value. The higher-signal cancer strongly contrasts against the very-low-signal cervical stroma.

Adnexal masses. Fat-suppressed contrast-enhanced dynamic T1-weighted GRE images delineate enhancing septations, papillary projections, and other solid components in neoplastic cystic lesions. A mass extending outside the capsule will be offset against the low signal intensity of the suppressed pelvic fat. If the fluid is bright on T1-weighted images because of hemorrhage or proteinaceous content, post-processing subtraction is needed to demonstrate the enhancing components (see Fig. 9.44). *Subtraction* is a post-processing technique whereby the pre-contrast images are subtracted from the post-contrast-enhanced images. On subtracted images the high-signal-intensity non-enhancing components show low signal, allowing enhancing tissue to become more clearly visible. Dynamic contrast-enhanced sequences well demonstrate the presence of necrosis and neoplastic peritoneal and omental implants.

Teratomas and *endometriomas* rarely undergo malignant degeneration. *Endometriosis* is associated with endometrioid and clear cell carcinoma. Enhancing components within these otherwise avascular structures are worrisome for malignancy.

Large extrauterine masses may invade the pelvic musculature. The edema from large tumors is difficult to differentiate from the tumor mass itself. Post-contrast-enhanced sequences demonstrate enhancement of the tumor invading muscle.

Leiomyomas show variable enhancement and may enhance less or more than the myometrium. Small leiomyomas tend to homogeneously enhance and those greater than 3 to 5 cm are usually heterogeneous. Necrosis within leiomyomas is well demonstrated on post-contrast-enhanced images.

Congenital anomalies. Contrast material administration is generally not needed in the evaluation of congenital anomalies.

ANATOMY

PELVIC PERITONEAL REFLECTIONS AND SUPPORTING LIGAMENTS

The true pelvis is bounded superiorly by the pelvic brim and contains the uterus, ovaries and fallopian tubes, bladder, and rectum. The true pelvis is divided into anterior and posterior spaces by the broad ligament, which extends laterally between the uterus and pelvic sidewalls. The false pelvis is defined superiorly by an anatomic plane drawn between the superior iliac spines and the inferior edge of vertebral body L5. The false pelvis extends inferiorly to the superior border of the true pelvis.

The uterus and cervix are supported by the levator ani muscles of the pelvic floor and supporting ligaments (Fig. 9.5). The uterosacral, cardinal, and pubocervical ligaments attach the cervix and lower uterine segment to the sacrum, ischial spine, and pubic symphysis, respectively. The vesicouterine ligament extends from the anterior uterine wall to the bladder. These ligaments serve as pathways for neoplastic spread. The round ligaments are fibromuscular cords that insert onto the uterus just below the fallopian tubes and extend through the inguinal canal to end in the labia majora. They are the homolog of the gubernaculum testis and help maintain the position of the uterus.

The ovaries usually lie near the bifurcation of the internal and external iliac arteries. The *ligament of the ovary* is a fibrous ligament within the broad ligament that extends from the ovary to the lateral aspect of the uterus just posterior and inferior to the fallopian tube. The *suspensory ligament of the ovary,* or *infundibulopelvic ligament*, is actually a fold of peritoneum extending between the ovary and the lateral pelvic wall. The suspensory ligament envelops the ovarian blood vessels and lymphatics and serves as a channel for the spread of ovarian and endometrial cancer to the para-aortic lymphatics.

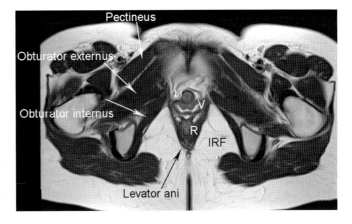

Figure 9.5 *Anatomy of the pelvic floor.* Axial MR image shows the vagina (*V*) with the urethra (*U*) coursing in its anterior wall. The rectum (*R*) is posterior. The *levator ani* serves as the muscular floor of the pelvis and defines the medial boundary of the ischiorectal fossa (*IRF*) of the perineum. The *obturator internus* is the important muscle that lines the true pelvis. External to the bony pelvic ring are the *obturator externus* and *pectineus* muscles.

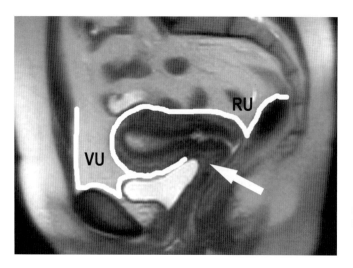

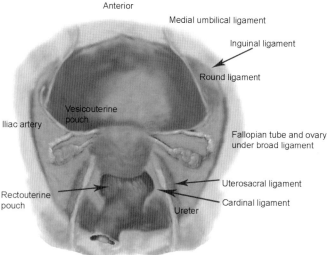

Figure 9.6 *Peritoneal coverings.* The *thick white line* outlines the peritoneal covering of the uterus and the peritoneal lining of the posterior rectouterine (*RU*) pouch of Douglas and the anterior vesicouterine recess (*VU*). The *arrow* indicates the anterior fibrofatty stroma that allows direct spread of cervical carcinoma to the bladder because there is no intervening peritoneum.

Figure 9.7 *Supporting ligaments and peritoneal coverings.* The broad ligament is a double-layered fold of peritoneum that extends from the sides of the uterus to the lateral pelvic wall. The broad ligament covers the fallopian tubes. The parametrium is the connective tissue and smooth muscle between the layers of the broad ligament. Two supporting uterine ligaments, the uterine artery and vein, lymphatics, and the ureters course through the parametrium. The ureters course within 2 cm of the cervix and can become obstructed as cervical cancer extends into the parametria.

Anteriorly to posteriorly, the peritoneal lining covers the superior aspect of the bladder, the uterine fundus and posterior body, and the anterior rectum. The remaining portion of the bladder and the cervix are separated by fibrofatty fascia, not by peritoneal lining (Fig. 9.6). This has importance in the spread of cervical cancer when deep anterior stromal invasion in these tissues serves as a relative contraindication to surgery. The peritoneal lining folds over the lateral uterus, tubes, ovaries, and round ligament. The individual folds are the mesometrium, mesosalpinx, mesovarium, and mesoteres, respectively. Together they make up the *broad ligament*, a thick shelf-like fold of peritoneum extending between the lateral aspect of the uterus and the lateral pelvic walls. The broad ligaments carry the respective supporting ligaments, nerves, and vessels.

Reflections of the peritoneal lining form recesses (Fig. 9.7). The vesicouterine pouch is between the uterus and bladder, with the vesicouterine ligament at its base and the paravesical fossae anterolaterally. The rectouterine pouch (also termed pouch of Douglas, rectovaginal pouch, or cul-de-sac) is the lowest portion of the peritoneal cavity and is a common location for intraperitoneal seeding of ovarian or gastrointestinal malignancies. The pararectal fossae are the lateral recesses between the rectum and the lateral abdominal cavity.

The *parametrium* is the connective tissue under the broad ligament, which extends laterally from the cervix and extends from the sacrouterine ligament superiorly and the cardinal ligaments inferiorly. It surrounds these ligaments, the cervical lymphatics, the uterine artery, and the ureter. The ureters course 2 cm lateral to the cervix just under the uterine artery. Cervical cancer frequently spreads into the parametria, where it can easily obstruct the ureters.

PELVIC ORGANS

The *uterus* is anatomically divided into the fundus (the part above the cornua), the body; the lower uterine segment

(isthmus), and the cervix (Fig. 9.8). The uterus may normally be anteflexed or retroflexed, terms that describe the angle between the cervix and uterine body. The external os demarcates the visible portion of the cervix, the exocervix, from the internal portion or endocervix.

The squamocolumnar junction divides the glandular mucin-secreting columnar epithelium proximally from the squamous epithelium distally. The junction between the glandular and squamous epithelium approximates the junction between the endocervix and exocervix, respectively. However, the location varies with age and hormonal status, and it may be located just within the endocervix.

The uterus displays homogeneously low signal intensity on T1-weighted images. The endometrium displays high signal intensity and the myometrium shows intermediate signal on T2-weighted images. The cervical stroma is lower in signal than myometrium because of its higher elastic fibrous content. The junctional zone is the low-signal-intensity rim of myometrium surrounding the endometrium. Its characteristic low signal on T2-weighted images is due to lower water content and more closely packed muscle cells than adjacent myometrium. Though clearly visible on MR, the junctional zone is not well defined histologically. The normal junctional zone myometrium is 2 to 8 mm in thickness on MR. In premenarchal girls and postmenopausal women, the uterus is small, the endometrium is thin (less than 4 mm), and the junctional zone is indistinct or absent.

The *vagina* is a fibromuscular tube supported by the levator ani and urogenital diaphragm and surrounded by the paravaginal connective tissue (paracolpium) and extends from

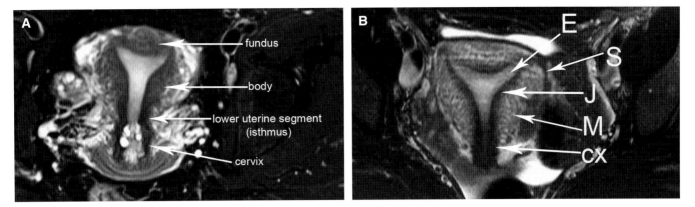

Figure 9.8 *Anatomy of the uterus.* (**A**) The uterine corpus is composed of the *fundus* (portion above cornua), the *body*, and the lower uterine segment (*isthmus*). The corpus and *cervix* make up the uterus. Numerous nabothian cysts are seen in the endocervical canal. (**B**) The myometrium (*M*) displays intermediate signal and is bounded by the low-signal-intensity outer serosa (*S*) and the low-signal-intensity junctional zone (*J*). The endometrium (*E*) is high signal. The cervical junctional zone (*CX*) is usually thicker than the uterine junctional zone because of its higher collagen content.

the cervix to the hymen. The rectal and bladder pillars attach the vagina to the rectum and bladder, respectively. The pillars are fibrovascular bundles with extensive vascular and lymphatic channels that allow for spread of cervical and vaginal neoplasia.

The outer cortex of the *ovary* contains maturing follicles, and the inner medulla contains stroma and most of the ovarian lymphatics and vasculature. If the follicle does not involute, an estrogen-producing follicular cyst can result. If the corpus luteum fails to involute, a progesterone-producing corpus luteal cyst can result. The prominent vascularity of a corpus luteum predisposes to intracystic hemorrhage.

On T2-weighted images, the ovaries are easily identifiable in women of reproductive age because of the presence of the fluid-filled follicles displaying high signal intensity. T2-weighted images show the zonal anatomy of the lower-signal ovarian cortex and the intermediate-signal medulla. The ovaries display homogeneously low signal on T1-weighted images unless hemorrhagic follicles are present (Fig. 9.9).

Follicles with hemorrhage are typically high in signal on T1-weighted images and intermediate or low in signal on T2-weighted images. Involuting follicles or cysts may have a serpiginous enhancing vascularized border that should not be confused with neoplasm (Figs. 9.9 and 9.10). Normal postmenopausal ovaries are difficult to identify because they lack the landmark follicles.

The *fallopian tubes* extend from the cornua and are suspended by the mesosalpinx, which carries the blood supply and lymphatics. The tubes are about 10 cm in length. The short interstitial (intramural) segment is contained within the myometrium of the uterus. The isthmus begins at the cornua and is the thickened 3-cm-long muscular portion of the tube. The ampulla is the tortuous thin-walled midportion, where fertilization usually occurs. The infundibulum is the end of the tube, with its ostium surrounded by 20 to 30 fimbriae, one of which is the elongated single large ovarian fimbria which attaches to the ovary. The fimbriae are open to the peritoneum and serve to trap the ovum at ovulation.

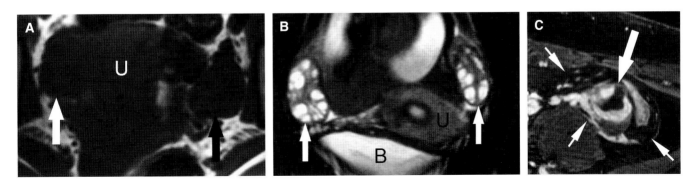

Figure 9.9 *Normal ovaries.* (**A**) Normal ovaries (*arrows*) appear as homogeneously low signal intensity structures on T1-weighted images unless hemorrhagic follicles are present. (**B**) On a paracoronal T2-weighted image, the ovarian follicles (*arrows*) are high signal intensity and stand out against the intermediate–signal-intensity medulla. (**C**) An involuting corpus luteum (*large arrow*), shown on a gadolinium contrast-enhanced axial T1-weighted image with fat saturation, typically has high vascularity and may show hemorrhagic components. The lesion should not be confused with neoplasia. The outline of the ovary is indicated by the *small arrows*. *U*, uterus. *B*, bladder.

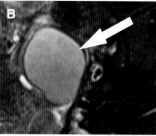
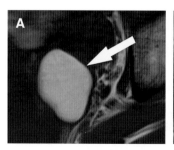

Figure 9.10 *Hemorrhagic ovarian cyst.* (**A**) On an axial T1-weighted image the 4-cm hemorrhagic cyst (*arrow*) displays high signal intensity. (**B**) On the corresponding T2-weighted image with fat suppression, the cyst (*arrow*) remains high in signal intensity. However, the signal is lower than that of a typical cyst because of the presence of hemosiderin.

BLOOD SUPPLY

The aorta bifurcates into the common iliac arteries at approximately the level of the L4 vertebra. The common iliac arteries bifurcate at the pelvic brim. The external iliac artery travels laterally along the pelvic sidewall to become the femoral artery distal to the inguinal ligament. The internal iliac artery travels posteriorly along the pelvic sidewall. Its anterior division supplies all pelvic organs except the ovaries (supplied by the ovarian artery) and the upper third of the rectum (supplied by the inferior mesenteric artery). Branches of the internal iliac artery are the obturator, inferior gluteal, umbilical, uterine, vaginal, inferior vesical, middle rectal, and internal pudendal arteries (Fig. 9.11).

The *uterine artery* courses in the parametria, enters the lower uterine segment, and divides. The descending branch supplies the cervix and upper two thirds of the vagina. The ascending branch supplies the lower uterine segment and uterine body and anastomoses with the ovarian artery to perfuse the uterine fundus. Vaginal artery branches supply the middle

and inferior vagina. The internal pudendal artery supplies the lower vagina and external genitalia.

The *ovarian artery* arises directly from the aorta just below the origin of the renal arteries and courses caudally beneath the peritoneum, resting on the psoas muscle, to the pelvic brim, where it passes medially between the layers of the suspensory ligament of the ovary to supply the ovary and the uterine fundus. The ovarian and uterine arteries both supply the round ligament and uterine fundus.

Venous drainage parallels the arteries.

PELVIC LYMPH NODES

The nodal chains of concern in gynecology are named in relation to the adjacent vessels: para-aortic, common iliac, internal iliac (often called hypogastric), external iliac, obturator, and inguinal lymph nodes. The obturator nodes lie adjacent to the obturator internus muscles and the distal external iliac vein. Though the obturator vessels arise from the internal iliac vessels, the obturator nodes are sometimes grouped as part of the external iliac chain based on their location (Figs. 9.12 and 9.13).

Most of the pelvic cavity drains into the external, internal, and common iliac lymph nodes. The common iliac nodes drain to the para-aortic nodes. From the para-aortic nodes, drainage can reach the supraclavicular nodes via the thoracic duct. Drainage also occurs along the ovarian vein directly to the para-aortic nodes or via the round ligament to the superficial inguinal nodes.

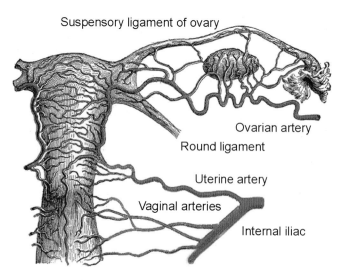

Figure 9.11 *Arterial supply.* The ovarian artery travels along the suspensory ligament of the ovary to supply the ovary and entire fallopian tube entirely as well as to contribute flow to the round ligament and uterine fundus. The uterine artery branch of the internal iliac artery courses in the parametrium to supply the lower uterine segment, cervix, and upper two thirds of the vagina. (Drawing from *Gray's Anatomy*.)

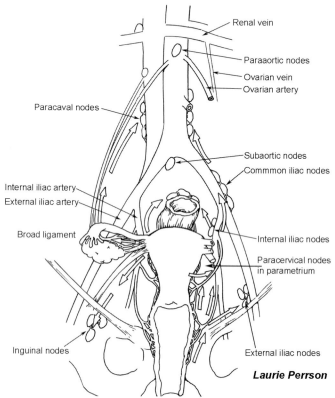

Figure 9.12 *Lymphatic drainage of the pelvis.* Line drawing indicates the location and nomenclature of the major lymph node groups that drain the pelvis. (Drawing by Laurie Perrson, Department of Radiology, University of Virginia.)

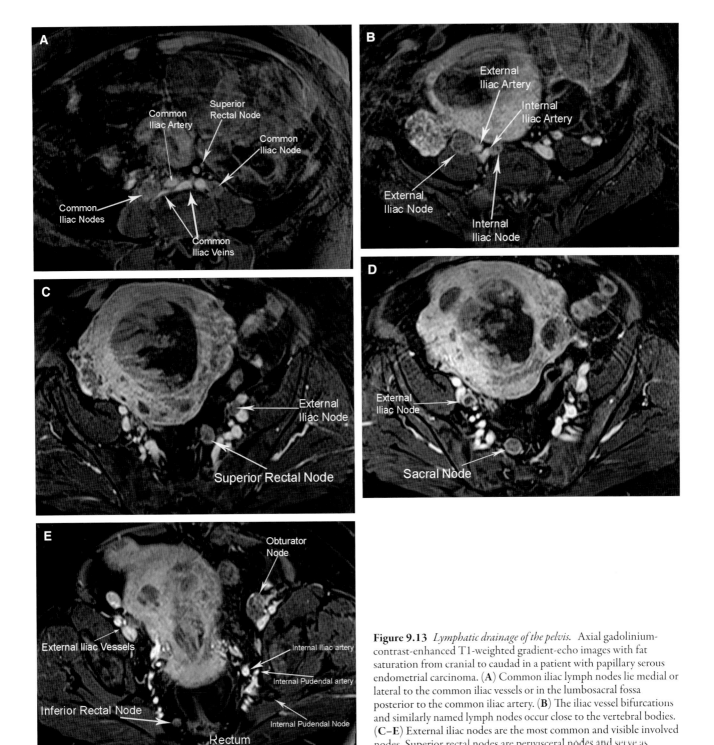

Figure 9.13 *Lymphatic drainage of the pelvis.* Axial gadolinium-contrast-enhanced T1-weighted gradient-echo images with fat saturation from cranial to caudad in a patient with papillary serous endometrial carcinoma. (**A**) Common iliac lymph nodes lie medial or lateral to the common iliac vessels or in the lumbosacral fossa posterior to the common iliac artery. (**B**) The iliac vessel bifurcations and similarly named lymph nodes occur close to the vertebral bodies. (**C–E**) External iliac nodes are the most common and visible involved nodes. Superior rectal nodes are perivisceral nodes and serve as regional drainage for the uterus, cervix, vagina, and ovary.

Common iliac lymph nodes lie medial or lateral to the common iliac vessels and in the lumbosacral fossa. The latter is a less conspicuous location posterior to the iliac vessels and adjacent to the psoas muscle and vertebral body (Fig. 9.13A). The external iliac lymph nodes may lie medial or lateral to the external iliac vessels. The internal iliac lymph nodes are posteriorly located near the vertebrae and sacrum. They include the lateral sacral and presacral nodes (which lie anterior to the mid-sacrum) and the inferior and superior gluteal lymph nodes.

Perivisceral nodes are those immediately adjacent to the pelvic viscera and are considered part of the regional drainage for those viscera. The perirectal nodes are also considered perivisceral nodes for the uterus, cervix, vagina, and ovary as well as the rectum and are included as regional drainage.

The fallopian tubes, ovaries, and upper uterine body have lymphatic drainage along three pathways: predominantly along the suspensory ovarian ligament to the para-aortic nodes and less frequently along the parametrium to the internal, external, and common iliac nodes or along the round ligament to the superficial inguinal lymph nodes.

The lower uterine body and cervix drain laterally through the parametrium to the external, obturator, and internal iliac nodes, followed by drainage to the common iliac and para-aortic nodes. Isolated common iliac node involvement is infrequent. However, posterior cervical drainage can also follow rectal drainage into the perirectal nodes and along the rectouterine fold to first involve the sacral, common iliac, and para-aortic lymph nodes.

Regional lymph nodes for the cervix are only the internal, external, and common iliac lymph nodes. Regional lymph nodes for the endometrium and ovary are the internal, external, and common iliac and the para-aortic lymph nodes. The inguinal nodes do not drain the cervix, endometrium, and ovaries.

Regional nodal drainage of the vagina is to the internal and external iliac nodes and the inguinal nodes. Only drainage to the superficial inguinal lymph nodes is considered regional nodal drainage for the external genitalia, including the vulva and perineum. The upper two thirds of the vagina tends to drain predominantly through the parametrium to the internal and external lymph nodes and the lower vagina to the superficial inguinal lymph nodes. The posterior vaginal wall at any level may drain to the inferior gluteal, presacral, and perirectal lymph nodes, similar to rectal drainage; these are still considered regional drainage.

Lymph nodes may be seen on T2-weighted images with fat saturation or T1-weighted images without fat saturation. Spatial detail and assessment of internal architecture are highest on thin-section contrast-enhanced dynamic T1-weighted sequences. Lymph nodes can be assessed in terms of size, shape, and internal architecture.[5] There is lack of consensus about the upper limit that is considered normal in terms of the size of pelvic lymph nodes by imaging, given considerable variation in the size of normal and tumor-involved lymph nodes. The likelihood of involvement based on size also varies according to the histology of the primary tumor. Knowledge of pathways of regional nodal spread is important for assessing borderline lymph nodes as possibly involved.

Upper limit sizes in most patients are 7 mm, 8 mm, and 10 mm for internal, obturator, and external iliac nodes, respectively. A short-axis size threshold of 8 mm for pelvic lymph nodes and 10 mm for retroperitoneal nodes can also be used.[5]

Normal lymph nodes are oval and shaped like a kidney bean, with a fatty hilum. A lymph node that has become more rounded or has an irregular border is more likely involved by tumor. Internal heterogeneity on T2-weighted or dynamic contrast-enhanced images and loss of the fatty hilum are features of tumor involvement.

For tumor staging, *regional lymph nodes* are the first sites of lymphatic drainage and tumor involvement. Tumor spread beyond the regional lymph nodes may be classified as metastatic disease.

CONGENITAL ANOMALIES

MR is the optimal imaging study in evaluating congenital anomalies and is used if hysterosalpingography and sonography are inconclusive. Congenital anomalies are associated with infertility, repeated spontaneous abortion, intrauterine growth restriction, malpresentation, premature labor, and urinary tract and axial skeletal abnormalities. MR may be included in the workup for infertility or repeated spontaneous abortions and in the evaluation of adolescent girls with amenorrhea or vaginal atresia.

Box 9.1 **ESSENTIALS TO REMEMBER**

- The uterus and upper two thirds of the vagina are linked embryologically and share common pathways for blood supply and lymphatic drainage.

- The lower vagina is embryologically linked with the perineum and external genitalia, with lymphatic spread of tumor to the superficial inguinal nodes possible.

- A "bare area" of fibrofatty tissue exists between the bladder and the anterior aspect of the cervix that allows for contiguous spread of tumor without intervening peritoneum. Deep tumor involvement into the anterior cervical stroma may preclude surgical resection.

- The ureters course through the parametria in close proximity to the cervix and may be involved early by direct spread of tumor from the cervix or lower uterine segment.

- The ovarian follicles, showing high signal intensity on T2-weighted images, serve as prominent landmarks for identification of the ovaries.

- The suspensory ligament of the ovary, extending from the tubal end of the ovary to the posterolateral pelvic side wall and enveloping the ovarian vessels, serves as an anatomic landmark to identify the ovary, which is especially important in postmenopausal women and premenarchal girls, whose ovaries lack follicles, and in instances when the ovary is replaced by tumor.

- The ligament of the ovary, extending from the uterine aspect of the ovary through the broad ligament to the lateral angle of the uterus, serves as a similar though less prominent landmark for identification of the ovary.

- The round ligaments, extending from the superior lateral aspect of the uterus through the inguinal canal to the labia majora, serve as anatomic markers of the uterus and are useful in confirming uterine origin of large pelvic masses.

Though the most familiar congenital anomalies are the isolated Müllerian anomalies, MR plays a critical role in the diagnosis of less frequent but very complex anomalies. These complex Müllerian anomalies are nearly always associated with a congenital renal anomaly, usually unilateral renal agenesis. Conversely, the incidental discovery of a renal anomaly has a high association with Müllerian anomalies and warrants evaluation of the reproductive tract.

On MR imaging, the external contour of the uterus and the contour and distribution of the endometrium must be delineated. Field of view and sequences must be adequate to detect and characterize fluid in obstructed anomalies (hydrosalpinx, hydrometros, hydrocolpos).

EMBRYOLOGY

The development of the genital tract is closely related to that of the urinary tract, and knowledge of embryology is necessary to elucidate the complex obstructed anomalies affecting multiple embryologic paths.

Most organs of the genitourinary system are derived from the urogenital ridge, a mesoderm precursor that gives rise to the kidneys, ovaries, uterus, and upper two thirds of the vagina. Caudally, the urorectal septum divides the cloaca into the urogenital sinus and the anorectal canal. The urogenital sinus is the endoderm-derived precursor of the lower third of the vagina, urethra, and urinary bladder.

Urogenital ridge

The *urogenital ridge* differentiates into four separate tissue structures. The gonadal ridge, nephrogenic cord, and mesonephric (Wolffian) ducts form at 4 to 5 weeks and the paramesonephric (Müllerian) ducts form at 6 weeks. Normal differentiation of the nephrogenic cord, Wolffian duct, and Müllerian ducts depends on the normal development of each. The *gonadal ridge* differentiates into the ovaries. It develops independently from the other systems, and therefore the ovaries are usually present in urogenital malformations. However, they may be malpositioned or elongated.

Kidneys

The *nephrogenic cord* differentiates into the kidneys after the ureteric bud (under Wolffian influence) contacts it and induces renal development.

Wolffian ducts

The paired *Wolffian ducts* form the male organs and regress in the female. However, they influence normal development of the kidneys, uterus, and lower vagina. Caudally, they open into the urogenital sinus and allow the ureteric bud to spout from the urogenital sinus and induce renal development. They also serve as scaffolding for subsequent normal development of the uterus and cervix. If the Wolffian ducts do not form normally, renal agenesis or hypoplasia and Müllerian anomalies occur. The sinovaginal bulbs of the urogenital sinus are of lower Wolffian duct origin and are precursors for the lower third of the vagina. Incomplete regression of the Wolffian duct is responsible for Gartner's duct cysts which parallel the vagina and uterus.

Müllerian structures

The paired Müllerian ducts develop along the regressing Wolffian ducts. Superiorly the unfused ducts form the fallopian tubes. Caudally, the Müllerian ducts undergo *lateral fusion*, becoming the uterovaginal primordium. The uterovaginal primordium and Müllerian tubercle together result in the uterus, cervix, and upper vagina. The uterovaginal primordium fuses with the Wolffian-derived sinovaginal bulbs of the urogenital sinus by *vertical fusion*, forming the Müllerian tubercle. The upper part of the Müllerian tubercle forms the cervix and the caudal part (vaginal plate) elongates to form the upper vagina.

Isolated or type I Mayer-Rokitansky-Kuster-Hauser syndrome is a combination of lack of development of both the Müllerian tubercle and ducts, resulting in a rudimentary uterus and upper vaginal agenesis.[6] Lack or incomplete fusion at the level of the Müllerian tubercle can result in cervico-upper vaginal atresia (Fig. 9.14) or rarely isolated upper vaginal atresia. *Vertical fusion defects* (at the vaginal plate) result in vaginal aplasia, transverse vaginal septum, and imperforate hymen.

Once lateral fusion is complete, the midline vertical septum in the uterus and upper vagina is resorbed segmentally from the isthmus and progresses in both directions. The intervening transverse vaginal septum also breaks down for a completely canalized vagina.

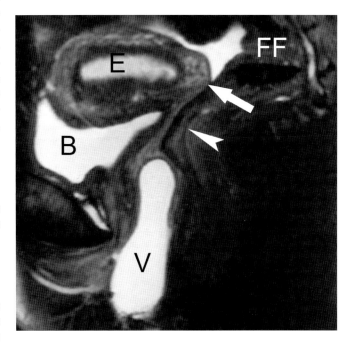

Figure 9.14 *Cervical and vaginal agenesis.* Sagittal T2-weighted FSE/TSE image performed with vaginal gel in a 13-year-old girl with amenorrhea and cyclic pain shows agenesis of the cervix (*arrow*) and 3 cm of the upper vagina (*arrowhead*). The bladder (*B*), gel within the vagina (*V*), secretory-phase endometrial canal (*E*), and small amount of cul-de-sac fluid (*FF*) are high in signal intensity.

Lower vagina

The uterovaginal primordium fuses with the urogenital sinus through vertical fusion and will induce the lower vagina to develop. Differentiation of the uterovaginal primordium itself is not necessary for vaginal development (as in the case with Mayer-Rokitansky-Kuster-Hauser syndrome).

ABSENCE OF THE UROGENITAL RIDGE

If the urogenital ridge is absent on one side, the ipsilateral ovary, kidney, and half the uterus does not form. A unicornuate uterus is present on the contralateral side. Axial skeletal anomalies (vertebral fusion or absence) also often occur because an insult at this early stage of development may easily affect adjacent developing mesoderm.

ISOLATED MÜLLERIAN ANOMALIES

Isolated Müllerian defects are the common uterine malformations resulting from lack of formation (agenesis), lack of development after formation (aplasia/hypoplasia), lack of fusion, and lack of septal resorption. Agenesis is rare and often associated with non-Müllerian anomalies (usually renal).

Table 9.1 AMERICAN FERTILITY CLASSIFICATION OF MÜLLERIAN ANOMALIES RELATED TO AGENESIS AND HYPOPLASIA (CLASS 1) AND LATERAL FUSION ANOMALIES (CLASS 2–6)

LACK OF DEVELOPMENT

I	Segmental or complete agenesis or hypoplasia	Agenesis or hypoplasia of the upper vagina, cervix, fundus, tubes or any combination. Complete Müllerian aplasia (Mayer-Rokitansky-Kuster-Hauser syndrome) is the most common.	
II	Unicornuate uterus with or without a rudimentary horn	Simple unicornuate or unicornuate with a rudimentary horn. Rudimentary horn may contain endometrium which may or may not communicate with the remainder of the endometrium. Ipsilateral renal agenesis is often present.	

Fusion anomalies

III	Didelphys uterus	Complete duplication of the uterus and cervix.	
IV	Complete or partial bicornuate uterus	Fusion has occurred at least caudally. Large fundal cleft variably extends down the body and cervix.	

Lack of septal resorption

V	Complete or partial septate uterus	Uterus completely fused; fundal contour is normal. A complete or partial midline septum is present.	
VI	Arcuate uterus	A small septum is present at the fundus.	

Other

VII	DES-related abnormalities	A T-shaped uterine cavity with or without dilated horns.	

Segmental or complete *hypoplasia or agenesis* of the Müllerian ducts can involve any level between the upper vagina and fallopian tubes. Unilateral aplasia or hypoplasia of one duct results in the variations of unicornuate uterus. Total or partial aplasia of both ducts results in the Mayer-Rokitansky-Kuster-Hauser syndrome, the most common anomaly of this group. Lack or incomplete fusion of the caudal segments of the paired ducts results in cervico-upper vaginal atresia.

Lateral fusion defects are the most common Müllerian anomalies and include the didelphys, bicornuate, septate, and arcuate uterus. Partial or complete failure of fusion results in the bicornuate and didelphys uterus, respectively. After fusion, the midline septum in the uterus, cervix, and upper vagina is resorbed segmentally to form a single uterine cavity and cervix. Failure of septal resorption results in the septate uterus, the most common anomaly, and arcuate uterus.

Transverse fusion defects result from lack of canalization of the transverse tissue between the upper Müllerian-derived vagina and the lower urogenital-derived vagina. A transverse vaginal septum or imperforate hymen can result.

The 1988 American Fertility Classification (AFC)[7] (Table 9.1) is most commonly used in the United States to categorize Müllerian anomalies related to time of failure and includes aplasia and hypoplasia (class 1 and 2) and lateral fusion anomalies (classes 3 to 6). Non-Müllerian-derived anomalies are not included in the classification.

Mayer-Rokitansky-Kuster-Hauser syndrome (Fig. 9.15) is one of the most common causes of primary amenorrhea in a sexually developed adolescent. Type I is an isolated Müllerian defect resulting in an absent or rudimentary uterus, and lack of the upper two thirds of the vagina. The ovaries and fallopian tubes are normal and two symmetric rudimentary uterine horns are present. Since type I is of Müllerian etiology, renal anomalies are not present. Type II has a different genetic and embryologic etiology and is associated with renal, skeletal, cardiac, otologic, and ovarian anomalies in addition to the presenting complaint of primary amenorrhea. The uterine aplasia also has characteristic features differing from type I.

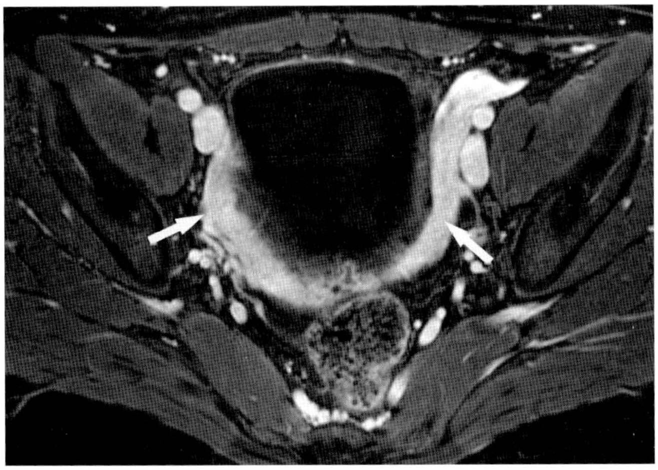

Unicornuate uterus occurs in four variations (Fig. 9.16). All have similar increased rates of spontaneous abortion, premature labor, and intrauterine growth restriction. Most (90%) occur with incomplete arrest in growth of one of the Müllerian ducts, resulting in the presence of a rudimentary horn that may or may not communicate with the uterine cavity and may or may not contain functioning endometrium. If the rudimentary horn contains endometrial tissue (a "cavitary" or "functioning" horn), it is important to assess whether the endometrium communicates with the remainder of the endometrium or is isolated by intervening myometrium (Fig. 9.17). The rudimentary horn associated with unicornuate uterus is small, while the horns are similar in size in a bicornuate or nonobstructed didelphys uterus. A functioning rudimentary horn may be displaced and appear detached from the unicornate uterus, connected by only a thin fibrous attachment.[8] MRI findings with unicornuate uterus:

- The key finding is a small, laterally deviated uterus.

- A simple unicornuate uterus has a single laterally deviated uterine horn with no rudimentary horn on the opposite side.

- Unicornuate uterus with a rudimentary horn does not communicate with the uterine cavity and does not contain functioning endometrium.

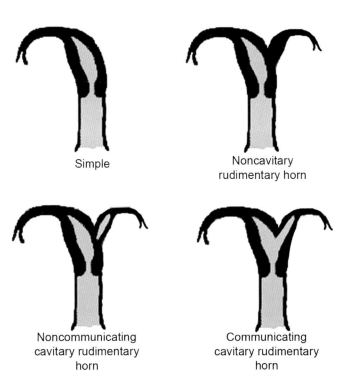

Figure 9.15 *Mayer-Rokintasky-Kuster-Hauser syndrome.* The uterus is absent and the proximal vagina is atretic. Both ovaries and kidneys were normal. Axial T1-weighted post-contrast-enhanced image demonstrates an avidly enhancing rim of tissue (*arrows*) lining the posterior pelvic wall that may occur. This represents arrested development of the urogenital ridge normally located along the posterior pelvic peritoneum. A sling of tissue was palpable at the level of the peritoneal reflection on rectal examination.

Simple

Noncavitary rudimentary horn

Noncommunicating cavitary rudimentary horn

Communicating cavitary rudimentary horn

Figure 9.16 *Variations of unicornate uterus.* (**A**) Simple unicornuate uterus. (**B**) Unicornuate uterus with a noncavitary rudimentary horn. (**C**) Unicornuate uterus with a noncommunicating cavitary rudimentary horn. (**D**) Unicornuate uterus with a communicating cavitary rudimentary horn.

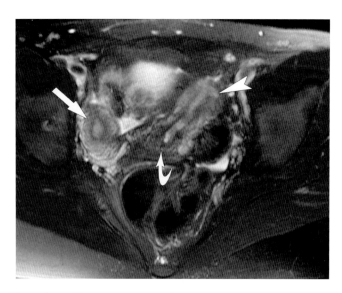

Figure 9.17 *Unicornuate uterus with a noncommunicating cavitary rudimentary horn.* Axial T2-weighted FSE/TSE image with fat-saturation demonstrates a unicornuate uterus on the left with the uterine body (*arrowhead*) communicating with the cervix (*curved arrow*) and a widely separated rudimentary horn with functioning endometrium on the right (*arrow*).

- Unicornuate uterus with a rudimentary horn may have functioning endometrium. If present, determine whether the endometrial lining of the rudimentary horn communicates with the endometrium of the unicornuate portion. Retrograde menstruation from endometrial tissue contained within a non-communicating rudimentary horn can result in extensive endometriosis (Fig. 9.18). Inflammatory obstruction at the fimbria can result in unilateral hematometros. A finding of hydrosalpinx in a menarchal-age female is likely due to a non-communicating functional unicornuate uterus. Fertilization from sperm arriving from the contralateral tube can result in ectopic pregnancy. This is specifically referred to as a cornual ectopic and is to be distinguished from an interstitial ectopic.

- All types of unicornuate uterus can be associated with urinary tract anomalies. The incidence is approximately 40% to 50%, and anomalies include renal agenesis, horseshoe kidney, ectopic kidney, and renal dysplasia.[9] The absent kidney is always on the same side as the rudimentary or absent horn. Though the unicornuate uterus is classified as a Müllerian anomaly, the absent kidney is a consequence of a combined non-Müllerian factor.

Didelphys uterus and bicornuate uterus represent a continuum in incomplete fusion, and thus there is a fundal cleft. A normal fundal contour signifies that fusion is complete and excludes a didelphys or bicornuate uterus. A midline structure would be the septum of a septate uterus.

Didelphys uterus (Fig. 9.19) is a completely duplicated uterus with two uteri and two cervices. A duplicated upper 2/3 of the vagina occurs in 75% of the cases. In essence there are two adjacent unicornuate uteri. Thus, the clinical problems from a didelphys uterus are similar to those associated with a

unicornuate uterus. The longitudinal vaginal septum can trap and collect menstrual blood as it bulges inferiorly. There is usually some opening that allows egress of menstrual fluid.

Bicornuate uterus (Fig. 9.20) is further along on the continuum of partial fusion of the uterus. At least some fusion has occurred in the region of the cervix. A vaginal septum is seen in approximately 25% of cases. Patients have two divergent uterine horns. After repeated abortions, surgical repair may be attempted by open metroplasty to form a more normal uterine morphology.

The cleft of a bicornuate configuration is of variable length in the uterine body. It can extend to the internal cervical os (bicornuate unicollis) or close to the external os to give the appearance of a nearly duplicated cervix (bicornuate bicollis). In the latter, the uterus can resemble a didelphys uterus. It may not be possible, and is not important, to distinguish between a didelphys and the extreme bicornuate bicollis uterus since they are nearly the same entity, with similar outcomes and treatment.

Septate uterus (Fig. 9.21) is the most common anomaly. Fusion is complete and the septate uterus has a normal external contour and dimensions as a normal uterus. A midline septum variably extends through the uterine body, cervix, and vagina, depending on the degree of resorption. The septum can result in an appearance similar to that of the presence of two cervices. The septum can appear quite prominent and the anomaly can be misdiagnosed as bicornuate uterus. Differentiation is important because septate uterus is treated by transvaginal hysteroscopic resection of the septum, whereas surgical repair of the bicornuate uterus involves metroplasty from an abdominal approach. Incidental diagnosis of septate uterus requires consideration of the low-risk prophylactic resection of the septum to avoid subsequent spontaneous abortions. Important points for MR diagnosis of congenital anomalies include:

- Differentiation of didelphys, bicornuate, and septate uterus by MRI (Figs. 9.19A, 9.20A, and 9.21A) starts with evaluation of the fundal contour, not the appearance of the septum. If the fundal contour is normal, the uterus is not a didelphys or bicornuate uterus.

- One cannot rely on the MR signal intensity of the intervening septum, myometrium, number of cervices, length of septation, or extension into the vagina to distinguish the three types. All three (didelphys, bicornuate, and septate) can have the appearance of two cervices, and all can have a vaginal septum.

Near-complete resorption of the fibrous uterine septum causes an **arcuate uterus**, which should be considered a normal variant and has no effect on fertility. Arcuate uterus is considered a mild form of septate uterus. The uterus may have a broad configuration (less than 1.5 cm) of the fundal myometrium (Fig. 9.22).

Diethylstilbestrol (DES)-related anomalies are Müllerian anomalies that resulted from use of synthetic estrogen, which was prescribed from 1945 to 1971 to prevent miscarriage. Anomalies included a T-shaped uterus, uterine or cervical cavity stenosis, uterine hypoplasia, and diverticula of the fallopian tubes. This drug was also rarely associated with clear cell

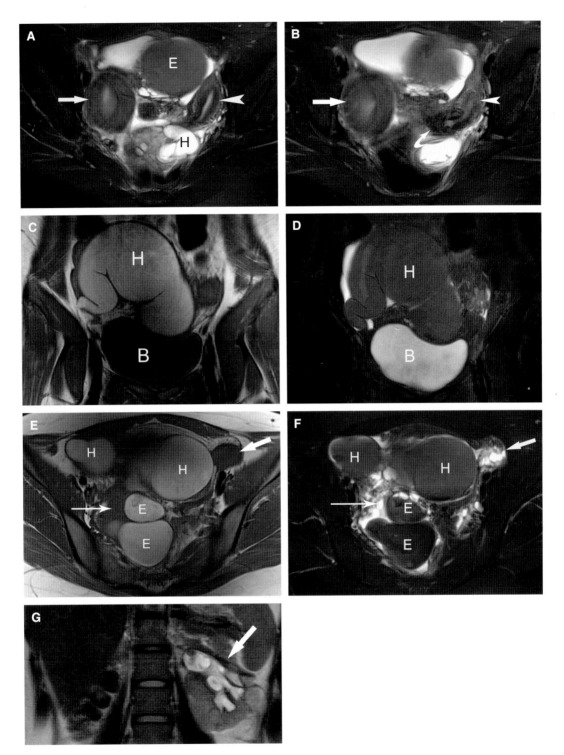

Figure 9.18 *Unicornuate uterus complicated by endometriosis.* (**A, B**) Axial T2-weighted fat-suppressed FSE/TSE images show widely displaced uterine horns containing high-signal-intensity functioning endometrium. The left horn (*arrowhead*) communicates with the cervix (*curved arrow* in image B), while the right horn (*arrow*) does not. Retrograde menstruation from the noncommunicating right horn has resulted in endometriosis (*E*) and scarring of the tube at the fimbrial end, with resultant right hematosalpinx (*H*). (**C, D**) A large right hematosalpinx (*H*) shows relatively high signal intensity on coronal T1-weighted image (**C**) and relatively low signal intensity on the corresponding T2-weighted image (**D**). The low signal intensity on the T2-weighted imaging is the result of the high ferritin and hemosiderin concentration within this chronic hemorrhagic collection. The hematosalpinx resulted from lack of communication of the right uterine horn with the cervix and scarring of the tube at the fimbrial end with retrograde menstruation into the tube. Endometriosis results from retrograde menstruation into the pelvic cavity from the incompletely obstructed tube. *B*, bladder. (**E, F**) The chronic right hematosalpinx (*H*) and several pelvic endometriomas (*E*) are shown on axial T1-weighted (**E**) and T2-weighted images with fat saturation (**F**). Note that both the chronic hematosalpinx and the endometriomas display intermediate signal intensity on T1-weighted and relatively low signal intensity on T2-weighted images, reflecting chronic hemorrhage within the cystic masses. Follicles of the right ovary (*skinny arrows*) with implanted endometrioma and of the anteriorly displaced left ovary (*fat arrows*) displaced anteriorly are high in insignal intensity on the T2-weighted image, providing landmarks for identification of the ovaries on these complex images. (**G**) Coronal T2-weighted image shows absence of the right kidney, a common associated finding with a unicornuate uterus. The left kidney (*arrow*) shows hydronephrosis caused by the endometriomas.

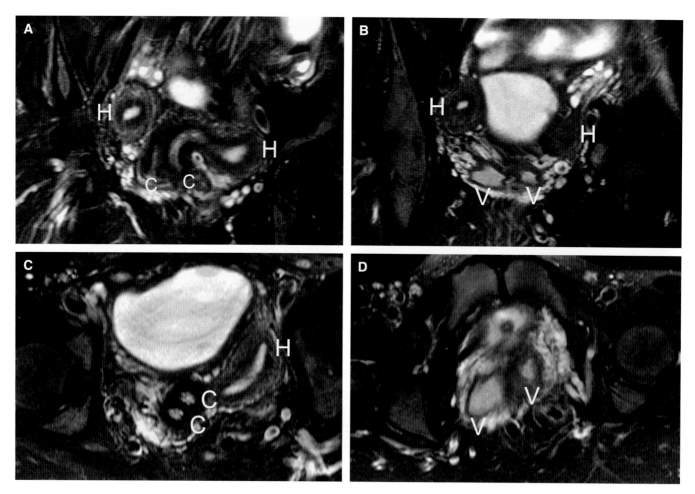

Figure 9.19 *Didelphys uterus.* Coronal (**A, B**) and axial (**C, D**) T2-weighted FSE/TSE image with fat saturation show widely divergent uterine horns (*H*), two cervices (*C*), and two vaginas (*V*). Fluid is present within the two vaginas separated by a vaginal septum, which is found in two thirds of patients with a didelphys uterus. Uterus didelphys results from nonfusion of the Müllerian ducts.

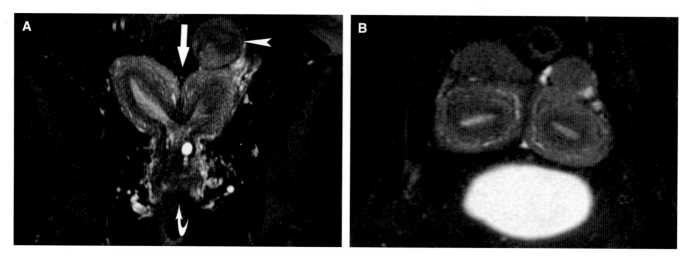

Figure 9.20 *Bicornuate uterus.* Coronal oblique T2-weighted FSE/TSE images with fat saturation through the long axis of the uterus (**A**) and the short axis of the uterus (**B**) provide optimal depiction of the uterus for characterization of developmental anomalies. The deep indentation (more than 1 cm) (*arrow* in image A) in the uterine fundus characterizes this uterus as bicornuate. A single cervix (*curved arrow* in image A) is present. A hemorrhagic ovarian cyst (*arrowhead* in image A) is noted.

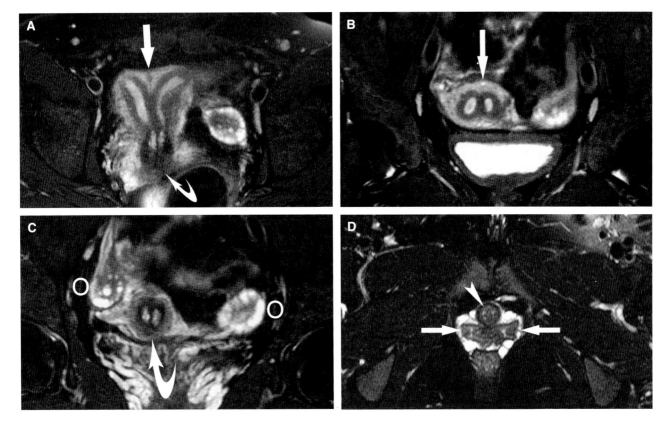

Figure 9.21 *Septate uterus.* (**A**) Although this plane on T2-weighted FSE/TSE imaging is axial to the pelvis, it is oblique axial in relationship to the uterine body and best demonstrates that the external contour has normal morphology (*straight arrow*). Therefore this cannot be a didelphys or bicornuate uterus. There is a long midline septum extending through the body and cervix (*curved arrow*). This is a complete septate uterus. (**B**) Image perpendicular to the long axis of the uterus shows the septum (*arrow*) dividing the lower uterine segment. (**C**) The septum is seen through the cervix (*curved arrow*) on the image obtained just inferior to image B. Both ovaries (*O*) are identified by the abundant small follicles. (**D**) A longitudinal septum can be variably present in the vagina. In the septate uterus of this patient, image obtained inferior to C shows the two vaginas (each indicated with arrow). The urethra (*arrowhead*) is evident coursing within the anterior wall of the vagina.

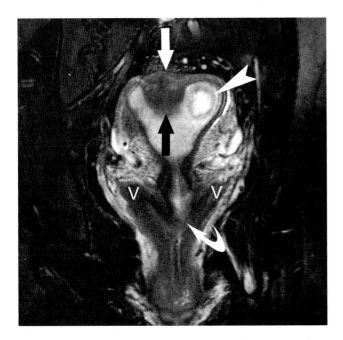

Figure 9.22 *Pregnancy in an arcuate uterus.* Coronal T2-weighted image demonstrates a normal fundal contour (*white arrow*) and a deep myometrial extension (*black arrow*). The early pregnancy (*arrowhead*) is in the left portion of the divided uterus within the intermediate high signal intensity endometrium. The cervix (*curved arrow*) and vaginal fornices (*V*) are normal.

adenocarcinoma of the vagina. These anomalies are currently seen infrequently on MR, given the remote use of this estrogen.

COMPLEX COMBINED ANOMALIES

A coexistent Müllerian and renal anomaly indicates a combined Müllerian and non-Müllerian anomaly. These anomalies are among the most complex (Fig. 9.23).[10] Dysgenesis of the entire or the distal part of a single Wolffian duct occurs early in embryologic development, prior to formation of the Müllerian ducts. Since the Wolffian duct helps direct renal, uterine, and vaginal development, dysgenesis may result in coexistent ipsilateral renal anomalies (almost always renal agenesis) and Müllerian duplication anomalies (usually didelphys). Upper and/or lower vaginal aplasia are also associated.

The classic anomaly of this group is obstructed hemivagina and ipsilateral renal anomaly (OHVIRA) syndrome (also called uterus didelphys with obstructed hemivagina).[11] The Wolffian duct does not open into the urogenital sinus and the uterine bud does not form to induce formation of the kidney, and therefore ipsilateral renal agenesis is almost always present. A uterine duplication anomaly is present, nearly always uterus didelphys. The affected side has a blind-ending upper vagina and absent lower vagina. The lower vagina is aplastic since it develops from the sinovaginal bulbs of the Wolffian

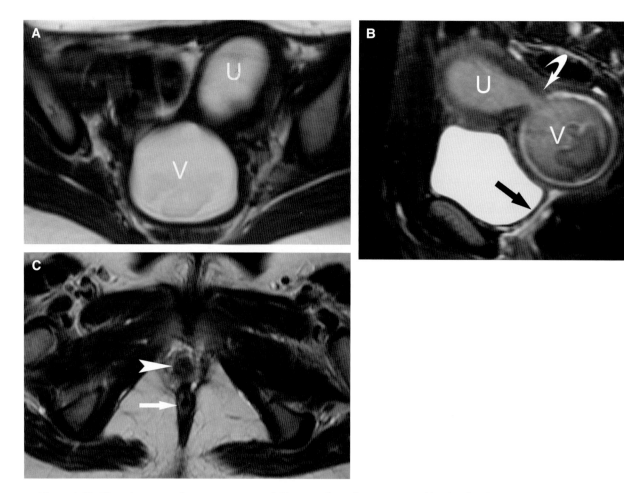

Figure 9.23 *Vaginal atresia and unicornuate uterus.* MR was performed on a 13-year-old girl with pelvic pain, amenorrhea, and absence of the lower vagina on physical examination. (**A**) Axial T1-weighted image shows high-signal-intensity fluid in the markedly dilated upper vagina (*V*) and distended uterus (*U*). (**B**) Sagittal T2-weighted image shows T2-shading effect with lowered signal intensity of the fluid in the uterus (*U*) and vagina (*V*) indicating chronic hemorrhage. The upper two thirds of the vagina is distended and filled with bloody fluid, and the lower third (*black arrow*) is atretic. This reflects the independent embryologic origins of the upper two thirds and lower third of the vagina. The uterus appears small with the cervix (*curved arrow*) open to the vagina. Additional imaging showed absence of the right kidney. (**C**) Axial T2-weighted image shows absence of the lower vagina from its normal location between the urethra (*arrowhead*) and the rectum (*arrow*). Surgery confirmed atresia of the lower vagina, unicornuate left uterine horn, and absence of the cervix, right uterine horn, fallopian tube, and uterine vasculature. Normal ovaries were present bilaterally, as would be expected given that their development is independent of that of the uterus.

duct. Since this anomaly results from dysgenesis of only one Wolffian duct, the contralateral vagina develops normally and clinically a normal vagina appears to be present.

Typically, the entity presents in an adolescent girl with pelvic pain or dysmenorrhea, and on examination a bulge in a vaginal sidewall and a cervix are present. The typical anomaly is uterus didelphys with obstructed hemivagina. On the side of the affected Wolffian duct, one horn of a didelphys uterus communicates with a blind-ending obstructed hemivagina, resulting in hematometrocolpos and hematosalpinx. Ipsilateral renal agenesis is typically also present.

Complex Müllerian and urologic variations can occur in this syndrome. The duplicated horns may be asymmetric and may communicate with each other. Other duplication anomalies include bicornuate uteri or single obstructed horn with cervical atresia and hemivagina. The obstructed hemivagina can decompress into large Gardner's duct cysts, the latter related to persisting remnants of the abnormal Wolffian duct. Communication can occur with the vagina through a small ori-

fice. Rarely, an ectopic ureteric bud may have been able to arise from a Wolffian remnant. If it ends ectopically into the hemivagina or a Gartner's duct cyst it may be able to induce some renal development, resulting in a dysplastic or polycystic kidney.[10]

A uterus didelphys with obstructed hemivagina is a different entity from that of the isolated Müllerian-related uterus didelphys with a partially obstructed longitudinal vaginal septum. In the former, an upper hemivagina does not canalize with the lower vagina. Menstrual fluids secreted by a functioning horn of a uterus didelphys are completely trapped. In a uterus didelphys with a partially obstructed longitudinal vaginal septum, the septum traps the menstrual fluid and surgical correction is done by simple clipping of the thin septum.

Unicornuate uteri are also frequently associated with renal agenesis and other renal anomalies (40% to 50%). Although unicornuate uterus has been classified as an isolated Müllerian anomaly by the AFC, unicornuate uterus with renal anomaly is the result of an early embryologic dysgenesis of a Wolffian duct. Embryologically the aforementioned complex anomalies and the unicornuate uterus are related. Instead of OHVIRA syndrome occurring, the cervix, hemiuterus, and hemivagina on the obstructed side did not develop at all, resulting in only a unicornate uterus on the contralateral side.

VAGINAL ANOMALIES

Upper vaginal atresia occurs in Mayer-Rokitansky-Kuster-Hauser syndrome (lack of or complete fusion of both the lower ducts and Müllerian tubercle), cervico-vaginal atresia (Müllerian tubercle only) (see Fig. 9.14), or rarely as an isolated upper vaginal atresia. Typically, with isolated upper vaginal atresia, a pubescent girl presents with abdominal or pelvic pain, amenorrhea, and with a mass in the lower vagina bulging with retained blood. MR reveals absence of the upper vagina and hematocolpos. With upper vaginal atresia and cervical agenesis, hysterectomy is the standard treatment, given the high incidence of peritonitis after attempted cervical canalization; however, uterovaginal anastomosis may be an option for perseveration of fertility.[12] Evaluation for the presence of a cervix by MR can sometimes be difficult, especially when the existing uterine canal is distended with blood.

Lower vaginal atresia occurs with normal upper structures and the lower vagina composed only of fibrous tissue.

Complete lack of a vagina is rare and may be due to agenesis of the uterovaginal primordium or related to chromosomal or genetic defects, the most common of which is androgen insensitivity syndrome (vaginal agenesis). The uterus is absent.

Transverse vaginal septum. Though the lower vagina may be canalized, the transverse tissue between the upper and lower vagina may not break down. A transverse vaginal septum can persist at several levels, and hydrometrocolpos, hematometra, or hematocolpos can result.

UTERINE MYOMETRIAL PATHOLOGY

LEIOMYOMAS

Smooth muscle tumors of the uterus are mesenchymal tumors classified according to the World Health Organization/International Society of Gynecologic Pathologists as benign leiomyomas and variants, which include the atypical, cellular, myxoid, and lipoleiomyoma; smooth-muscle tumor of uncertain malignant potential (STUMP); and leiomyosarcomas (typical, epithelioid, myxoid). The majority of smooth muscle tumors are typical leiomyomas that can be confidently diagnosed as benign by MR imaging. The atypical leiomyoma is a benign leiomyoma with nuclear atypia and no other worrisome features. STUMP tumor is a term applied to leiomyomas with indeterminate histologic features of malignancy. Use of the term is currently discouraged as a nondiagnostic term. Leiomyosarcomas are rare and the diagnosis is usually suggested when a uterine mass lacks one or more features diagnostic of a leiomyoma; in such case further workup is needed. A small group of benign leiomyomas demonstrate features that overlap with leiomyosarcomas and need histologic confirmation or close follow-up. They include the myxoid and cellular (so-called "hydropic") leiomyoma variants and typical leiomyomas with extensive cystic or myxoid change.

Benign leiomyomas are well-circumscribed, firm, rubbery masses composed of tightly packed aggregates of smooth muscle cells with varying amounts of intervening collagen. The muscle cell aggregates swirl and intersect at right angles to one another to give the characteristic whorled appearance. The term "leiomyoma" is preferred over fibroid, given their predominant smooth muscle composition. A pseudo-capsule composed of a separate layer of connective tissue sharply demarcates the tumor from the surrounding myometrium and allows them to be relatively easily shelled out at surgery. The absence of this cleavage plane indicates possible infiltration, a characteristic of leiomyosarcoma.[13]

Leiomyomas are believed to arise from estrogen-stimulated mutagenesis and growth of a single myometrial cell. A large percentage of reproductive-age women have small asymptomatic leiomyomas. They regress after menopause unless hormone replacement therapy is used. Leiomyomas are more common in obese women and in African American women and show familial clustering. They often increase in size in early pregnancy and degenerate in late pregnancy.

Symptoms occur in 20% of patients and are related to the number, size, and location of leiomyomas. Mass effect, resulting in dilatation of the adjacent venules, accounts for

---

Box 9.2 **ESSENTIALS TO REMEMBER**

- Anomalies of the genital tract may be isolated or associated with developmental anomalies of the urinary tract. Absence of a kidney is associated with either any of the unicornuate uterus variations or with very complex anomalies.

- Unicornate uterus may be simple or associated with a smaller rudimentary horn. If the rudimentary horn contains endometrial tissue, it is imperative to determine whether it communicates with the remainder of the endometrium. A rudimentary horn containing endometrium may be displaced considerably from the unicornate part and connected by only a thin fibrous attachment. Endometriosis or a cornual ectopic may occur if not diagnosed.

- Fusion anomalies result in the spectrum of arcuate, septate, bicornuate, and didelphys uterus. These anomalies are best characterized by obtaining angled T2-weighted MR images aligned with the long axis of the uterus.

- Upper and lower vaginal anomalies are associated with different spectrums of anomalies, given their differing embryologic origin. Atresia or septation may occur as isolated anomalies or in association with uterine anomalies.

menorrhagia. Pressure symptoms include urinary frequency, pain, and infertility. Hemorrhagic degeneration causes abdominal pain, low-grade fever, and leukocytosis. Certain locations are particularly problematic. MR enables classification of leiomyomas as submucosal, intramural, or subserosal:

- *Submucosal* leiomyomas arise adjacent to the endometrium and protrude into the endometrial canal. Submucosal leiomyomas may cause excess bleeding or infertility caused by distortion or inflammation of the endometrial lining. They may be broad-based or pedunculated. Those with a narrow stalk can prolapse, resulting in hematocolpos, pyocolpos, or even uterine inversion (Fig. 9.24). Submucosal leiomyomas simulate endometrial polyps by location but can usually be distinguished by their characteristic low signal and heterogeneity at MR imaging.

- *Intramural* leiomyomas are located within the myometrium. An intramural leiomyoma with a submucosal component partially borders on the endometrial lining.

- *Subserosal* leiomyomas have an epicenter beyond the outer uterine wall. They may be broad-based or pedunculated. Pedunculated subserosal leiomyomas may degenerate or torse, causing acute pain. Pedunculated leiomyomas demonstrate the typical imaging features of intrauterine leiomyomas. MR defines the origin of the mass. The stalk of a pedunculated leiomyoma is detected by recognizing uterine vessels that extend from the myometrium to the leiomyoma, the "bridging vascular sign." Vessels are best seen on T2-weighted images and gadolinium-contrast-enhanced T1-weighted images. A separate ovary should be sought. If an ovary cannot be found, the differential includes a fibrous ovarian tumor.

- *Adnexal* leiomyomas are extrauterine, arising from subserosal leiomyomas that parasitize blood supply from adnexal structures. Leiomyomas may also arise from embryonic rests in extrauterine structures such as the broad ligament or round ligament. Broad-ligament leiomyomas can cause ureteral obstruction through mass effect.

- *Cervical* leiomyomas constitute 1% to 2% of leiomyomas and are almost always solitary.

As leiomyomas enlarge they commonly outgrow their blood supply, resulting in hyaline degeneration, cystic change, and "red" degeneration.

Leiomyomas are prone to *hyaline degeneration* because they lack the dual blood supply of the normal uterus, have lower arterial density, and have a disorganized vascular pattern compared with normal myometrium. As a result, the majority of leiomyomas over 3 to 5 cm in size have variable hyaline degeneration. Smooth muscle cells and blood vessels are replaced by a proteinaceous acellular hyaline matrix of collagen, giving a characteristic diffuse speckled pattern of higher-signal foci in an otherwise low-signal intensity background (Fig. 9.25C).

With increasing ischemia, small foci of *cystic degeneration* may occur. A small amount of cystic change within an otherwise solid firm typical leiomyoma can be confidently diagnosed as benign (Fig. 9.26). A greater extent of cystic degeneration can create a problem in diagnosis.

Marked ischemia rarely also results in extensive *myxoid (or mucoid) degeneration*. Although pathologists do not consider either cystic or myxoid degeneration a notable quality in the diagnosis of benign leiomyoma, myxoid degeneration is usually striking by MR, and the imaging findings can be similar to that of a sarcoma.

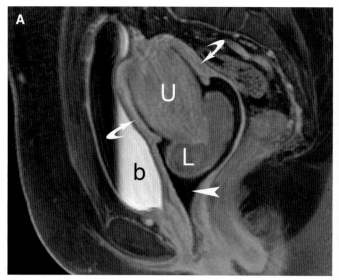 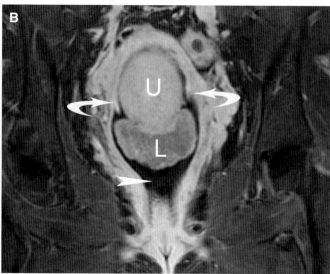

Figure 9.24 *Uterine prolapse.* Sagittal (**A**) and coronal (**B**) post-gadolinium-contrast-enhanced T1-weighted images show prolapse of the uterus (*U*) through the cervix (*curved arrows*) led by a submucosal broad-based cellular leiomyoma (*L*). The fundal leiomyoma acted as a lead point with uterine contractions causing prolapse. The inverted uterine body is contained within the walls of the cervix. The vagina is filled with gel (*arrowhead*) showing low signal intensity on this T1-weighted image, and providing good definition of the mass protruding into the vagina. The bladder (*b*) is partially filled with contrast agent showing high signal intensity.

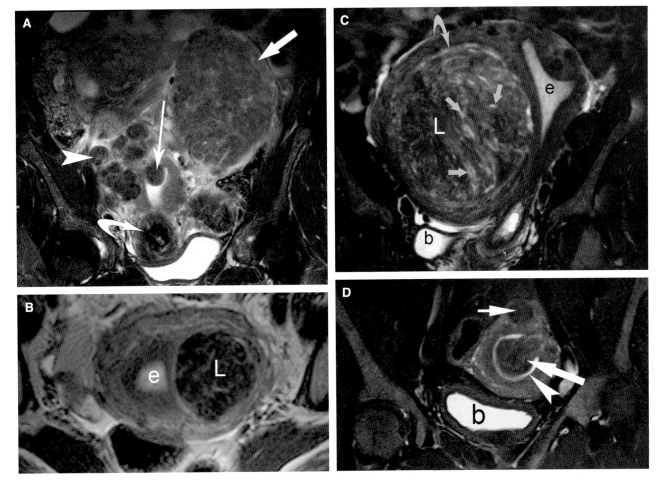

Figure 9.25 *Classic features of leiomyomas.* Typical leiomyomas are characteristically low in signal intensity on T2-weighted sequences. (**A**) Numerous leiomyomas greatly enlarge the uterus and include large subserosal (*fat arrow*), intramural (*arrowhead*), and lower uterine segment (*curved arrow*) leiomyomas as well as a submucosal leiomyoma extending into the endometrial canal (*skinny arrow*). (**B**) T2-weighted image shows that leiomyomas (*L*) tend to be display lower signal intensity than adjacent myometrium. *e*, endometrium. (**C**) Hyaline degeneration in a large leiomyoma (*L*) appears as speckled foci of high signal intensity (*arrows*) and is considered part of the normal spectrum of appearance of a benign leiomyoma. A high-signal-intensity rim (*curved arrow*) is common and reflects edema and dilated lymphatics. *b*, bladder; *e*, endometrium. (**D**) A pedunculated submucosal leiomyoma (*long arrow*) bulges into the high-signal-intensity endometrial canal (*arrowhead*). It can be distinguished from an endometrial polyp by its low signal on all sequences. A smaller leiomyoma is also noted (*short arrow*). *b*, bladder.

Red or carneous (hemorrhagic) degeneration (Fig. 9.27) is a consequence of massive hemorrhagic infarction caused by venous thrombosis in the periphery of the leiomyoma. Hemorrhagic infarction characteristically occurs during pregnancy and occasionally with oral contraceptive use, causing self-limiting symptoms of pain, low-grade fever, and leukocytosis.

Nearly all leiomyomas can be diagnosed as benign leiomyomas on ultrasound examination by the characteristic sonographic features of whorled shadowing round masses and lack of concerning clinical findings. MR may be indicated because of:

- Lack of the characteristic imaging findings of a leiomyoma on ultrasound

- Increase in size of the uterus, or in the size of a uterine mass thought to be leiomyoma, especially with new onset of bleeding and a nondiagnostic ultrasound

- Difficulty differentiating an exophytic or pedunculated leiomyoma from an adnexal mass. MR better demonstrates

the attachment as well as the typical features diagnostic of leiomyoma or fibrous ovarian tumor.

- Use with treatment planning with respect of selection of patients for hysterectomy, embolization, or hysteroscopic or open myomectomy

- Assessment of the leiomyomas before and after uterine artery embolization.

Nearly all leiomyomas have classic features, enabling confident diagnosis. The tightly packed muscle cells, the sparse compressed vessels, and the variable amount of collagen account for the lower signal in leiomyomas than in normal myometrium on T1- and T2-weighted images. MR features of benign leiomyomas (see Fig. 9.25) include:

- A well-circumscribed mass with sharply defined borders and predominantly low signal on all sequences, with or without a bright rim, are findings pathognomonic for a leiomyoma.

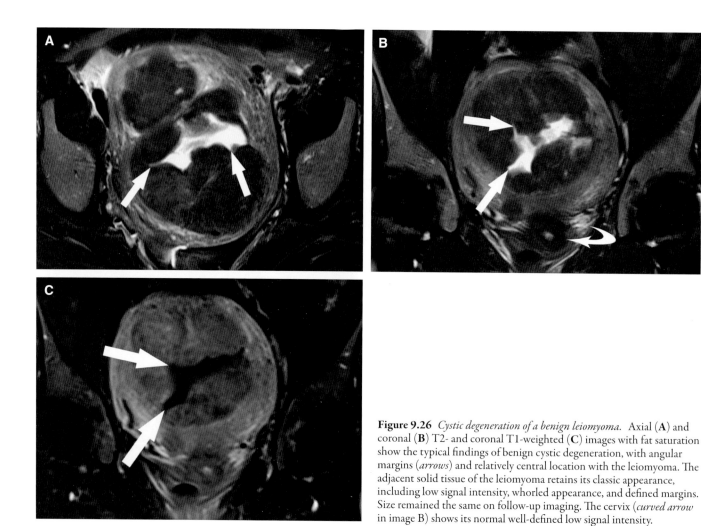

Figure 9.26 *Cystic degeneration of a benign leiomyoma.* Axial (**A**) and coronal (**B**) T2- and coronal T1-weighted (**C**) images with fat saturation show the typical findings of benign cystic degeneration, with angular margins (*arrows*) and relatively central location with the leiomyoma. The adjacent solid tissue of the leiomyoma retains its classic appearance, including low signal intensity, whorled appearance, and defined margins. Size remained the same on follow-up imaging. The cervix (*curved arrow* in image B) shows its normal well-defined low signal intensity.

Figure 9.27 *Red (carneous) degeneration.* A 32-year-old woman presented with acute pelvic pain. T1- (**A**) and T2-weighted (**B**) images with fat saturation show intermediate diffuse increased signal intensity of the leiomyoma (*L*), reflecting subacute hemorrhage. The leiomyoma did not enhance on post-contrast-enhanced images (not shown). A distinct peripheral rim (*arrows*) displays high signal intensity on T1-weighted images and low signal intensity on T2-weighted images. This rim is caused by thrombosis of the veins surrounding the infarcted leiomyoma.

- Leiomyomas are firm and compress the adjacent myometrium, creating a characteristic pseudo-capsule.

- Benign leiomyomas have "compressive force." In addition to the pseudo-capsule, they hold a rounded shape, bulging into the endometrium or beyond the uterine border.[13]

- On T1-weighted images, typical leiomyomas have signal intensity similar to that of the myometrium. A slightly higher signal than myometrium may occur as a result of hyaline degeneration (Fig. 9.25C).

- On T2-weighted images small leiomyomas display homogeneously low signal, whereas leiomyomas larger than 3 to 5 cm have a characteristic speckled or cobblestone pattern of higher-signal foci resulting from hyaline degeneration. Overall low signal predominates within the lesion, however.

- A high-signal-intensity rim on T2-weighted images is common and results from edema and dilated lymphatics (Fig. 9.25A). The rim may enhance with intravenous gadolinium contrast material administration.

- Cystic degeneration occurs centrally, and characteristically the fluid shows angular margins (Fig. 9.26). The solid portion of the leiomyoma retains its low signal intensity, whorled appearance, and pseudo-capsule.

- Red or carneous degeneration appears as intermediate to high signal intensity on T1- and T2-weighted images (Fig. 9.27). Internal high signal intensity on T1-weighted images reflects the presence of subacute hemorrhage. A distinct peripheral rim of acutely thrombosed peripheral veins surrounds the infarcted leiomyoma. The rim is high in signal intensity on T1-weighted images and very low on T2-weighted images due to the T1- and T2*-shortening effect of methemoglobin. A leiomyoma that does not enhance reflects total infarction.

- Intravenous contrast enhancement is usually not needed in the diagnosis of typical leiomyomas, but dynamic contrast-enhanced sequences can be of use in the workup for UAE or for evaluating the atypical leiomyoma or possible leiomyosarcoma. If contrast material is administered, enhancement tends to be heterogeneous and less than that of the myometrium. Contrast enhancement improves demonstration of necrosis.

- Peripheral or internal focal areas of signal void reflect coarse calcification, typical of degenerated leiomyoma.

Intervention is often undertaken for the treatment of bleeding, anemia, pressure on adjacent organs, pain, or infertility caused by the lesions. Medical therapy, myomectomy, and myolysis (focused ultrasound, radiofrequency ablation, and cryoablation) may be attempted in lieu of hysterectomy. Selective UAE is used to treat symptomatic leiomyomas in women who may desire subsequent pregnancy. Nonselective bilateral UAE is a less invasive option when pregnancy is not desired.

Gonadotropin-releasing analogs (GnRHa) are often used to diminish size prior to surgery. They are usually not effective alone, as the treated leiomyomas generally return to their original size after a year due to an increase in estrogen receptors. When treated with GnRHa, regions of the tumor may undergo coagulative necrosis through ischemia or infarction, simulating the MR appearance of leiomyosarcoma (Fig. 9.28). Knowledge of the effects of treatment with GnRHa is essential for making the correct imaging diagnosis.

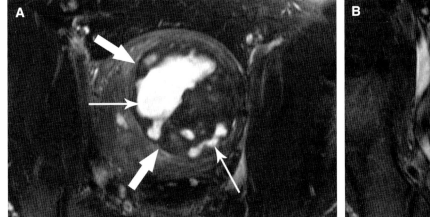 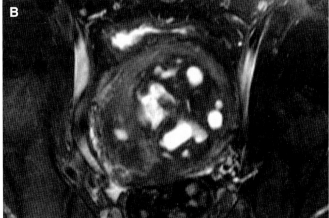

Figure 9.28 *Atypical cystic degeneration in a benign leiomyoma.* (**A, B**) Axial T2-weighted fat-saturation images at different levels of large leiomyoma show extensive cystic degeneration (*skinny arrows*) with peripheral involvement. These findings are unusual for benign cystic change, and tumoral necrosis or treatment with GnRH analogs should be considered. The fluid showed low signal intensity on T1-weighted (not shown) and high signal intensity on T2-weighted images, indicating non-hemorrhagic fluid. The borders of the fluid are well defined (*fat arrows*) and the surrounding tissue of the leiomyoma is low in signal with presence of a pseudo-capsule. These findings indicate a likely benign leiomyoma. New symptoms of pain or bleeding would be concerning for malignancy. Close imaging follow-up should be considered.

Uterine artery embolization selectively devascularizes leiomyomas because the lesions have a lower vessel density and lack of collateral blood supply compared to the myometrium. MR is used in pre- and post-embolization evaluation. Dynamic contrast-enhanced thin-section T1-weighted images allow assessment of alternative vascular supply in large exophytic leiomyomas. Some pedunculated subserosal and submucosal leiomyomas may be a relative contraindication for performing uterine artery embolization, as these tumors may detach and move into the peritoneal cavity to cause peritonitis, or may detach from the endometrium into the uterine canal to cause acute uterine obstruction (Fig. 9.29)

The goals of pre-embolization MR assessment are as follows:

- Delineate the size and location of large leiomyomas for comparison following treatment

- Identify exophytic pedunculated leiomyomas and leiomyomas that are parasitized to the adnexa to delineate their arterial supply

- Determine the presence of unexpected pathology such as endometrial lesions or leiomyomas with features worrisome for malignancy. Atypical appearance of leiomyomas on MR may simulate a leiomyosarcoma. If so, it may be more prudent to perform hysterectomy.

- Determine whether UAE is unlikely to be effective. Leiomyomas with little or no enhancement or with preexisting hemorrhagic infarction are unlikely to respond to the treatment.

- Differentiate adenomyosis from leiomyomas. UAE is less effective in treating adenomyosis.

The goals of the post-embolization MR assessment are as follows:

- Assess size and persistence of enhancement of treated leiomyomas. Successfully treated leiomyomas undergo devascularization and hemorrhagic infarction, depicted as homogeneously high signal intensity on T1-weighted images, decreased signal on T2-weighted images, and lack of contrast enhancement.

- If there is continued growth of a leiomyoma after a technically successful embolization, leiomyosarcoma should be considered.

Lipoleiomyoma is a benign leiomyoma variant that contains a mixture of mature fat and smooth muscle cells. The fat within the lesion follows the signal intensity of subcutaneous fat on all MR sequences. They are high in signal on T1-weighted images and low in signal on fat-suppressed T1- and T2-weighted images.

Leiomyomatosis represents a rare aggressive growth pattern of benign leiomyomas within or beyond the uterus. The masses still display imaging features similar to those of smooth muscle and may shrink after anti-estrogen treatment. Other features include:

- *Diffuse uterine leiomyomatosis* involves the replacement of nearly all of the myometrium by innumerable poorly defined leiomyomas that coalesce and almost completely

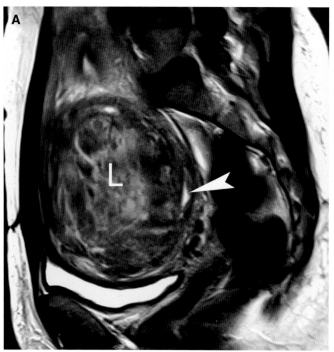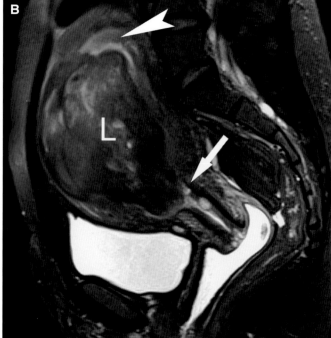

Figure 9.29 *Sloughing of a treated leiomyoma.* (**A**) Pretreatment sagittal T2-weighted image shows a large intramural leiomyoma (*L*) impinging on and compressing and distorting the endometrial canal (*arrowhead*). (**B**) The patient presented with pain, fever, and vaginal discharge several weeks after uterine artery embolization. The now smaller, deformable, devascularized mass (*L*) sloughed into the uterine cavity, occluding the internal os (*arrow*) of the cervix and trapping complex fluid in the upper uterine canal. Note the excellent demonstration of the cervix with use of vaginal gel.

replace the myometrium. Patients present with uterine enlargement, pain, and abnormal uterine bleeding not controlled by hormone therapy.

- *Benign metastasizing leiomyomas.* Benign uterine leiomyomas can spread hematogenously to the lungs, presenting as cavitary nodules.

- In *disseminated peritoneal leiomyomatosis*, small leiomyomas are studded along the peritoneal surfaces due to estrogen-induced metaplasia in pregnancy or oral contraceptive use and less frequently after hysterectomy, or along the surgical tract following laparoscopic myomectomy. They regress spontaneously with withdrawal of the estrogen stimulus. The tumors can be differentiated from peritoneal carcinomatosis by the patient's history, lack of ascites and the uniform appearance of the tumors, and MR signal intensities similar to leiomyomas.

- In *intravenous leiomyomatosis*, rubbery wormlike leiomyomas may grow into the myometrial veins and rarely further into pelvic veins to reach the right heart and pulmonary arteries.

Benign leiomyomas with unusual imaging features can be worrisome for malignancy. Some of the rare leiomyoma variants or benign leiomyomas with extensive cystic or myxoid degeneration may share features with leiomyosarcomas and should be followed at very short intervals to determine growth or should be removed for histologic confirmation.

Benign cystic degeneration typically occurs over time as a focal ischemic process near the center of a leiomyoma, where vessel density is decreased (Fig. 9.26). Variable host response accompanies cystic change with inflammation, hyaline change, and a graded transition from viable to nonviable tissue (Fig. 9.30). It may be difficult to distinguish a benign leiomyoma from a leiomyosarcoma during this acute phase. As the process becomes stable, nonviable tissue is resorbed, leaving behind well-defined viable portions of the leiomyoma. The tissue bordering the cystic areas maintains the classic low-signal-intensity whorled appearance of benign leiomyoma (Fig. 9.28). It displays a firm composition by demonstrating well-demarcated round margins where the firm tissue "pushes" into the fluid.

MR features of benign cystic degeneration of leiomyomas are as follows:

- The central dominant, usually solitary area of cystic degeneration is relatively small compared with noninvolved tissue. Fluid spaces are typically angular and well demarcated.

- The fluid is typically low in signal on T1-weighted and high in signal on T2-weighted images. Hemorrhagic fluid is a finding worrisome for malignancy.

- Nondegenerated tissue retains its classic low-signal intensity and whorled appearance.

- The outer border of the mass retains the pseudo-capsule typical of benign leiomyoma.

- Borders between the focus of cystic degeneration and unaffected myomatous tissue are well demarcated. Margins of the firm tissue are rounded and "pushing" into the cystic space.

Coagulative necrosis in a leiomyosarcoma is extensive, multifocal, irregularly distributed, and geographically complex (Fig. 9.31). Hemorrhage is frequent, resulting from rapid tumor growth and ischemia. On imaging, the borders between

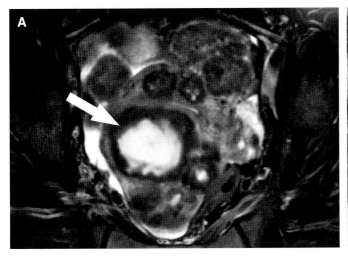 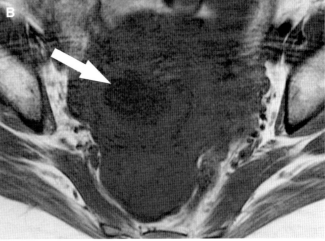

Figure 9.30 *Extensive atypical cystic degeneration.* (**A**) Axial T2-weighted fat-saturated image shows the largest of numerous uterine leiomyomas to have extensive cystic degeneration (*arrow*) with poorly defined margins between the fluid and the solid tissue. This finding is concerning for malignancy. (**B**) The fluid (*arrow*) shows low signal intensity on T1-weighted images. The patient was asymptomatic and imaging follow-up showed improved definition of the fluid interface with solid tissue, consistent with benign cystic degeneration in the acute phase.

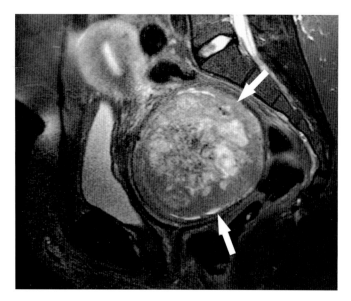

Figure 9.31 *Cystic degeneration in a leiomyosarcoma.* Cystic degeneration in this tumor (*arrows*) arising from the cervix, shown on a sagittal T2-weighted image, is extensive and poorly defined and involves peripheral regions of the lesion, not expected to be areas of low blood vessel density most subject to ischemia. Most of the mass is involved and there is no normal-appearing tissue between the cystic regions. Leiomyosarcoma was confirmed at surgery.

the degeneration and adjacent edematous neoplastic tissue are poorly defined. The intervening edematous tissue is deformable in appearance and is higher in signal intensity on T2-weighted images than noninvolved myomatous tissue, given its higher fluid content.

Cellular leiomyomas are composed of densely concentrated compact smooth muscle cells with little or no intervening collagen. They are internally homogeneous, lacking the whorled appearance of typical leiomyomas. They are characteristically soft and therefore appear elongated and deformable on imaging. They often have focal extensions into the adjacent myometrium, appearing infiltrative with loss of the pseudo-capsule on imaging.[13] They display relatively high signal intensity on T2-weighted imaging and enhance more avidly than the typical leiomyoma (Figs. 9.32 and 9.33).

Atypical leiomyomas have cellular atypia as the dominant histologic characteristic but do not meet the histologic criteria for a leiomyosarcoma. On imaging they are usually indistinguishable from a typical leiomyoma. However, they are more likely to be softer and thus deformable-appearing, and more likely to show areas of hemorrhage and cystic or myxoid change.

A *myxoid leiomyoma* has extensive myxoid change. Smooth muscle cells are scattered within an abundant amorphous

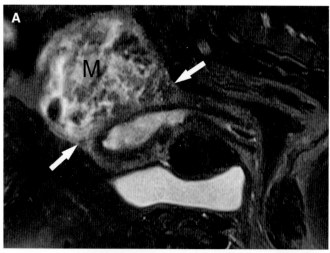

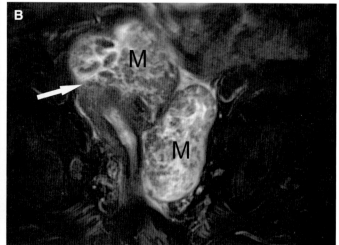

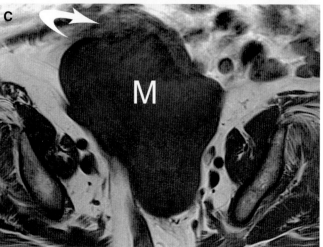

Figure 9.32 *Cellular leiomyoma with extensive myxoid degeneration.* (**A, B**) Sagittal and coronal T2-weighted images with fat saturation demonstrate a large bilobed mass (*M*) with extensive areas of high signal intensity, much greater than the typical speckled pattern of hyaline degeneration in a benign leiomyoma. The margins of the mass with the myometrium are poorly defined (*arrows*) with deep infiltration of tumor into the myometrium. The outer margin is lobulated and appears deformable, findings suggesting a leiomyosarcoma. (**C**) Axial T1-weighted image shows the mass (*M*) to be lower in signal intensity than the myometrium (*curved arrow*). Final pathologic diagnosis was a cellular leiomyoma with extensive myxoid degeneration.

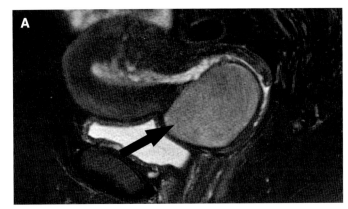

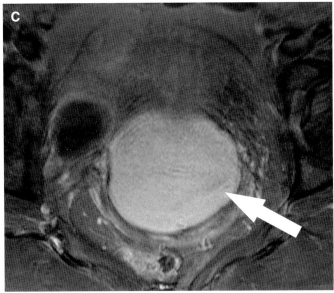

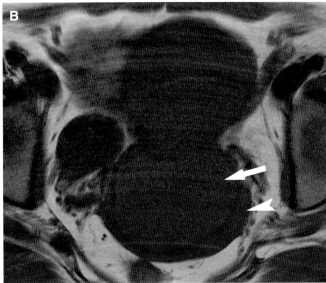

Figure 9.33 *Cellular leiomyoma of the cervix.* (**A**) Sagittal T2-weighted image with fat saturation shows a large, homogeneous, relatively high-signal-intensity mass (*arrow*) replacing the anterior lip of the cervix. The mass does not appear to involve the endocervical canal, making a cervical carcinoma unlikely. (**B**) On the T1-weighted axial image the mass (*arrow*) is slightly higher in signal intensity than the cervix (*arrowhead*). (**C**) Avid enhancement of the mass (*arrow*) is evident on the post-contrast-enhanced T1-weighted image. Pathology revealed a cellular cervical leiomyoma. The slightly higher signal intensity on T1-weighted images is due to the relatively high protein content of a cellular leiomyoma.

gelatinous matrix. Focal accumulation of myxoid matrix creates a soft gelatinous area. The ischemia in leiomyosarcomas can also result in similar-appearing myxoid degeneration, and therefore the two lesions may not be distinguishable by imaging. Both are soft masses that display elongated and deformable margins. Both are likely to have coexistent hemorrhage and cystic change. Although borders help in differentiation, this may not be reliable. A benign myxoid leiomyoma and a leiomyosarcoma may both have defined borders.

Myxoid change demonstrates variable and geographic T1-weighted signal, depending on protein content. It displays usually high signal intensity on T2-weighted images (Fig. 9.32). On dynamic contrast-enhanced imaging, the myxoid regions usually demonstrate minimal initial enhancement with prolonged predominantly peripheral enhancement at delayed imaging. The intervening internal stroma enhances with a mesh-like quality, and enhancement is greater than the minimally enhancing lakes of myxoid material.

LEIOMYOSARCOMAS

Leiomyosarcomas are rare and are believed to arise *de novo* from a single myometrial cell unrelated to a preexisting leiomyoma. They are most frequent in women over age 40, most of whom present with new or abnormal vaginal bleeding. Less frequently, patients present with pelvic pain or a rapidly expanding mass. Tumors are nearly always larger than 5 cm. Endometrial sampling may identify leiomyosarcomas if they involve the endometrial canal. Rapid growth may be a sign of leiomyosarcoma; however, leiomyomas are much more prevalent, and rapid growth more commonly represents benign degenerative changes. Histologic diagnosis is based on nuclear atypia, increased mitotic activity, and infiltrative margins. The International Federation of Gynecology and Obstetrics (FIGO) adopted a new staging system for uterine sarcomas in 2009 (Table 9.2). Previously, uterine sarcomas were staged in the same way as endometrial carcinomas.

Mitotic index, cytologic atypia, and the presence or absence of coagulative necrosis distinguish leiomyosarcomas from leiomyomas and serve as important predictors of behavior. Tissue types include the typical leiomyosarcoma, and the rare epithelioid and myxoid variants. All have similar unfavorable prognosis. Myxoid leiomyosarcoma has low cellularity, with few mitoses and little atypia, simulating a benign leiomyoma, but it has other diagnostic features, including an infiltrative margin.[14]

Table 9.2 TNM STAGING OF UTERINE SARCOMA STAGING—LEIOMYOSARCOMA AND ENDOMETRIAL STROMA SARCOMA

AJCC TNM STAGE	FIGO STAGE	DESCRIPTION
T Stage		**Tumor extent**
TX		Primary tumor cannot be assessed
T0		No evidence of primary tumor
T1	I	Tumor limited to the uterus
T1a	IA	Tumor ≤ 5 cm
T1b	IB	Tumor > 5 cm
T2	II	Tumor extends beyond the uterus but is limited to pelvis
T2a	IIA	Tumor involves adnexa
T2b	IIB	Tumor involves other pelvic tissues
T3	III	Tumor infiltrates abdominal tissues
T3a	IIIA	One site
T3b	IIIB	More than one site
T4	IVA	Tumor invades bladder or rectum
N Stage		**Lymph node spread**
NX		Regional lymph node cannot be assessed
N0		No regional lymph node metastasis
N1	IIIC	Regional lymph node metastasis (iliac, paraaotic)
M Stage		**Distant spread**
M0		No metastases
M1	IVB	Distant metastasis (excludes spread to adexa, pelvic and abdominal tissue and regional lymph nodes)

Adapted from International Federation of Gynecology and Obstetrics (FIGO) new sarcoma staging system, 2009, and American Joint Committee on Cancer. *AJCC Cancer Staging Manual,* 7th ed. New York, Springer, 2010. Uterine sarcomas were previously staged using endometrial carcinoma staging.

Grossly and on imaging, tumors are soft and deformable and lack the round shape of a typical leiomyoma. They infiltrate rather than displace the myometrium and usually have regions of necrosis and hemorrhage. Tumor necrosis in leiomyosarcomas is complex and multifocal and is randomly distributed throughout the tumor (Figs. 9.31 9.34). MR imaging features are as follows:

- The mass is predominantly intermediate or high in signal intensity on T2-weighted images, as opposed to the low signal typical of benign leiomyomas.

- The pseudo-capsule is absent and the mass has infiltrative margins with the myometrium or infiltrates into the endometrium rather than displacing it.

- Tumors lack the characteristic whorled pattern expected in a leiomyoma.

- Cystic degeneration is pronounced, multifocal, and irregularly distributed.

- Hemorrhagic degeneration (high-signal fluid on T1-weighted images) is worrisome for malignancy.

- Malignant tumors are soft and lack the "compressive force" of benign leiomyomas. On imaging, the mass appears soft and deformable. The mass is elongated rather than round and has outer undulating margins.

- Tissue bounding cystic regions is poorly defined, heterogeneous, and high in signal intensity and lacks the convex "pushing" nature otherwise seen in a benign leiomyoma.

ADENOMYOSIS

Adenomyosis refers to non-neoplastic benign invasion of endometrium into myometrium, resulting in reactive overgrowth of smooth muscle. Aggregates of endometrial glands and stroma extend into the myometrium without a proportionate increase in vascularity. The greatest involvement is in the junctional zone and adjacent myometrium. Cyclic bleeding of the ectopic endometrium results in myometrial hypertrophy and decreased efficiency of the normal menstrual contractions that act to diminish bleeding. Increased pain (dysmenorrhea) and increased bleeding (menorrhagia) during menstruation are the dominant symptoms. Marked hypertrophy results in a tender, globular, and boggy-feeling uterus. Infertility may result.

Although usually a diffuse abnormality (Fig. 9.35), focal aggregates of endometrial glands and smooth muscle, called *adenomyomas* (Fig. 9.36), may occur, resulting in marked tenderness and cramping during normal menstrual contractions or intercourse. Infrequently, focal cystic adenomyomas occur (Fig. 9.35). These are round and well defined and composed predominantly of hemorrhage in different stages of evolution. A dark rim may be present on T2-weighted images, reflecting increased hemosiderin.

Leiomyomas, adenomyosis, and endometriosis are likely to occur concurrently in late child-bearing years. The conditions have similar symptoms but differing treatment. The standard treatment for symptomatic adenomyosis is hysterectomy. Curettage or endometrial ablation can be effective if involvement is superficial. Combination oral contraceptives, progesterone-releasing intrauterine devices (IUDs), and GnRHa may also control symptoms.

Ultrasound may suggest the diagnosis of adenomyosis, with findings of heterogeneous myometrium most marked centrally, posterior wall myometrial thickening, and lack of a focal defined mass. Echogenic poorly defined nodules and echogenic striations may be present; cysts in the myometrium

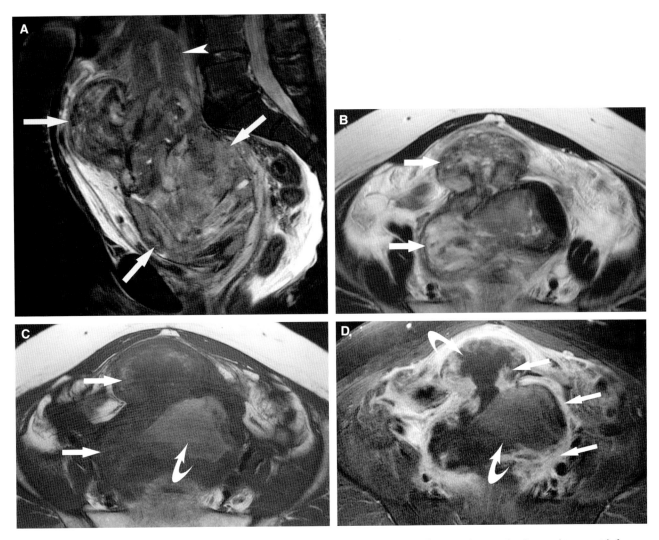

Figure 9.34 *Uterine leiomyosarcoma.* This patient presented with pain and a rapidly growing pelvic mass. T2-weighted sagittal image with fat saturation (**A**) and axial T1-weighted image without fat saturation (**B**) show a large heterogeneous mass (*arrows*) extending from the lower uterine segment. The uterine fundus (*arrowhead*) is normal. (**C**) Axial T1-weighted image shows a high-signal-intensity area (*curved arrow*) within the mass (*straight arrows*) that did not enhance on post-contrast-enhanced images and represents hemorrhagic necrosis. (**D**) Post-contrast-enhanced T1-weighted image shows enhancement of viable tumor (*straight arrows*) and extensive tumor necrosis (*curved arrows*) without enhancement. Pathology confirmed a leiomyosarcoma.

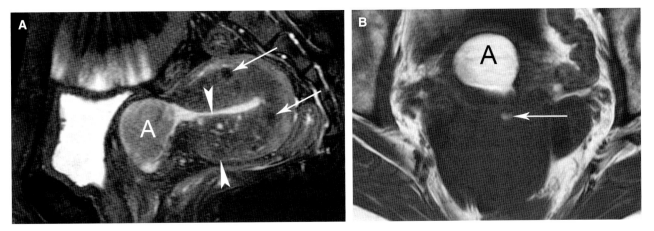

Figure 9.35 *Diffuse adenomyosis and cystic adenomyoma.* (**A**) Sagittal fat-saturated T2-weighted image demonstrates a retroflexed uterus with a markedly thickened junctional zone. The 22-mm thickness (between *arrowheads*) exceeds the 12-mm threshold and is diagnostic for diffuse adenomyosis. The low-signal-intensity foci (*arrows*) on the T2-weighted image correspond to high-signal foci (*arrow*) on the axial T1-weighted image (**B**). These findings indicate hemorrhagic intramural foci, pathognomonic for adenomyosis. The well defined structure (*A*) is an intrauterine cystic adenomyoma contained within the uterine canal.

are most specific. Hysterosalpingography may demonstrate multiple cavities in the uterine wall, but this method of examination is not sensitive. MR is both sensitive and specific for diagnosing adenomyosis and allows for differentiation of diffuse and focal adenomyosis from leiomyomas. Findings reveal the severity of involvement, help in directing treatment, and predict the likelihood of response. MR is used to monitor disease progression and the response to conservative therapy. MR features are as follows:[15]

- Poor definition of the junctional zone with the adjacent myometrium

- Hemosiderin deposition from chronic bleeding results in low signal intensity in the involved areas on T2-weighted images (Figs. 9.35 to 9.37).

- A dark junctional zone measuring 12 mm or more in thickness, focally or diffusely, is highly predictive of adenomyosis (Fig. 9.35). If the junctional zone thickness is less than 8 mm, the diagnosis is excluded. During menstruation, particularly the first two days, the junctional zone may normally thicken. Imaging is best avoided during menstruation to decrease the risk of false-positive diagnosis.

- A globular or enlarged uterus. The posterior wall is often asymmetrically thickened.

- Myometrial cysts are frequent. On T2-weighted images, high-signal foci interspersed within abnormally low-signal myometrium correspond to focal aggregates of endometrium with subacute hemorrhage or cystic dilatation of endometrial glands. These foci may be high or low in signal intensity on T1-weighted images. High signal intensity on T1-weighted images indicates subacute hemorrhagic fluid and is pathognomonic for adenomyosis.

- Fine linear striations emanating from the endometrium on MR represent direct radial extensions of heterotopic endometrium from the uterine canal. They display high signal intensity on T2-weighted images relative to adjacent myometrium. The striations can be extensive, blending in with the endometrium and infrequently simulating myometrial invasion from endometrial carcinoma.

- Adenomyomas appear as localized, usually oval, ill-defined masses that are low in signal intensity on both T1- and T2-weighted images. The masses are continuous with and are oriented in the long axis of the junctional zone and cause little mass effect (Fig. 9.36). Associated myometrial thickening is usually present.

- A pseudo-capsule is not present because adenomyosis interdigitates into the myometrium rather than displacing it like a leiomyoma. A pseudo-capsule is characteristically present around a leiomyoma and is frequently high in signal intensity due to associated dilated vessels.

- The appearance of adenomyosis on both T1- and T2-weighted imaging can vary during the menstrual cycle. Hemorrhage occurring during menstruation causes high-signal foci within the adenomyosis on both T1- and T2-weighted images, reflecting hemorrhagic cystic dilation of glands.

Pitfalls with MR imaging of adenomyosis are as follows:

- Focal myometrial contraction versus an adenomyoma. A myometrial contraction shows low signal intensity on T2-weighted images as the contraction lowers the water content within the contracting myometrium. Contractions bulge into the endometrial cavity in distinction to an adenomyoma, which has minimal mass effect. Further, a contraction is a transient phenomenon that is therefore

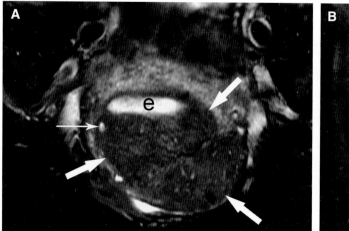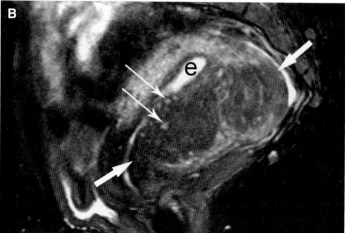

Figure 9.36 *Focal adenomyoma.* Axial (**A**) and sagittal (**B**) T2-weighted images with fat saturation show a large, low-signal-intensity mass (*fat arrows*) in the posterior myometrium that is contiguous with the junctional zone myometrium and extends to the endometrium (*e*). The sagittal view shows that the mass is elongated (between *fat arrows*) and aligned with the junctional zone. High-signal-intensity foci (*skinny arrows*) within the mass are cystic deposits of endometrium. These features are typical of an adenomyoma and distinguish it from a leiomyoma. The adenomyoma displays low signal intensity because of fibrosis induced by recurrent bleeding in the myometrium.

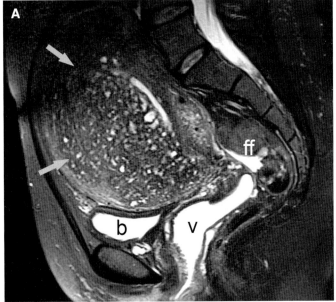

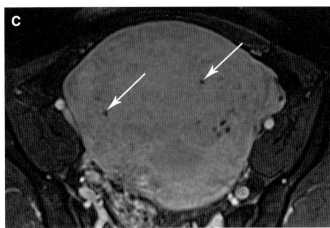

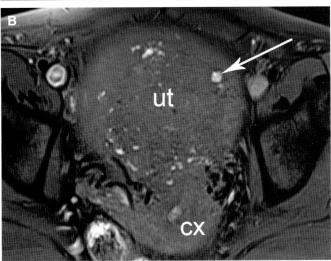

Figure 9.37 *Large adenomyoma.* (**A**) Sagittal T2-weighted image with fat saturation demonstrates a markedly thickened anterior myometrium (*arrows*) with innumerable small high-signal-intensity foci representing heterotopic islands of endometrium with associated acute or subacute hemorrhage. The endometrial canal is deviated posteriorly. The bladder (*b*), vaginal gel used to delineate the vagina (*v*), and small amount of free pelvic fluid (*ff*) are well delineated. (**B**) On the T1-weighted fat-saturated image, many small foci (*arrow*) with the uterus (*ut*) remain high in signal intensity, indicating more acute hemorrhage. As the hemorrhage becomes chronic, hemosiderin accumulation results in decrease of signal intensity on T1-weighted images. Though infrequent, the high signal intensity of the foci on the T1-weighted image is pathognomonic for adenomyosis. *cx*, cervix. (**C**) Axial post-contrast-enhanced T1-weighted image with fat saturation reveals no enhancement of the foci (*arrows*), confirming they are non-neoplastic lesions.

not likely to be seen on all imaging sequences of the same study.

- Adenomyosis and leiomyomas are frequently associated. Focal adenomyomas are distinguished from leiomyomas by their minimal mass effect, their location involving the junctional zone, the orientation along the long axis of the junctional zone, oval rather than spherical shape, indistinct margins, presence of highly characteristic cysts in the myometrium, and lack of a pseudo-capsule.

- Focal cystic adenomyosis simulates a degenerated leiomyoma. The former is suggested by its location adjacent to the junctional zone, its small size relative to the degree of cystic change (cystic change is unusual in small leiomyomas), and signal characteristics showing hemorrhage in various stages of evolution (also unusual in small leiomyomas).

- A cavitary rudimentary horn (containing endometrial tissue) may be confused with focal cystic adenomyosis.

A unicornuate uterus with a rudimentary horn has a characteristic morphology, including a deep fundal indentation.

ENDOMETRIAL-ORIGIN MASSES

The endometrium is composed of glandular tissue (epithelial origin) and its supporting stroma (mesenchymal origin). Most benign endometrial masses are polyps arising from the glandular tissue. The most common endometrial malignancy is epithelial endometrial cancer derived from the epithelial glandular tissue. Most epithelial endometrial cancer is the low-grade estrogen-dependent endometrial carcinoma. The rare endometrial sarcomas are derived from the endometrial stromal mesenchymal tissue. They are classified as low-grade and high-grade (or undifferentiated) sarcoma.

For endometrial-origin neoplasms, women usually present with postmenopausal or abnormal intermenopausal bleeding.

Box 9.3 ESSENTIALS TO REMEMBER

- The classic MR appearance of leiomyoma is a well-defined solid mass with predominantly low signal intensity relative to normal myometrium on all image sequences. Hyaline degeneration (giving a speckled background) is present in most larger ones and is considered part of the normal spectrum of findings.

- Leiomyomas are classified by location as submucosal (most likely to cause menorrhagia), intramural, subserosal, and penduculated (most likely to present as an adnexal mass).

- Benign myxoid and cellular leiomyoma variants and typical leiomyomas with extensive cystic or myxoid degeneration are uncommon and may share features of a leiomyoscaroma on imaging.

- Leiomyosarcomas are rare and may be suspected by rapid growth, abnormal bleeding, and the finding of a uterine mass lacking one or more features diagnostic of a leiomyoma.

- Adenomyosis is characterized by thickening of the junctional-zone myometrium of at least 12 mm, with associated tiny myometrial cysts representing focal deposits of endometrium.

- A focal adenomyoma can be distinguished from a leiomyoma by its elongated shape, location along the axis of the junctional zone, indistinct margins, lack of a pseudo-capsule, and presence of highly characteristic cysts in the myometrium.

Postmenopausal bleeding is caused by endometrial atrophy (70%), polyps and hyperplasia (20%), and cancer (10%). However, when stratified by age, a 60- to 70-year-old woman with new onset of vaginal bleeding has a higher likelihood of having cancer than a benign cause. Ultrasound demonstration of thin endometrium (less than 5 mm) in a postmenopausal woman indicates endometrial atrophy and essentially excludes endometrial cancer.

The goal of imaging of endometrial canal masses includes determination of the depth of myometrial invasion, cervical extension, and extrauterine extent. For a large bulky mass, another imaging goal is to determine whether the tumor originated from the endometrium, myometrium, cervix, or ovary. Most epithelial endometrial cancers and low-grade endometrial stromal sarcomas appear as endometrial thickening. High-grade endometrial malignancies often appear as large bulky masses, with extrauterine spread common.

Endometrial polyps are seen in 10% of perimenopausal women, are multiple in 20%, and undergo malignant transformation in 1% to 2%. Smaller polyps often regress. Polyps are typically smooth-walled, possess a fibrous stalk or core (Fig. 9.38), and may be sessile or pedunculated. Larger polyps are more likely to cause bleeding or prolapse into the cervix.

Malignant transformation is more frequent with increasing age, tamoxifen use, polyp size greater than 1.5 cm, and symptoms (bleeding). Polyps are usually distinguishable from leiomyomas and endometrial cancer not associated with a polyp. However, malignant transformation in a polyp is not reliably identified by imaging, and polyps are removed in patients with increased-risk factors, including age, for symptoms such as bleeding and when they are large in size. Polyps less than 1.5 cm in asymptomatic premenopausal women can be observed; many of these will spontaneously involute. MR imaging features are as follows:[16,17]

- Small polyps are often difficult to distinguish from adjacent endometrium on non-contrast-enhanced MR, as both have similar high signal on T2-weighted images.

- Large polyps are more visible on MR, given their heterogeneity on T2-weighted images and demonstration of a stalk on dynamic contrast-enhanced T1-weighted images imaging (Fig. 9.38). They usually enhance less than the normal endometrium.

- Polyps are typically homogeneous smooth-walled oval lesions with a fibrous stalk or core and often contain characteristic intratumoral cysts. Focal endometrial cancers characteristically have a relatively broad base and are heterogeneous, poorly defined lesions. Detection of necrosis, a papillary or irregular surface, or myometrial invasion is highly predictive of carcinoma.

- Dynamic gadolinium contrast-enhanced sequences are best for demonstrating whether a mass is sessile or pedunculated. This helps guide the surgical approach.

- Submucosal leiomyomas are distinguished from endometrial polyps by low signal intensity and heterogeneity on T2-weighted images, similar to that of typical myometrial leiomyomas (see Fig. 9.25).

Epithelial endometrial cancer is the most common female genital malignancy, with a bimodal peak in the perimenopausal years and in women in their 60s and 70s. Hereditary nonpolyposis colorectal syndrome (Lynch syndrome) carries an extremely high lifetime risk of developing endometrial and colon cancer, accounting for 5% to 10% of endometrial cancer cases overall. Nearly all patients present with postmenopausal or abnormal intermenopausal bleeding when the cancer is still in an early stage. In 75% of cases the disease is confined to the uterus.

Endometrioid adenocarcinoma is the most common cell type (80% to 90%). The high-risk subtypes (10%), uterine papillary serous carcinoma and clear cell carcinoma, account for most of the remainder. Adenosquamous and squamous cell types are infrequent. The clear cell and papillary serous carcinomas are aggressive cell types, spread like ovarian cancer,

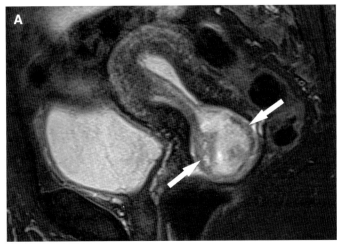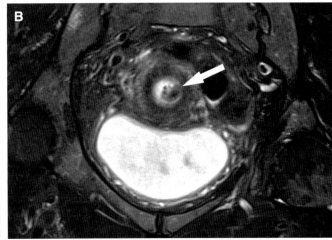

Figure 9.38 *Prolapsed endometrial polyp.* (**A**) Sagittal T2-weighted fat-saturated image shows a large endometrial polyp (*arrows*) originating from the endometrium of the lower uterine segment and prolapsing through the cervix on a long stalk. (**B**) Oblique coronal T2-weighted image through the transverse axis of the lower uterine segment shows the low-signal-intensity origin (*arrow*) of the stalk of the polyp. The surrounding endometrium displays higher signal intensity. The polyp contained adenocarcinoma, a finding found more frequently in large polyps.

and are commonly metastatic when detected. Like ovarian cancer, both respond to platinum-based chemotherapy, and CA-125 can be used to gauge treatment response or recurrence. Endometrial cancers are divided into groups based on pathophysiology and prognosis:

- **Low-risk subtype (estrogen-associated)**: Most endometrial carcinomas (80%) are indolent, well-differentiated estrogen-dependent endometrioid adenocarcinomas with cell growth in differentiated patterns simulating glands. These cancers arise from chronically estrogen-stimulated endometrium with a continuum of hyperplasia, atypical hyperplasia, and well-differentiated adenocarcinoma. Most occur in hyperestrogenic perimenopausal, often obese, women. Other hyperestrogenic states that confer risk include unopposed estrogen replacement therapy, tamoxifen therapy, and chronic anovulation, as in the polycystic ovarian syndrome. Tumors usually present with bleeding in an early, treatable stage. Low-grade endometrioid carcinomas grow as a localized single mass or multiple sessile polypoid masses or as an infiltrative process diffusely involving the endometrium. Spread occurs contiguously to the myometrium and eventually through the serosa to involve adjacent pelvic structures. Spread may also occur caudally to involve the cervix. The adnexal and pelvic iliac lymph nodes are common early sites of spread.

- **High-risk subtype (estrogen-independent)**: The high-risk endometrial cancers are estrogen-independent, poorly differentiated tumors with unfavorable histology and include clear cell carcinoma, papillary serous carcinoma, and grade 3 endometrioid carcinoma. These tumors are believed to arise from a spontaneous mutation occurring in older women with atrophic endometrium and without risk factors. All are likely to have deep myometrial invasion and to metastasize early, accounting for the disproportionately high mortality from endometrial malignancy. The papillary

serous carcinoma is very likely to have extrauterine spread with little myometrial invasion.[18]

- **Sarcomatoid carcinomas**: In 2003 the World Health Organization reclassified malignant mixed mesodermal tumors (MMMT) as sarcomatoid carcinomas. These are metaplastic carcinomas with sarcomatous metaplasia. The epithelial carcinoma component, which usually has endometrioid histology, determines the behavior of this tumor.[19] The epidemiology, risk factors, poor prognosis, and highly aggressive behavior parallel those of high-grade endometrial carcinoma, and classification and treatment of the tumors is the same. Patients are usually postmenopausal and present with extrauterine spread. Five-year survival rates are 30% overall and 50% for stage I disease, respectively. Up to 40% of patients have a prior history of pelvic radiation.

Regional lymph nodes involved in endometrial cancer are the internal, external, and common iliac nodes and para-aortic lymph nodes. Involvement of nonregional nodes is considered metastatic disease (M1). For the low-risk subtypes, there is an extremely low likelihood of para-aortic lymph node involvement if there is no iliac lymph node involvement. Thus, in the case of endometrial carcinoma without involvement of the iliac lymph nodes, para-aortic lymphadenectomy can be avoided. Spread to the vagina may occur. Ovarian metastases are common. Hematogenous spread is uncommon, with the lungs, liver, and bones most often involved.

Staging of endometrial cancer includes transabdominal hysterectomy, bilateral salpingo-oophorectomy, selective pelvic and para-aortic lymphadenectomy, peritoneal biopsies and washings, omentectomy, and tumor debulking if disseminated disease is present (Table 9.3). Because surgical staging is standard, MR has had less of a role for staging endometrial cancer than for staging cervical cancer. Extended-field radiation therapy is given after surgery if the para-aortic nodes are positive.

For the endometrioid type, the depth of myometrial invasion is the most important predictor of lymph node involvement, extrauterine disease, and eventual tumor recurrence. When the disease is confined to the endometrium (stage T1a) (Fig. 9.39), extrauterine disease is present in only 1% of patients, obviating the need for extensive surgery. Deep myometrial invasion correlates with higher-risk histology (grade 3), a larger tumor size (more than 2 cm), and a higher likelihood of cervical extension, extrauterine disease, and involvement of pelvic lymph nodes. When deep myometrial invasion is present, pelvic and para-aortic lymphadenectomy is generally performed. Endometrioid carcinoma may grow as a single mass or

Table 9.3 TNM STAGING OF ENDOMETRIAL CANCER (includes sarcomatoid carcinomas)

STAGE		FINDINGS	MR IMAGING STAGING
AJCC TNM Stage	FIGO Stage		
T stage		Extent of tumor	
TX		Primary tumor cannot be assessed	
T0		No evidence of primary tumor	Normal appearance of the endometrium
T1	I	Tumor is confined to the body of the uterus	
T1a	Ia	Tumor is confined to the endometrium or invades < 1/2 of the myometrium	Confined to endometrium: Continuous noninterrupted low signal intensity junctional zone myometrium and continuous subendometrial enhancement. Early invasion: Disruption of the junctional zone myometrium and disruption of subendometrial enhancement by tumor signal intensity up to inner half of myometrium
T1b	Ib	Tumor is confined to the uterus with invasion ≥ ½ thickness of the myometrium	Tumor signal intensity extends to outer half myometrium
T2	II	Tumor has spread to the stroma of the cervix but not beyond the uterus (Endocervical glandular involvement only is stage I)	Higher signal intensity tumor invading the normal low signal intensity stroma of the cervix
T3A	IIIA	Tumor invades the serosa and/or the fallopian tubes and ovaries	Irregular contour of the uterine surface. Tumor signal intensity in the adnexa and on the ovaries
T3B	IIIB	Tumor invades the vagina and/or the parametrium	Disruption of the normal low signal intensity of the vaginal wall by the higher signal intensity of the tumor
T4	IVA	Tumor has spread to the bladder mucosa and/or the rectal mucosa	Disruption of the normal low signal intensity of the bladder and/or rectal wall by the higher signal intensity of the tumor
N Stage		Tumor involvement of lymph nodes	
NX		Regional lymph nodes not evaluated	
N0		No regional lymph node metastases	Regional iliac lymph nodes larger than 8 mm in short axis diameter
N1	IIIC1	Regional lymph node metastases to pelvic nodes	Regional iliac lymph nodes larger than 8 mm in short axis diameter
N2	IIIC2	Regional lymph node metastases to para-aortic nodes	Para-aortic lymph nodes larger than 10 mm in short axis diameter.
M stage		Distant metastases	
M0		No distant metastatic disease	
M1	IVB	Distant metastases	Tumor in inguinal lymph nodes, extrapelvic organs or tissues. Excludes spread to vagina, pelvic serosa, adnexa

(Adapted from American Joint Committee on Cancer. Kidney. AJCC Cancer Staging Manual. 7th ed. New York, NY. Springer. 2010, and FIGO–International Federation of Obstetrics and Gynecology-2009)

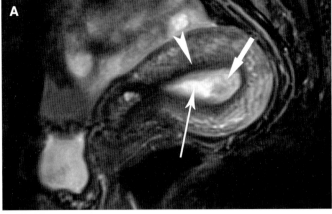

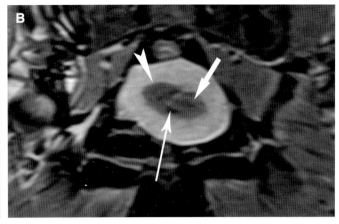

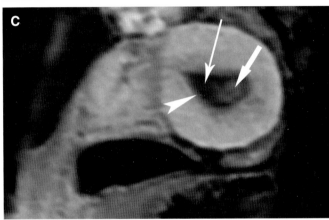

Figure 9.39 *Endometrial carcinoma confined to the endometrial cavity, stage IA.* (**A**) Sagittal T2-weighted fat-saturated image of a retroflexed uterus shows an endometrial carcinoma confined to the uterine cavity. The tumor (*fat arrow*) is slightly lower in signal intensity than the normal endometrium (*skinny arrow*). The low-signal-intensity junctional-zone myometrium (*arrowhead*) is intact. Dynamic T1-weighted post-contrast images axial (**B**) and sagittal to uterine body (**C**) reveal a lobulated enhancing intraendometrial mass (*fat arrow*) within low-signal-intensity fluid (*skinny arrow*). Fluid and normal-enhancing endometrial lining are much better differentiated on the dynamic contrast-enhanced images. Preservation of continuous uninterrupted subendometrial enhancement (*arrowhead*) is consistent with a mass confined to the cavity. Surgical pathology confirmed a stage 1A tumor confined to the endometrium without myometrial invasion.

multiple masses or as diffuse endometrial thickening. The lesion is usually a papillary or irregular mass, often with ulceration. Indications for MR are as follows:

- To exclude myometrial invasion in patients desiring fertility-sparing treatment (curettage, hormonal therapy)

- In poor-operative-risk patients, MR is used to determine the extent of myometrial invasion to plan radiation fields or to ascertain if limited surgery (transvaginal hysterectomy) is an alternative. Radiation fields are extended to the para-aortic lymph nodes when there is deep (more than 50%) invasion of the myometrium, and limited pelvic or no radiation is given for less than 50% involvement.

- Surgical and radiation planning in advanced disease

MR findings are as follows (Table 9.3):[2, 20–23]

- On T1-weighted images, endometrial carcinoma is iso-intense with normal endometrium.

- On T2-weighted images, endometrial carcinoma shows lobular or irregular focal or diffuse thickening of the endometrium. The tumor is usually slightly lower in signal intensity and more heterogeneous than the normal endometrium (Fig. 9.39). Dynamic contrast-enhanced T1-weighted sequences may better demonstrate necrosis

and multiple heterogeneous irregular masses, which differentially enhance against normal endometrium and the nonenhancing fluid or debris.

- A neoplasm confined to the uterine cavity (intraendometrial) shows a continuous noninterrupted, low-signal-intensity junctional zone on T2 weighted images and a continuous line of subendometrial enhancement on dynamic post-gadolinium-contrast-enhanced T1-weighted images (Fig. 9.39). If the junctional zone is not visible, the interface between the endometrium and the myometrium is sharp on T2-weighted and dynamic post-contrast-enhanced T1-weighted images.

- Superficial invasion of the myometrium shows disruption and irregularity of the junctional zone on T2-weighted (Fig. 9.40) and dynamic post-contrast-enhanced T1-weighted images. The junctional zone is often poorly visible in postmenopausal women. Use of dynamic post-contrast-enhanced T1-weighted images improves contrast by demonstrating a differential enhancement of the late-enhancing cancer invading the early-enhancing myometrium.

- Deep invasion of the myometrium shows tumor extending to the outer half of the myometrium, with a preserved outer rim of myometrium (Fig. 9.41).

- Transmural invasion of the myometrium is indicated by higher signal intensity of tumor (relative to the myometrium) on T2-weighted images extending to

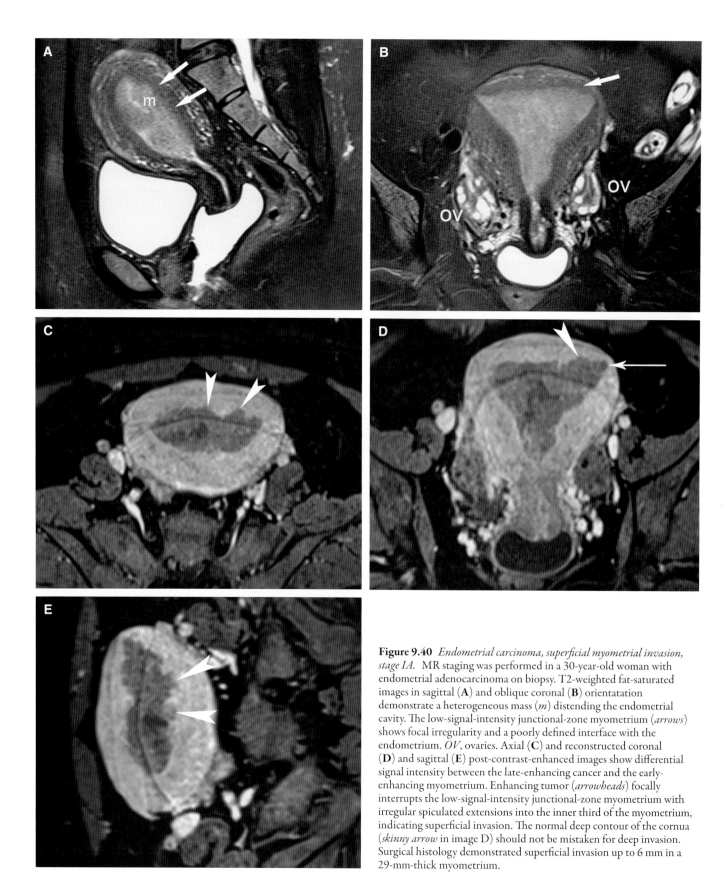

Figure 9.40 *Endometrial carcinoma, superficial myometrial invasion, stage IA.* MR staging was performed in a 30-year-old woman with endometrial adenocarcinoma on biopsy. T2-weighted fat-saturated images in sagittal (**A**) and oblique coronal (**B**) orientatation demonstrate a heterogeneous mass (*m*) distending the endometrial cavity. The low-signal-intensity junctional-zone myometrium (*arrows*) shows focal irregularity and a poorly defined interface with the endometrium. *OV*, ovaries. Axial (**C**) and reconstructed coronal (**D**) and sagittal (**E**) post-contrast-enhanced images show differential signal intensity between the late-enhancing cancer and the early-enhancing myometrium. Enhancing tumor (*arrowheads*) focally interrupts the low-signal-intensity junctional-zone myometrium with irregular spiculated extensions into the inner third of the myometrium, indicating superficial invasion. The normal deep contour of the cornua (*skinny arrow* in image D) should not be mistaken for deep invasion. Surgical histology demonstrated superficial invasion up to 6 mm in a 29-mm-thick myometrium.

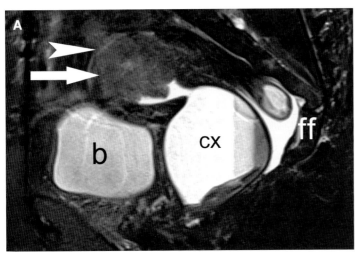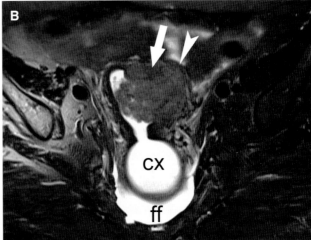

Figure 9.41 *Endometrial carcinoma, deep myometrial invasion, stage this is Stage IB on the new staging system.* A 70-year-old woman with a past history of cervical cancer treated with radiation therapy developed new hydrometrocolpos secondary to a new endometrial carcinoma, exposing a previously asymptomatic cervical stenosis. Sagittal (**A**) and axial (**B**) T2-weighted images with fat saturation show the intermediate-signal-intensity tumor (*arrow*) expanding the uterine cavity and extending deeply (*arrowhead*) into the myometrium and involving the serosa. Because of preexisting cervical stenosis, blood and fluid secreted from the tumor massively distends the cervical canal (*cx*). Free fluid (*ff*) is present in the cul-de-sac. *b*, bladder.

the serosa. The uterine surface additionally may be irregular with extension into the serosa.

- Invasion of the cervix is evidenced by the presence of a higher-signal-intensity mass disrupting the normally low signal intensity cervical stroma on T2-weighted images. This should be differentiated from endocervical glanular involvement only (Fig. 9.42).

- Invasion of the vagina is indicated by tumor disrupting the low-signal-intensity muscular wall.

- Regional lymph nodes that are enlarged in the short axis and possess internal heterogeneity, rounded morphology, irregular borders, or loss of the fatty hilum are likely involved by tumor (Fig. 9.43).

- Tumor involvement of the ovary may be differentiated from a hemorrhagic cyst by demonstration of tumor enhancement on post-intravenous-contrast-enhanced images using image subtraction (see Fig. 9.44).

- Invasion of the bladder or rectum is indicated by disruption of the normal tissue planes and loss of the normal low signal intensity of the bladder wall or rectal wall on T2-weighted images.

- For bulky masses of unclear origin (Fig. 9.45), determine the epicenter or greatest area of tumor bulk to determine its likely origin (cervical, endometrial, myometrial, or ovarian).[24]

Pitfalls of MR are as follows:

- A bulky tumor confined to the endometrial canal may thin out the myometrium, simulating deep invasion. Uniform thinning of the entire myometrium favors lack of

invasion—in contrast to focal thinning, which indicates focal invasion. Tumor extending to the cornua may simulate deep invasion. MPR images would demonstrate the normal deep contour of the uterine cavity at the cornua.

- Sensitivity for detecting endometrial cancer invading the myometrium is lowered in the presence of extensive adenomyosis. Myometrial invasion by endometrial carcinoma is likely to be underestimated on T2-weighted images. Invasion may not be visualized as a typical high-signal intensity mass. Dynamic contrast-enhanced sequences are essential for increasing sensitivity.[25]

- Metastases to the adnexa are common, especially in the high-grade endometrial cancers. These can easily be mistaken for a hemorrhagic ovarian follicle. Standard T1- and T2-weighted images allow determination of a simple non-hemorrhagic follicle based on characteristic signal for simple fluid. However, a hemorrhagic follicle and an adnexal metastasis can have similar signal intensity, and dynamic contrast administration with post-processing subtraction is essential to visualize enhancement.

HIGH-GRADE MALIGNANCIES WITH SPECIFIC IMAGING FEATURES

Papillary serous endometrial carcinoma is a high-grade and aggressive cancer that arises in atrophic endometrium. The histology, biologic behavior, and imaging appearance of both papillary serous endometrial and serous ovarian carcinoma are similar (Figs. 9.43 and 9.45). Unlike other endometrial cancers, the tumor leads to early paratubal spread, resulting in extensive cystic and solid adnexal and intraperitoneal metastases and pelvic and para-aortic lymphadenopathy

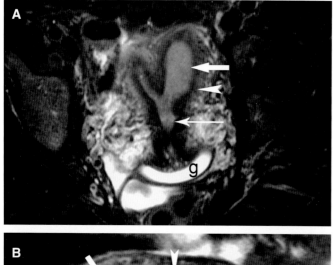

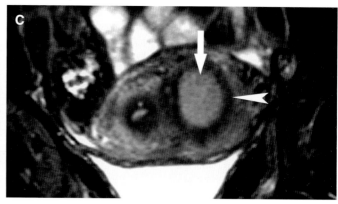

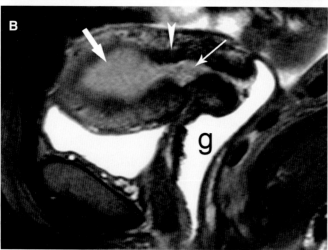

Figure 9.42 *Endometrial carcinoma, endocervical glanular involvement only, stage IA.* T2-weighted fat-saturated images in the oblique coronal plane through the long axis of the uterus (**A**), in the sagittal plane through the left moiety of the septated uterus (**B**), and in the oblique plane through the short axis of the uterus (**C**) show moderately high-signal-intensity tumor tissue distending the endometrial cavity (*fat arrow*) and extending to involve endocervical glands (*skinny arrow*) in the upper cervix. The junctional-zone myometrium (*arrowhead*) is intact, indicating the absence of myometrial invasion. Th e vagina is distended with vaginal gel (*g*) and is clearly demonstrated to be uninvolved by tumor.

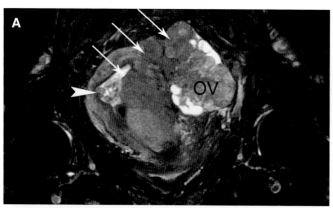

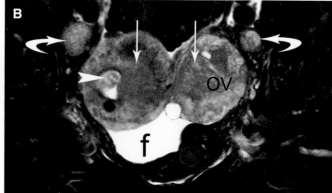

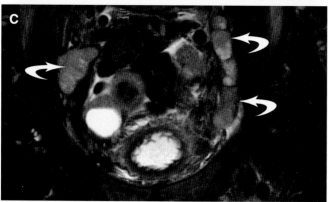

Figure 9.43 *Endometrial carcinoma, direct extension and lymph node involvement, stage IIIC.* T2-weighted fat-saturated images in coronal (**A**), axial (**B**), and oblique coronal short axis of the uterus (**C**) planes show a large endometrial mass (*straight arrows*) invading deeply through the myometrium to involve the left fallopian tube and left ovary (*OV*) as a confluent mass. The endometrial mass is multicentric with additional polypoid components (*arrowhead*). Bilateral lymph node metastases (*curved arrows*) are present. Free fluid (*f*) is seen in the cul-de-sac. Pathologic diagnosis was endometrial serous papillary carcinoma.

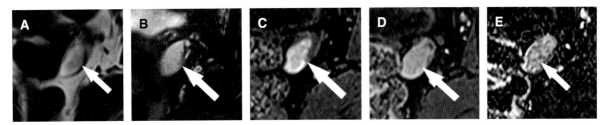

Figure 9.44 *Tumor involvement of the ovary.* Follow-up MR on a woman who had a hysterectomy for endometrial cancer demonstrates a left ovarian cystic mass (*arrows*) that is high in signal intensity on both T1- (**A**) and T2-weighted (**B**) images. Intravenous gadolinium-based contrast material was administered to assess for tumor enhancement using T1-weighted fat-saturated gradient-echo sequences before (**C**) and after contrast enhancement (**D**). High signal intensity is present within the lesion (*arrows*) on both sequences and enhancement is not obvious. Subtraction image (**E**) created by subtracting the pre-contrast image from the post-contrast image shows persistent high signal intensity within the lesion (*arrow*), definitively indicating enhancement. The enhancing ovarian mass represents recurrent tumor in the ovary, not a hemorrhagic cyst.

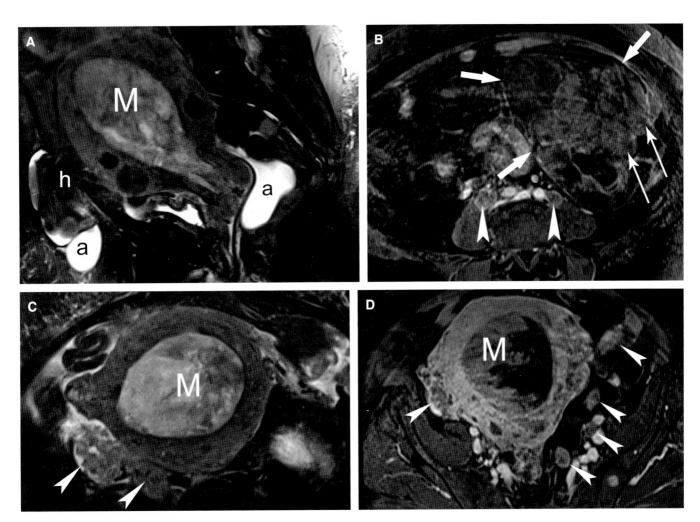

Figure 9.45 *Endometrial or ovarian primary?* MR was requested to determine uterine or ovarian origin of a large left abdominopelvic mixed cystic/solid mass. (**A**) T2-weighted fat-saturated image shows a heterogeneous mass (*M*) that markedly dilates the endometrial cavity and extends into the cervix. Small low-signal-intensity leiomyomas are present in the myometrium. The patient also has an abdominal wall hernia (*h*) containing bowel. Ascites (*a*) is present both in the hernia sac and in the cul-de-sac. (**B**) Subtraction image from post-gadolinium-contrast-enhanced T1-weighted gradient-echo sequence through the lower abdomen shows a huge cystic mass (between *fat arrows*) with solid components (*skinny arrows*) that extended from the left upper quadrant to the pelvis. Low-grade enhancement of the solid tumor components is seen against the dark background of fluid. Enlarged iliac lymph nodes are also evident. The intrauterine mass (*M*) displays heterogeneous high signal intensity on the T2-weighted image (**C**) and is shown to consist of solid components and hemorrhagic fluid on T1-weighted post-gadolinium-contrast-enhanced gradient-echo image (**D**). Lymphadenopathy and tumor (*arrowheads*) outside the uterus are evident. Pathology revealed poorly differentiated high-grade papillary serous adenocarcinoma, a tumor that may be either endometrial or ovarian in origin. Tumor marker analysis favored ovarian origin.

Box 9.4 **ESSENTIALS TO REMEMBER**

- Tumor invasion of the myometrium by endometrial carcinoma is recognized on T2-weighted images by visualization of higher-signal-intensity tumor within the normally low-signal-intensity junctional zone or myometrium. A non-interrupted low-signal junctional zone indicates the absence of myometrial invasion.

- Dynamic contrast-enhanced sequences distinguish between an enhancing mass and fluid within the endometrial canal and best depict subtle invasion of endometrial carcinoma beyond the junctional zone.

- Adnexal involvement is frequent with the high-grade malignancies. Differentiation of an ovarian metastasis from a hemorrhagic follicle is done with post-gadolinium-contrast-enhanced subtraction images.

with little or no myometrial invasion. A key to differentiation is determining the epicenter of the mass. A very large intraendometrial component favors endometrial origin.

Sarcomatoid carcinoma and ***undifferentiated endometrial stromal sarcoma*** have similar imaging appearances as the high-grade endometrial malignancies, and distinction by imaging is immaterial. These tumors are usually very large at presentation, replacing and considerably enlarging the endometrial cavity. Bulky polypoid masses deeply invade the myometrium and often protrude through the external cervical os. Hemorrhage and cystic necrosis are common. The uterus may be distorted by the large masses and become completely unrecognizable.

CERVICAL CANCER

Cervical cancer has a bimodal peak at age 30 and age 60, with most tumors (more than 90%) being caused by the human papilloma virus. A long preinvasive state allows for effective screening and treatment. Cancers detected by screening Pap smears tend to be small (volume less than 1 cc) compared with those detected clinically with bleeding or pain. Cervical cancer originates from the squamous epithelium of the exocervix or the glandular epithelium of the cervical canal (the endocervix). Most (about 85%) cervical cancers are squamous cell carcinomas that arise from the exocervix and are visible on physical examination. Adenocarcinomas (15%) arise from the mucin-producing columnar glandular epithelium of the endocervix and are more likely to be advanced, given their clinically occult location. Rare subtypes are adenosquamous carcinomas and neuroendocrine tumors.

Local spread of cervical cancer occurs by direct extension into the vagina, the endometrium, and the parametria. Spread to the vagina is common. Surgery may still be possible if extension is limited to the upper two thirds of the vagina (stage T2a). Insertion of vaginal gel for MR imaging provides distention and thinning of the vaginal wall to better delineate tumor involvement. The ureters run through the parametria 2 cm lateral to the cervix and are commonly involved (Fig. 9.48). Ureteral obstruction is classified as pelvic sidewall involvement. Cervical cancer can spread anteriorly along the vesicouterine ligament and through the fibrofatty fascia between the bladder and cervix. Deep extension into the

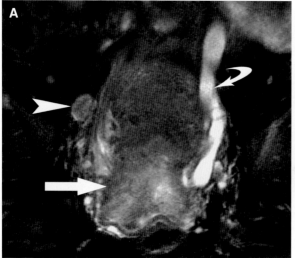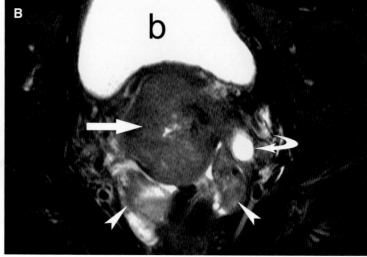

Figure 9.46 *Cervical cancer involvement of ureter, FIGO stage IIIB, AJCC T3b.* Coronal (**A**) and axial (**B**) T2-weighted images demonstrate a cervical mass (*straight arrows*) circumferentially involving the outer cervical stroma. The normal peripheral low signal intensity of the cervix is lost, indicating spread of tumor into the parametrium. Extension of the mass into the left parametrium obstructs the left ureter (*curved arrow*), resulting in hydroureter. An enlarged lymph node (*arrowhead* in A) containing metastatic tumor is evident. The ovaries (*arrowheads* in B) are uninvolved. *b*, bladder. Parametrial spread of cervical cancer frequently involves the nearby coursing ureter. Involvement of the ureter is classified as stage T3, FIGO III.

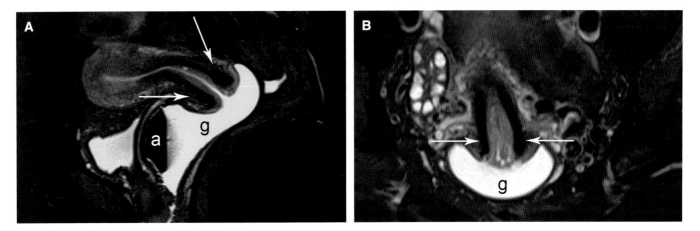

Figure 9.47 *Cervical cancer, normal on MR, FIGO stage IA, AJCC T1a.* Biopsy of the squamocolumnar junction of the cervix demonstrated adenocarcinoma. Sagittal (**A**) and axial (**B**) T2-weighted images appear normal, with the cervix (*arrows*) well outlined by vaginal gel (*g*). The patient is a surgical candidate. The nondependent low-signal-intensity region in the vagina in image A is air (*a*).

anterior cervical stroma is a relative contraindication to surgery as adequate tumor free margins may be difficult to achieve. Posterior spread to the rectum is less likely to occur because of the presence of the intervening rectouterine pouch.

Lymphatic spread is fairly orderly. The cervical lymphatics drain first into the paracervical and parametrial lymph nodes contained within the parametrium. The parametrium is thus removed as part of a radical hysterectomy. Drainage next occurs to the external iliac and obturator lymph nodes and less frequently to the internal iliac nodes. Drainage then occurs to the common iliac nodes and may continue to involve the para-aortic nodes and eventually the mediastinal and supraclavicular nodes via the thoracic duct. A posterior cervical cancer may follow rectal lymphatic drainage along the rectouterine fold or the uterosacral ligaments to involve the sacral and preaortic lymph nodes. Inguinal, para-aortic, and mediastinal involvement is classified as metastasis (stage M1).

Hematogenous spread is infrequent in cervical cancer, with the most common sites of involvement being the lungs, liver, bones, ovaries, and peritoneal cavity.

Surgery and radiation therapy (external beam and/or brachytherapy) with concurrent chemotherapy afford similar survival rates for stage 1 disease. Limited surgery is a generally more desirable option than radiation therapy because the latter has greater short- and long-term consequences than the former, including loss of ovarian function (unless the ovaries are transposed to remove them from the radiation field), shortening/fibrosis of the vagina, and radiation enteritis.

Microinvasive cancer (American Joint Committee on Cancer [AJCC] stage T1a, FIGO stage IA) (Fig. 9.47) can be treated by conization or simple hysterectomy. Women with limited non-bulky disease (FIGO stage IA2 through IIA and size less than 4 cm) (Figs. 9.49 and 9.50) are candidates for radical hysterectomy with lymph node dissection. In some centers,

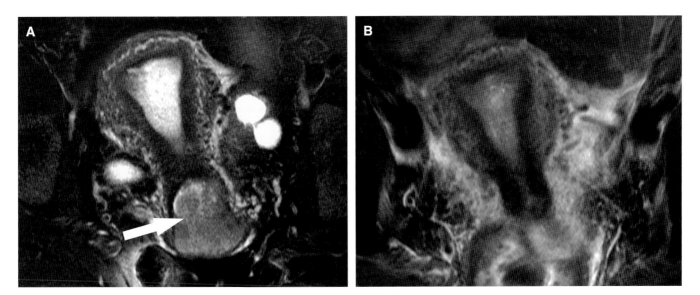

Figure 9.48 *Cervical cancer, confined to the cervix, FIGO stage Ib1, AJCC T1b1.* (**A**) Intermediate-signal-intensity 3.5 cm carcinoma (*arrow*) replaces the low-intensity stroma of the cervix but does not extend beyond the cervix on this T2-weighted oblique axial image through the long axis of the uterus. (**B**) Four months after radiation treatment, there was no evidence of residual disease by imaging or on subsequent Pap smears.

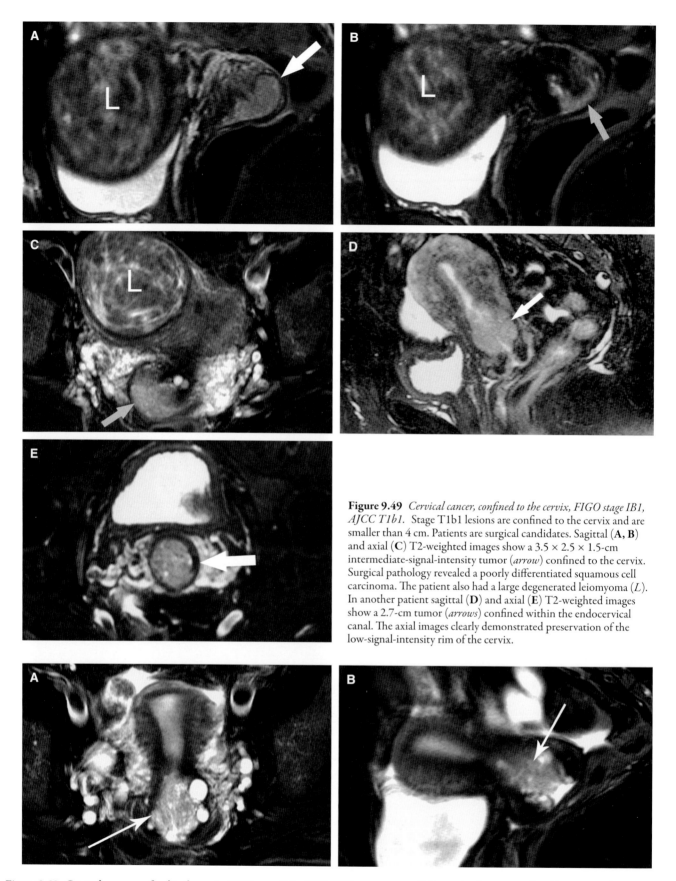

Figure 9.49 *Cervical cancer, confined to the cervix, FIGO stage IB1, AJCC T1b1.* Stage T1b1 lesions are confined to the cervix and are smaller than 4 cm. Patients are surgical candidates. Sagittal (**A, B**) and axial (**C**) T2-weighted images show a 3.5 × 2.5 × 1.5-cm intermediate-signal-intensity tumor (*arrow*) confined to the cervix. Surgical pathology revealed a poorly differentiated squamous cell carcinoma. The patient also had a large degenerated leiomyoma (*L*). In another patient sagittal (**D**) and axial (**E**) T2-weighted images show a 2.7-cm tumor (*arrows*) confined within the endocervical canal. The axial images clearly demonstrated preservation of the low-signal-intensity rim of the cervix.

Figure 9.50 *Cervical cancer, confined to the cervix, FIGO stage IB2, AJCC T1b2.* Fat-saturated T2-weighted images in the oblique axial plane obtained in the long axis of the uterus (**A**) and in the sagittal plane (**B**) show a 5.2 cm endocervical tumor (*arrows*) expanding the cervical canal. The cervix is invaded but a clear rind of preserved low-signal-intensity stroma confirms that the tumor is confined to the cervix. Visible tumor larger than 4 cm makes the stage FIGO IB2. Biopsy showed well-differentiated adenocarcinoma of the endocervical type. The patient was treated with chemotherapy, external-beam radiation, and brachytherapy and remains disease-free 6 years after diagnosis. Several nabothian cysts are evident in the endocervical canal.

candidates with favorable stage 1b1 disease (favorable histology and size less than 2 cm and the tumor at an adequate distance from the internal os) may be offered fertility-sparing surgery (trachelectomy) in lieu of hysterectomy. The cervix, parametrium, and upper 2 cm of the vagina are then removed and the uterus is attached to the remaining vagina.[26] In these cases a cerclage is used during pregnancy. Tumor recurrence is similar to that following standard surgery. Trachelectomy is a difficult procedure and is limited to few candidates and institutions.

Stage IB2 tumors with size greater than 4 cm, FIGO stage IIA and IIB tumors (Figs. 9.49 and 9.50) are usually treated with radiation therapy and cisplatin-based chemotherapy. Some centers may treat bulky tumors with chemotherapy and follow with surgery if a response has occurred. Parametrial invasion usually necessitates radiation therapy where available.

Reportable staging of cervical cancer by both FIGO and AJCC is determined by physical examination, colposcopy, hysteroscopy, biopsy, conization, cystoscopy, and proctosigmoidoscopy, procedures that are available in most countries (Table 9.4). Information from CT and MR imaging are invaluable for subsequent treatment planning.

Clinical staging is limited in evaluating parametrial invasion, a critical assessment in determining whether the tumor is resectable. The probability of parametrial invasion is high if the tumor is endocervical or is larger than 2 cm. MR allows assessment of tumor size, parametrial invasion, and pelvic lymphadenopathy. When the tumor is smaller than 1 cm and exophytic, clinical staging alone is usually sufficient. In these cases the likelihood of parametrial invasion and iliac lymph node metastases is low and the patient can undergo radical hysterectomy without imaging. If advanced disease such as pelvic sidewall involvement is diagnosed at physical examination or by imaging, radiation is the best option.

Indications for MR include the following:

- Determining whether a patient is a surgical candidate when the size and extent of a large or endocervical tumor is difficult to determine clinically

- Determining whether a patient with clinically very-early-stage disease is a candidate for fertility-sparing surgery. MR helps determine suitability by demonstrating the extent of endocervical involvement.

- Determining the extent of advanced disease for surgical or radiation therapy planning

MR findings are as follows (Table 9.4):[27,28]

- Cervical cancer is usually best assessed on T2-weighted images rather than dynamic contrast-enhanced images because the intermediate- to high-signal intensity tumor contrasts against the very-low-intensity cervical stroma.

- Preservation of the low signal intensity stromal ring excludes parametrial invasion (Figs. 9.47 to 9.51).

- Parametrial invasion is indicated by loss of the low signal of the lateral stromal margin and is best seen on axial or coronal fat-suppressed T2-weighted images (Figs. 9.52 and 9.53). Additional findings of parametrial invasion include visualization of tumor tissue in the parametrium, obliteration of parametrial vessels, asymmetrical bulging or irregularity of the cervical border, thickening of the uterosacral ligaments, and ureteral obstruction.

- Vaginal invasion is evidenced by disruption of the low signal intensity vaginal wall by high signal intensity tumor on T2-weighted images or by enhancing tumor on post-contrast-enhanced T1-weighted images.

- *Adenoma malignum* (minimal-deviation adenocarcinoma) is an uncommon unique subtype of mucinous adenocarcinoma of the cervix characterized by multicystic lesions with solid components extending from the endocervical glands (Fig. 9.53). When small, this tumor can mimic clustered nabothian cysts, as both may demonstrate well-defined-mucin-filled-cysts displaying

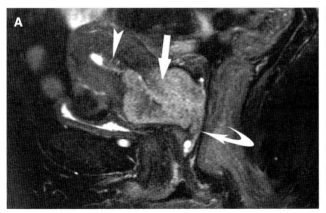
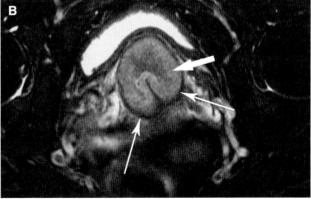

Figure 9.51 *Cervical cancer, extending into the upper vagina.* T2-weighted sagittal (**A**) and axial (**B**) fat-saturated images show a large, intermediate-signal intensity mass (*fat arrows*) replacing the cervix and involving the anterior vaginal wall. The tumor deeply invades the cervical stroma but the low-signal ring (*skinny arrows*) is preserved, excluding parametrial involvement. On exam the tumor measured larger than 6 cm and no vaginal invasion was detected, yielding FIGO IB2. MRI was consistent with a T2a tumor based on upper vaginal extension. An likely incidental endometrial polyp (*arrowhead*) was also noted. Surgical pathology was a poorly differentiated squamous cell carcinoma. Based on MRI findings, a vaginal brachytherapy implant was in addition to whole pelvic radiation and chemosensitization prior to hysterectomy.

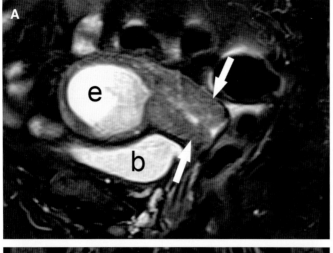

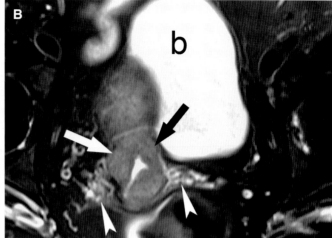

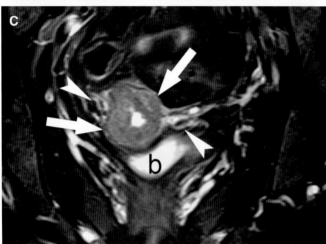

Figure 9.52 *Cervical cancer, early parametrial invasion, FIGO stage IIB, AJCC T2b.* Sagittal (**A**), oblique axial (**B**), and oblique coronal (**C**) T2-weighted fat-saturated images show an intermediate-signal-intensity tumor (*arrows*) circumferentially replacing the cervix stroma. The low-signal-intensity stromal ring is no longer present, indicating parametrial invasion. Fluid has accumulated within the endometrial canal (*e*) because of cervical obstruction. The close relationship of the parametria with the lateral cervix is illustrated here. The vessels (*arrowheads*) and their associated lymphatics in the parametria enter the cervix inferiolaterally. *b*, bladder.

high signal intensity on both T1- and T2-weighted images. Intravenous contrast enhancement of the solid tumor components will be demonstrated. The tumor spreads early and has a poor response to treatment and an overall poor prognosis.

- More advanced cancers can easily obstruct the ureter by parametrial invasion causing hydronephrosis (Figs. 9.46 and 9.54).

- Involvement of the vagina, bladder, and rectum involvement is evident from the segmental disruption of the low-signal-intensity wall of these structures, often associated with thickening or nodularity of the wall. Smooth-walled thickening of the posterior bladder wall, which displays increased signal intensity on T2-weighted images, is suggestive of bullous edema rather than invasion.

- Lymph nodes are considered to be involved by tumor based on size, margins, and internal structure. Irregular margins, internal heterogeneity, and loss of the fatty hilum are strong predictors of tumor involvement.

Critical assessments are as follows:

- Tumor size

- Depth of anterior stromal involvement (distance from bladder wall) and parametrial extension

- Distance of an endocervical lesion from the internal os

- Lymphadenopathy: regional (internal, external, and common iliac) and nonregional (inguinal, para-aortic)

Pitfalls of MR imaging are as follows:

- Cone biopsy: Distortion and edema of the stroma on T2-weighted images following cone biopsy may cause a false-positive diagnosis of a cervical mass. The use of contrast-enhanced T1-weighted images may help differentiate between edema and true tumor enhancement.

- When an exophytic cervical neoplasm extends into the vagina, caution must be taken to interpret it for

Table 9.4 TNM STAGING OF CERVICAL CANCER

AJCC TNM STAGE	FIGO STAGE	DESCRIPTION	MR IMAGING STAGING
T Stage		**Tumor extent**	
Tx		Primary tumor cannot be assessed because of lack of information	
T0		No evidence of primary tumor	
Tis	0	Carcinoma *in situ*	Tumor not visible
	I	Tumor confined to cervix	
T1a	*IA*	Invasive carcinoma diagnosed only by microscopy. All clinically visible lesions, even with superficial invasion, are T1b/1B.	
T1a1	IA1	Confined to the cervix, diagnosed only by microscopy with invasion < 3 mm in depth and lateral spread < 7 mm	No visible tumor
T1a2	IA2	Confined to the cervix, diagnosed only by microscopy with invasion > 3 mm and < 5 mm in depth and lateral spread < 7 mm	Small enhancing tumor possible
T1b	IB	Tumor is clinically visible, confined to the cervix	Tumor is visible, confined to the cervix, low signal intensity stromal ring is intact
T1b1	IB1	Clinically visible lesion, or greater than IA2, < 4 cm in greatest dimension	Visible tumor < 4 cm, confined to cervix
T1b2	IB2	Clinically visible lesion, > 4 cm in greatest dimension	Visible tumor > 4 cm, confined to cervix
	II	Tumor invades beyond cervix but not to pelvic wall or lower third of vagina	
T2a	*IIA*	Tumor without parametrial invasion	
T2a1	IIA1	Involvement of the upper two-thirds of the vagina, without parametrial invasion, < 4 cm in greatest dimension	Tumor, < 4 cm, disrupts the low-signal intensity wall of the vagina
T2a2	IIA2	>4 cm in greatest dimension	Tumor, > 4 cm, disrupts the low-signal intensity wall of the vagina
T2b	IIB	With parametrial involvement	Tumor interrupts the low signal intensity stromal ring of the cervix
	III	Tumor extends to pelvic wall and/or involves lower third of vagina and/or causes hydronephrosis	
T3a	IIIA	Tumor extends to lower third of vagina without extension to pelvic side wall	Tumor invades the lower third of the vagina
T3b	IIIB	Tumor extends to pelvic sidewall and/or obstructs one or both ureters causing hydronephrosis	Tumor extends to pelvic sidewall and/or obstructs one or both ureters
	IVA	Tumor invades mucosa of bladder* or rectum and/or extends to pelvic side walls, or extends beyond the pelvis	Tumor disrupts the low signal intensity wall of the bladder and/or the rectum
N stage		**Lymph node spread**	
NX		Regional lymph nodes cannot be assessed because of lack of information	
N0		No spread to lymph nodes	
N1		Cancer has spread to regional lymph nodes	
M Stage		**Distant spread**	
M0		No cancer spread to distant lymph nodes, organs, or tissues	
M1	IVB	Cancer has spread to distant lymph nodes, distant organs, and/or to the peritoneum	

* True mucosal involvement designates a T4 lesion but bullous edema may simulate mucosal involvement; this can be differentiated with cystoscopy and biopsy.

Adapted from American Joint Committee on Cancer. *AJCC Cancer Staging Manual*, 7th ed. New York, Springer, 2010, and FIGO, 2009.

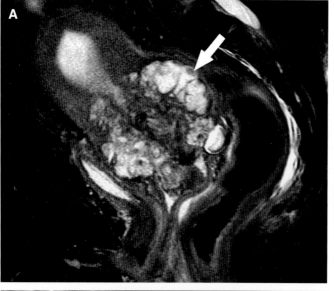

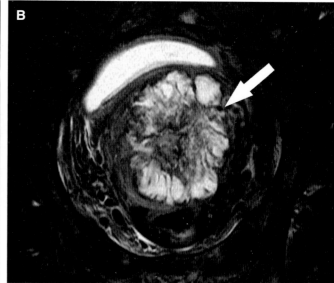

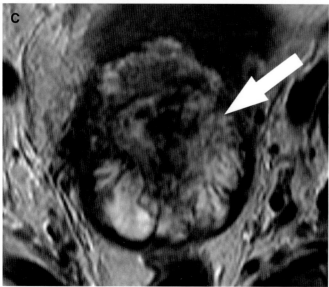

Figure 9.53 *Adenoma malignum, parametrial invasion.* Fat-saturated sagittal (**A**) and axial (**B**) T2-weighted images and axial T1-weighted image (**C**) demonstrate a multilocular circumferential cystic mass (*arrows*) replacing the cervix Tumor signal interrupts the low-signal-intensity stromal margin of the cervix, indicating parametrial invasion (best seen on the T1-weighted image). This lesion was staged FIGO IIIB on the basis of obstruction of the ureter resulting from parametrial invasion. *R*, rectum.

parametrial involvement. Use MPR images or reference lines to determine the relationship of the parametria with the mass.

- In advanced disease, pelvic sidewall edema can be mistaken for tumor, and contrast-enhanced imaging can help differentiating between the two.

ADNEXAL MASSES

Transvaginal ultrasound is the primary imaging modality for adnexal imaging, given its availability, spatial detail, and overall high specificity. The vast majority of cystic lesions are functional cysts that can be confidently diagnosed with this technique as benign simple or hemorrhagic cysts. For the less frequent complex mass, transvaginal ultrasound is also usually diagnostic. Gray-scale ultrasound demonstration of a cystic ovarian mass with papillary excrescences is diagnostic and the patient is often taken directly to surgery.

MR provides spatial detail, tissue characterization, and complete multiplanar pelvic coverage. The morphology and relationship of the adnexal mass to other structures is visualized, and the mass can be characterized as containing fat, mucin, blood, fibrous tissue, and calcium. Malignancy is unlikely if an ovarian origin is excluded. The majority of simple and hemorrhagic cysts, endometriomas, fibrous lesions, mature teratomas, hydrosalpinx, and peritoneal inclusion cysts can be accurately characterized by MR. Indications for MR are as follows:

- Evaluation of adnexal pathology after a nondiagnostic ultrasound showing an unusual or incompletely characterized adnexal mass

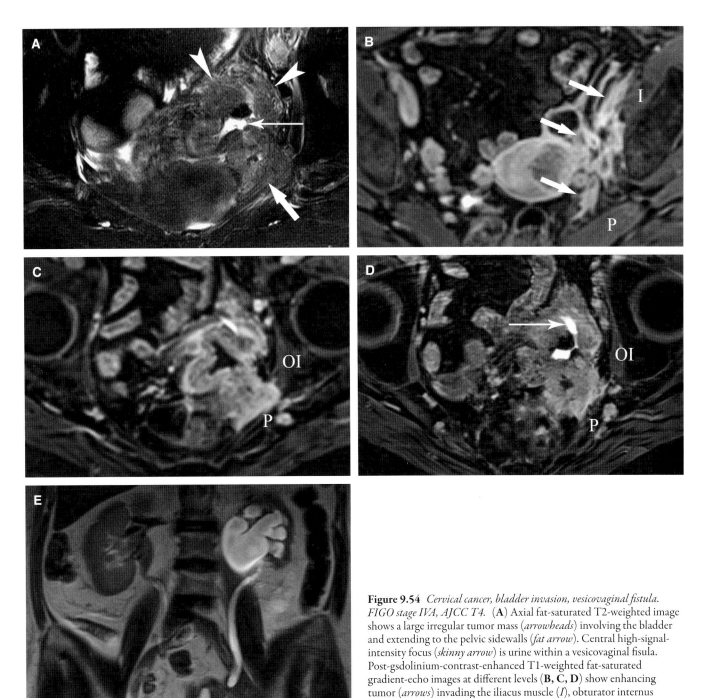

Figure 9.54 *Cervical cancer, bladder invasion, vesicovaginal fistula. FIGO stage IVA, AJCC T4.* (**A**) Axial fat-saturated T2-weighted image shows a large irregular tumor mass (*arrowheads*) involving the bladder and extending to the pelvic sidewalls (*fat arrow*). Central high-signal-intensity focus (*skinny arrow*) is urine within a vesicovaginal fisula. Post-gsdolinium-contrast-enhanced T1-weighted fat-saturated gradient-echo images at different levels (**B, C, D**) show enhancing tumor (*arrows*) invading the iliacus muscle (*I*), obturator internus muscle (*OI*), and piriformis muscle (*P*). Gadolinium contrast-enhanced urine (*skinny arrow*) is seen in the fistula. Urine not containing gadolinium would be low in signal intensity on this sequence. (**E**) Coronal T2-weighted image demonstrates marked left hydronephrosis and hydroureter. The atrophy of the renal parenchyma indicates chronic obstruction from the pelvic tumor.

- Evaluation of adnexal masses in pregnancy when ultrasound is nondiagnostic

- Surveillance of a likely benign large cystic adnexal mass in a poor-operative-risk patient

- Characterization of solid-appearing adnexal masses where the differential includes endometrioma, dermoid, adnexal leiomyomas, or solid ovarian mass

NON-NEOPLASTIC ADNEXAL MASSES WITH CLASSIC FEATURES

Functional cysts are common incidental findings. Nearly all are diagnosed as benign by transvaginal ultrasound, and MR is seldom indicated.[29] However, they may present as incidental findings that should be appropriately characterized. Follicular ovarian cysts have simple fluid and a thin wall. Corpus luteal cysts occur at the site of ovulation and have thick walls with

Box 9.5 ESSENTIALS TO REMEMBER

- A small cervical carcinoma on T2-weighted images is recognized as disruption of the normally uniform low-signal-intensity stromal ring of the cervix by the intermediate high-signal-intensity tumor.

- The anterior stroma between the anterior cervix and the bladder is a critical area to assess for bladder wall involvement as the interface is not covered by peritoneum.

- Parametrial invasion of cervical cancer is indicated by at least disruption of the low signal intensity outer cervical stroma. Invasion of parametrial fat is best seen on axial or coronal fat-suppressed T2-weighted images.

- Ureteral obstruction in cervical cancer is caused by parametrial invasion and is considered pelvic sidewall invasion.

- Tumor invasion of the bladder or rectum by cancer of the cervix is indicated by tumor disruption of the normally uniform low-signal-intensity muscular wall of the organs.

- Adenoma malignum is a mucinous adenocarcinoma of the cervix appearing as a multicystic tumor with solid components extending from the endocervix. Small tumors may mimic the appearance of multiple nabothian cysts.

---

increased vascularity that often leads to intracystic hemorrhage, rupture, and intrapelvic hemorrhage. Corpus luteal cysts tend to have thicker walls than follicular cysts. All borderline or malignant neoplasms have mural nodules or septations. A borderline tumor may appear deceptively simple. However, it is typically a large cystic lesion with at least minimal wall nodularity. Careful search of the entire cyst wall must be diligently performed by ultrasound examination and on MR images. MR findings are as follows:[30]

- Uncomplicated functional cysts contain simple fluid that shows with low signal intensity on T1-weighted images and high signal intensity on T2-weighted images.

- Hemorrhagic functional or corpus luteal cysts contain bloody fluid that displays higher signal intensity than simple fluid on T1-weighted images (Figs 9.9 and 9.55).

- Most functional cysts are unilocular and 3 to 8 cm in size.

- The thin wall of a follicular cyst or the thicker wall of a corpus luteal cyst may show contrast enhancement.

- Functional cysts usually regress within 2 months.

Para-ovarian cysts usually occur close to but separate from the ovary. Para-ovarian cysts arise from embryonic rests within the folds of the broad ligament. Imaging features are similar to those of typical functional ovarian cysts and this should not present a diagnostic dilemma.

Peritoneal inclusion cysts. Normal ovaries cyclically secrete fluid that is resorbed by the peritoneal lining. Pelvic inflammatory disease, endometriosis, or pelvic surgery cause the adjacent pelvic peritoneal lining to lose its normal resorptive capacity and scar down around an ovary to form a

confined space trapping the ovarian fluid. A loculated fluid collection around the ovary builds up to a specific threshold and causes pressure symptoms and pain. The fluid usually recurs after attempted aspirations. Percutaneous sclerosis can be attempted when surgery is precluded due to extensive adhesions and hormonal therapy has failed.[31] Surgical resection that includes removal of the ovary is usually curative. MR findings are as follows:

- The ovary is surrounded by fluid that conforms to the peritoneal recesses between structures, creating angular margins (Fig. 9.56).

- The contained ovary is usually eccentrically positioned.

- Pseudo-septations are formed by fluid tracking around adhesions.

- Papillary or other solid components are absent.

- The contained fluid has signal intensity of simple fluid: low signal intensity on T1-weighted imaging and high signal intensity on T2-weighted imaging. Particulate matter may be present.

- Very large peritoneal inclusion cysts can appear mass-like with rounded margins.

Pelvic congestion syndrome is a recognized cause of chronic pelvic pain. Vascular congestion and pain are a consequence of venous valvular incompetence resulting from the dilatation of the gonadal veins that occurs during pregnancy. Portal hypertension or an extrinsically compressed left renal vein ("nutcracker syndrome") are other causes. MR criteria for this diagnosis in a patient with chronic pelvic pain include numerous and tortuous para-uterine and pelvic veins that

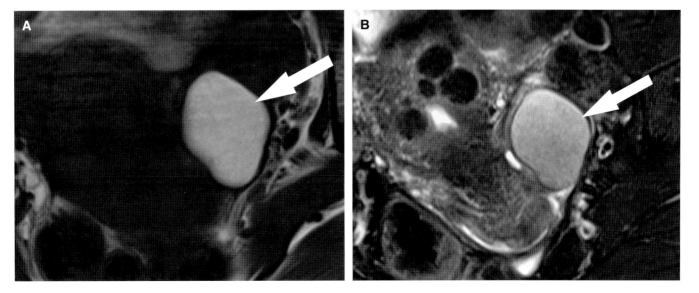

Figure 9.55 *Hemorrhagic functional ovarian cyst.* (**A**) Axial T1-weighted image reveals a well-defined homogeneous left ovarian mass (*arrow*) with uniform high-intensity internal signal. (**B**) T2-weighted fat-saturated image also shows uniform high signal intensity within the lesion (*arrow*), confirming a hemorrhagic ovarian cyst. Fat-saturation or chemical-shift sequences are needed to exclude internal fat content characteristic of benign cystic teratoma. Several small low-signal-intensity leiomyomas are seen in the uterus.

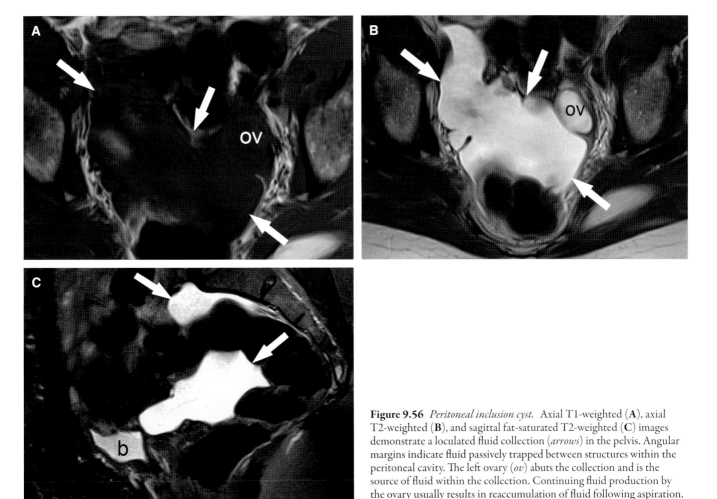

Figure 9.56 *Peritoneal inclusion cyst.* Axial T1-weighted (**A**), axial T2-weighted (**B**), and sagittal fat-saturated T2-weighted (**C**) images demonstrate a loculated fluid collection (*arrows*) in the pelvis. Angular margins indicate fluid passively trapped between structures within the peritoneal cavity. The left ovary (*ov*) abuts the collection and is the source of fluid within the collection. Continuing fluid production by the ovary usually results in reaccumulation of fluid following aspiration. Effective treatment generally requires removal of the ovary. *b*, bladder.

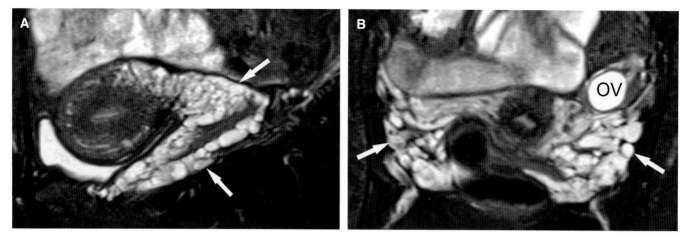

Figure 9.57 *Pelvic congestion syndrome.* T2-weighted fat-saturated images in sagittal (**A**) and coronal (**B**) planes demonstrate numerous enlarged extrauterine vessels (*arrows*) in a patient with chronic pelvic pain. The left ovary contains a dominant follicle (*OV*).

communicate with dilated arcuate veins in the myometrium (Fig. 9.57). The veins are enlarged with a diameter of more than 5 to 6 mm. Doppler sonography may demonstrate reversal of flow in the ovarian vein, and dynamic contrast-enhanced imaging may demonstrate early filling of the ovarian veins.

Hydrosalpinx is a dilated fallopian tube filled with fluid that is usually simple. Pelvic inflammatory processes can seal the fimbriae. Hydrosalpinx is more likely to occur if the proximal tube is already sealed from prior inflammation or tubal ligation. Pyosalpinx (pus-filled tube) and hematosalpinx (blood-filled tube) are precursors of chronic hydrosalpinx.

The ampullary (distal) portion of the tube, with its less muscular wall, is usually asymmetrically more dilated than the proximal portion of the tube which has a more muscular wall. The mucosal lining may be chronically inflamed and thickened. Infrequently, a very small or very large hydrosalpinx may be difficult to differentiate from an ovarian tumor. MR findings are as follows:

- The fluid-filled mass is tubular, sausage-shaped, or C-shaped (Fig. 9.58).

- A "cogwheel" appearance of incomplete polypoid invaginations into the lumen, representing the thickened mucosal folds, is characteristic.

- Signal intensity of fluid within a hydrosalpinx is that of simple fluid. The presence of proteinaceous material, pus, or blood within the tube will lead to an increase of the signal on T1-weighted images.

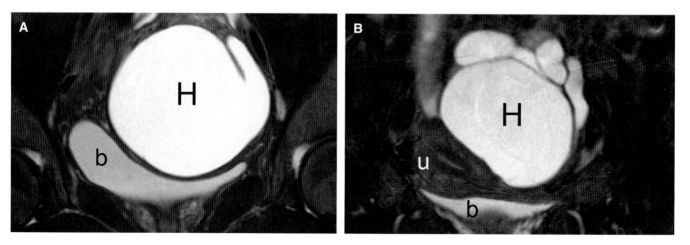

Figure 9.58 *Hydrosalpinx.* Coronal (**A, B**) fat-saturated T2-weighted images obtained at different levels show a large cystic pelvic mass (*H*). Review of serial images, preferably on a workstation allowing scrolling through sequential images, confirms massive dilatation of the fimbriated end of the fallopian tube, and fusiform dilatation and tortuosity of the remainder of the tube. *u*, uterus. *b*, bladder.

- Hematosalpinx may show imaging features similar to those of endometriomas, including the T2-shading effect of chronic hemorrhage.

Tubo-ovarian abscess is identified when a dilated fallopian tube is seen in a symptomatic patient. The walls of the tube are thickened and the fluid often contains debris. With increasing inflammation, the tube and ovary become less well defined. The fluid itself varies in signal, depending on the presence of hemorrhagic and proteinaceous content. MR findings are as follows:[30]

- Lesions appear as complex fluid-filled masses, usually high in signal intensity, on both T1- and T2-weighted images (Fig 9.59).

- Edema and other inflammatory changes surround the inflamed tube.

- Involvement of pelvic fat and the wall of adjacent bowel is manifest by ill-defined high signal intensity on T2-weighted images.

- Post-gadolinium-contrast-enhanced images typically show a thick wall with avid enhancement of inflamed tissue bounding the lesion.

- If air is present within the abscess, foci of intense signal void are seen on T2*-weighted gradient-echo images.

- A dark peripheral rim in the fluid represents protein or hemorrhage in different stages of evolution (Fig. 9.59).

Endometriosis refers to the implantation of endometrial tissue outside the uterus. It is theorized to occur as a result of implantation during retrograde menstruation in some patients, metaplasia of peritoneal cells, or hormonal induction of peritoneal Müllerian remnants into functioning endometrial glands. Further spread of endometrial cells can occur through lymphatic and hematogenous routes. The cyclic bleeding from the hormonally responsive extrauterine endometrial tissue results in a chronic inflammatory reaction. Endometriosis predominantly involves the pelvis and usually includes the ovaries, cul-de-sac, and broad ligaments. Less frequently involved are the uterosacral ligament, rectum, sigmoid colon, bladder, and distal ureter. Distant sites may include the pleura, spinal canal, and solid organs. Although occasionally asymptomatic, most women have cyclic and worsening pelvic pain and infertility.

Endometriosis implants usually are tiny non-mass-like surface coatings that are difficult to visualize by imaging and are usually detectable only by laparoscopy. Specific serum markers have relatively high sensitivity and specificity for determining the presence of tumor.

An **endometrioma** ("chocolate cyst") results from chronic cyclical bleeding over years producing a particulate, highly viscous cystic mass with high concentrations of iron and protein. MR findings are as follows:[28]

- Endometriomas, given the presence of hemorrhage, typically display high signal intensity on T1-weighted images. Signal on T2-weighted images is variable and depends on the amount of hemosiderin (Figs. 9.18 and 9.60).

- The T2-shading effect, caused by dependent layering of hemosiderin, reflects a chronic process and helps to differentiate a chronic endometrioma from an acute hemorrhagic functional cyst.

- If a very high concentration of hemosiderin is present, the fluid may have extremely low signal intensity ("signal void") on T2-weighted images.

- The cyst wall itself displays low signal intensity on both T1- and T2-weighted images due to its fibrous nature and

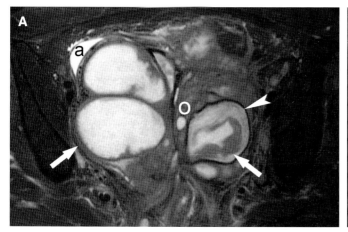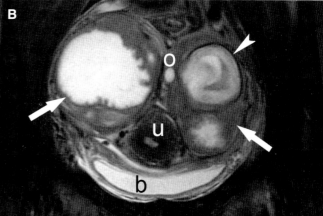

Figure 9.59 *Bilateral tubo-ovarian abscesses.* Axial (**A**) and coronal (**B**) T2-weighted fat-saturated images show complex high-signal-intensity masses (*arrows*) in both adnexa. Review of sequential images confirms bilateral markedly dilated fallopian tubes, and the ovary (*o*) and uterus (*u*) being enveloped by the mass. The low-signal rim (*arrowhead*) and the mixed-signal-intensity shading of the fluid in the left tube indicate complex fluid and a chronic process. Surgical resection of the fallopian tubes demonstrated hemorrhage, pus, and mucoid material within the tubes. *a*, ascites. *b*, bladder.

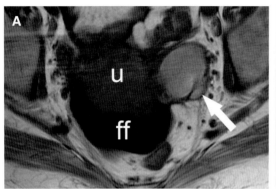
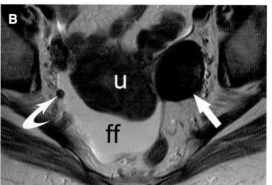
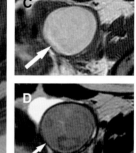

Figure 9.60 *Endometriomas.* Axial T1- (**A**) and T2-weighted (**B**) images show a well-marginated left adnexal mass (*arrow*) with intermediate internal signal intensity on the T1-weighted image and very low internal signal intensity on the T2-weighted image characteristic of chronic blood products within an endometrioma. A moderate volume of free fluid (*ff*) in the cul-de-sac posterior to the uterus (*u*) is evidence of endometrial deposition (*curved arrow* in image B) on peritoneal surfaces. Axial T1- (**C**) and T2-weighted (**D**) images obtained in another patient with endometrioma, shows different signal intensity of the lesions than in **A** and **B** resulting from the differences in the internal iron and protein content. These differences in composition of the lesion contents lead to variations in signal intensity of the contained fluid.

the abundance of hemosiderin-laden macrophages in the wall. The wall thickens over time (Fig. 9.60D).

- Inflammation from the endometrioma may cause adjacent dense adhesions with obscuration of the fat planes and poor definition of the endometrioma. Small endometrial implants may eventually become solid and fibrotic and enhance similar to other fibrotic tissue. Low signal intensity on both T1- and T2-weighted images helps distinguish endometrial implants from malignancy.

- Endometriomas are frequently multiple, especially in the cul-de-sac. The ovaries are most commonly involved.

- In distinction to endometriomas, hemorrhagic functional cysts are usually solitary; hemoglobin is less concentrated and T2 shading is rare. Bloody fluid in a hemorrhagic functional cyst is high in signal intensity on T1-weighted images and remains high in signal intensity on T2-weighted images. Acute hemorrhagic cysts typically resolve within 2 months, whereas endometriomas are chronic and remain present on serial imaging.

- Endometriomas may be distinguished from subacute hematomas in the pelvis or musculature. On fat-saturated T1-weighted images, a subacute hematoma may demonstrate the concentric ring sign, where a low-signal wall (due to ferritin in macrophages) is adjacent to a high-signal rim of fluid with extracellular methemoglobin. This is absent in endometriomas and functional cysts.

- A large functional cyst or an endometrioma may similarly stretch out the involved ovary. After contrast enhancement, this distorted and enhancing ovarian tissue should not be confused with malignancy. The crescent shape and presence of follicles can characterize this tissue as normal ovarian parenchyma.

- Endometriomas display relatively high signal intensity on T1-weighted images, so enhancing internal components may be difficult to detect. Post-contrast-enhanced subtraction images must be performed to visualize enhancement of mural nodules.

- With malignant transformation, the portion of the endometrioma that underwent malignant transformation typically secretes serous fluid. This low-signal-intensity fluid on T1-weighted images dilutes the thick hemorrhagic fluid, thereby lowering the signal intensity on T1-weighted images and increasing the signal intensity of part or all of the endometrioma on T2-weighted images.

- *Caveat:* In pregnancy, detection of enhancing solid peritoneal nodules or an abdominal cystic mass with enhancing components should include extrauterine deciduosis in the differential diagnosis.

About 1% of endometriomas give rise to ovarian endometrioid and clear cell adenocarcinomas, similar to the two subtypes found in endometrial cancer (Fig. 9.65). Conversely, both occur with coexistent endometriosis in a large percentage of women. These usually occur in women over 45 and in endometriomas larger than 9 cm in size.[32,33]

With malignant transformation, rapid growth of an endometrioma typically occurs. Neoplastic mural nodules secrete fluid, diluting the thick hemorrhagic fluid of a chocolate cyst so that the cyst enlarges and becomes more liquefied.

When evaluating endometriosis, care must be taken to look for enhancing components that may represent foci of degeneration within neoplasms. When intravenous contrast enhancement is used, dynamic contrast-enhanced sequences with post-processing subtraction are essential for differentiating enhancing solid components from adjacent blood.

Ectopic decidua (extrauterine deciduosis) is an infrequent, histologically benign condition that can be mistakenly diagnosed as peritoneal carcinomatosis. It most often occurs during late pregnancy but can be related to other progesterone-altered states. Progesterone induces vascularization and growth of ectopic endometrial tissue.

Tiny (1 to 5 mm) serosal nodules are composed of glandular tissue with little fibrosis and the implants most frequently occur on the ovaries or cervix but may also arise on bowel serosa, peritoneum, lungs, pleura, or retroperitoneal lymph nodes. They display high signal intensity on T2-weighted images and enhance on post-gadolinium-contrast-enhanced T1-weighted images, both features mimicking malignancy. Less frequently, large decidualized ovarian endometriomas may demonstrate enhancing papillary masses simulating malignancy especially in pregnancy, the differential diagnosis should include ectopic deciduosis. The lesions resolve spontaneously within 6 weeks postpartum.[34]

OVARIAN NEOPLASMS

Ovarian cancer in the United States accounts for more deaths than the combined mortality from all other gynecologic malignancies. Epithelial ovarian carcinomas account for 90% to 95% of ovarian cancer deaths. Patients have no or only nonspecific symptoms in early disease. Most women have stage III or IV disease at diagnosis. Screening with CA-125 is not effective in non-high-risk women given its poor specificity (positive predictive value of 5%). CA-125 is normal in 50% of women with early ovarian cancer. CA-125, however, has good specificity and sensitivity in detecting ovarian cancer recurrence after treatment.

WHO/FIGO classifies primary ovarian tumors according to the ovarian components from which the tumors arise:

- Surface epithelial-stromal tumors constitute 70% of all ovarian neoplasms. The majority of malignant ovarian tumors (90%) are of epithelial origin. Subtypes are serous (50%), mucinous, endometrioid, clear cell, and transitional cell carcinomas. Each can be of benign, borderline, or have malignant histology.

- Germ cell tumors make up 20%. Nearly all are benign dermoids.

- Sex cord-stromal tumors (10%) are rarely malignant.

- Non-ovarian-origin tumors, including lymphoma and metastases, constitute 5% of ovarian neoplasms. Most ovarian metastases are gastrointestinal in origin.

Ovarian malignancies characteristically spread by intraperitoneal seeding (Table 9.5). Peritoneal tumor implants usually cause ascites. Within the peritoneum, mucinous tumors generally form larger masses while serous tumors spread more diffusely. Lymphatic spread follows ovarian blood supply along the infundibulopelvic ligament to the para-aortic nodes. Other lymphatics pass laterally through the parametrium, similar to cervical cancer, to involve the external, internal, and common iliac nodal chains. Infrequently, metastases follow the round ligament to the inguinal nodes (nonregional spread). Regional lymph node involvement includes the internal, external, and common iliac nodes and para-aortic nodes, and involvement of these will classify the tumor as at least FIGO stage IIIC. FIGO/AJCC staging classifies growth confined to one ovary as stage I with or without malignant ascites. Higher stages are differentiated by confinement of implants to the pelvis (stage II) and extrapelvic peritoneal implants or positive retroperitoneal or inguinal nodes (stage III). Transdiaphragmatic spread leads to pleural metastases with malignant pleural fluid. Hematogenous spread is rare, occurring in only a few percent of patients.

Box 9.6 ESSENTIALS TO REMEMBER

- Thin-walled ovarian cysts containing simple or hemorrhagic fluid found in a woman of menstrual age are very likely to be functional follicular or corpus luteal cysts that will spontaneously resolve within one or two menstrual cycles.

- Peritoneal inclusion cysts envelop the ovary in a fluid collection that characteristically extends into peritoneal recesses, producing an angular shape.

- Hydrosalpinx can produce complex adnexal masses that mimic ovarian neoplasms.

- Endometriomas commonly implant on the ovary, mimicking an ovarian-origin mass.

- The appearance of endometriomas on MR overlaps with that of acute hemorrhagic functional ovarian cysts. Findings of chronic hemorrhage, including T2 shading, are strongly indicative of endometriomas.

- The presence of two or more hemorrhagic adnexal cysts suggests endometriosis as a possible diagnosis.

- In pregnancy, when enhancing solid peritoneal nodules are encountered, the diagnosis of extrauterine deciduosis should be included in the differential diagnosis.

Table 9.5 TNM STAGING OF OVARIAN CANCER

AJCC TNM STAGE	FIGO STAGE	DESCRIPTION
T Stage		Tumor extent
Tx		Primary tumor cannot be assessed because lack of information
T0		No tumor evident in the ovary
T1	I	Growth limited to the ovaries
T1a	IA	Growth limited to one ovary, no ascites, no tumor on external surface, capsule intact
T1b	IB	Growth limited to both ovaries, no ascites, no tumor on external surface, capsule intact
T1c	IC	Tumor either stage IA or IB but with tumor on surface of one or both ovaries, ruptured capsule, ascites with malignant cells or positive peritoneal washings
T2	II	Growth involving one or both ovaries, with pelvic extension
T2a	IIA	Extension and/or metastases to the uterus or fallopian tubes
T2b	IIB	Extension to other pelvic tissues
T2c	IIC	Stage IIA or IIB but with tumor on surface of one or both ovaries, ruptured capsule, ascites with malignant cells or positive peritoneal washings
T3	III	Tumor involving one or both ovaries, with peritoneal implants outside the pelvis and/or retroperitoneal or inguinal nodes; superficial liver metastases constitute stage III disease
T3a	IIIA	Tumor grossly limited to pelvis, negative lymph node but histological proof of microscopic disease on abdominal peritoneal surfaces
T3b	IIIB	Confirmed implants outside of pelvis in the abdominal peritoneal surface; no implant exceeds 2 cm in diameters and lymph nodes are negative
T3c	IIIC	Abdominal implants larger than 2 cm in diameter and/or positive lymph nodes
N Stage		Lymph node spread
N0		No spread to lymph nodes
N1		Cancer has spread to pelvic lymph nodes
M Stage		Distant spread
M0		No cancer spread to distant lymph nodes, organs, or tissues
M1	IV	Distant metastases; pleural effusion must have a positive cytology to be classified as stage IV; parenchymal liver metastases constitute stage IV disease

Adapted from American Joint Committee on Cancer. *AJCC Cancer Staging Manual*, 7th ed. New York, Springer, 2010, and FIGO, 2009.

Germ cell tumors are mostly (95% to 97%) benign mature cystic teratomas (dermoids). Most are diagnosed in relatively young women. Ten percent are bilateral. These tumors are lined by squamous epithelium and contain mature epithelial elements (skin, hair, teeth, sebum). Malignant degeneration to invasive squamous cell carcinoma is rare and typically occurs postmenopausal in large dermoids. Torsion and rarely rupture can occur. A chronically leaking dermoid can lead to chronic granulomatous peritonitis causing mesenteric infiltration, bowel wall thickening, and occasionally ascites. This can mimic carcinomatosis or tuberculous peritonitis. Rupture of a benign dermoid containing neural elements can lead to

peritoneal gliosis, a very unusual condition in which benign proliferative masses grow in the peritoneum. Repeated resections may be necessary.

The remaining 3% to 5% of germ cell tumors are immature malignant teratoma, dysgerminoma, yolk sac tumor, embryonal carcinoma, polyembryoma, choriocarcinoma, and mixed tumors. These usually affect young women, with mean age of 20 years. Alpha-fetoprotein (AFP), human chorionic gonadotropin (beta-hCG), and other tumor markers may be elevated. The dysgerminoma is similar to the testicular seminoma and is the most common malignant ovarian tumor in children. Most malignant germ cell tumors are stage I (confined to the ovary) at diagnosis. Ovarian germ cell malignancies metastasize intra-peritoneally, lymphatically, and hematogenously. MR findings are as follows:[30,35,36]

- Macroscopic (adipose) fatty material is typically seen within a dermoid tumor. Only a few have little or no macroscopic fat. The diagnosis of fat is made as its signal intensity parallels that of subcutaneous fat on all image sequences (Fig. 9.61). Frequency-selective fat suppression helps differentiating macroscopic fat from hemorrhage.

- A dermoid without macroscopic fat may instead contain a component with intracellular fat. The latter is still diagnostic of a dermoid and the addition of in-phase and out-of-phase gradient-echo sequences can help with detection of these components.

- A generally non-enhancing solid nodule (the Rokitansky nodule or dermoid plug) within the cystic lesion is characteristic and often contains some variation of calcification, fat, dental material, or hair. It is a common site of malignant transformation, which is suspected when there is marked enhancement.

- Layering debris is common.

- Ossified bone and teeth show very low signal intensity.

- An enhancing soft tissue component within or adjacent to a fat-containing cystic tumor can indicate malignant degeneration or the presence of a histologically distinct second tumor (collision tumor). The most common ovarian collision tumors are dermoid, mucinous cystadenoma, or cystadenocarcinoma.

Sex-cord stromal tumors usually present in middle age, are usually benign or of low grade, are confined to the ovary, and are nearly always solid masses. They may be hormonally active, producing estrogens and/or androgens. Specific sex

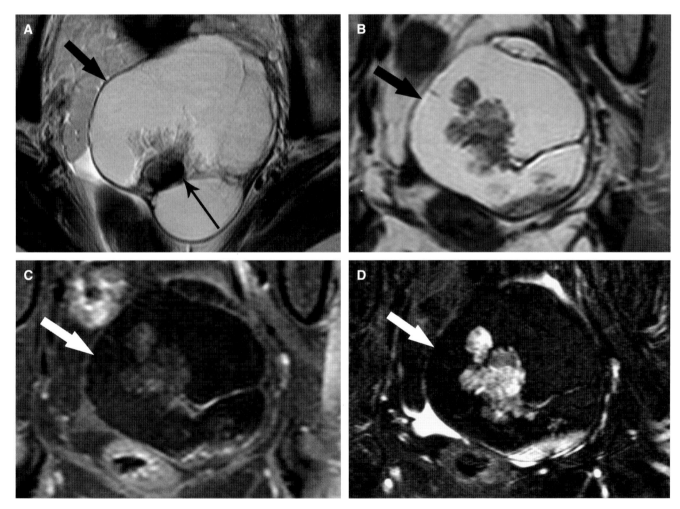

Figure 9.61 *Benign mature cystic teratoma.* Axial (**A**) T2-weighted and coronal (**B**) T1-weighted images show a large, well-defined pelvic mass (*fat arrows*) with homogeneous high signal intensity surrounding low-signal-intensity internal components. The focus of particularly low signal (flow void) corresponds to calcium (*skinny arrow*). The curvilinear low-signal-intensity strands emanating from it are from hair. Coronal T1- (**C**) and T2-weighted (**D**) fat-saturated images show marked reduction in signal intensity of most of the mass (*arrows*), indicating fat content of sebum. Higher signal intensity is evident in the solid components, which proved to be a mixture of tissue, fat, and hair.

cord-stromal tumors occur more frequently in Peutz-Jeghers, Cushing, Meigs, and nevoid basal cell carcinoma syndromes. These tumors constitute 8% to 10% of ovarian neoplasms. Two thirds are fibromas. The remainder include thecomas, fibrothecomas, granulosa cell tumors, Sertoli-Leydig cell tumors, and steroid cell tumors.

Meigs syndrome occurs in 10% of fibromas. Meigs syndrome is the association of a benign ovarian fibroma with benign ascites and pleural fluid; these fluids resolve with surgical resection of the fibroma. The secretion of the fluid may be from the mass itself or from a mechanical effect resulting from irritation or torsion. Fibromas and fibrothecomas are solid tumors and composed of abundant collagen, and therefore appear as very-low-signal-intensity masses on T1- and T2-weighted images. Dense calcifications producing signal voids may be present. Areas of edema or cystic degeneration within the lesions produce high-signal-intensity areas on T2-weighted images. These fibrous ovarian lesions must be differentiated from exophytic and pedunculated leiomyomas. An edematous fibroma may simulate ovarian edema.

Sertoli-Leydig tumors are also predominantly solid and may contain small cysts or focal hemorrhage. They occur in young women (under age 30) and produce virilizing hormones.

Granulosa cell tumors are commonly malignant but are usually confined to the ovary. They frequently produce high levels of estrogen, resulting in endometrial hyperplasia in 50% of cases. Granulosa cell tumors (Fig. 9.62) are highly variable in MR appearance, with some appearing solid, others with prominent areas of hemorrhage and necrosis, and others as a multicystic mass.[30] Unlike epithelial ovarian tumors, these tumors are much less likely to seed the peritoneum with tumor.

Metastases to the ovaries are most commonly adenocarcinomas of the colon and stomach, followed by breast, lung, and tumors from the contralateral ovary. Gastrointestinal-origin mucin-producing metastases are referred to as Krukenberg tumors. On MR, metastases are predominantly solid or mixed tumors with solid and cystic areas.[37] Krukenberg tumors[38] usually are bilateral and have a characteristic and striking appearance. Signet ring cells easily penetrate the ovaries and cause a collagenous stromal reaction peripherally and in scattered areas centrally. The ovaries enlarge and maintain their oval shape. The signet ring cells may secrete abundant mucin centrally. As the ovarian mass enlarges, non-enhancing focal cystic, myxoid, or hemorrhagic necrosis also occurs. On MR, the periphery is characteristically low in signal intensity and the central region is predominantly intermediate or high in signal on T2-weighted images, depending on amount of mucin within the collagenous stroma. After gadolinium contrast material administration, the periphery and central septa typically avidly enhance.

Epithelial ovarian cancers may have a hereditary predisposition. Hereditary breast-ovarian cancer syndrome is related to the autosomal dominant BRCA1 and BRCA2 tumor-suppressor gene mutations and is responsible for 10% of ovarian cancers and 5% of breast cancers. Hereditary nonpolyposis colorectal cancer (Lynch II syndrome) carries a high risk of colorectal, endometrial, gastric, small bowel, breast, pancreas, and ovarian cancers. Bilateral salpingo-oophorectomy performed after childbearing age reduces the risk for developing these cancers in carriers of the BRCA mutations. Non-hereditary risk is possibly related to the cumulative effect of uninterrupted ovulatory cycles, which is hypothesized to have a chronic mutagenic effect.

Five major histologic subtypes of epithelial ovarian neoplasms (WHO/FIGO) account for 95% of epithelial tumors: serous, mucinous, endometrioid, clear cell, and transitional cell (Brenner) tumors. Additional primary cancers include

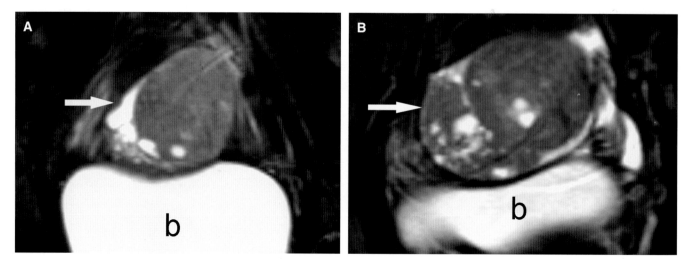

Figure 9.62 *Granulosa cell tumor.* A 21-year-old woman presented with pelvic pain and irregular menstrual bleeding. (**A, B**) Two coronal images from a fat-saturated T2-weighted MR sequence shows a predominantly solid mass (*arrows*) demonstrating intermediate signal intensity and cystic components demonstrating high signal intensity. Cystic components containing simple or hemorrhagic fluid occur commonly in stromal tumors. Surgical pathology revealed granulosa cell carcinoma. *b*, bladder.

undifferentiated, squamous cell, and mixed epithelial tumors. The serous type resembles the epithelium of the fallopian tube. Endometrioid and clear cell types resemble the endometrium and endocervix, respectively, and are associated with endometriosis. The mucinous and transitional cell types morphologically resemble the epithelium of the gastrointestinal tract and urinary bladder, respectively.

Each epithelial subtype is histologically characterized as benign, as of low malignant potential, or as malignant adenocarcinomas. Thus, a serous tumor may be a serous cystadenoma, a serous cystic tumor of low malignant potential, or a serous cystadenocarcinoma. A borderline serous or mucinous tumor is usually indistinguishable from a benign tumor. Either can have features of a simple cysts as well as papillary projections. Carcinomas, however, will demonstrate solid components and are more likely to demonstrate a greater proportion of papillary and solid areas than benign or borderline tumors.[13,39]

Epithelial tumors are primarily cystic and may be unilocular or multilocular.

Serous tumors are 60% benign, 15% are of low malignant potential, and 25% are malignant. A unilocular or multilocular tumor with thin uniform walls and septations containing simple fluid (by MR imaging) is likely a benign serous cystadenoma.

Mucinous tumors tend to be larger lesions; 80% of these are benign, 10% to 15% have low malignant potential, and 5% to 10% are malignant. Mucinous cystadenomas typically appear as large multilocular cysts with thin septations. The overall

low signal intensity on T1-weighted images and high signal on T2-weighted images is related to the high water content of the mucin. However, the locules contain mucinous fluid of differing viscosity, resulting in variations in signal intensity on both T1- and T2-weighted images. Some locules are lower or higher in signal than others on T1- and T2-weighted images, respectively.[3] The septated collections of fluid of differing signal intensity have been termed the "stained glass" appearance (Fig. 9.63).[30]

Endometrioid and clear cell carcinomas represent 15% and 5%, respectively, of ovarian carcinomas. Both tumor types are nearly always malignant, but more than half of either are stage I at the time of diagnosis, offering a better prognosis than most ovarian cancers.

The endometrioid ovarian carcinoma has a growth pattern similar to that of the neoplastic proliferations of the endometrial lining. Although concurrent endometriosis is diagnosed in 40% of cases, nearly all endometrioid ovarian cancers are believed to arise from endometriosis. One third of ovarian endometrioid carcinomas is associated with synchronous endometrial carcinoma or endometrial hyperplasia, and one third is bilateral. The clear cell subtype is believed to arise from Müllerian remnants and can occur in the ovary, endometrium, fallopian tube, cervix, and vagina. It also has a very high association with endometriosis.[13]

Both typically present as a large unilocular cyst (15 to 20 cm) with solid protrusions and variable necrosis and hemorrhage; fluid is usually hemorrhagic, in contrast to serous and mucinous tumors. They are less frequently solid with necrosis

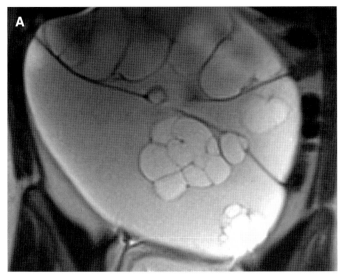

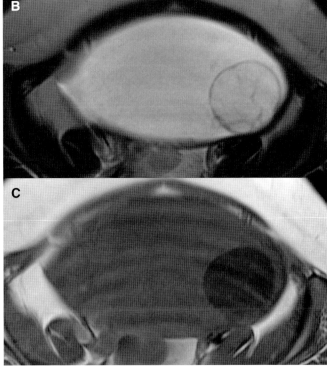

Figure 9.63 *Mucinous ovarian tumor of low malignant potential.* Coronal (**A**) and axial (**B**) T2-weighted and axial T1-weighted (**C**) images demonstrate a large cystic mass arising from the pelvis and extending into the abdomen. The wall is uniformly thin. Numerous thin septations form cystic locules containing fluid of differing signal intensity. This is an example of the "stained glass" appearance characteristic of mucinous tumors and caused by mucin content of varying viscosity.

or hemorrhage. If either arose within an endometriotic cyst, an enhancing mass is typically seen within a thick-walled endometrioma containing the typical MR features of chronic hemorrhage.[40]

Brenner tumors represent 2% to 3% of ovarian tumors and consist of nests of transitional cells surrounded by dense collagenous stroma. They are rarely malignant but one third is associated with other ovarian tumors, especially mucinous cystic neoplasms, in the same ovary. Most are small (less than 2 cm), and are solid lesions that display very low signal intensity on T2-weighted images, given their fibrous nature. Mild or moderate enhancement is usually evident. Small cysts are common and focal calcifications may occur.[30]

Overall, 15% to 35% of epithelial ovarian neoplasms are of low malignant potential *(borderline tumor)*. They have proliferating epithelial cells with nuclear abnormalities but without demonstrating stromal invasion. The majority are of serous or mucinous origin. Borderline tumors can spread within the abdomen and pelvis without invasion. They have an excellent prognosis even when extraovarian disease is encountered. As may be expected given the continuum of histology, most epithelial neoplasms in women under 40 years are borderline tumors, while only 10% are borderline in women over 40 years. The 5-year survival is 95%. The tumors can recur with extensive peritoneal involvement. Surprisingly, peritoneal involvement usually shows low-malignant-potential tumor histology.

There are two distinctive categories of epithelial ovarian cancer based on genetic abnormalities and behavior. *Type I* is a more genetically stable, indolent group, with a long continuum from a benign cystic lesion to an intermediary stage of tumor of low malignant potential to low-grade malignancy. This group includes low-grade serous, endometrioid, clear cell, mucinous, and transitional carcinomas. They usually grow slowly and are generally confined to the ovary at diagnosis. Serous tumors in this group tend to be well-differentiated with defined papillary structures and frequent presence of pathognomonic psammoma bodies. Type II highly aggressive cancers have distinct mutations and are nearly always advanced when diagnosed. The lesions are the high-grade serous carcinoma and the undifferentiated carcinoma. Tumors with moderate to poor differentiation show progressive reduction in gland formation with solid sheets of tumor cells. MR indications are as follows:

- Determine the origin of an adnexal mass as uterine, ovarian, or nongenital

- Assess the character of the lesion to determine whether the lesion is likely to be benign (leiomyoma, fibroma, endometrioma, dermoid)

- Characterize a pelvic cystic mass as benign (thin walls and septations and all walls free of nodules), as indeterminate (needing surveillance or a tissue diagnosis), or as a likely malignant ovarian neoplasm (identification of enhancing mural nodules)

MR criteria for a neoplastic lesion are:[28,34]

- Large solid components (Figs. 9.64 and 9.65)

- Irregular, nodular thickening of the wall or a septation with thickness greater than 3 mm

---

***Box 9.7* ESSENTIALS TO REMEMBER**

- The primary MR findings of an ovarian neoplasm are solid (enhancing) components along the ovarian wall, or septations or septal thickening exceeding 3 mm in thickness.

- Unilocular cystic masses with thin walls (less than 3 mm) containing simple fluid are almost always benign.

- Mucinous cystadenomas have locules of variable signal intensity on T2-weighted images because of variable viscosity of the mucin. Locules within a cystic mass containing fluid of differing signal intensity suggest a mucinous neoplasm (the "stained glass sign").

- Benign cystic teratomas vary widely in appearance but can confidently be diagnosed by the presence of fat, indicated by fat-suppression or chemical-shift MR sequences.

- Well-defined ovarian tumors with uniform very low signal intensity on T1- and T2-weighted images and minimal contrast enhancement are likely fibroma-thecomas or Brenner tumors. They may contain small cystic areas and edema, resulting in focal regions of increased signal intensity on T2-weighted images.

- Enhancing solid components within endometriomas suggest degeneration into endometrioid or clear cell carcinomas.

- Bilaterally enlarged defined ovoid masses with a low-signal periphery and central higher signal intensity on T2-weighted images suggest Krukenburg tumors.

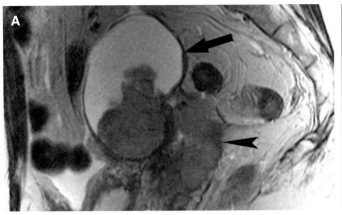

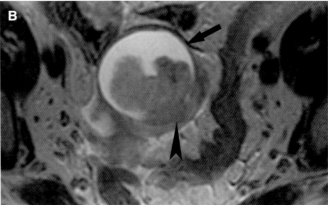

Figure 9.64 *Serous cystadenocarcinoma of the ovary.* Sagittal (**A**) and oblique axial (**B**) T2-weighted images of a 63-year-old woman demonstrate a cystic tumor (*arrows*) with prominent solid components of intermediate signal intensity. Solid tumor (*arrowheads*) extends beyond the ovary and into the cul-de-sac.

- Nodularity, papillary projections, and vegetations projecting from the walls or septations of the mass. These solid components typically enhance (Fig. 9.64).

- Although papillary excrescences within the cyst or along the outside wall may be seen in a benign, borderline, or malignant ovarian mass, an increased relative volume of the solid components favors a higher likelihood of malignancy.

- Additional findings of malignancy include ascites; lymphadenopathy; metastatic disease involving the peritoneum, mesentery, or omentum; and extension of tumor to pelvic sidewalls or other pelvic organs.

- Tumors of low malignant potential are typically large and contain papillary excrescences. The presence of papillary excrescences and enhancing components places the cystic

lesion in a neoplastic category. Solid components may extend internal or external to the cyst wall.

- Malignant implants are common on the surface of the contralateral ovary. These can be differentiated from hemorrhagic ovarian follicles by use of subtraction post-contrast-enhanced images.

- Assess for para-aortic, iliac, and inguinal lymphadenopathy and serosal implants

FALLOPIAN TUBE CARCINOMA

Although much rarer than epithelial ovarian cancer, fallopian tube carcinomas have many clinical similarities with ovarian cancer and risk factors, histologic types, surgical staging, pattern of spread, treatment, and prognosis are comparable. To be considered a primary carcinoma of the fallopian tube, the tumor must be located macroscopically within the tube or its fimbriated end. Primary peritoneal carcinomas, fallopian tube cancers, and serous ovarian cancers are similar and all are now theorized to arise from malignant transformation within the fallopian tube.[13,41,42] Imaging features are similar to those of papillary serous ovarian carcinomas.

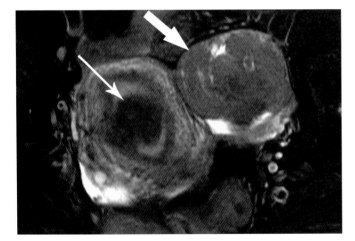

Figure 9.65 *Clear cell ovarian carcinoma arising in an endometrioma.* Fat-saturated coronal T2- weighted image reveals a predominantly solid left adnexal mass (*fat arrow*) with small amount of peripheral fluid. Differential diagnosis would include stromal tumors and acute degeneration of a pedunculated or detached leiomyoma. A submucosal leiomyoma (*skinny arrow*) with its characteristic low signal intensity is also present in the uterine cavity.

VAGINAL CANCER

Primary vaginal cancer is rare. Most vaginal cancers (80%) are squamous cell carcinomas and 10% are adenocarcinomas. The remainder consist of a clear cell variant of adenocarcinoma related to diethylstilbestrol exposure *in utero*, melanoma (very rare), and sarcoma.

Most primary vaginal cancers occur in the upper third of the vagina (Fig. 9.66). Primary vaginal cancers are defined as arising solely from the vagina, with no involvement of the external cervical os or vulva. A vaginal lesion involving the external os of the cervix is classified and treated as cervical cancer per FIGO criteria. A lesion involving both the vulva and vagina is considered a vulvar cancer.

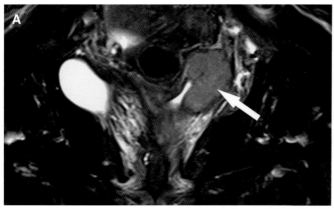

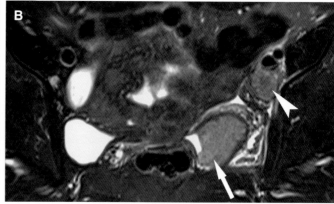

Figure 9.66 *Squamous cell carcinoma of the vagina.* In a patient who had previous radical hysterectomy for benign causes a multilobulated intermediate-signal-intensity solid mass (*arrows*) is seen at the apex of the vaginal vault on T2-weighted coronal (**A**) and axial (**B**) images. The tumor invades the adjacent structures directly and there is metastatic spread to a left external iliac lymph node (*arrowhead*).

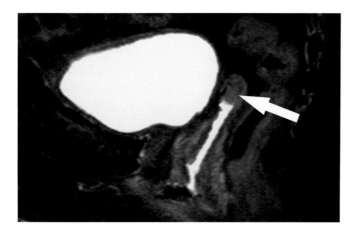

Figure 9.67 *Cervical cancer recurrence in the vagina.* Vaginal gel enables visualization of a solid mass (*arrow*) at the apex of the vaginal vault in a patient who had undergone hysterectomy for cervical carcinoma. The T2-weighted fat-saturated image was obtained in the sagittal plane.

Metastatic vaginal lesions are far more common than primary tumors, accounting for the majority of all vaginal malignancies. These are usually metastatic from cervical or endometrial primaries (Fig. 9.67).

For MR imaging, vaginal gel is very helpful in delineating the extent of vaginal involvement. Vaginal distention provided by the gel better delineates a mass from the normal vaginal wall. The tumor shows with intermediate signal intensity against the vaginal gel. On dynamic post-gadolinium-contrast-enhanced T1-weighted images, the vaginal gel displays low signal intensity and the tumor stands out as a high-signal-intensity lesion. Thin-section axial T1-weighted sequences without fat suppression or with weak fat suppression are particularly helpful in depicting the relationship of small vaginal tumors with the levator ani and urethra.

REFERENCES

1. Brown MA, Mattrey RF, Stamato S, Sirlin CB. MR of the female pelvis using vaginal gel. *AJR Am J Roentgenol.* 2005;185: 1221–1227.

2. Whitten C, deSouza N. Magnetic resonance imaging of uterine malignancies. *Topics in Magnetic Resonance Imaging.* 2006;17: 365–377.

3. Siegelman ES, Outwater EK. Tissue characterization in the female pelvis by means of MR imaging. *Radiology.* 1999;212:5–18.

4. Frei KA, Kinkel K, Bonel HM, et al. Prediction of deep myometrial invasion in patients with endometrial cancer: clinical utility of contrast-enhanced MR imaging—a meta-analysis and bayesian analysis. *Radiology.* 2000;216:444–449.

5. McMahon CJ, Rofsky NM, Pedrosa I. Lymphatic metastases from pelvic tumors: anatomic classification, characterization and staging. *Radiology.* 2010;254:31–46.

6. Morcel K, Camborieux L, Guerrier D. Mayer-Rokitansky-Küster-Hauser (MRKH) syndrome. *Orphanet Journal of Rare Diseases.* 2007. Available at: http://www.OJRD.com/content/2/1/13

7. American Fertility Society. The American Fertility Society classifications of adnexal adhesions, distal tubal occlusion, tubal occlusion secondary to tubal ligation, tubal pregnancies, müllerian anomalies and intrauterine adhesions. *Fertil Steril.* 1988;49:944–955.

8. Falcone T, Gidwani G, Paraiso M, et al. Anatomical variation in the rudimentary horns of a unicornuate uterus: implications for laparoscopic surgery. *Hum Reprod.* 1997;12:263–265.

9. Fedele L, Bianchi S, Agnoli B, et al. Urinary tract anomalies associated with unicornuate uterus. *J Urol.* 1996;155:847–848.

10. Acién P, Acién M, Sánchez-Ferrer M. Complex malformations of the female genital tract. New types and revision of classification. *Hum Reprod.* 2004;19:2377–2384.

11. Smith NA, Laufer MR. Obstructed hemivagina and ipsilateral renal anomaly (OHVIRA) syndrome: management and follow-up. *Fertil Steril.* 2007;87:918–922.

12. Deffarges JV, Haddad B, Musset R, Paniel BJ. Utero-vaginal anastomosis in women with uterine cervix atresia: long-term follow-up and reproductive performance. A study of 18 cases. *Hum Reprod.* 2001;16: 1722–1725.

13. Robboy SJ, Bentley RC, Russell P, et al. *Robboy's Pathology of the Female Reproductive Tract.* Edinburgh: Churchill-Livingstone/Elsevier, 2008.

14. D'Angelo E, Prat J. Uterine sarcomas: A review. *Gynecol Oncol.* 2010;116:131–139.

15. Tamai K, Togashi K, Ito T, et al. MR imaging findings of adenomyosis: correlation with histopathologic features and diagnostic pitfalls. *Radiographics.* 2005;25:21–40.

16. Grasel RP, Outwater EK, Siegelman ES, et al. Endometrial polyps: MR imaging features and distinction from endometrial carcinoma. *Radiology.* 2000;214:47–52.

17. Wolfman DJ, Ascher SM. Magnetic resonance imaging of benign uterine pathology. *Top Magn Reson Imaging.* 2006;17: 399–407.

18. Faratian D, Stillie A, Busby-Earle RM et al. A review of the pathology and management of uterine papillary serous carcinoma and correlation with outcome. *Int J Gynecol Cancer*. 2006;16:972–978.

19. McCluggage WG. Malignant biphasic uterine tumours: carcinosarcomas or metaplastic carcinomas? *J Clin Pathol*. 2002;55:321–325.

20. Rechichi G, Galimberti S, Signorelli M, et al. Myometrial invasion in endometrial cancer: diagnostic performance of diffusion-weighted MR imaging at 1.5-T. *Eur Radiol*. 2010;20:754–762.

21. Frei KA, Kinkel K. Staging endometrial cancer: role of magnetic resonance imaging. *J Magn Reson Imaging*. 2001;13:850–855.

22. Manfredi R, Mirk P, Maresca G, et al. Local-regional staging of endometrial carcinoma: role of MR in surgical planning. *Radiology*. 2004;231:372–378.

23. Torricelli P, Ferraresi S, Fiocchi F, et al. 3-T MRI in the preoperative evaluation of depth of myometrial infiltration in endometrial cancer. *AJR Am J Roentgenol*. 2008;190:489–495.

24. Saksouk FA, Johnson SC. Recognition of the ovaries and ovarian origin of pelvic masses with CT. *Radiographics*. 2004;24: S133–S146.

25. Utsunomiya D, Notsute S, Hayashida Y, et al. Endometrial carcinoma in adenomyosis: assessment of myometrial invasion on T2-weighted spin-echo and gadolinium-enhanced T1-weighted images. *AJR Am J Roentgenol*. 2004;182:399–404.

26. Olawaiye A, Del Carmen M, Tambouret R, et al. Abdominal radical trachelectomy: Success and pitfalls in a general gynecologic oncology practice. *Gynecol Oncol*. 2009;112:506–510.

27. Okamoto Y, Tanaka YO, Nishida M, et al. MR imaging of the uterine cervix: imaging-pathologic correlation. *Radiographics*. 2003;23: 425–445.

28. Hricak H, Gatsonis C, Coakeley FV, et al. Early invasive cervical cancer: CT and MR imaging preoperative evaluation-ACRIN/GOG comparitive study of diagnostic performance and interobserver variability. *Radiology*. 2007;245:491–498.

29. Levine D, Brown DL, Andreotti RF, et al. Management of asymptomatic ovarian and other adnexal cysts imaged at US. *Radiology*. 2010;256:943–954.

30. Imaoka I, Wada A, Kaji Y, et al. Developing an MR strategy for diagnosis of ovarian masses. *Radiographics*. 2006;26:1431–1448.

31. Lim HK, Cho JY, Kim SH. Sclerotherapy of peritoneal inclusion cysts: a long-term evaluation study. *Abdom Imaging*. 2010;35: 431–436.

32. Kobayashi H, Sumimoto K, Kitanaka T, et al. Ovarian endometrioma—risks factors of ovarian cancer development. *Eur J Obstet Gynecol Reprod Biol*. 2008;138:187–193.

33. Takeuchi M, Matsuzaki K, Uehara J, et al. Malignant transformation of pelvic endometriosis: MR imaging findings and pathologic correlation. *Radiographics*. 2006;26:407–417.

34. Machida S, Matsubara S, Ohwada M, et al. Decidualization of ovarian endometriosis during pregnancy mimicking malignancy: report of three cases with a literature review. *Gynecol Obstet Invest*. 2008;66:241–247.

35. Rha SE, Byun JY, Jung SE, et al. Atypical CT and MRI manifestations of mature ovarian cystic teratomas. *AJR Am J Roentgenol*. 2004;183:743–750.

36. Park SB, Kim JK, Kim KR, Cho KS. Imaging findings of complications and unusual manifestations of ovarian teratomas. *Radiographics*. 2008; 28:969–983.

37. Brown LB, Qou KH, Tempany CM, et al. Primary versus secondary ovarian malignancy: imaging findings of adnexal masses in the Radiology Diagnostic Oncology Group Study. *Radiology*. 2001;219: 213–218.

38. Ha HK, Baek SY, Kim SH, et al. Krukenberg's tumor of the ovary: MR imaging features. *AJR Am J Roentgenol*. 1995;164:1435–1439.

39. Jung SE, Lee JM, Rha SE, et al. CT and MR imaging of ovarian tumors with emphasis on differential diagnosis. *Radiographics*. 2002;22:1305–1325.

40. Matsuoka Y, Ohtomo K, Araki T, et al. MR imaging of clear cell carcinoma of the ovary. *Eur Radiol*. 2001;11:946–951.

41. Crum CP, Drapkin R, Miron A, et al. The distal fallopian tube: a new model for pelvic serous carcinogenesis. *Curr Opin Obstet Gynecol*. 2007;19:3–9.

42. Kurman RJ, Shih I. The origin and pathogenesis of epithelial ovarian cancer: a proposed unifying theory. *Am J Surg Pathol*. 2010;34: 433–443.

10.

CARDIAC MR IMAGING

Patrick T. Norton, MD

In the past decade, rapid and successive advances in MR hardware and sequence development have led to MRI becoming a robust modality for imaging cardiac pathology. Initially used as a complement to other imaging modalities, cardiac MR (CMR) has now become the first step in the diagnosis of many disease processes of the heart. It is an effective tool for the evaluation of both acquired and congenital heart disease, providing the ability to evaluate abnormalities of both anatomy and physiology in one setting.

MAGNETIC RESONANCE IMAGING TECHNIQUE

Due to the technical demands of imaging a moving structure, the equipment requirements to perform an adequate CMR examination are greater than those for imaging static structures. A 1.5T imaging system with strong, fast gradients is currently the state-of-the-art system for CMR. A dedicated cardiac multi-element phased-array coil provides optimal image quality and permits parallel imaging, which reduces imaging time to reasonable breath-hold durations. The imaging system must also have an integrated cardiac gating system to compensate for cardiac motion by coordinating the acquisition of *k*-space data to the electrocardiogram (ECG) signal.

Basic sequences. A variety of different pulse sequences have been tailored for CMR depending on the goal of imaging. Broadly, these can be broken down into black-blood and bright-blood techniques. Spin-echo sequences used for cardiac imaging are typically black-blood and gradient-echo sequences are typically bright-blood techniques.

Spin-echo sequences often have longer acquisition times than gradient-echo images. T1-weighted spin-echo imaging is currently used for creating high-resolution anatomic images, whereas T2-weighted spin-echo imaging is used for assessing myocardial edema and identifying cystic structures. Compared to gradient-echo images, spin-echo images tend to be less sensitive to susceptibility artifacts induced by metallic structures, which can be beneficial, particularly when imaging the

mediastinum in a patient who had sternal wires placed at a prior sternotomy.

Gradient-echo imaging has relatively fast acquisition times and is the workhorse of cardiac imaging due to its versatility. Gradient-echo imaging, in its different forms, can be employed for the assessment of ventricular function, blood velocity and flow measurements, assessment of valvular disease, myocardial perfusion, delayed contrast-enhanced imaging, and magnetic resonance angiography (MRA).

Steady-state free precession (SSFP) is an imaging sequence that has become the backbone of cardiac cine imaging (in which a series of images is played as a movie) due to its fast acquisition and excellent contrast between myocardium and blood pool, making it well suited for the evaluation of wall motion and volumetric measurements (Fig. 10.1). Acquisitions are performed during a breath hold, and cine loops can be produced providing a temporal resolution of 40 ms per cardiac phase. In patients who cannot hold their breath for an appropriate duration or who have significant cardiac arrhythmias, real-time SSFP can be performed at lower spatial and temporal resolution without ECG gating. The drawback of SSFP sequences is that they are dependent on a homogenous magnetic field, creating difficulties when using the sequence at higher field strength, such as at 3T.

Tagged cine imaging is a variation of the gradient-echo cine sequence in which tissue is nulled in either parallel lines or a grid pattern at the beginning of each heart cycle. The tag lines move with the myocardium over the heart cycle, providing a method for visual assessment of tissue displacement and deformation. This sequence is useful for detecting regional abnormalities in myocardial contraction and for determining if two adjacent tissues are adherent or move independent of each other.

Inversion-recovery sequences are used to null the signal of a target tissue to accentuate surrounding pathology, which is bright. This technique is employed for late gadolinium contrast-enhanced imaging and T2-weighted short-tau inversion-recovery (STIR) imaging. In late gadolinium contrast enhanced imaging, the signal from the myocardium is nulled by selecting an inversion time (TI) such that the longitudinal magnetization

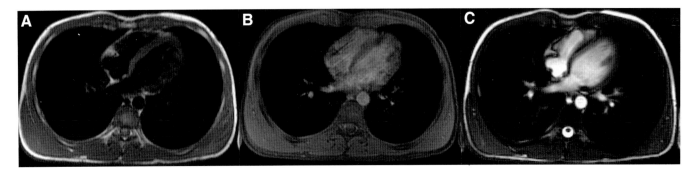

Figure 10.1 *Cardiac sequences.* Axial spin-echo (**A**), gradient-echo (**B**), and steady-state free precession (**C**) images of the heart. In cardiac imaging, spin-echo sequences create static imaging with a dark blood pool. Gradient-echo sequences can be used to acquire static images or cines. Steady-state free-precession (SSFP) is the primary sequence used for functional cine imaging as it provides high contrast between the blood pool and the myocardium.

of normal myocardium is zero at the time of readout. The desired TI required for late gadolinum enhanced imaging depends on multiple factors, including the design of the sequence, time of imaging after injection of gadolinium contrast media, and patient-specific clearance characteristics of contrast material. The appropriate TI is determined using a TI scout sequence in which each image in the series has a progressively larger TI (Fig. 10.2). Using a typical gradient-echo inversion-recovery technique, a TI of 300 to 320 ms for nulling the signal of the myocardium is expected when imaging 12 to 15 minutes after injection of gadolinium contrast media. An alternative to this approach is the semi-automated phase-sensitive

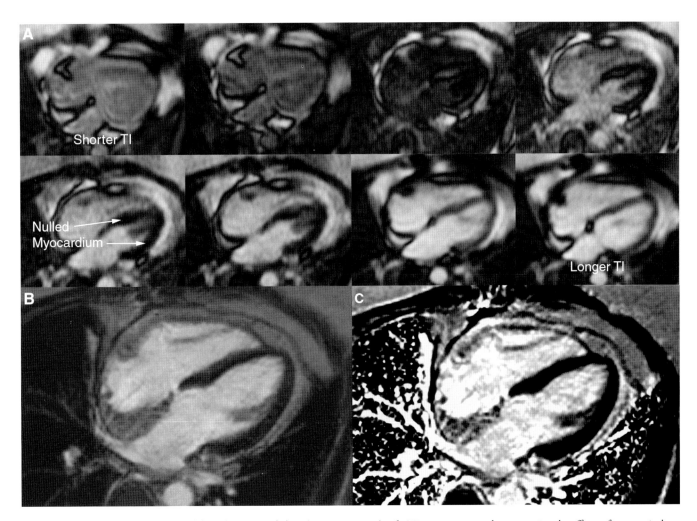

Figure 10.2 *Late gadolinium-enhanced (LGE) imaging.* (**A**) Eight-image example of a TI scout sequence demonstrating the effects of progressively longer inversion times (TI). The first TI in which the myocardium is nulled is selected for high-resolution imaging. (**B**) High-resolution inversion-recovery gradient-echo image of normal myocardium with proper nulling. (**C**) Phase-sensitive inversion recovery (PSIR) is performed without the manual selection of an inversion time. Note the unique appearance of the lung parenchyma that is characteristic in phase-reconstructed images.

inversion-recovery (PSIR) technique, which does not require a pre-selected TI value.

Cardiac gating. The fundamental challenge of CMR is preventing imaging artifacts caused by cardiac motion. This is overcome using cardiac gating, in which the acquisition of the *k*-space data is synchronized to the ECG. Static ECG-gated images are obtained by acquiring data only during a specified portion of the cardiac cycle, typically during diastole when the heart is not moving. The R wave of the ECG is used as a reference point, with data acquisition being initiated following a specified delay after the R wave. Images are created from data collected over a series of heartbeats (Fig. 10.3A).

In cine imaging, multiple images are obtained throughout the cardiac cycle and are displayed as a short looped movie. Using ECG-gated segmented imaging, the *k* space of each image is built up over multiple heartbeats and synchronized to the R-wave trigger (Fig. 10.3B). Cine loops are typically composed of 10 to 25 images (or views) and require breath-hold durations of 10 to 20 seconds, depending on the sequence and temporal resolution required. In functional imaging, as the heart rate increases, the temporal resolution needs to increase to allow accurate imaging at end-systole. As with all gated imaging, cines are susceptible to variability in the heart rate, such as occurs with arrhythmias, which results in artifacts (blurring) in the images.

Cardiac gating requires placement of ECG leads over the patient's left chest, using either a three- or four-lead configuration. The goal of lead placement is to maximize the R wave while minimizing the T wave, as a common obstacle to ECG gating is triggering off an enlarged T wave. ECG gating may be impaired in people with low ECG signals, which can occur in patients with chronic obstructive pulmonary disease (COPD),

due to increase in the anteroposterior (AP) diameter of the chest, or in patients with large pericardial effusions. Occasionally, placing the ECG leads on the posterior side of the patient's thorax can increase the signal in such cases. The *magnetohydrodynamic effect* is a physical property that compromises ECG gating and occurs when ions in the flowing blood, particularly the thoracic aorta, are transported through a magnetic field and induce an electric charge that distorts the ECG in a time-varying way. This distortion can be overcome using vectorcardiogram gating (VCG), which differentiates the electrical signal of flowing blood from the electrical activity of the heart. In cases where gating is severely limited by poor ECG signal, pulse oximetry gating can be used to synchronize imaging to the systolic upstroke of the pulse. However, this is rarely used as real-time imaging can be performed on state-of-the-art MR systems and is the technique of choice when ECG gating is severely limited.

Contrast media. In the United States the use of gadolinium contrast media for CMR is off-label. However, gadolinium chelates are an integral component of the CMR examination and are used for myocardial perfusion imaging, tissue characterization, and MRA. Extracellular gadolinium contrast media, the most common type of agent, contains small molecules that diffuse freely between the blood pool and the extracellular space. Dosing of contrast media depends on the application. A single dose refers to 0.1 mmol/kg, and using the typical preparation of gadolinium contrast agents (0.5 mmol/cc) this results in 0.2 cc/kg of contrast media. Single dosing (0.2 cc/kg) is used for qualitative myocardial perfusion imaging. Single to double dosing (0.2 to 0.4 cc/kg) is used for LGE imaging. Single-dose administration is usually sufficient for MRA of the thoracic aorta and its branches.

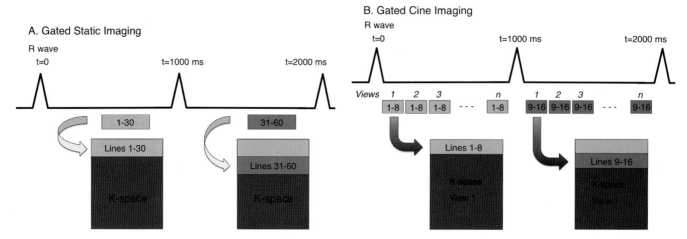

Figure 10.3 *Cardiac gating.* (**A**) Electrocardiogram (ECG)-gated static imaging produces a single image for each breath hold by building up *k* space over multiple heartbeats. The acquisition period (rectangular box under the ECG) can be positioned as desired within the R–R interval (beginning of R wave to next R wave) but most often is performed in mid-diastole, prior to atrial contraction, when the heart is quiescent. In this example, the R–R interval is 1,000 ms, equating to a heart rate of 60 bpm. (**B**) ECG-gated cine imaging produces a series of multiple images (views) by building up *k* space for each view over multiple heartbeats. The total number of views is represented by *n*, which is typically 10 to 25. In this example, the first eight lines of *k* space for each view are acquired during the first heartbeat. The next eight lines are acquired for each view in the next heartbeat, continuing in this way until all lines of *k* space are acquired for each view. In the diagram, the temporal resolution of the cine is inversely proportional to the length of the box (time during each R–R interval when data are acquired) for each view. Increased temporal resolution is achieved by increasing the number of views, which requires acquisition of fewer lines of *k* space for each view during a given heartbeat, imaging over more heartbeats, and a longer breath hold.

Late gadolinium enhanced imaging is used in the detection of myocardial necrosis, fibrosis, and infiltrative processes. Myocardial pathology alters the size of the extracellular space and the diffusion kinetics of MR contrast media. In the case of normal myocardium, there is very little extracellular volume relative to the intracellular volume of the densely packed myocytes, and MR contrast media concentrations between blood pool and extracellular space equilibrate rapidly. After an acute myocardial infarction, lysis of myocytes results in an increase of the extracellular spaces, into which gadolinium contrast media freely diffuses. At late gadolinium enhanced imaging, which is performed 12 to 15 minutes after injection MR contrast media remains in the abnormal extracellular spaces due to relatively slow diffusion resulting from cellular injury. Similarly, myocardial scar shows late gadolinium enhancement due to increased extracellular space between the collagen fibers combined with slower diffusion kinetics than normal myocardium. Late gadolinium enhancement is also present in non-ischemic injuries including infiltrative disorders and cardiomyopathies. The pattern of late gadolinium enhancement is used to differentiate between different pathologic conditions, as will be discussed later.

Coronary artery imaging. Imaging of the coronary arteries is technically difficult due to the small size of the vessels. As a result, long acquisition times are required to produce adequate signal for high-resolution imaging. This can be achieved using single-slice spin-echo or gradient-echo imaging during a breath hold. However, this method requires the anatomy of interest to lie within a single plane, which is not ideal for imaging the entire coronary vasculature. Due to this limitation, 3D acquisition techniques were developed, which require longer acquisition times necessitating combined respiratory and cardiac gated techniques for free-breathing imaging. With these combined techniques, images are obtained only while the diaphragm is located within a specified range, typically at end-expiration, and during mid-diastole when heart motion is minimal. Both unenhanced and enhanced methods can be performed with the 3D techniques. New rapid techniques are being developed that will allow acquisition of a full 3D volume in a single breath hold.

NORMAL ANATOMY

The heart is situated in the mediastinum of the thorax, contained by the fibrous pericardium, and is composed of four chambers: right atrium (RA), right ventricle (RV), left atrium (LA), and left ventricle (LV).

Right atrium Deoxygenated blood is delivered to the RA via the superior vena cava (SVC) and the inferior vena cava (IVC). The eustachian valve, more of a tissue flap than a true valve, limits reflux of blood into the IVC and is located at the IVC junction with the RA. When this tissue has a trabeculated appearance, it is called a *Chiari network*. The RA also receives deoxygenated blood from the coronary circulation via the coronary sinus, which also has a tissue flap covering its ostium, referred to as the thebesian valve. The RA is derived from tissue of two distinct embryologic origins: trabeculated

tissue anteriorly and smooth tissue posteriorly. The interface between these two tissues forms the crista terminalis and runs from the SVC to IVC ostia; it is notable because it can be mistaken for a mass when prominent and can be a nidus for thrombus formation. The right atrial appendage arises from the trabeculated portion of the RA, just anterior to the insertion of the SVC.

Right ventricle Blood flows from the RA through the tricuspid valve into the RV. The RV is usually smaller and more trabeculated than the LV. A distinguishing characteristic of the RV is the presence of the moderator band, which is present 75% of the time. This muscular band extends from the apical free wall to the intraventricular septum. Blood leaves the RV via the right ventricular outflow tract (RVOT), through the pulmonic valve, and into the pulmonary artery. The pulmonary valve, a tricuspid valve, separates the RVOT from the pulmonary artery. The pulmonary artery, a great vessel of the heart, bifurcates within the pericardium, delivering blood to left and right lungs.

Left atrium. After passing through the pulmonary capillaries, oxygenated blood returns to the heart via four pulmonary veins inserting on the LA. There is some normal variability in the configuration of these veins, but typically there are bilateral, superior and inferior pulmonary veins. The most common variation is the presence of a right middle pulmonary vein.

Left ventricle. During diastole, blood passes from the LA into the LV through the mitral valve. The mitral valve is a bicuspid valve composed of an anterior and a posterior leaflet. The LV is responsible for generating pressures required to propel the blood through the systemic circulation. Thus, the myocardium of the LV is the thickest within the heart and is very compacted, with fewer trabeculations than the RV. During systole, the mitral valve closes and the blood of the LV is forced through the left ventricular outflow tract (LVOT) and subsequently through the tricuspid aortic valve into the ascending aorta. The coronary arteries arise from the sinuses of the aortic root, which are named from their corresponding artery (e.g., left, right, non-coronary).

Aorta. The tubular portion of the ascending aorta begins just above the sinuses and continues to the level of the supra-aortic branch vessels. The normal configuration of the arch (left arch) is anterior and to the left of the trachea with supra-aortic branches arising from proximal to distal as follows: brachiocephalic (innominate) artery in the first position, left common carotid artery in the second position, and left subclavian artery in the third position. The most common variation is a common brachiocephalic trunk, in which the brachiocephalic artery and right common carotid artery arise from a common origin (so-called "bovine arch"). The descending aorta courses inferiorly through the posterior mediastinum, passing posterior to the posterior wall of the LA.

Coronary artery anatomy and perfusion territories The coronary arteries arise from sinuses of Valsalva, just superior to the aortic valve (Fig. 10.4). The right coronary artery arises from the right sinus of Valsalva and descends anteriorly in the right atrioventricular groove, spawning the acute marginal branches that supply the RV myocardium. In the case of right

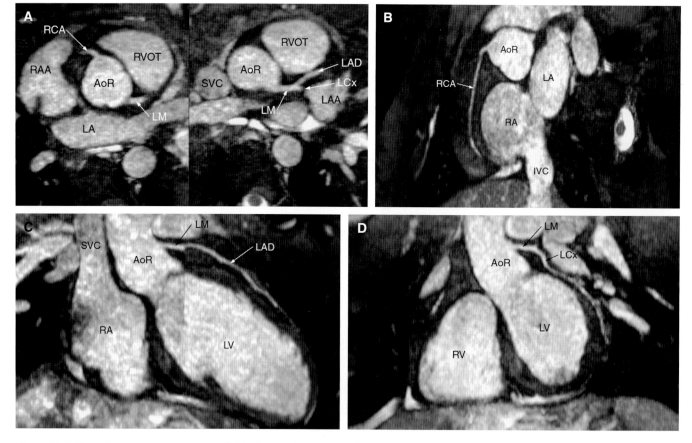

Figure 10.4 *Normal coronary artery anatomy.* (**A**) Left image demonstrates the origin of the right coronary artery (*RCA*) arising anteriorly from the right sinus of Valsalva and the left main (*LM*) coronary artery arising from the left sinus of Valsalva. Right image shows the bifurcation of the LM into left anterior descending (*LAD*) and left circumflex (*LCx*) coronary arteries. (**B**) The *RCA* descends in the right atrioventricular (*AV*) groove anteriorly supplying the right ventricle and the inferior wall of the left ventricle via the posterior descending artery (PDA), which is not shown. (**C**) The LAD courses in the anterior interventricular groove to the apex of the heart, supplying the anterior wall of the left ventricle. (**D**) The LCx courses in the left atrioventricular grove, under the left atrial appendage (*LAA*) proximally, supplying the lateral wall of the left ventricle. *AoR*, aortic root; *LA*, left atrium; *LV*, left ventricle; *RA*, right atrium; *RAA*, right atrial appendage; *RV*, right ventricle; *RVOT*, right ventricular outflow tract; *SVC*, superior vena cava; *IVC*, inferior vena cava.

coronary dominance (90% of people), the right coronary artery branches into posterior lateral branches and the posterior descending artery that travels in the inferior interventricular groove. The posterior descending artery supplies blood to the majority of the inferior wall of the LV. The left main coronary artery arises from the left sinus of Valsalva and courses in a horizontal fashion posterior to the RVOT. It divides to become the left anterior descending artery and the left circumflex artery. The left anterior descending artery courses in the anterior interventricular groove and supplies the anterior wall, septum and the apex of the LV. The left circumflex artery descends in the left atrioventricular groove, supplying the lateral wall of the LV (Fig. 10.5).

Basic imaging planes. The ability to image in any desired plane makes MR particularly suited for cardiac examination, where standard planes are obliqued relative to transverse, coronal, and sagittal planes. Imaging typically begins with a set of scout images through the heart that includes transverse imaging of the LV (Fig. 10.6). The two-chamber long-axis view is composed by imaging in a plane perpendicular to the transverse plane and is aligned along the LV long axis, a line passing through the center of the mitral valve and LV apex. The horizontal long-axis (four-chamber) view is created from a plane perpendicular to the two-chamber long-axis view that is oriented to intersect the bottom third of the mitral valve and the LV apex. The short-axis views are oriented perpendicular to the four-chamber plane and perpendicular to the long axis of the LV. A three-chamber view is in the plane of the long axis of the LV and LVOT. The easiest way to obtain this view is from a coronal view that is in the plane of the aortic valve. An imaging plane is then prescribed perpendicular to the coronal plane and oriented perpendicular to the aortic valve annulus (Fig. 10.7). Alternatively, a three-chamber view can be created from a plane perpendicular to the short-axis plane and the angle between the four-chamber and two-chamber long-axis views (Fig. 10.8).

ASSESSMENT OF CARDIAC FUNCTION

The ability of CMR to provide accurate, precise, and reproducible measurement of ventricular volumes, global and region

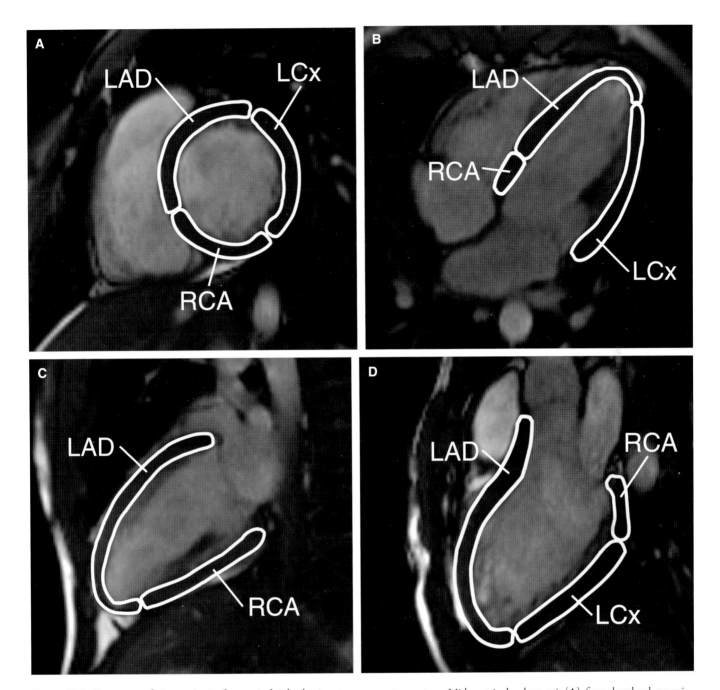

Figure 10.5 *Coronary perfusion territories for a typical right-dominant coronary artery system.* Mid-ventricular short-axis (**A**), four-chamber long-axis (**B**), two-chamber long-axis (**C**) and three-chamber long-axis (**D**) views delineating typical coronary artery perfusion territories for right coronary artery (*RCA*) and left anterior descending (*LAD*) and left circumflex (*LCx*) coronary arteries. Note that there can be considerable variability of territories, particularly how much the distal extent of the LAD wraps around the apex of the heart.

function, and myocardial mass makes it now considered the reference standard for these measurements. CMR is used routinely in pathologic states where measurements are critical for monitoring disease progress.

Regional assessment of function. Regional ventricular function is most commonly assessed qualitatively using a combination of long- and short-axis views. Function is characterized as normal, hypokinetic, akinetic, or dyskinetic; making this distinction requires excellent delineation of the myocardium from adjacent structures. Assessment should be directed at wall thickening and not just movement of the endocardial border toward the center of the ventricle, as abnormal myocardium can be pulled inward by surrounding normal myocardium, giving the appearance of normal function. Normal segments of myocardium should thicken at least 30% between end-diastole to end-systole; for instance, if the wall is 10 mm at end-diastole, then it should be at least 13 mm at end-systole. Hypokinetic segments demonstrate thickening that is less than the normal 30%, whereas akinetic segments demonstrate no perceivable thickening. Dyskinetic segments do not thicken, demonstrate movement away from the center of the ventricle during systole, and can be aneurysmal (Fig. 10.9).

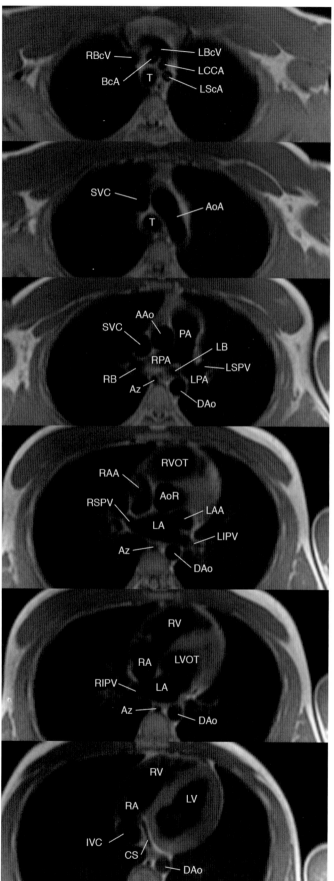

A pitfall of characterizing regional wall-motion abnormalities is characterizing a dyssynchronous segment as dyskinetic. Dyssynchronous segments typically contract at a later time in the cardiac cycle compared to normal segments, due to an abnormality in electrical conduction of the myocardium. This results in the appearance of movement away from the center of the ventricle while the normal myocardium is contracting, similar to dyskinesis. However, dyssynchronous segments eventually thicken, in contradistinction to dyskinetic segments.

Measurement of cardiac indices. Ventricular indices, including end-diastolic volume (EDV), end-systolic volume (ESV), stroke volume (SV), and ejection fraction (EF), can accurately and reproducibly be calculated from standard SSFP cine imaging. LV volumes are calculated from adjacent short-axis cines covering the entire ventricle. For EDV, a tracing is made around the endocardial border at end-diastole for each slice, including the papillary muscle and trabeculation as part of the blood pool by convention. End-diastole is measured at the largest ventricular volume, which is usually the first image in the series, occurring at the initiation of the R wave. The EDV of the slice is obtained by multiplying the area of the end-diastolic endocardial tracing by slice spacing. The volume of each slice is then added together to obtain the overall EDV of the LV. The same procedure is performed at end-systole to calculate ESV. From these measurements, EF and SV can be calculated according to the following equations:

$$SV = EDV - ESV$$

$$EF = SV/EDV$$

For the RV, imaging is performed in the transverse (axial) plane from the base of the RV to the top of the RVOT, as measurement in this plane has been shown to be more reproducible.

The method of disc summation, referred to as "Simpson's Rule", can also be used to measure myocardial mass by measuring the area of myocardium in each slice (area defined by the epicardial tracing minus the area defined by the endocardial tracing), multiplying it by the slice spacing, and summing the volume of each slice. The total myocardial volume is multiplied by the density of myocardium (1.06 g/cc) to achieve myocardial mass.

Figure 10.6 *Axial plane anatomy of the mediastinum. AAo*, ascending aorta; *AoA*, aortic arch; *AoR*, aortic root; *Az*, azygos vein; *BcA*, brachiocephalic artery; *CS*, coronary sinus; *DAo*, descending aorta; *IVC*, inferior vena cava; *LA*, left atrium; *LAA*, left atrial appendage; *LB*, left mainstem bronchus; *LBcV*, left brachiocephalic vein; *LCCA*, left common carotid artery; *LPA*, left pulmonary artery; *LScA*, left subclavian artery; *LIPV*, left inferior pulmonary vein; *LSPV*, left superior pulmonary vein; *LV*, left ventricle; *LVOT*, left ventricular outflow tract; *PA*, main pulmonary artery; *RA*, right atrium; *RAA*, right atrial appendage; *RB*, right mainstem bronchus; *RBcV*, right brachiocephalic vein; *RPA*, right pulmonary artery; *RIPV*, right inferior pulmonary vein; *RSPV*, right superior pulmonary vein; *RV*, right ventricle; *SVC*, superior vena cava; *T*, trachea.

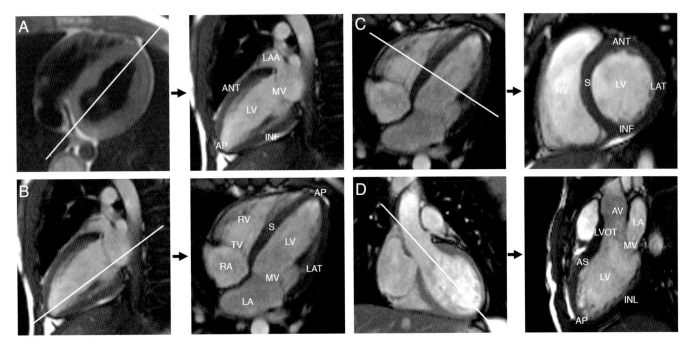

Figure 10.7 *Image acquisition, cardiac anatomy, and basic imaging planes.* (**A**) Vertical long-axis (two-chamber) view derived from the axial scout image. (**B**) Horizontal long-axis (four-chamber) view derived from the vertical long-axis view. (**C**) Short-axis view derived from the horizontal long-axis view. (**D**) Three-chamber view derived from a coronal scout image. *White lines* in figure represent perpendicular intersection of resultant plane. *LV*, left ventricle; *AP*, apex; *ANT*, anterior wall; *LAT*, lateral wall; *INF*, inferior wall; *S*, septal wall; *AS*, anteroseptal wall; *INL*, inferolateral wall; *LA*, left atrium; *LAA*, left atrial appendage; *LVOT*, left ventricular outflow tract; *RA*, right atrium; *RV*, right ventricle; *AV*, aortic valve; *MV*, mitral valve; *TV*, tricuspid valve.

Figure 10.8 *Relationship of basic imaging planes.* The horizontal long-axis view (right upper), three-chamber view (right lower), and vertical long-axis view (left lower) are common to the long axis of the left ventricle and can be created from a plane (*white lines*) perpendicular to the short axis plane (left upper).

ISCHEMIC HEART DISEASE

Heart disease is the most common cause of death in the United States, and ischemic heart disease accounts for approximately two thirds of all deaths related to heart disease. Ischemic heart disease has a variety of clinical presentations, including asymptomatic, stable angina, and sudden death, a feared consequence that can represent the initial presentation of the disease. Due to its widespread prevalence, ischemic heart disease results in a significant cost to health-care systems of the Western world. Currently, cardiac MRI offers the most complete evaluation of ischemic heart disease with one modality, which includes evaluation of global as well as regional cardiac function, detection of acute and chronic infarcts, determination of areas of ischemia and viability in chronic disease, and delineation of areas at risk and microvascular obstruction in acute myocardial infarction.[1]

Pathophysiology of ischemic heart disease. Myocardial ischemia refers to insufficient delivery of oxygen to the myocardium, which can occur as a result of partial or total occlusion of a coronary artery. Ischemia leads to dysfunction of the myocardium and, if it is severe and sustained, results in infarction of the myocardium. Myocardial infarction typically is initiated by rupture of an unstable coronary atherosclerotic plaque, leading to abrupt arterial occlusion. The tissue perfused by the obstructed coronary artery experiences varying degrees of ischemia based on location, with the subendocardium being most vulnerable to ischemia. After 15 minutes of total occlusion of coronary blood flow, cellular necrosis will

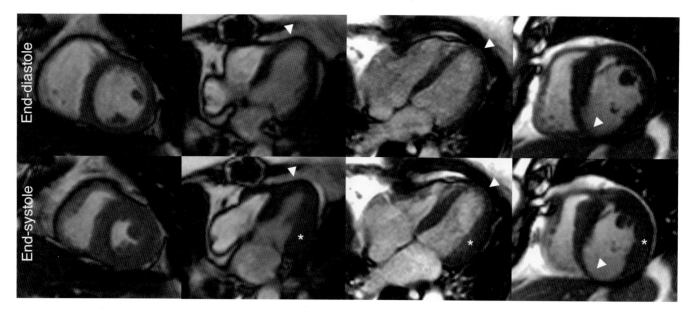

Figure 10.9 *Descriptors of regional wall motion.* **First column:** Normal wall motion. There is uniform thickening, greater than 30%, of the ventricular wall during systole. **Second column:** Hypokinesis. Reduced myocardial thickening (*arrowhead*) is seen at the left ventricular apex compared to the normal segment (*). **Third column:** Akinesis. No myocardial thickening (*arrowhead*) at the ventricular apex is evident between end-diastole and end-systole. Normal thickening occurs in the lateral wall (*). **Fourth column:** Dyskinesis. The dyskinetic wall (*arrowhead*) moves outward during systole. Normal thickening is present in the lateral wall (*).

expand from the subendocardium to the subepicardium in the so-called wave front of injury, with the greatest damage to the subendocardium.

Patients experiencing ischemia may have symptoms of pressure, squeezing, or pain in the chest. This pain may radiate to the arms or the jaw. Pain that does not resolve is suggestive of infarction. Additional symptoms of ischemia/infarction include light-headedness, dyspnea, sweating, and nausea.

After an acute ischemic event, reperfusion may occur spontaneously or secondary to intervention. The goal of current therapeutic strategies is rapid restoration of coronary flow using mechanical or thrombolytic methods in an effort to salvage the ischemic myocardium and prevent adverse LV remodeling. Following reperfusion, the myocardium responds depending on the type of injury: cells in the periphery of the "area at risk" have experienced hypoxia but can be improved by reperfusion (salvage), and the deeper core of myocardium has experienced sustained ischemia leading to cellular necrosis. This core of infarct is further subdivided into areas of solely myocyte necrosis and areas of more severe damage with necrosis of both myocytes and blood vessels, termed microvascular obstruction, where reperfusion is impossible. Over time, the heart replaces the necrotic myocytes with fibrotic tissue, leading to increased hemodynamic load on the normal myocardium and ultimately to adverse LV remodeling—progressive ventricular dilatation and dysfunction. Additionally, this scar tissue becomes a potential substrate for the development and propagation of fatal cardiac arrhythmias. The presence of microvascular obstruction is an independent predictor of death and adverse LV remodeling, with more microvascular obstruction resulting in worse prognosis.

Acute ischemia leads to immediate myocardial contractile dysfunction that may be reversible if reperfusion occurs rapidly. However, after the restoration of the blood flow, the myocardium can remain dysfunctional for days to weeks before normalization; this is referred to as *stunned myocardium*. Return of the myocardium to normal contractile function can be accelerated with the administration of inotropes. In the case of less severe, longstanding ischemia, the myocytes respond by downregulating energy-consumptive processes and become dysfunctional. This process results in a protective state referred to as *hibernating myocardium*, which can be reversed with revascularization.

Detection of coronary artery disease. The presence of coronary artery disease (CAD) can be assessed through either morphologic interrogation of the coronary arteries or ischemia testing.

Coronary artery imaging with MRI has been extensively researched and results have been promising; however, the modality has not yet been integrated into the routine cardiac examination due to the relatively long time that it takes to acquire the images. Additionally, the rapid advancement of coronary CT angiography offers a relatively easy noninvasive assessment of the coronaries, albeit at the added cost of radiation exposure. Nevertheless, ischemia testing combined with late gadolinium contrast enhancement has become the mainstay of detection of CAD with MRI.

Due to the autoregulatory function of the coronary arteries, a stenosis as great as 85% may not produce any symptoms at rest. Therefore, ischemia testing is performed during the stressed state, when myocardial oxygen demand and/or coronary blood flow is significantly increased by the administration of pharmacologic agents. A stenosis of about 45% becomes critical when the coronary blood flow is raised to four times above the resting state.

There are two approaches to functionally determine the presence of significant coronary artery stenosis with MRI: wall-motion analysis during the administration of an inotropic stress agent (e.g., dobutamine) or perfusion analysis during administration of a vasodilator (e.g., adenosine). Both methods require continuous physiologic monitoring and the ability to perform cardiovascular resuscitation at the scanner should an emergency occur.

During dobutamine stress MR, the contractility of the heart is increased, which in turn increases oxygen demand and increases coronary blood flow. If a stenosis is present in a coronary artery, the myocardial oxygen demand outstrips oxygen delivery and the underperfused myocardium becomes dysfunctional. Cine MR is acquired during the intravenous administration of increasing rates of continuous dobutamine infusion. An abnormality is detected when a wall segment demonstrates decreased function relative to other wall segments at increasing levels of stress. To detect CAD with a high level of sensitivity and reproducibility, the defined endpoint of submaximal stress must be achieved. Submaximal stress is defined as 85% of a patient age-predicted maximal heart rate, as below:

Target heart rate (bpm) = 0.85 (220 – age [in years])

A commonly used dobutamine stress MR protocol begins with 10 µg/kg body weight dobutamine infusion for 3 minutes; the dosage is increased by 10 µg/kg body weight every 3 minutes until 40 µg/kg body weight is reached. If submaximal stress is not reached at this point, then 1 mg atropine is added in 0.25-mg steps. SSFP imaging is acquired at each level of stress, with a temporal resolution of 40 ms or less required for the accurate detection of end-systole. Typically, imaging is performed at three short-axis views along the LV (basal, mid, apical) in addition to long-axis (two- and four-chamber) views (Fig. 10.10). The study is terminated when submaximal stress is reached, blood pressure drops from baseline more than 20 mmHg systolic or 40 mmHg diastolic, blood pressure increases to above 240/120 mmHg, unremitting symptoms occur (e.g., chest pain), new or worsening wall-motion abnormalities occur, or complex cardiac rhythms are detected. Dobutamine stress MR is contraindicated in cases of severe arterial hypertension (above 220/120 mmHg), unstable angina pectoris, significant aortic stenosis, complex cardiac arrhythmias, significant hypertrophic obstructive cardiomyopathy, or the presence of myocarditis, endocarditis, or pericarditis.[2]

An alternative approach to ischemia testing with MRI is first-pass myocardial perfusion imaging. Compared to dobutamine stress MR, this is a technically easier method for detecting flow-limiting coronary stenosis. The goal of stress perfusion imaging is to maximally vasodilate all coronary arteries to unmask differences in regional myocardial blood flow caused by significant epicardial coronary stenoses. Maximal pharmacologic vasodilation is achieved with adenosine or dipyridamole during perfusion imaging with gadolinium contrast media. Imaging is performed at both stress and rest states to allow for accurate detection of hypoperfused territories. Typically, three slices can be obtained during each heartbeat of a perfusion acquisition and are allocated to short-axis (basal, mid, apical) views. If the heart rate is slow enough, an

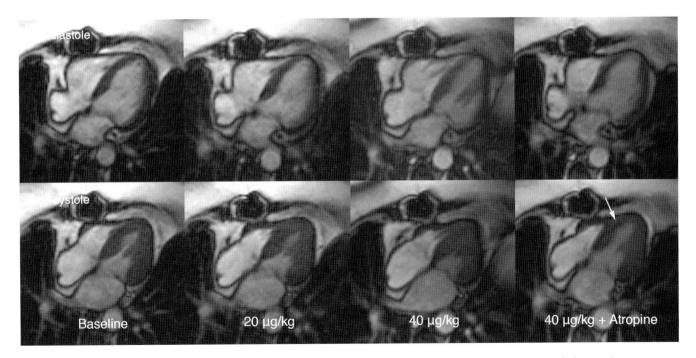

Figure 10.10 *Dobutamine stress MR.* Study of a 65-year-old woman with progressive exertional angina and prior bypass grafting (left internal mammary artery to left anterior descending coronary artery). End-diastole (**top row**) and end-systole (**bottom row**) demonstrate difference in contraction at doses of dobutamine. At maximum dobutamine dose (40 µg/kg), submaximal heart rate was not reached and atropine was added. A wall-motion abnormality was revealed in the apical septum due to ischemia (*arrow*). VENC MR revealed no flow in the left internal mammary artery bypass graft.

additional view such as a four-chamber long-axis view can be added. Image analysis is performed at each slice, comparing rest and stress images (Fig. 10.11). An area of pure ischemia is identified as an area of delayed subendocardial hypoenhancement on stress imaging that is not present on rest imaging. A pitfall of perfusion imaging is a dark subendocardial ring artifact that can mimic a perfusion defect. Characteristically, this artifact covers a large portion of the ventricle, persists for a shorter time as compared to a true perfusion defect, is present on both sides of the ventricle in the phase-encoding direction, and is present on both rest and stress imaging. Accuracy for the detection of CAD can be further improved using late gadolinium-enhanced imaging, such that imaging suggesting prior myocardial infarction implies the presence of CAD.[3]

Acute myocardial infarction. Cardiac MR can be performed within the first 24 hours after a myocardial infarction without safety concerns, if the patient is stable. Recent coronary stent placement is not a contraindication to imaging and with current stents there are not significant problems with susceptibility artifacts. Using a comprehensive imaging protocol that includes functional imaging, T2-weighted edema imaging, and perfusion CMR with late gadolinium contrast enhancement, prognostic information can be gained to direct therapy.

Late gadolinium-enhanced imaging performed in the acute phase of a myocardial infarction accurately reflects the size and distribution of necrosis. The characteristic appearance of late gadolinium enhancement in acute myocardial infarction is an area of enhancement that extends from the subendocardium toward the epicardial surface in a distribution correlating with a coronary artery perfusion territory (see Fig. 10.5). The thickness and extent of the enhancement are determined by the severity of the infarct. This pattern is in distinction to

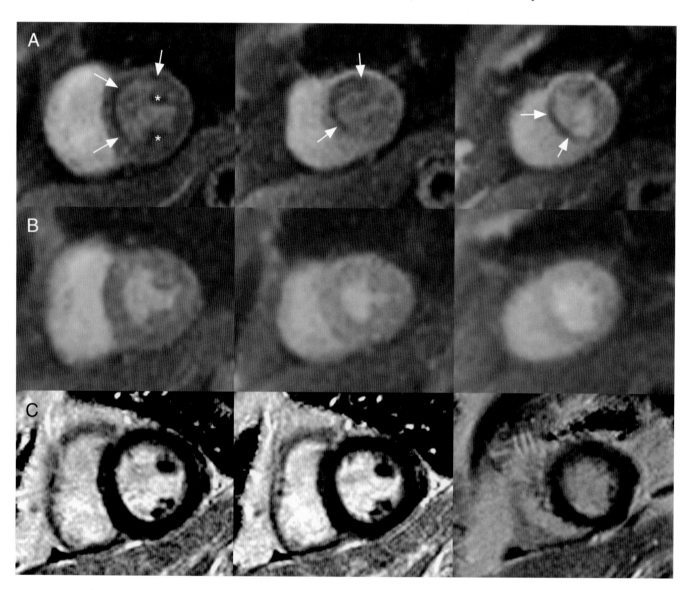

Figure 10.11 *Adenosine perfusion imaging of pure ischemia.* (**A**) First-pass (stress) perfusion imaging during the adenosine infusion reveals subendocardial defects (*arrows*) in the septum and anterior wall at the base and mid-ventricle (left and middle, respectively) and in the septum at the apex (right). Note that the papillary muscles (*) often appear hypoperfused during adenosine administration and this should not be confused with ischemia. (**B**) Rest perfusion imaging performed 10 minutes after termination of adenosine infusion is without defects, validating that the defects during stress are not artifacts. (**C**) Late gadolinium-enhanced imaging shows no evidence of myocardial infarction. Cardiac catheterization showed a 70% left main coronary artery stenosis.

non-ischemic causes of late gadolinium enhancement, which have mid-wall or epicardial involvement and are independent of the coronary perfusion territories. Microvascular obstruction is present in large infarcts and is represented by a dark subendocardial core surround by transmural enhancement, portending a worse prognosis (Fig. 10.12).

Injured myocardium has increased free water content compared to normal myocardium and can be identified using T2-weighted imaging. Edema can be seen for at least 1 week following myocardial infarction and is sometimes detectable at 1 month. Both infarcted myocardium and the jeopardized myocardium surrounding the infarction will be bright on T2-weighted images relative to normal myocardium due to increased interstitial fluid. Thus, the total edematous tissue after a myocardial infarction represents the myocardial *area at risk*, which is the myocardium within the perfusion bed that is distal to the culprit lesion of the infarct-related coronary artery. By comparing the volume of the area at risk to that of myocardial infarction (using late gadolinium enhanced images), the volume of salvaged myocardium after intervention can be calculated, which provides clinical information regarding the efficacy of treatment and may be useful for guiding subsequent therapies. In addition to identifying areas of edema, T2-weighted images identify hemorrhagic areas within infarcts as areas of dark signal within the bright area at risk. Hemorrhagic areas appear dark due to the paramagnetic properties of blood resulting in shortening of the T2 relaxation time. Myocardial hemorrhage tends to occur in larger infarcts that have a significant amount of microvascular obstruction. Preliminary studies suggest that myocardial hemorrhage may be an independent marker of adverse ventricular remodeling after infarction (Fig. 10.13).

Acute myocardial infarction often results in complications that can be easily identified by CMR. Mural LV thrombus after acute myocardial infarction is associated with akinetic walls, particularly in the apex of the heart. Thrombi are differentiated from cardiac masses in that they do not demonstrate enhancement. Thrombi are best imaged after administration of contrast

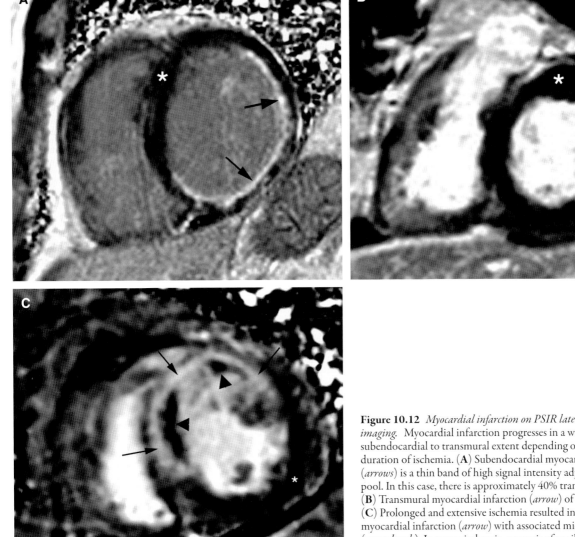

Figure 10.12 *Myocardial infarction on PSIR late gadolinium-enhanced imaging.* Myocardial infarction progresses in a wavefront manner from subendocardial to transmural extent depending on the degree and duration of ischemia. (**A**) Subendocardial myocardial infarction (*arrows*) is a thin band of high signal intensity adjacent to the blood pool. In this case, there is approximately 40% transmural involvement. (**B**) Transmural myocardial infarction (*arrow*) of the lateral wall. (**C**) Prolonged and extensive ischemia resulted in a transmural myocardial infarction (*arrow*) with associated microvascular obstruction (*arrowheads*). In severe ischemia, necrosis of capillaries prevents delivery of contrast media to the subendocardium, resulting in islands of low signal (*arrowheads*) surrounded by areas of myocardial necrosis with intact blood vessels (*arrows*). Asterisk indicates normal myocardium.

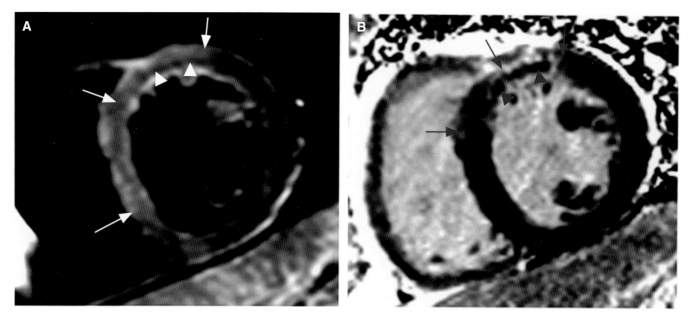

Figure 10.13 *Myocardial infarction.* T2-weighted imaging in a 55-year-old man who was diagnosed clinically with ST-elevation myocardial infarction (STEMI) and subsequently underwent percutaneous intervention to re-establish flow in the left anterior coronary artery. (**A**) High signal (*arrows*) in anterior and septal walls represents edema and delineates the area at risk. Low signal intensity within the subendocardium (*arrowhead*) represents intramural hemorrhage. (**B**) Late gadolinium-contrast-enhanced image shows transmural infarct of the anteroseptum (*arrows*) with areas of microvascular obstruction (*arrowheads*). There is significant myocardial salvage of the septum due to the intervention, as represented by the area at risk shown in image A less the transmural myocardial infarction shown in image B. The extent of intramyocardial hemorrhage in image A correlates with the extent of microvascular obstruction in image B.

media with SSFP or late gadolinium enhanced imaging. When using SSFP imaging, both unenhanced and enhanced imaging should be at the same slice location and orientation. Normal myocardium will demonstrate enhancement whereas thrombus will not. On late gadolinium enhanced images, thrombi will be black. On occasion, thrombi and microvascular obstruction can be difficult to differentiate. In these cases, reference to the wall thickness on SSFP functional images may be helpful, as microvascular obstruction is within the myocardium and thrombi are within the LV cavity (Fig. 10.14). Additionally, other complications, including valvular dysfunction, pericardial effusion, pericarditis, aneurysm formation, and ventricular free wall or septal rupture, can be identified using a comprehensive CMR protocol.

Determining myocardial viability. In patients with ischemic heart disease and viable myocardium, LV dysfunction can improve with coronary revascularization. A 2002 meta-analysis[4] showed that patients with viable myocardium who underwent successful revascularization had better outcomes than those receiving medical therapy alone. Viability is defined as the presence of living myocytes and can be present in the absence of contractility. Both hibernating myocardium, which represents chronically hypoperfused myocytes, and stunned myocardium, which can occur after periods of transient ischemia, are viable myocardium that is dysfunctional.

Using late gadolinium enhanced imaging, CMR can identify nonviable myocardium and guide revascularization in the setting of ongoing myocardial ischemia. Chronic myocardial infarctions appear as areas of thin myocardium in which the non-viable myocardium (fibrous scar) is present as a subendocardial

or transmural area of enhancement (bright) compared to the normal myocardium (dark). CMR is the only imaging modality that can accurately differentiate subendocardial from transmural myocardial infarctions. The likelihood of recovery of contractile function after revascularization of a dysfuctional segment is related to the degree of transmural late gadolinium enhancement of the segment, such that the chance of recovery decreases with increasing transmurality of enhancement. Segments in which there is abnormal wall motion at rest without late gadolinium contrast enhancement represent hibernating myocardium and are most likely to recover function after revascularization. Regions with wall-motion abnormalities and late enhancement ranging from 1% to 25% transmural thickness are likely to regain function after revascularization. Regions with 25% to 50% transmural late contrast enhancement may recover function. Regions with 50% to 100% transmural late enhancement are unlikely to recover function.

It is important to recognize that only the dysfunctional ischemic myocardium can recover function after revascularization. Thus, in the absence of angina, determining the appropriateness of revascularization should include ischemia testing. Furthermore, the decision to revascularize and the type of revascularization to be performed (percutaneous vs. surgical) should be based on the transmurality and distribution of late contrast enhancement, the complexity of the CAD, and the patient's surgical risk. CMR is an attractive modality due to its ability to assess the myocardial function, the presence of ischemia, and viability all in one examination.

Anomalous coronary arteries. Young patients who present with chest pain suggestive of coronary ischemia and who

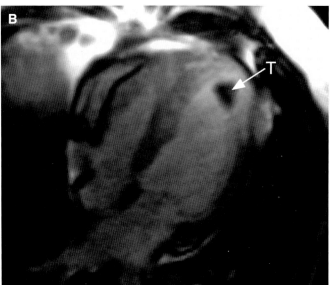

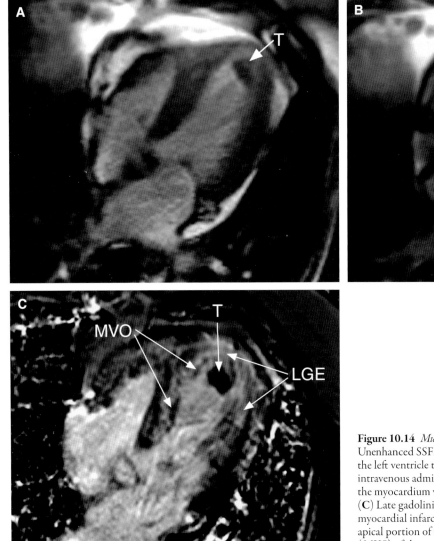

Figure 10.14 *Mural thrombus and microvascular obstruction.* (**A**) Unenhanced SSFP imaging demonstrates a structure (*T*) in the apex of the left ventricle that is iso-intense to myocardium. (**B**) After intravenous administration of contrast media, there is enhancement of the myocardium without enhancement of the mural thrombus (*T*). (**C**) Late gadolinium-enhanced imaging reveals a large transmural myocardial infarction involving most of the septum, the apex, and the apical portion of the lateral wall (*LGE*) with microvascular obstruction (*MVO*) of the septum and apex. Note that compared with images **A** and **B**, microvascular obstruction is within the myocardium, whereas the mural thrombus (*T*) is within the cavity.

are unlikely to have significant coronary atherosclerosis should be evaluated for the presence of anomalous coronary arteries. MRI is a superior modality for this patient population due to the noninvasive nature, lack of ionizing radiation, and excellent ability to identify the origins of the coronary arteries and their proximal course without the administration of contrast media. Current techniques use 2D breath-hold sequences or 3D free-breathing acquisitions, neither requiring the use of contrast media. Most often, 3D free-breathing sequence are employed because they are easier to use, as they do not require that the breath-hold position between planning imaging and coronary acquisition be exactly the same—a difficulty with performing 2D imaging. Current 3D free-breathing techniques employ SSFP acquisition with navigator pulses that track the diaphragm and acquire image data only at end-expiration. However, in some cases the diaphragm is difficult to track or breathing is irregular, necessitating the use of 2D techniques.

Coronary anomalies are categorized as malignant or nonmalignant configurations. In the malignant type, the

anomalous coronary artery follows an intra-arterial course, passing between the aorta and the pulmonary artery. This includes left main coronary artery arising from the right sinus of Valsalva and right coronary artery arising from the left sinus of Valsalva. In malignant anomalies, the coronary artery is compressed by the aorta and pulmonary artery, resulting in stenosis and myocardial ischemia. This is most concerning in the case of an anomalous left main coronary artery due to the majority of the LV perfusion territory being at risk. Consequently, this anomaly is treated even when discovered incidentally. In addition to being compressed between the great arteries, intra-arterial coronary arteries have abnormal ostia that are slit-like or have an intramural course, both contributing to decreased coronary flow. Nonmalignant coronary anomalies do not course between the great arteries. For example, the left main coronary artery can arise from the right sinus of Valsalva separate from the right coronary artery or as a branch of the right coronary artery, then course posterior to the aorta to resume the appropriate course (Fig. 10.15).

HEART FAILURE AND CLASSIFICATION OF CARDIOMYOPATHIES

Heart failure is a significant burden to the health-care system in terms of morbidity and mortality as well as financial resources. The general treatment of heart failure is common to many patients; however, early diagnosis and identification of the underlying etiology are of clinical importance because some causes of heart failure have specific treatments and may be reversible. CMR with late gadolinium enhancement imaging has revolutionized the evaluation of heart failure patients, allowing identification of the etiology in the majority of cases.

Cardiomyopathy can easily be separated into ischemic and non-ischemic causes with late gadolinium enhancement imaging. As discussed previously, myocardial infarctions appear as late gadolinium enhancement extending from the subendocardium outward and following a coronary artery distribution. This is in distinction to non-ischemic etiologies, which typically result in mid-wall or epicardial late gadolinium enhancement and are often patchy in distribution without regard to coronary distribution. Often, the pattern of late gadolinium enhancement in non-ischemic cardiomyopathies can lead to a specific diagnosis or limit the differential significantly.[5]

Dilated cardiomyopathy is a process of progressive dilatation of the heart and loss of contractile function. The host of inciting factors includes prior myocarditis, exposure to toxins (e.g., anthrocyclines, alcohol), autoimmune disorders, or genetic factors. In approximately half of the cases, the cause is idiopathic. Histologically, the course of the disease is typified by progressive interstitial fibrosis. Diffuse wall thinning is the hallmark of the end stage of the disease.

Classically, patients with heart failure have been evaluated with echocardiography to assess function and coronary angiography to exclude CAD as a cause of heart failure. However, a normal coronary angiogram does not exclude the possibility of CAD as an etiology of the disease. About 10% of patients diagnosed with dilated cardiomyopathy show late contrast enhancement consistent with prior myocardial infarction. This situation may occur as a result of spontaneous recanalization of an occlusive coronary event, as a result of embolic

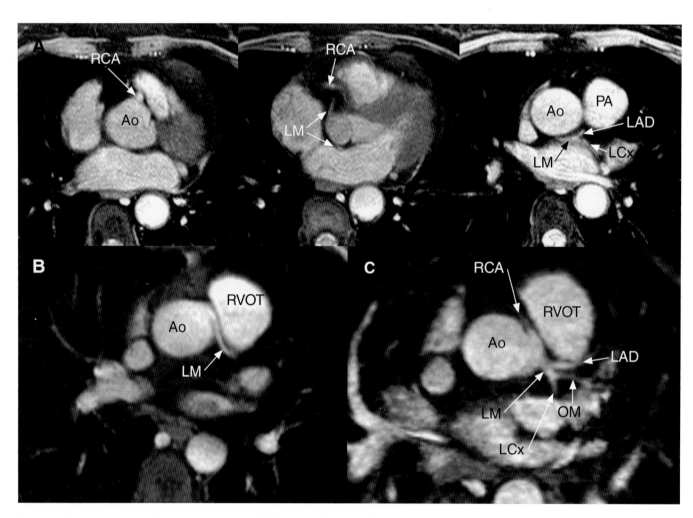

Figure 10.15 *Coronary anomalies.* Respiratory-gated SSFP imaging. (**A, top row**) Nonmalignant coronary anomaly: Left main (*LM*) coronary artery arises from the right coronary artery (*RCA*) and courses posterior to the aorta (*Ao*) to divide in the normal location and give rise to the left anterior descending (*LAD*) and left circumflex (*LCx*) coronary arteries. Malignant coronary anomalies: (**B**) Interarterial course of the left main coronary artery (*LM*), arising from the right sinus of Valsalva. (**C**) Interarterial course of the right coronary artery (*RCA*), arising from a common ostium with the left main coronary artery (*LM*) from the left sinus of Valsalva. *OM*, obtuse marginal artery; *Ao*, aorta; *RVOT*, right ventricular outflow tract.

Box 10.1 ESSENTIALS TO REMEMBER

- MRI testing for CAD and myocardial ischemia is performed by pharmacologic stress testing or by first pass myocardial perfusion imaging and late gadolinium contrast enhancement.

- Areas of pure ischemia are identified by subendocardial hypoenhancement at stress perfusion imaging that is not present at rest imaging.

- Low signal intensity subendocardial ring artifact can mimic a perfusion defect. The artifact is identified by noting that it covers a large portion of the ventricle, persists for a shorter time than perfusion defect, is present on both sides of the ventricle in the phase-encoded direction, and is present on both rest and stress images.

- Acute myocardial infarction is identified as an area of contrast enhancement that extends from the subendocardium toward the epicardial surface in a distribution that correlates with the perfusion territory of a coronary artery. The thickness and extent of the enhancement reflect the severity of the infarction.

- Non-ischemic causes of late gadolinium enhancement have mid-wall or epicardial involvement and affect myocardium that does not correspond to a coronary artery perfusion territory.

- Edema, seen as high signal intensity myocardium on T2-weighted images, is present for at least one week following myocardial infarction and identifies both the infarcted myocardium and the jeopardized myocardium.

- Microvascular obstruction associated with myocardial infarction appears as a subendocardial area of hypointensity surrounded by high signal on late gadolinium enhanced imaging and portends a poor outcome.

disease from a non-critical ruptured atherosclerotic plaque, or caused by prior coronary vasospasm. About 20% of dilated cardiomyopathy patients without subendocardial enhancement will show patchy or longitudinal, nonspecific mid-wall late gadolinium enhancement, which corresponds to fibrosis histologically. These areas of scarring are of prognostic value as their presence represents an increased risk of ventricular arrhythmias and poor response to optimal medical therapy in terms of recovery of systolic function. The lack of late gadolinium enhancement does not exclude the possibility of ischemic heart disease, as in the rare case of global myocardial hibernation, and thus ischemia testing should be included in patients who have a high likelihood of CAD and have not undergone cardiac catheterization.

Myocarditis. In the acute or fulminant case of heart failure, viral myocarditis should be considered, particularly in the setting of a recent viral-like illness. During the acute and subacute phases, myocarditis can be diagnosed by the presence of a late contrast enhancement pattern with subepicardial to mid-wall involvement, sparing the subendocardium. Late gadolinium enhancement of myocarditis is most often present within the inferolateral wall of the LV; however, involvement of the septum or patchy involvement of the ventricle can also be seen (Fig. 10.16). CMR imaging studies correlated with endomyocardial biopsy have shown inferolateral wall late gadolinium enhancement correlating with parvovirus infections and septal late gadolinium enhancement correlating with herpesvirus infections.[6]

As the myocardium heals, the area of late gadolinium enhancement may completely resolve. Large areas of late gadolinium enhancement may persist indefinitely, causing distinctive linear medial striae of hyperenhancement, a pattern appreciated in dilated cardiomyopathy. This finding suggests myocarditis as the underlying etiology of dilated cardiomyopathy in a proportion of cases.

The typical pattern of late gadolinium enhancement is specific for myocarditis, but the absence of late enhancement does not exclude myocarditis. In patients with suspected myocarditis, the presence of edema within the mid-wall and

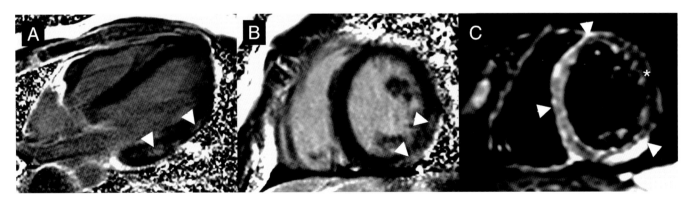

Figure 10.16 *Myocarditis.* Images of a 36-year-old man with new-onset heart failure and recent upper respiratory infection. (**A**) Late gadolinium-horizontal long-axis view shows typical findings of patch subepicardial hyperenhancement in the lateral wall (*arrowheads*). (**B**) Short-axis late gadolinium enhanced image shows classic inferolateral enhancement that is associated with infection by parvovirus serotypes. (**C**) T2-weighted image reveals extensive edema in the septal and inferior walls (*arrowheads*) compared to the normal signal in the lateral wall (*).

epicardium on T2-weighted images is sufficient for the diagnosis. For this reason, Abdel-Aty and coworkers have advocated a combined imaging approach using T2-weighted images and late gadolinium contrast-enhanced images to increase sensitivity.[7]

Hypertrophic cardiomyopathy (HCM) is characterized as abnormal hypertrophy of the myocardium that results in diastolic dysfunction. There are many different phenotypes, but the most common is asymmetric hypertrophy of the intraventricular septum. In a subgroup of patients, septal hypertrophy is associated with LVOT obstruction and is denoted *hypertrophic obstructive cardiomyopathy (HOCM)*. This condition is of clinical importance because it is a cause of sudden death in young patients. Histologically, hypertrophic cardiomyopathy results in disarray of myofibrils and patchy myocardial necrosis due to abnormal tissue perfusion.

CMR currently is the best imaging modality for diagnosis of hypertrophic cardiomyopathy due to its high spatial resolution, resulting in a better ability to detect and quantify hypertrophy compared to echocardiography. CMR is particularly useful for visualizing other hypertrophic patterns, including symmetric, apical, mass-like, and sole involvement of papillary muscles. Imaging should include SSFP functional imaging to define the LV morphology. Tagged cine imaging demonstrates decreased deformation in the area of hypertrophy, which is useful for delineating borderline cases. In cases of asymmetric hypertrophy with LVOT obstruction, velocity-encoded imaging can be performed to calculate peak velocity and, thus, the pressure gradient across the obstruction. The mitral valve should be carefully evaluated in the case of hypertrophic cardiomyopathy, as there is often mitral regurgitation. This can be due to underlying structural abnormalities of the valve associated with hypertrophic cardiomyopathy or due to LVOT obstruction resulting in Venturi or drag forces moving the anterior leaflet of the mitral valve into the LVOT, which is denoted as systolic anterior motion of the mitral valve. Late gadolinium enhancement imaging is performed to detect areas of confluent fibrosis that is present in severely hypertrophied myocardium and occasionally can be identified in normal-thickness myocardium. The pattern of late enhancement is patchy and typically mid-wall, and tends to occur at the insertion of the RV on the LV[8] (Fig. 10.17). The presence of late gadolinium enhancement in hypertrophic cardiomyopathy is an independent risk factor for developing nonsustained

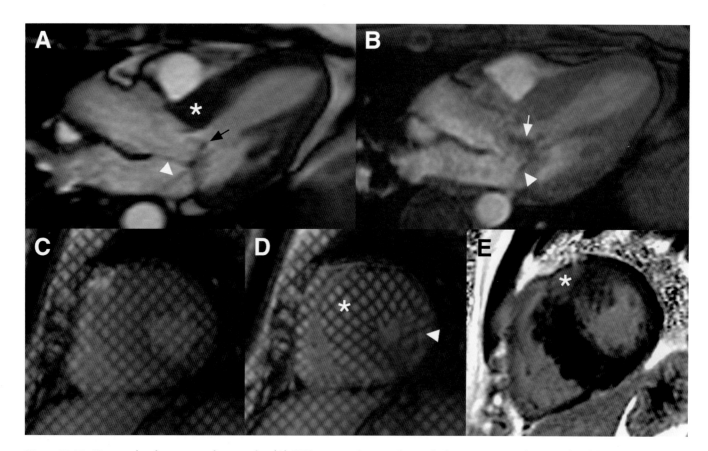

Figure 10.17 *Hypertrophic obstructive cardiomyopathy.* (**A**) SSFP imaging during early systole shows asymmetric hypertrophy of the basal anteroseptum (*). Partial obstruction of the left ventricular outflow tract results in flow acceleration and deflection of the tip of the anterior leaflet of the mitral valve (*arrow*) into the left ventricular outflow tract. Mild mitral regurgitation (*arrowhead*) is present, a common associated finding in hypertrophic obstructive cardiomyopathy. (**B**) Gradient-echo imaging shows turbulence in the left ventricular outflow tract (*arrow*), not appreciated on SSFP imaging, suggesting significant obstructive features. Mild mitral regurgitation (*arrowhead*) is present. (**C**) Tagged gradient-echo imaging at end-diastole. (**D**) End-systolic image showing normal deformation and thickening in the lateral wall (*arrowhead*). Abnormally decreased deformation of tag lines is present in the thickened septum (*). (**E**) Subepicardial and mid-wall late gadolinium enhancement in the anteroseptum (*), at the insertion of the right ventricle on the left ventricle, is a classic location for hypertrophic cardiomyopathy and histologically corresponds to the presence of fibrosis.

ventricular tachycardia, but more studies are needed to determine if it predicts sudden death or heart failure.[9]

Arrhythmogenic right ventricular cardiomyopathy (ARVC) is a genetic disorder characterized by progressive degeneration of the RV myocardium, and to a much lesser extent the LV myocardium, that can present with ventricular arrhythmias of left bundle branch block pattern, right heart failure, or sudden death. Both sporadic and familial forms of arrhythmogenic RV cardiomyopathy exist, with familial forms demonstrating predominantly autosomal dominant inheritance. The disease affects approximately 1:5,000 people in the United States, with presentation typically in adolescence or early adulthood and more commonly in males and athletes. Arrhythmogenic RV cardiomyopathy accounts for 5% of all sudden death cases in subject less than 35 years of age.

Morphologic changes include fibrous and/or fatty replacement of myocardial tissue, extensive wall thinning or thickening, RVOT enlargement, and atypical arrangement of the trabecular muscle. Functional changes include focal aneurysms, regional wall-motion abnormalities, and RV dilatation and dysfunction. The diagnosis of arrhythmogenic RV cardiomyopathy is made on the basis of imaging, electrophysiologic, and historical criteria. Major imaging criteria of the RV include localized aneurysms, severe global/segmental dilatation, and severe global dysfunction with no (or only mild) LV impairment. Detection of fibrous/fatty replacement using T1-weighted images is usually not possible due to its poor sensitivity and specificity. That being said, late gadolinium enhancement correlates well with fibrous/fatty replacement and predicts inducible ventricular tachycardia during electrophysiologic studies (Fig. 10.18).[10]

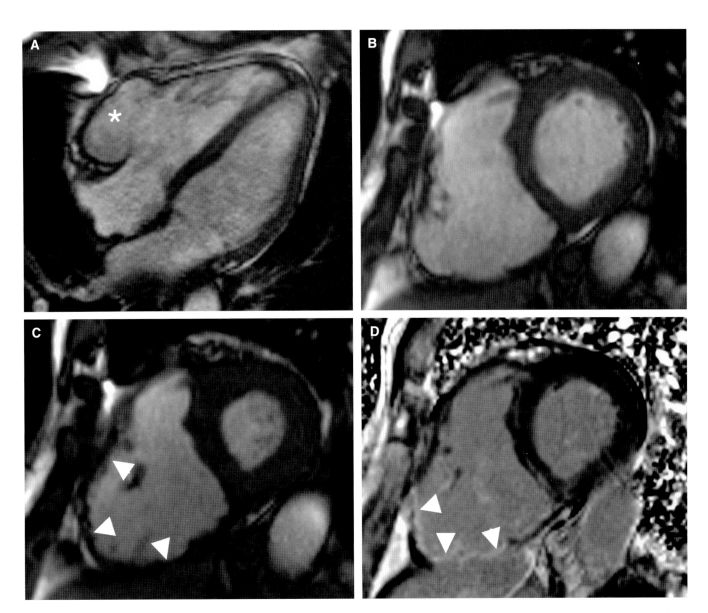

Figure 10.18 *Arrhythmogenic right ventricular cardiomyopathy.* (**A**) A major imaging criterion of arrhythmogenic right ventricular cardiomyopathy is the presence of focal aneurysms of the right ventricular wall, as shown here (*) in this SSFP horizontal long-axis image. Short-axis view at end-diastole (**B**) and at end-systole (**C**) reveals the dyskinetic function of the aneurysm (*arrowheads*), which enlarges in systole while the rest of the right ventricle contracts. (**D**) Late gadolinium enhancement of the wall of the aneurysm of the right ventricle (*arrowheads*) correlates well with the extent of fibrous/fatty replacement of the myocardium in arrhythmogenic right ventricular cardiomyopathy.

Sarcoidosis. Approximately 5% of patients with sarcoidosis will develop cardiac involvement that may present as acute cardiac failure, ventricular arrhythmias or bradyarrhythmias, or sudden death. However, 30% of patients will have evidence of cardiac involvement at autopsy, suggesting that screening may be appropriate to assess the risk of sudden death from arrhythmias, which is the most common cause of death in this population. CMR can image the three separate histologic stages of cardiac sarcoidosis that progress from initial edema to granulomatous infiltration to post-inflammatory scarring. T2-weighted images can identify areas of myocardial edema, which is present in the first two stages. Late gadolinium enhancement identifies active granulomas as patchy areas of subepicardial or mid-wall enhancement most commonly involving the LV lateral wall, basal septum, and RV free wall. Granulomas may also have a focal nodular appearance on cine imaging. Subepicardial late enhancement with wall thinning and hypokinesis typify scarring. Late contrast enhancement may appear transmural and rarely in a subepicardial pattern, but the non-coronary distribution of the enhancement allows differentiation from ischemic heart disease (Fig. 10.19).[11]

Amyloidosis is a result of deposition of malformed proteins in the extracellular compartment of tissue, occurring in both isolated organ and multisystem disease states. Multiple forms of the disease are possible; however, cardiac involvement is most commonly present in systemic (primary) amyloidosis, in which up to 90% of patients are affected, and senile systemic amyloidosis. Patients with cardiac involvement are typically over 65 years of age and have a poor prognosis after the onset of heart failure, with a median survival of less than 6 months if untreated.

Deposition of amyloid proteins in the myocardial interstitium results in concentric wall thickening with normal or reduced contractility, diastolic dysfunction, and restrictive physiologic features, including bi-atrial enlargement. Involvement of all four cardiac chambers is common with amyloid, and thickening of the interatrial septum and free wall of the RA is highly specific for the disease. Both a diffuse subendocardial enhancement pattern and a more patchy transmural pattern can be seen at late contrast enhancement imaging, the prior being highly specific for cardiac amyloid (Fig. 10.20). Selecting the appropriate inversion time for late gadolinium enhancement imaging can be technically challenging due to an atypically dark blood pool, secondary to rapid blood pool washout, combined with the diffuse subendocardial involvement. These factors lead to difficulty differentiating normal from abnormal myocardium on TI-weighted scout sequences suggesting that amyloidosis may be present.[12]

PERICARDIAL DISEASE

The pericardium is composed of two layers, a visceral and a parietal pericardium, that surround and contain the heart in the mediastinum. The visceral pericardium is a thin mesothelial layer covering the epicardium of the heart. The parietal pericardium is a thicker, fibrous layer that constrains the heart, provides a barrier to the spread of infection, and limits the degree to which the heart can distend acutely. Under normal conditions, approximately 50 mL of clear serous fluid resides between the two layers, acting as a lubricant, allowing the heart to contract and distend normally. The normal thickness of the pericardium on MRI is less than 3 mm, and it appears

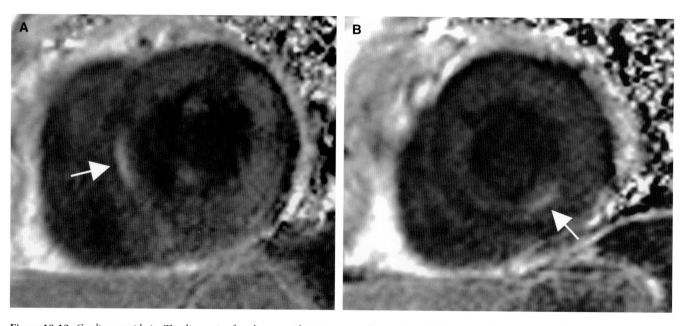

Figure 10.19 *Cardiac sarcoidosis.* The diagnosis of cardiac sarcoidosis is suspected in patients with known pulmonary sarcoidosis who present with new heart failure, bradyarrhythmias, or sudden death. Short-axis left ventricular imaging from a patient in the granulomatous phase of the disease demonstrates patchy mid-wall (*arrows*) late gadolinium enhancement in the basal septum (**A**) and the apical inferolateral wall (**B**), representing active granulomas.

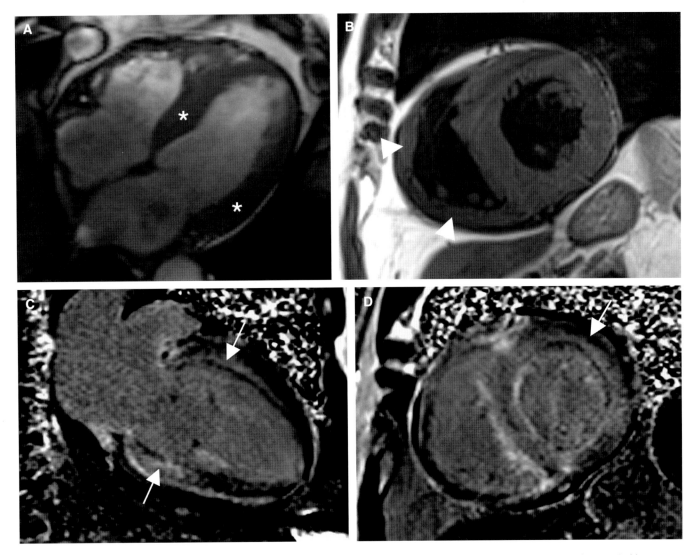

Figure 10.20 *Cardiac amyloidosis.* (**A**) Amyloid protein deposition leads to abnormal thickening of the basal portion of the left ventricle (*) as demonstrated by SSFP imaging. Note that the apical portion of the left ventricle is normal in thickness. (**B**) Involvement of multiple cardiac chambers is common in cardiac amyloidosis, evidenced by both left and right (*arrowheads*) ventricular thickening, as shown in this short-axis high-resolution T1-weighted spin-echo image acquired at the base of the heart. (**C**) Diffuse subendocardial and transmural late gadolinium enhancement mirrors the extent of the abnormal wall thickening. The non-coronary distribution of the enhancement (isolated to the base of the ventricle) differentiates amyloidosis from late gadolinium enhancement associated with myocardial infarction. (**D**) Diffuse, circumferential late gadolinium enhancement is a hallmark finding in cardiac amyloidosis. In this short-axis image, only a sliver of normal nulled myocardium (*arrow*) is present.

Box 10.2 ESSENTIALS TO REMEMBER

- Dilated cardiomyopathy refers to progressive dilatation of the heart with loss of contractile function. About 20% of patients have fibrosis indentified by patchy mid-wall late gadolinium enhancement. Scarred fibrotic areas of myocardium are associated with increased risk of ventricular arrhymthmias and poor response to medical therapy.

- Acute myocarditis is identified by late gadolinium contrast enhancement of the subepicarial to mid wall, sparing the endocardium. In patients suspected of myocarditis, edema in the absence of late gadolinium enhancement is sufficient for diagnosis.

- Hypertrophic cardiomyopathy results in diastolic dysfunction caused by abnormal hypertrophy of areas of myocardium. The most common patern of abnormality is asymmetric hypertrophy of the intraventricular septum. In more severe cases, late gadolinium enhancement may be present in a patchy midwall distribution, increasing the risk of ventricular arrythmia.

- Arrhythmogenic right ventricular cardiomyopathy is histologically characterized by fibrous or fatty replacement of the RV myocardium. The presence of localized RV aneurysms, severe global/segmental RV dilatation, or severe global RV dysfunction with no (or only mild) LV impairment suggests the presence of disease.

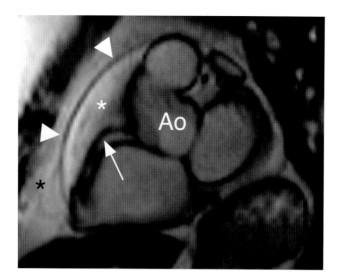

Figure 10.21 *Normal pericardium.* Short-axis SSFP image showing the low-signal normal pericardium (*arrowheads*) surrounded by pericardial fat (*black* *) anteriorly and epicardial fat (*white* *) located between the pericardium and myocardium. The right coronary artery (*arrow*) is also surrounded by epicardial fat. The normal thickness of the pericardium is 3 mm or less. *Ao,* aortic root.

as a thin low-intensity line on both cine and static imaging techniques (Fig. 10.21).

Pericardial cysts are benign lesions arising from the pericardium during embryologic development and do not communicate with the pericardial cavity. They are most commonly found in the right cardiophrenic sulcus but can occur anywhere along the pericardium. The imaging characteristics are similar to those of other simple cysts, displaying low signal intensity on T1-weighted and high signal intensity on T2-weighted images. The structure is usually unilocular, and they do not enhance

(Fig. 10.22). In rare cases, the cysts can become infected and hemorrhage.

Acute pericarditis is typically a clinical diagnosis that does not require imaging, but it may be discovered during an imaging workup for the etiology of chest pain. Most cases of acute pericarditis are either viral or idiopathic in origin. Imaging may reveal a new small pericardial effusion with mild pericardial thickening. Significant pericardial thickening implies a chronic process. T2-weighted images may show edema in the pericardial fat secondary to the adjacent inflammation. Occasionally, pericardial enhancement, caused by hyperemia, can be observed after administration of gadolinium contrast media.

Pericardial effusion. Any process that causes pericardial inflammation may result in the development of a pericardial effusion. Echocardiography is typically the first choice for imaging pericardial effusion; however, MRI is better at detecting small and loculated effusions. Additionally, MRI is excellent at characterizing hemorrhagic effusions and detecting pericardial masses responsible for an effusion.

Simple pericardial effusions are lower than myocardium in signal intensity on T2-weighted images, are similar in intensity to cerebral spinal fluid, and are without internal septations or structures. On SSFP imaging, the effusion will also be bright, with the pericardium appearing dark. Epicardial fat may undulate in a large pericardial effusion resulting from heart motion; however, this is readily characterized as fat by the presence of a dark line at the fat/fluid interface on SSFP cine imaging (Fig. 10.23). Hemorrhagic or proteinaceous material within the effusion causes an increase in the signal on T1-weighted images. Hemorrhage or infection should be suspected when the effusion is complicated by internal structures or is loculated, or if there is pericardial enhancement.

Cardiac tamponade. Because of the fibrous nature of the pericardium, an acute increase in the volume of the pericardial

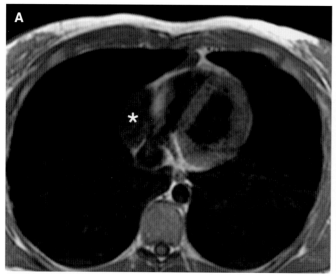

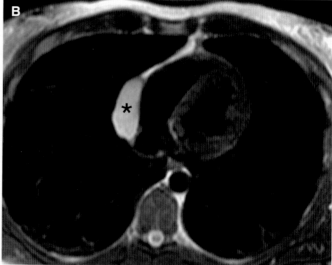

Figure 10.22 *Pericardial cyst.* T1-weighted (**A**) and T2-weighted (**B**) spin-echo images show a pericardial cyst (*) located in the right cardiophrenic sulcus, the most common location of this entity. These lesions typically follow signal intensity of water on all MR sequences. Note the unilocular, uncomplicated, and homogenous appearance of fluid on both T1- and T2-weighted imaging. This is the most common imaging appearance. Pericardial cysts always have an attachment to the pericardium.

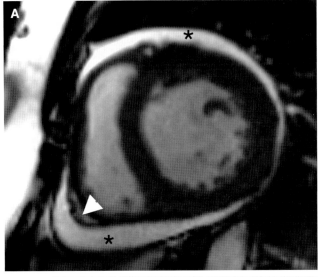

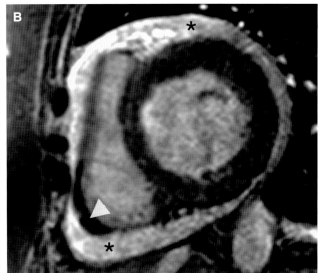

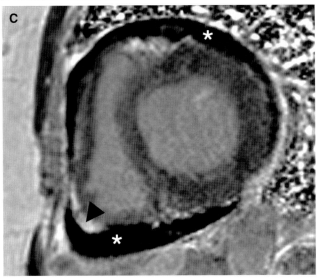

Figure 10.23 *Pericardial effusion.* Short-axis SSFP (**A**), T2-weighted image with fat saturation (**B**), and phase-sensitive inversion-recovery image (**C**) showing a simple pericardial effusion (*). In image A, fluid is brighter than the blood pool and the epicardial fat (*arrowhead*). A dark band around the periphery of relatively bright epicardial fat results from the phase cancellation observed in SSFP imaging when fat and fluid share the same voxel. In image B, the fluid is again brighter than the blood pool and the epicardial fat is dark caused by the fat saturation of this sequence. In image C, the pericardial effusion is darker than the normal myocardium and epicardial fat is bright.

fluid beyond a certain point results in a rapid increase in intrapericardial pressure. The elevated pressure compromises filling of the cardiac chambers, affecting the atria first, and with further increase in pressure decreased ventricular filling results. This state of compromised filling is referred to as cardiac tamponade and can occur with rapid accumulation of as little as 100 mL of fluid. The rate of accumulation of fluid is the key factor in the development of cardiac tamponade, as patients with slow accumulation of fluid can tolerate extremely large pericardial effusions because the pericardium can stretch over time.

Cardiac tamponade is typically a clinical diagnosis that is augmented with echocardiographic findings when hemodynamic compromise is present, as an MRI scanner is not a place for an unstable patient. However, in nonemergent cases in which echocardiographic imaging is not optimal, CMR can detect the presence of altered physiology caused by an effusion. Cardiac tamponade most commonly occurs in the presence of a large circumferential effusion resulting in diastolic collapse of the RA and RV, the latter being more specific for hemodynamic compromise (Fig. 10.24). Additionally, real-time imaging may be useful to demonstrate that the pericar-

dium has reached the limit of distensibility. In this state, short-axis imaging during deep inspiration shows flattening or inversion of the intraventricular septum toward the LV, a consequence of augmented RV filling (due to inspiration) compromising LV filling in a nondistensible compartment (pericardium).[13]

Constrictive pericarditis is the result of chronic pericardial inflammation that results in a thickened, fibrotic, and/or calcified pericardium with decreased compliance. Physiologically, this limits distention of the heart and impairs ventricular filling. Elevated systemic venous pressures and low cardiac output are presenting features of the disease. The most commonly identified etiologies are prior cardiac surgery and radiation-induced pericarditis; however, most cases are idiopathic. Clinical differentiation between constrictive pericarditis and restrictive cardiomyopathy can be difficult. Comprehensive evaluation with CMR can help distinguish between the two by identifying specific morphologic and hemodynamic characteristics.

The primary morphologic feature of constrictive pericarditis is thickening of the pericardium. A pericardium measuring

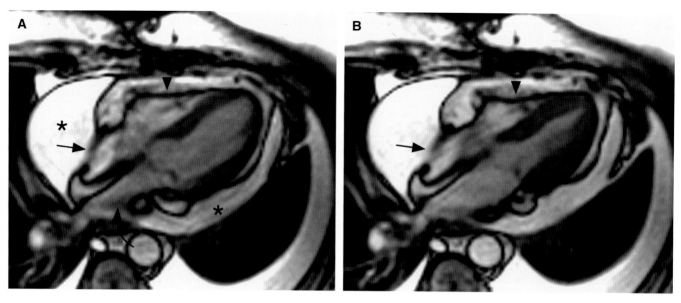

Figure 10.24 *Pericardial tamponade.* (**A**) End-diastolic SSFP imaging shows the effect of increased pressure in the pericardial cavity caused by a large circumferential pericardial effusion (*) resulting in diastolic collapse of the right (*arrow*) and left atrium (*curved arrow*). There is also partial diastolic collapse of the right ventricle (*arrowhead*) as evidenced by its small size and the concavity of the free wall. (**B**) End-systolic imaging reveals poor right ventricular ejection fraction (*arrowhead*) and poor filling of the right atrium (*arrow*), worrisome for impending hemodynamic collapse.

4 mm in thickness is suggestive of pericardial constriction, with thicknesses greater than 6 mm being highly specific for the disease process. The thickening is most commonly diffuse, but focal thickening can occur, usually involving the right side of the heart (RV and anterior atrioventricular groove); however, in 5% of cases the pericardium is normal in thickness. Thus, in cases of suspected constrictive pericarditis, a thorough evaluation of the pericardium in multiple imaging planes is required. The heart chambers may have a distorted tubular appearance caused by the abnormal pericardium. Secondary finding of unilateral or bilateral enlargement of the atria, hepatomegaly, ascites, and IVC distention may be present with restrictive cardiomyopathy as well as constrictive pericarditis.

Functional abnormalities resulting from constrictive pericarditis can be imaged with CMR and further support the diagnosis. Due to the fixed pericardial volume resulting from the fibrotic pericardium, the filling pressure in the ventricles becomes dependent on one another (ventricular interdependence), resulting in an early diastolic septal flattening or inversion ("septal bounce"). This feature distinguishes pericardial constriction from restrictive cardiomyopathy and is accentuated by respiration, where RV filling is augmented by inspiration and LV filling is augmented by expiration. Using real-time imaging in the short axis, there is a marked shift of the intraventricular septum toward the LV during inspiration, as is also present in cardiac tamponade (Fig. 10.25).[14]

CARDIAC MASSES

Known or suspected cases of cardiac masses are often referred to CMR for further evaluation. In many cases, CMR can characterize the type of tumor or at least significantly limit the differential diagnosis. In situations where the tumor type cannot be identified, CMR is useful for defining the extent and physiologic consequence of the mass, and for planning therapy.

Suspected cardiac masses can be separated into pseudo-masses and true cardiac masses. Pseudo-masses represent non-neoplastic lesions that mimic a significant cardiac or pericardiac mass, including prominent crista terminalis, eustachian valve, or Chiari network. External compression of the cardiac chambers from large hiatal hernias can also mimic masses, creating confusion at echocardiography.

Lipomatous hypertrophy of the interatrial septum likely should be grouped as a pseudo-mass, as it is not a neoplastic process and is typically referred to as an atrial mass seen on echocardiography. Lipomatous hypertrophy of the interatrial septum represents hyperplasia, not hypertrophy, of normal adipocytes within the interatrial septum. MRI characterization is relatively straightforward, employing T1-weighted images with and without fat saturation, as the lesion follows the appearance of fat on all sequences. The process typically spares the fossa ovalis, creating a typical dumbbell-shaped lesion. Diagnosis requires the interatrial septum to be greater than 2 cm thick. Lipomatous hypertrophy of the interatrial septum appears to be associated with increasing age and obesity, and has been shown to be an etiology of atrial arrhythmias. Surgery is performed if there is SVC obstruction or intractable atrial arrhythmias.[15]

Intracardiac thrombi represent the most common cardiac mass. Thrombi are often located within the left atrial appendage (in patients with atrial fibrillation) or in the LV (in patients with prior large myocardial infarctions). The decreased function leading to the stasis of blood in such settings allows for the formation of thrombus. Another common location is the RA in the setting of a central venous catheter. Fibrin sheaths develop around chronic indwelling central venous catheters, providing a nidus

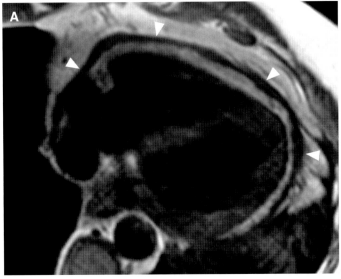

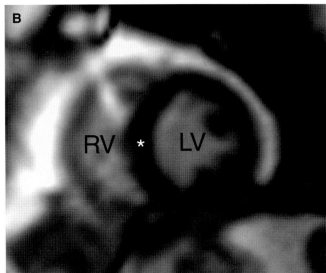

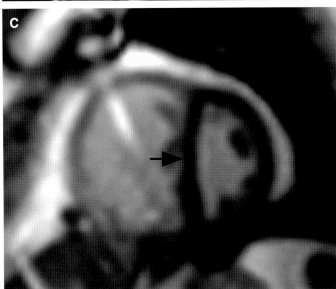

Figure 10.25 *Constrictive pericarditis.* The hallmark of pericardial constriction is a thickened pericardium greater than 4 mm. (**A**) T1-weighted FSE/TSE image demonstrates an irregularly thickened pericardium with signal intensity iso-intense to myocardium. Ventricular interdependence occurs in the setting of pericardial constriction due to the decreased compliance of the fibrotic pericardium. Real-time short-axis SSFP imaging can be employed to detect interdependence by imaging throughout the respiratory cycle. (**B**) At end-expiration, there is a normal appearance of the right ventricle (*RV*), interventricular septum (*), and left ventricle (*LV*). (**C**) During inspiration, the intrathoracic pressure is decreased, resulting in increased blood return to the right heart. Due to the fixed volume of the fibrotic pericardium, left ventricular filling is limited by right ventricular filling, resulting in a shift of the interventricular septum to the left (*arrow*).

for thrombus formation. Thrombus can then become adherent to right atrial structures, particularly the crista terminalis.

Overall, cardiac neoplasms are exceedingly rare. Metastatic involvement of the heart is most frequently encountered, occurring approximately 30 times more often than primary tumor involvement. Primary cardiac neoplasms are characterized as either benign or malignant, with benign tumors representing 75% of all primary cardiac neoplasms.[13,16,17]

BENIGN PRIMARY CARDIAC TUMORS

Myxomas account for approximately 50% of all benign cardiac neoplasms. They have a female predominance and occur between the fourth and seventh decades. The clinical presentation can be varied but usually includes at least one of the classic triad of constitutional symptoms (fever, malaise, weight loss), valvular obstruction, or embolic events. Cardiac myxomas are gelatinous in nature, are often covered with

---

Box 10.3 ESSENTIALS TO REMEMBER

- Pericardial cysts appear as thin-walled unilocular simple cysts containing fluid that is low in signal intensity on T1-weighted and high in signal intensity on T2-weighted images.

- The signal intensity patterns of pericardial effusions will differentiate simple transudative effusions from proteinaceous or hemorrhagic exudative or post-traumatic effusions.

- Constrictive pericarditis is evidenced by thickening of the pericardium exceeding 4 mm.

thrombus, and may contain calcifications. Morphologically, they are always intracavitary and typically solitary, and are most often located in the LA. On MRI, myxomas are well-defined masses that demonstrate high signal on T2-weighted images due to the gelatinous nature, often are dark and heterogeneous on cine gradient-echo images due to thrombus and calcifications, and appear heterogeneous on late gadolinium enhancement imaging. Myxomas are often pedunculated, arising from the fossa ovalis. Cine SSFP images may reveal valvular obstruction as the mass passes through the mitral or tricuspid valve (Fig. 10.26).

Rhabdomyoma is the most common primary tumor of infancy and childhood, is associated with tuberous sclerosis in 50% of cases, and accounts for 20% of all primary cardiac tumors. Most tumors are discovered incidentally and will regress spontaneously. Morphologically, rhabdomyomas are multiple and have an intramural ventricular location, often involving the intraventricular septum. When not associated with tuberous sclerosis, they are more likely to be single and less likely to spontaneously regress. CMR reveals intramural masses that distort the normal ventricular morphology, alter focal contraction, and are homogenously iso-intense to slightly

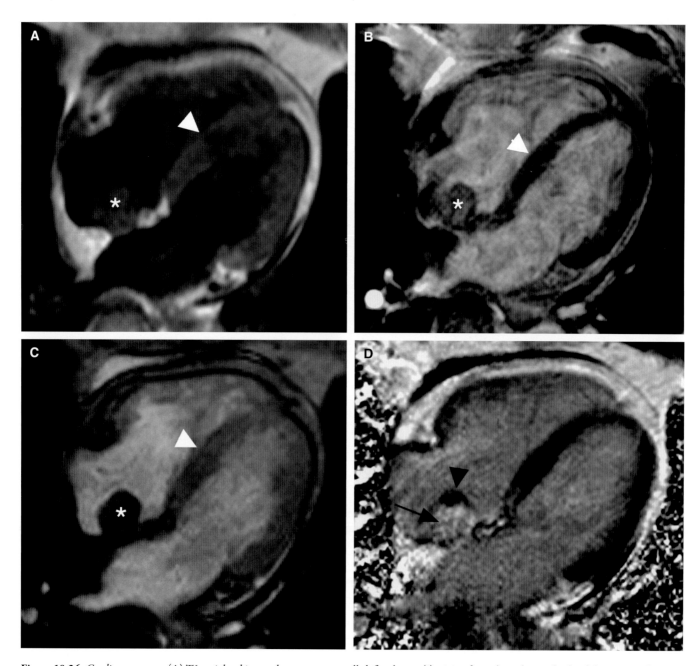

Figure 10.26 *Cardiac myxoma.* (**A**) T1-weighted image demonstrates a well-defined mass (*) arising from the right atrial side of the interatrial septum in the region of the fossa ovalis. The myxoma (*) is relatively iso-intense to normal myocardium (*arrowhead*). On the T2-weighted image (**B**), the myxoma (*) is hyperintense to normal myocardium (*arrowhead*) and on gradient-echo imaging (**C**), it is hypointense to the normal myocardium, due to its composition of blood products and calcium. (**D**) Late gadolinium-enhanced imaging shows a heterogeneous enhancement mass (*arrow*) with a cap of bland thrombus (*arrowhead*), which is a risk for embolization.

hyperintense to normal myocardium on T1-weighted images and are hyperintense on T2-weighted images (Fig. 10.27).

Fibromas constitute the second most common primary cardiac tumor of childhood, with one third of cases presenting before 1 year of age. Histologically, the tumor is composed of a homogenous proliferation of fibroblasts. Presentation is often symptomatic due to arrhythmias, heart failure, or cyanosis; however, one third of cases are detected incidentally. Similar to rhabdomyomas, cardiac fibromas are intramural tumors that tend to be located in the intraventricular septum and present as a singular, focal mass. Calcifications are often present but may not be appreciated on MRI. Diagnosis of fibromas is fairly specific in that the tumors are iso-intense to myocardium on T1-weighted images and markedly hypo-intense on T2-weighted images due to the fibrous nature. Perfusion imaging demonstrates a hypovascular mass, which is strikingly hyperintense on late gadolinium enhancement images (Fig. 10.28).

Lipomas are rare tumors composed of an encapsulated mass of mature adipose tissue, similar to extracardiac lipomas. Cardiac lipomas tend to occur on the endocardial surface of the RA or within the interatrial septum. They are typically homogenous but may contain thin septations. The approach to imaging is similar to lipomatous hypertrophy of the interatrial septum, as they follow fat on all sequences.

MALIGNANT PRIMARY CARDIAC TUMORS

Malignant tumors make up 25% of primary cardiac tumors, with sarcoma representing about 95% of cases and primary cardiac lymphoma the next most common. Compared to benign tumors, malignant tumors are locally invasive and are clinically more aggressive, often resulting in rapid development of heart failure, bloody pericardial effusion, tamponade, SVC syndrome, and arrhythmias.

Angiosarcoma is the most common primary cardiac sarcoma and accounts for approximately 40% of cases. The tumors tend to occur in the RA and involve the pericardium, often resulting in right-sided heart failure or tamponade. Presentation is typically late in the course of the disease, with metastases present at diagnosis. Imaging reveals a bulky, infiltrating mass that has a relatively heterogeneous appearance on T1- and T2-weighted images, with nodular areas of increased signal intensity representing intratumoral hemorrhage. The tumor demonstrates marked heterogeneous enhancement after the administration of gadolinium-containing contrast media.

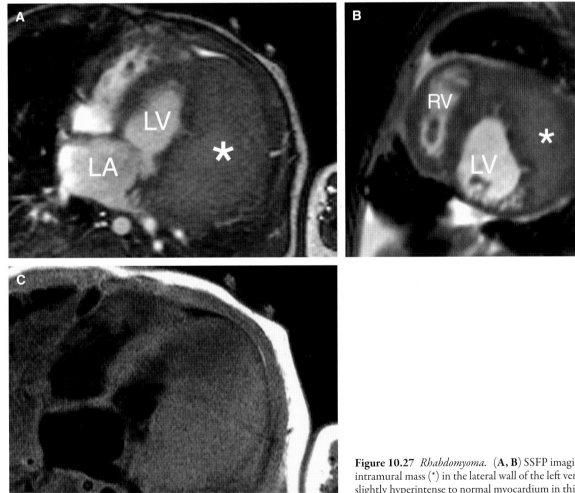

Figure 10.27 *Rhabdomyoma.* (**A, B**) SSFP imaging demonstrates an intramural mass (*) in the lateral wall of the left ventricle (*LV*) that is slightly hyperintense to normal myocardium in this 4-month-old patient. (**C**) On the T1-weighted image, the rhabdomyoma is iso-intense to normal myocardium. *RV*, right ventricle; *LA*, left atrium.

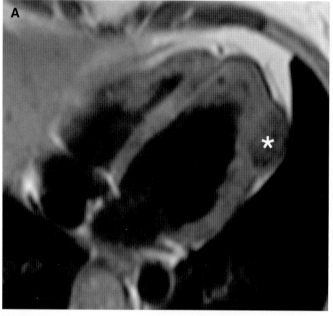

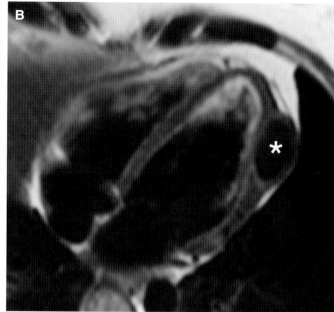

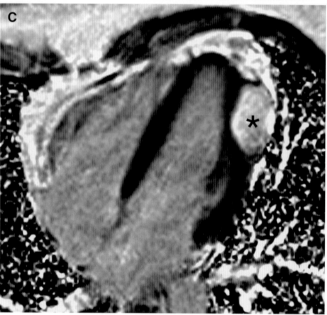

Figure 10.28 *Cardiac fibroma.* (**A**) Four-chamber view demonstrates a well-circumscribed intramural mass (*) that is slightly hypointense to myocardium on T1-weighted spin-echo imaging. (**B**) On T2-weighted spin-echo imaging, the tumor is very dark relative to myocardium due to its fibrous content. (**C**) The fibrous composition results in marked retention of gadolinium contrast media on late enhanced imaging (PSIR).

Diffuse pericardial infiltration is another presentation, where the tumor tends to grow along the perivascular spaces associated with the epicardial vessels, resulting in a "sunray" appearance on contrast-enhanced imaging.

Other sarcomas include malignant fibrous histiocytomas (representing the second most common cardiac sarcoma), undifferentiated sarcomas, osteosarcomas, leiomyosarcoma, fibrosarcoma, and rhabdomyosarcomas. These tumors appear as bulky, infiltrating masses that affect patients between 20 and 50 years of age, except for rhabdomyosarcoma, which has a mean age of occurrence of 14 years.

Primary cardiac lymphoma is a distinct entity, separate from systemic lymphoma, that involves the heart in up to 24% of cases. These tumors are almost always aggressive B-cell lymphomas and have an increased prevalence in patients who are immunocompromised, particularly patients with AIDS.

Patients typically present with shortness of breath, arrhythmias, SVC obstruction, or cardiac tamponade due to the frequent involvement of the pericardium. Imaging reveals tumor nodules that are relatively hypointense on T1-weighted images and hyperintense on T2-weighted images, but signal characteristics are variable. Enhancement is typical, but it may be homogenous or heterogeneous. Late gadolinium enhancement imaging can be useful in delineating the extent of myocardial tumor involvement.

METASTATIC DISEASE OF THE HEART AND PERICARDIUM

Metastatic disease involving the heart often affects the pericardium and is about 20 to 40 times more common than primary neoplasm involvement. Cardiac metastases are encountered in approximately 10% of malignant tumors, but they are often clinically silent.

The tumors that most frequently metastasize to the heart are lung, breast and esophageal carcinoma, lymphoma, and melanoma. Metastatic melanoma is most likely to involve the heart, occurring in 45% to 65% of patients. However, due to the low prevalence of melanoma, metastases from lung and breast carcinoma are more common. The epicardium is the most commonly affected site for metastases due to retrograde spread from mediastinal lymph nodes. Sarcomas and lymphomas metastasize via hematogenous spread, and lead to both myocardial and epicardial deposits. Hematogenous spread is often accompanied by metastases to other organs, particularly the lungs. Direct extension can occur in esophageal, thymic, bronchial, and lung malignancies. Tumor can also spread to the heart through the venous structures, as in lung cancer (via SVC and pulmonary veins) and liver and renal cancer (via the IVC).

Imaging with MR is often performed with standard sequences, for functional assessment and tissue characterization, and contrast-enhanced sequences. The goal of imaging is to differentiate tumor from thrombus, to delineate the involvement of tumor, and to determine the effect on myocardial and valvular function. In the case of primary tumors with direct extension to the pericardium, imaging may be performed to assess resectability. In these cases, tagged imaging may be helpful for determining if the tumor remains free of the epicardial surface. Melanoma may demonstrate characteristic nodular implants that are hyperintense to myocardium on T1-weighted images. Metastatic malignancies will demonstrate myocardial infiltration and abnormal enhancement, are often associated with pericardial effusion, and may have nodular pericardial implants. In the absence of a known primary malignancy, differentiating primary cardiac malignancy from a metastasis may be difficult, necessitating a biopsy to make the final diagnosis.

VALVULAR HEART DISEASE

Despite its low incidence in developed countries relative to ischemic heart disease, valvular heart disease continues to result in significant morbidity and mortality, necessitating over 100,000 valve surgeries every year in the United States. The presence of symptoms, including shortness of breath, dyspnea on exertion, exertional syncope, angina, palpitations, fatigue, or heart failure, combined with the findings at physical examination, including diastolic or systolic murmur, leads to the diagnosis.

Due to its low cost and wide availability, noninvasive imaging with echocardiography is the standard first-line approach to assessing the severity of disease and the effect on the cardiac function, which is used to determine the time of corrective surgery. The role of CMR in the management of valvular dysfunction has not been fully elucidated, and it is often reserved for patients with poor acoustic windows or when the clinical findings do not agree with echocardiographic results. However, CMR has advantages over echocardiography, as it allows to calculate the left and right ventricular volumes (end-diastolic, end-systolic, and stroke volumes) with high accuracy and to directly assess regurgitant flow, something that can be done only indirectly using echocardiography. These advantages are useful for determining the time of intervention, particularly in patients with congenital heart disease.

Normal-functioning heart valves serve to restrict the flow of blood to a single direction in the heart and do not impede the flow when open or allow reversal of flow when closed, except for a trivial amount of "physiologic" regurgitation (usually involving the tricuspid and pulmonary valves). When diseased, however, valve leaflet excursion may be reduced, resulting in valvular stenosis, or the valve leaflets may not coapt completely, resulting in regurgitation. The goal of imaging with CMR is to assess the following features: (1) valvular anatomy, including the number of leaflets, their thickness, and presence of vegetations or masses; (2) valvular function, including degree of stenosis and/or regurgitation; (3) effect of valvular dysfunction on atrial and ventricular volume, function, and mass; (4) effect of valvular dysfunction on aortic and pulmonary artery size; and (5) assessment of cardiac dysfunction not related to valvular heart disease (e.g., coronary disease, cardiomyopathy).

MR imaging of valve disease uses functional cine imaging and velocity-encoded cine MR imaging. Functional cine imaging is used to evaluate chamber function and size as previously described. It can also be used to visualize high-velocity jets caused by valvular stenosis or regurgitation (Fig. 10.29). High-velocity flow through a small orifice causes turbulence, leading to intravoxel dephasing of protons, which is visualized as a dark jet on cine imaging. Functional cine imaging cannot accurately determine the degree of disease, as the size of the jet is influenced by a number of variables, of which echo time (TE) is the most important. However, it can be used as a qualitative assessment of disease and is useful for determining the direction of the jet, which is needed when attempting to quantify peak velocity.

Velocity-encoded cine MR imaging (VENC), also known as velocity mapping or phase-contrast imaging, is a technique for quantifying the velocity of flowing blood. By measuring the phase shift that occurs as protons in the blood move through a spatially varying magnetic field, information about the velocity and direction of the blood flow can be obtained. The technique is analogous to duplex ultrasound in that a maximum imaging velocity is selected prior to acquisition; aliasing will occur when the velocity of the blood is greater than that of the selective imaging velocity. The VENC acquisition is set up such that the imaging plane is perpendicular to the direction of blood flow. The alignment of the acquisition plane is important because underestimation of velocity can occur if the flow is oblique to the imaging plane, similar to duplex ultrasound. The technique is gated and produces cine images at multiple time points throughout the cardiac cycle. Stationary tissue appears gray in these images, with blood moving through the plane appearing as shades of either white or black, depending on the direction and speed. Blood flow is determined by integating the blood velocities over a cross-sectional area, either a valve orifice or a blood vessel. Quantification of blood velocity and flow is performed by

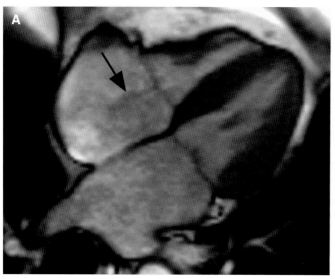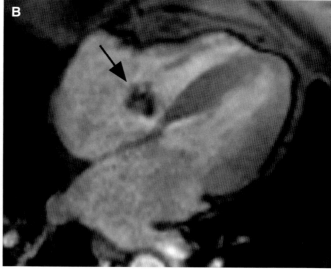

Figure 10.29 *Tricuspid regurgitation.* Intravoxel dephasing due to turbulence is apparent as a dark jet (*arrow*) on both (**A**) SSFP and (**B**) gradient-echo imaging. Due to the properties of the sequence, a gradient-echo sequence is typically more sensitive to dephasing (turbulence) than SSFP, as is demonstrated by the larger jet in this example of mild tricuspid regurgitation.

software that requires the user to outline the cross-section of interest for each image in the series. Time-velocity and time-flow curves can be produced from the data. The pressure gradient across a diseased valve is calculated by applying the modified Bernoulli equation:

$$\Delta P = 4\,V^2$$

where P is the pressure drop across the valve (in mmHg) and V is the velocity (in meters per second). In this manner, VENC MR imaging is used to qualitatively assess the degree of valvular disease.[18–20]

AORTIC VALVE

The aortic valve is a tri-leaflet valve located between the LVOT and the aortic sinuses. There are three valve leaflets or cusps, named left, right, and non-coronary, based on their relationship with the orifices of the coronary arteries. A bicuspid aortic valve results when there is some degree of fusion of two cusps (raphe) or when there is a morphologically two-leaflet valve. Bicuspid aortic valves can result in stenosis and/or regurgitation. Short-axis MR of the aortic valve using SSFP should be performed to assess the valve morphology. Three-chamber or coronal imaging through the center of the aortic valve is used to detect stenosis or regurgitation.

Aortic stenosis may be due to congenital (bicuspid) or acquired (degenerative or rheumatic heart disease) etiologies. The stenosis most commonly develops slowly as part of a degenerative process that includes calcification of the leaflets (fibrocalcific senile aortic stenosis); however, this process is accelerated in patients with bicuspid aortic valves. In subvalvular stenosis, another form of aortic stenosis, a tissue membrane limits ventricular outflow. Supravalvular stenosis, a rare

cause of aortic stenosis, can be isolated or associated with Williams syndrome. The hemodynamic result of aortic stenosis is increased LV afterload leading to concentric LV hypertrophy.

The degree of aortic stenosis is quantified either using planimetry or measuring the stenosis-related accelerated blood velocity. In planimetry, the maximum valve orifice area during systole is measured. Using SSPF, imaging is performed perpendicular to the aortic valve annulus (aortic valve short axis) at the tips of the leaflets. The valve area is outlined using a workstation and the area is measured directly. Using valve area, aortic stenosis is graded as mild, moderate, and severe using cutoff values of more than 1.5 cm², 1.0 to 1.5 cm², and less than 1.0 cm², respectively. Using VENC, aortic stenosis is graded by maximum velocity of the jet. Acquisition is performed using a combination of through-plane and in-plane measurement aligned perpendicular and parallel to the jet, respectively. Using peak velocity, aortic stenosis is graded as mild, moderate, and severe using cutoff values of less than 3.0 m/s, 3.0 to 4.0 m/s, and more than 4.0 m/s, respectively. It should be noted that these values apply only when there is normal LV function. In patients with LV dysfunction, valve area is a more accurate assessment of the degree of aortic stenosis.

Aortic regurgitation is caused by processes that affect proper coaptation of the valve leaflet, including abnormalities of the cusps or annulus or dilatation of the aortic root. Common etiologies include bicuspid aortic valve, bacterial endocarditis, Marfan's disease, aortic root dilatation due to hypertension, and aortic dissection. The speed of onset of aortic regurgitation determines the hemodynamic impact on the heart. Acute development of aortic regurgitation, as in aortic dissection, does not allow time for adaptation, and as a result, rapid increase in LV filling pressures and decrease in cardiac output occur, ultimately leading to cardiogenic shock.

In chronic aortic regurgitation, increase in wall stress leads to LV hypertrophy followed by LV dilation and eventual failure.

Aortic regurgitation can be measured directly using VENC, aligned perpendicular to flow in the tubular portion of the aorta to avoid artifact due to eddy currents near the regurgitant valve. In this manner, the regurgitant volume per stroke can be directly measured, and is calculated as the percentage of retrograde aortic flow to forward aortic flow. Aortic regurgitant fraction is graded as mild, moderate, and severe with values ranging 15% to 20%, 20% to 40%, and more than 40%, respectively. In addition to direct measurement of regurgitation, the etiology of regurgitation should be interrogated, including the valve and aortic root morphology. Measurement of LV function and size should be performed in the evaluation of aortic valvular disease to assess the impact on cardiac function and for planning the timing of therapeutic intervention.

MITRAL VALVE

The mitral valve is located between the LA and LV. It is composed of two leaflets: a short, broad posterior leaflet and a longer anterior leaflet. The posterior leaflet has three ridges denoted as P1 to P3, with P1 located anterolaterally. The anterior leaflet is smooth and segmented into A1 to A3, denoted by the coaptation points of the corresponding posterior segments. Atrial fibrillation develops in 20% to 50% of patients with marked mitral valve disease, significantly limiting evaluation with MRI. Qualitative assessment of mitral disease is best performed in the four-chamber horizontal view.

Mitral stenosis is the consequence of disease processes that limit the opening of the mitral valve, causing a diastolic pressure gradient between the LA and LV. Rheumatic heart disease is the most common cause of mitral stenosis, resulting in fusion of the commissures, thickening of the leaflets, and sclerosis of the chordae tendineae. Mitral stenosis is assessed by measuring the peak velocity of the stenotic jet and calculating the peak pressure gradient. Alternatively, the valve area can be measured directly from short-axis imaging, with an area less than 2.0 cm^2 being considered stenotic and an area less than 1.0 cm^2 being considered severe.

Mitral regurgitation results from abnormalities of the annulus, leaflets, chordae tendineae, or papillary muscles. Small LA and LV volumes, low cardiac output, and pulmonary congestion characterize acute mitral regurgitation. The most common etiologies of acute regurgitation are endocarditis or papillary muscle or chordal rupture from myocardial infarction. Chronic regurgitation can result from a primary process, such as mitral valve prolapse or myxomatous degeneration, or more commonly from secondary causes that result in mitral annular dilatation, including dilated cardiomyopathy, ischemic heart disease, hypertension, and atrial fibrillation.

Mitral regurgitation can be quantified as either the difference between LV stroke volume (measured volumetrically) and forward flow in the aorta (measured by VENC), or by using VENC alone in a short-axis plane parallel to the mitral valve annulus to directly measure the reversal of flow. The second method is technically more difficult due to the translation of the mitral valve during systole but is preferred in the presence of aortic regurgitation. Severity of disease is graded using regurgitant fraction as follows: mild 15% or less, moderate 15% to 25%, moderate to severe 26% to 48%, and severe more than 48%.

PULMONARY VALVE

Pulmonary valve disease can be assessed using the same methods applied to assess aortic stenosis and regurgitation. Standard SSFP imaging in the RV outflow longitudinal view are performed to identify stenotic or regurgitant jets. The hemodynamic consequence of pulmonary valvular disease is determined by RV volumes and ejection fraction.

Pulmonary stenosis can be valvular, supravalvular, or subvalvular and is most commonly congenital. Valvular stenosis is the most common form and results from fusion of the leaflet at the commissure, which is often tolerated for many years. In severe stenosis, the patient presents with symptoms of right heart failure. VENC is performed to assess the pressure gradient across the valve; however, there is no clear consensus on the grading of stenosis. One proposed grading system suggests peak gradients of 20 to 50 mmHg to be considered mild, 50 to 75 mmHg moderate, and more than 75 mmHg severe. Post-stenotic dilatation of the pulmonary artery is also evaluated with MR with the use of SSFP or contrast-enhanced MRA.

Pulmonary regurgitation is more often encountered in patients with congenital pulmonary valve disease who have undergone a valve operation, particularly patients with tetralogy of Fallot. The primary index of severity is the regurgitant fraction, which is measured with through-plane VENC at the pulmonic valve. Valvular regurgitation is graded as follows: mild less than 20%, moderate 20% to 40%, and severe more than 40%.

TRICUSPID VALVE

The tricuspid valve is a tri-leaflet valve with anterior, posterior, and septal leaflets. Tricuspid regurgitation from secondary causes is the most common form of tricuspid valve disease. Due to the relatively weak tricuspid annulus compared to the mitral annulus, it is more prone to dilatation when the RA or RV enlarges. Regurgitation can also occur as a result of endocarditis, particularly in the setting of intravenous drug abuse, or carcinoid syndrome, where serotonin degrades the valve. Tricuspid atresia is a congenital abnormality that occurs in the presence of RV hypoplasia. Tricuspid stenosis may occur when the valve is hypoplastic. Ebstein anomaly is a congenital heart defect in which the septal and, variably, the posterior leaflets are displaced apically, resulting in enlargement of the RA, decreased RV volume, and tricuspid regurgitation. Assessment of tricuspid disease is similar to that for evaluating the mitral valve, with the four-chamber long-axis view being best for determining the presence of stenosis or regurgitation, and a combination of VENC and volumetric imaging used to calculate the stenotic pressure gradient and regurgitant fraction.

CONGENITAL HEART DISEASE

Congenital cardiovascular abnormalities are the most common cause of fatal birth defects and occur in 1% of live births. The goal of imaging is to determine the cardiovascular anatomy and hemodynamics for treatment planning, post-treatment assessment of complications, and for planning the timing of repeat intervention. Echocardiography is the mainstay of imaging congenital heart disease, with MRI playing a complementary role, particularly in older patients, where the acoustic windows may be limited, or where echocardiography cannot provide all the diagnostic information to determine appropriate therapy.

INTRACARDIAC SHUNTS

The heart is a synchronized two-channel pump in which the cardiac output from the right side is equal to that from the left side. Intracardiac shunts arise from defects that allow blood to flow between the right and left sides, resulting in non-equal left and right cardiac outputs. Most commonly, intracardiac shunts arise from atrial septal defects, but they can also result from ventricular septal defects.

Atrial septal defects are the most common form of congenital heart disease, occurring in 1 out of 1,500 live births. They most commonly affect the secundum portion of the interatrial septum, in the region of the fossa ovale. Less commonly, they occur in the primum portion of the septum, which is located near the atrioventricular plane, or in the high posterior septum, in which case they are termed "sinus venous septal defects" and are associated with partial anomalous pulmonary venous return.

Ventricular septal defects may be isolated or may occur in the presence of complex congenital heart disease. The intraventricular septum is composed of a membranous septum, which is located nearest to the atrioventricular valves, and a muscular portion, which is made up of thick myocardium. Ventricular septal defects are classified as perimembranous, muscular, or supracristal. Perimembranous defects are most common, involving the region between the membranous and muscular portions of the ventricular septum, and are associated with aneurysms of the septal leaflet of the mitral valve. Muscular ventricular septal defects are contained completely within the muscular portion and are often multiple. Supracristal ventricular septal defects lie beneath the aortic valve, communicating with the RVOT, and are associated with aortic regurgitation due to prolapse of the right aortic cusp.

In simple congenital heart disease involving isolated intracardiac shunts, flow is typically from left to right, due to the higher left-sided pressures in both the atria and ventricles. An enlarged right heart raises the suspicion for the presence of a shunt. Detection and characterization of septal defects frequently require multiple MR sequences. Often, cine SSFP imaging is performed in multiple planes with the goal of visualizing a discontinuity in the septal wall. Thin slices (maximum 6 mm) are required to prevent volume averaging from obscuring a small defect. Gradient-echo imaging is used to detect turbulence caused by rapid flow through a shunt. First-pass perfusion, acquired during the rapid intravenous administration of contrast medium, is performed in multiple planes in the suspected region of a shunt to investigate flow across the septum. In left-to-right shunts, unenhanced blood from the left side streams into the right-sided chamber that is filled with contrast-enhanced blood before enhanced blood arrives on the left side of the heart (Fig. 10.30). The pulmonary-to-systemic flow ratio (Qp/Qs) is determined from velocity-encoded cine MR (VENC) of the main pulmonary artery and aorta (Fig. 10.31). Ideally, this should be validated by comparing stroke volumes of the left and right ventricles, which should approximate flow in the great arteries in the absence of significant valvular disease.[21,22]

TETRALOGY OF FALLOT

Tetralogy of Fallot is a conotruncal defect that that has a prevalence of 0.5 per 1,000 live births and is the most frequent form of cyanotic heart disease. Tetralogy of Fallot is the result of the conal septum being deviated anteriorly, superiorly, and leftward. This results in a varying degree of RVOT obstruction, consequential RV hypertrophy, an aorta that overrides the ventricular septum, and a perimembranous ventricular septal defect. Repair of tetralogy of Fallot involves relieving the RVOT obstruction and closing the ventricular septal defect. RVOT obstruction can be subvalvular and/or valvular and can be treated with patchplasty of the RVOT, balloon

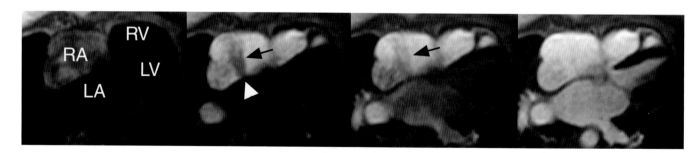

Figure 10.30 *Atrial septal defect.* Four time points from a first-pass perfusion imaging sequence demonstrate enhanced blood entering the right atrium (*RA*) from a peripheral vein injection and sequentially passing through the right ventricle (*RV*), left atrium (*LA*), and left ventricle (*LV*). In the second and third images, a jet (*arrow*) of unenhanced blood is present, originating from the left atrium and passing through the atrial septal defect (*arrowhead*). When both the right and left sides of the heart are enhanced, this defect no longer can be identified. The discontinuity in the atrial septum is never directly identified due to volume averaging, which is common for small defects.

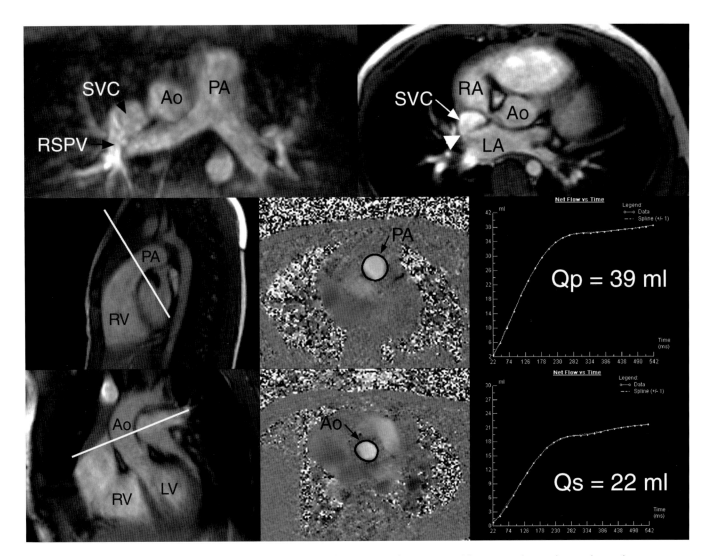

Figure 10.31 *Calculation of pulmonary-to-systemic blood flow (Qp/Qs).* Images are from a 2-year-old patient with partial anomalous pulmonary venous return and sinus venous atrial septal defect. **Top row:** The image on the left is from a contrast-enhanced MRA, showing the partial anomalous pulmonary venous return in which the right superior pulmonary vein (*RSPV*) enters directly into the superior vena cava (*SVC*) rather than the left atrium (*LA*). The image on the right demonstrates the high posterior defect in the atrial septum (*arrowhead*), which represents a sinus venous atrial septal defect. The degree of left-to-right shunting is quantified by the ratio of the pulmonary to systemic blood flow (*Qp/Qs*), which is calculated by measuring blood flow just distal to the pulmonary valve (**middle row**) and aortic valve (**bottom row**). **Middle and bottom rows:** The images on the left localize the velocity-encoded (VENC) imaging plane. The middle images are the resultant VENC images with the regions of interest drawn at the cross-sectional borders of the aorta (*Ao*) and pulmonary artery (*PA*). The graphs on the right are the respective net flow versus time curves. The resulting Qp/Qs is 1.8. *RA*, right atrium; *RV*, right ventricle; *LV*, left ventricle.

Box 10.4 ESSENTIALS TO REMEMBER

- In valvular heart disease CMR is used to assess valve anatomy, degree of stenosis or regurgitation, effect of valve disease on the size and function of atria and ventricles, impact on the size of the pulmonary artery and aorta, and overall cardiac function.

- High velocity blood flow caused by valvular stenosis or regurgitation causes turbulence and intravoxel dephasing of protons resulting in low signal intensity jets on cine imaging.

- Phase contrast velocity mapping is used to determine the velocity and direction of blood flow corresponding to the severity of valvular stenosis or regurgitation.

Box 10.5 ESSENTIALS TO REMEMBER

Rapid advances in MR over the past decade have made comprehensive cardiac evaluation in a single examination possible for patients with heart disease. CMR is now considered the "gold standard" for the assessment of regional and global systolic function, myocardial infarction and viability, and congenital heart disease. As further advances are made and referring physicians become familiar with the wide variety of examinations available, CMR will have a greater role in the diagnosis and monitoring of heart disease.

valvuloplasty, or pulmonary conduit creation. Pulmonary regurgitation is universally present after repair, necessitating imaging follow-up to monitor RV function for timing of pulmonary valve replacement. MR is the reference standard for quantitating RV size and function due to its high accuracy and reproducibility. VENC of the main pulmonary artery is performed to quantify the regurgitant fraction. Postoperative complications, including aneurysm of the RVOT patch, are easily characterized with MR imaging.[23]

TRANSPOSITION OF THE GREAT ARTERIES

Transposition of the great arteries, another conotruncal defect, occurs when the aorta and pulmonary artery are transposed, with the aorta arising from the RV and the pulmonary artery arising from the LV. In the most common form, d-TGA, this ventricular–arterial discordance results in separation of the pulmonary and systemic circuits, which is incompatible with life in the absence of an intracardiac shunt to allow mixing of the saturated and desaturated blood. Surgical corrections performed decades ago (Mustard and Senning procedures) focused on redirecting the inflow with atrial baffles that directed the systemic venous return to the LA and the pulmonary venous return to the RA. The RV remained the systemic ventricle, which over the long term resulted in RV dysfunction and failure. Today, perinatal intervention is performed with an arterial switch, where the aorta and the pulmonary artery are surgically exchanged to create normal ventricular–arterial concordance.

In patients repaired with atrial baffles, imaging is performed to assess RV size and function, baffle obstructions or leaks, LVOT and RVOT obstruction, tricuspid regurgitation, and descending aortic pulmonary collaterals. In arterial switch patients, complications include aortic root dilatation, aortic regurgitation, and pulmonary artery stenosis. A comprehensive imaging protocol includes SSFP for anatomic and functional assessment as well as baffle assessment; MRA for detection of stenosis, aneurysms, and collateral vessels; VENC for assessment of regurgitation; and late gadolinium enhancement imaging for detection of myocardial fibrosis.[24]

COARCTATION OF THE AORTA

Coarctation of the aorta is a congenital stenosis of the descending thoracic aorta that occurs in the region of the aortic isthmus. Its location is described as preductal, ductal, or postductal depending on its relation to the ligamentum arteriosum. The transverse aortic arch is often elongated and hypoplastic. Coarctation of the aorta is classified as simple,

when it is an isolated finding, or complex, when it occurs with other intracardiac abnormalities such as bicuspid aortic valve, atrial septal defect, ventricular septal defect, patent ductus arteriosus, and conotruncal abnormalities. As the severity of aortic coarctation and the presence of associated abnormalities varies, the age at which patients present is highly variable, with those having more severe disease presenting earlier.

The exact location and morphology of the coarctation, the location and size of collateral vessels, the degree of aortic stenosis, the presence of associated cardiac abnormalities, and the presence of complications after intervention can be evaluated with imaging. MR angiography is used to determine the location and morphology of the coarctation as well as the presence of collateral vessels, postoperative aneurysm, or restenosis. Gradient cine imaging is used to determine if there is turbulent flow at the level of the coarctation. VENC is used to determine the pressure gradient across the stenosis, which gives information about the severity in the absence of significant collateral vessels. This should be performed both with in-plane and through-plane measurement to determine the maximum velocity, similar to the method for assessing a stenotic valve. The pressure gradient across the coarctation will be low in the presence of well-developed collateral vessels, and quantification of collateral flow is a better method for determining severity in this case. Through-plane VENC is performed in the descending aorta just distal to the coarctation and at the diaphragm to determine flow. Normally, the flow should be about 5% *less* at the diaphragm due to flow out of the aorta through the intercostal arteries.[21]

REFERENCES

1. Wright J, Bogaert J. Role of cardiac magnetic resonance imaging in ischaemic heart disease. *Intern Med J.* 2009;39:563–573.
2. Nagel E. Left ventricular function in ischemic heart disease. In: Higgins CB, de Roos A, eds. *MRI and CT of the Cardiovascular System*, 2nd ed. Philadelphia: Lippincott Williams & Wilkins, 2005:215.
3. Klem I, Heitner JF, Shah DJ, et al. Improved detection of coronary artery disease by stress perfusion cardiovascular magnetic resonance with the use of delayed enhancement infarction imaging. *J Am Coll Cardiol.* 2006;47:1630–1638.
4. Allman KC, Shaw LJ, Hachamovitch R, Udelson JE. Myocardial viability testing and impact of revascularization on prognosis in patients with coronary artery disease and left ventricular dysfunction: a meta-analysis. *J Am Coll Cardiol.* 2002;39:1151–1158.
5. Karamitsos TD, Francis JM, Myerson S, et al. The role of cardiovascular magnetic resonance imaging in heart failure. *J Am Coll Cardiol.* 2009;54:1407–1424.
6. Olimulder MA, van Es J, Galjee MA. The importance of cardiac MRI as a diagnostic tool in viral myocarditis-induced cardiomyopathy. *Neth Heart J.* 2009;17:481–486.

7. Abdel-Aty H, Boye P, Zagrosek A, et al. Diagnostic performance of cardiovascular magnetic resonance in patients with suspected acute myocarditis: comparison of different approaches. *J Am Coll Cardiol.* 2005;45:1815–1822.

8. Hansen MW, Merchant N. MRI of hypertrophic cardiomyopathy: part I, MRI appearances. *AJR Am J Roentgenol.* 2007;189:1335–1343.

9. Hansen MW, Merchant N. MRI of hypertrophic cardiomyopathy: Part 2, Differential diagnosis, risk stratification, and posttreatment MRI appearances. *AJR Am J Roentgenol.* 2007;189:1344–1352.

10. Jain A, Tandri H, Calkins H, Bluemke DA. Role of cardiovascular magnetic resonance imaging in arrhythmogenic right ventricular dysplasia. *J Cardiovasc Magn Reson.* 2008;10:32.

11. Sparrow PJ, Merchant N, Provost YL, et al. CT and MR imaging findings in patients with acquired heart disease at risk for sudden cardiac death. *Radiographics.* 2009;29:805–823.

12. White JA, Patel MR. The role of cardiovascular MRI in heart failure and the cardiomyopathies. *Magn Reson Imaging Clin North Am.* 2007;15:541–564.

13. Grizzard JD, Ang GB. Magnetic resonance imaging of pericardial disease and cardiac masses. *Magn Reson Imaging Clin North Am.* 2007;15:579–607.

14. Bogaert J, Francone M. Cardiovascular magnetic resonance in pericardial diseases. *J Cardiovasc Magn Reson,* 2009;11:14.

15. O'Connor S, Recavarren R, Nichols LC, Parwani AV. Lipomatous hypertrophy of the interatrial septum: an overview. *Arch Pathol Lab Med,* 2006;130:397–399.

16. Kim EY, Choe YH, Sung K, et al. Multidetector CT and MR imaging of cardiac tumors. *Korean J Radiol.* 2009;10:164–175.

17. Fieno DS, Saouaf R, Thomson LE, et al. Cardiovascular magnetic resonance of primary tumors of the heart: A review. *J Cardiovasc Magn Reson.* 2006;8:839–853.

18. Didier D, Ratib O, Lerch R, Friedli B. Detection and quantification of valvular heart disease with dynamic cardiac MR imaging. *Radiographics.* 2000; 20:1279–1301.

19. Koskenvuo JW, Jarvinen V, Parkka JP, et al. Cardiac magnetic resonance imaging in valvular heart disease. *Clin Physiol Funct Imaging.* 2009;29:229–240.

20. Bogaert J, Dymarkowski S, Herregods M, Taylor AM. Valvular heart disease. In: Higgins CB, de Roos A, eds. *MRI and CT of the Cardiovascular System,* 2nd ed. Philadelphia: Lippincott Williams & Wilkins, 2005:183.

21. Reddy GP, Araoz PA, Ordovas K, Higgins CB. Congenital heart disease: magnetic resonance evaluation of morphology and function. In: Higgins CB, de Roos A, eds. *MRI and CT of the Cardiovascular System,* 2nd ed. Philadelphia: Lippincott Williams & Wilkins, 2005:385.

22. Valente AM, Powell AJ. Clinical applications of cardiovascular magnetic resonance in congenital heart disease. *Cardiol Clin.* 2007;25:97–110.

23. Krishnamurthy R. The role of MRI and CT in congenital heart disease. *Pediatr Radiol.* 2009;39(Suppl 2):S196-204.

24. Babar JL, Jones RG, Hudsmith L, et al. Application of MR imaging in assessment and follow-up of congenital heart disease in adults. *Radiographics.* 2010;30(4):1145.

11.

VASCULAR MR IMAGING

Patrick T. Norton, MD and Klaus D. Hagspiel, MD

Noninvasive imaging is the initial step in the diagnosis and differentiation of many vascular diseases. MR is well suited for imaging vascular pathology as it delivers high-resolution anatomic imaging of the vasculature and provides physiologic information with regard to blood flow and perfusion, all without exposing the patient to ionizing radiation. This section will explore the technical aspects of imaging the vascular system and review the imaging features of extracranial vascular pathology.

MR TECHNIQUES

State-of-the-art MR imaging of the vasculature requires a 1.5T system with fast gradients and dedicated phased-array coils, needed for parallel imaging techniques. Although 3T systems have the advantage of higher signal-to-noise (SNR) ratios compared to those of lower-field-strength systems, there has yet to be significant evidence that the incremental improvement in image quality leads to improved performance characteristics. A power injector for the intravenous delivery of contrast media is essential for high-quality gadolinium contrast-enhanced MR angiography (ceMRA). The ability to perform cardiac gating is a prerequisite for many unenhanced MRA techniques and significantly improves imaging of the vessels in regions prone to motion artifact, such as the ascending aorta. In addition to the hardware and software used for acquisition, a workstation capable of 3D post-processing, particularly with the ability to perform multiplanar reconstructions (MPR) and maximum intensity projection (MIP) reconstructions is essential for accurate interpretation of MRA data sets.

UNENHANCED MR ANGIOGRAPHY

Time-of-flight angiography (TOF) was one of the earliest techniques developed for MRA. This technique can be performed as either a 2D or 3D acquisition but is most often performed in the 2D form in the body and extremities. 2D TOF relies on saturating spins in the imaging slice and then imaging the slice after allowing blood with unsaturated spins to flow into the slice. An additional saturation band can be applied on either side of the imaging slice to selectively null arterial or venous blood entering the slice. TOF is best performed for vessels that course perpendicular to the slice (e.g., aorta in the body and the vessels in the extremities) as inflow of unsaturated spins is then strongest; however, the technique is less sensitive in depicting blood flowing parallel to the imaging slice and thus performs poorly at imaging tortuous vessels. The advantage of 2D TOF is that blood flow in a single direction can be isolated, which is often useful in venous-mapping applications in cases of chronic venous occlusion. The disadvantage of a TOF sequence is that it takes several minutes to acquire the images and thus is highly susceptible to motion artifacts when the patient is breathing. ECG gating is often used in conjunction with TOF to improve signal characteristics at the cost of longer acquisition times.

Balanced steady-state free precession (bSSFP) is an MR technique with high SNR that produces bright blood images due to the intrinsic properties of blood, rather than flow characteristics. bSSFP image contrast is proportional to T2/T1. Since blood has a long T2 and short T1 compared to most tissues, vessels appear bright on bSSFP. Multislice imaging can be performed in orthogonal planes for assessing the size of aneurysms. Cine versions are used routinely in cardiac imaging and can be employed for assessment of dissection flaps and valvular pathology. Recently, 3D respiratory and ECG-gated SSFP sequences have been developed that produce high-resolution MR data sets comparable to ceMRA of the abdominal and pelvic vessels without the need for breath holding. However, this technique is not as robust as ceMRA and requires additional experience of the technologist, and acquisition of the images takes 5 to 10 minutes, depending on the size of the slab (imaging volume) needed to cover the vasculature.

CONTRAST-ENHANCED MR ANGIOGRAPHY

Gadolinium contrast-enhanced MR angiography (ceMRA) is the workhorse of MR vascular imaging, providing high resolution and fast acquisition. ceMRA employs a 3D gradient-echo acquisition that is timed to peak enhancement of the target vascular territory for arterial imaging. Repeat acquisition, without additional contrast agent administration, provides venous-phase images. Parallel imaging techniques, which exploit spatially distributed receiver characteristics of multi-channel coils and undersampling of k space, reduce acquisition time and are used to produce 3D data sets composed of submillimeter voxels that can be obtained within a breath hold.

The extent of imaging coverage in the cranial-caudal direction of the patient for a single MR acquisition is typically limited to approximately 70 cm for most modern MR scanners. To image larger regions, such as required for the entire vasculature of the lower extremities, a multi-station approach is employed. A station is defined as a region of coverage for a single acquisition. Prior to multi-station imaging, the technologist defines the location of the stations, with some overlap between adjacent stations. Multi-station arterial-phase ceMRA is performed after intravenous administration of contrast material with acquisition of the first station. When this is completed, the scanner moves the table position to the next station, after which the next acquisition immediately begins. This process continues until all stations are acquired. With this approach, whole-body imaging in both arterial and venous phases with administration of one bolus of contrast material can be performed.

Arterial signal in ceMRA is based solely on the T1-shortening effect of the gadolinium in the contrast material bolus during its first pass through the vasculature. Therefore, correct timing of the gadolinium bolus is essential for obtaining images with high signal in the arteries, and use of an automated power injector is strongly preferred for optimal injection of the gadolinium contrast material bolus. The goal of arterial imaging is to have peak enhancement of the vasculature coincide with the acquisition of the center data of k space, where low spatial frequencies predominantly contribute to the contrast in the image. To achieve this goal, theoretically two independent durations need to be known: the time from the beginning of the injection to the time of peak arterial enhancement, and the time from the beginning of the MRA acquisition to the acquisition of the center of the k space. Thus, the time to the beginning of acquisition would occur at the time to peak arterial enhancement minus the time to the center of

k space (See also Figure 2.18 of Chapter 2). It is important to tailor the injection to the type of k-space mapping (e.g., sequential versus centric) as this determines when the center of k space is acquired. The peripheral k-space lines determine image detail, so it is not necessary to maximize arterial enhancement during this phase of data acquisition. For this reason, the effect of the gadolinium bolus needs to last for only part of the scan duration, which allows for a reduced contrast material dose and a higher injection rate. The injection rate should be adjusted to such level that the duration of the injection is approximately one half to two thirds of the scan duration. Typically, intravenous administration of the contrast material bolus for ceMRA is performed by injection into one of the antecubital veins, with an injection rate ranging from 1.5 to 2.5 mL/sec. While an injection with a high flow rate and short duration improves contrast-to-noise ratio and image quality, it does require precise timing.

There are two main strategies for achieving accurate bolus administration timing: the test bolus method and the automatic triggering method. With the test bolus method, the time to initial enhancement is determined by administering a small amount of contrast media (2 mL) during the serial acquisition of low-resolution 2D images planned at the inflow to the vascular territory of interest. Imaging is typically performed at 1- to 2-second intervals starting with the injection of contrast media and terminating after peak enhancement. The time delay is determined as above and contrast-enhanced MRA is performed following the injection of the full volume of contrast media, with imaging initiated after the determined delay. This method allows the operator to modify the delay in patients who have abnormally high or low cardiac output, but requires an additional timing step and additional contrast media.

The automated triggering method relies on monitoring the inflow to the vascular territory of interest during the injection of the entire contrast media volume, rather than a small volume as in the timing bolus method. Monitoring is performed similar to the timing bolus method, with low-resolution 2D imaging at 1- to 2-second intervals. When contrast-enhanced blood first enters the vessel of interest, imaging is initiated. Compared to the timing bolus method, the automated triggering method requires less contrast material and time to prepare, but has a greater risk for failure if an error is made in the monitoring setup, as no corrections can be made once the full volume of contrast material has been injected.

MRA image contrast can be improved by using background subtraction, in which an unenhanced mask data set is obtained and is subtracted from the resultant arterial- or venous-phase MRA images to produce the subtracted data set. Since subtraction removes background signal, the subtracted data sets are ideal for creating 3D MIP or volume-rendered (VR) images. However, subtracted data sets are prone to misregistration artifacts that occur when patients move between mask and enhanced acquisitions. For this reason, vascular lesions identified on subtracted datasets should be verified on the nonsubtracted source images.

Time-resolved MRA (trMRA) provides anatomic detail of the vessel lumen combined with temporal information on the flow of blood through the lumen, similar in appearance to digital subtraction angiography. Currently, all major equipment vendors offer variations of these sequences. In trMRA, rapid acquisitions of multiple 3D ceMRA data sets are obtained, which can then be displayed as 2D angiograms using MIP images. For most clinical applications, 90 seconds of total imaging time is sufficient. Imaging parameters are configured such that acquisition time for each 3D data set is on the order of 1 to 5 seconds. An individual trMRA 3D data set takes significantly less time to acquire compared to a high-resolution ceMRA, which would typically take 15 to 20 seconds for the same volume. To accurately represent rapidly changing flow patterns, the acquisition time of each data set should be short. trMRA techniques use several methods to reduce 3D data set acquisition time. A single 3D data set is composed of multiple slices. Increasing the slice thickness reduces the number of slices needed to image the same volume. Acquisition time, which is proportional to the number of slices acquired, is thus reduced. The use of k-space view-sharing techniques further reduces 3D data set acquisition time. During a trMRA acquisition, contrast in the imaging volume changes rapidly as the contrast media bolus flows through the vessels. However, there is little change in high spatial frequencies, representing the detail in the image. Thus, the periphery of k space can be shared between consecutive time points (views), allowing undersampling of the periphery of k space without image degradation.

In a comprehensive MR examination of the vasculature, trMRA is typically employed prior to high-resolution ceMRA. A small amount of contrast media (6 to 10 mL) is administered intravenously and the sequence is begun 3 to 5 seconds later. The first data set is acquired before enhancement of the blood and is used for subsequent image subtractions. Imaging is performed for an appropriate duration to capture the hemodynamics of interest. Time-resolved imaging is useful in pathologies with characteristic flow patterns, such as vascular malformations or arteriovenous fistulas. Additionally, territories that are prone to venous contamination (simultaneous arterial and venous enhancement), such as the calf when performing MRA of the lower extremity, benefit from trMRA performed prior to high-resolution ceMRA as a way to separate arteries from veins (Fig. 11.1)

ADDITIONAL SEQUENCES

In addition to the MRA techniques described above, comprehensive MR vascular examinations may include additional sequences for assessing tissue characteristics and blood flow. Black blood techniques employ a double-inversion-recovery approach to null flowing blood and are useful for assessing the wall of blood vessels and perivascular structures in the setting of aortic aneurysm, dissections, and inflammatory aneurysms. The typical black blood sequences use an ECG-gated fast/turbo spin-echo that can be either T1 or T2 weighted.

T1-weighted 3D gradient-echo fat-saturated sequences performed prior to and after administration of gadolinium contrast agent are excellent for detecting enhancement within tissues and assessing thrombi in the arterial and venous circulation. Additionally, this sequence is the primary sequence used to detect leaks associated with endografts.

2D phase-contrast MR, also known as velocity-encoded MR, allows for the quantitative assessment of blood flow velocity and direction. Protons flowing parallel to the encoding direction acquire a phase shift that is proportional to their velocity. Acquisition is performed over multiple heartbeats using ECG gating, producing a series (cine) of velocity images. Flow is quantified by integrating the flow over the cross-section of the vessel for each time point in the cine. Similar to Doppler ultrasound, a maximum velocity must be selected prior to acquisition, and measurements are subject to aliasing for velocities greater than the selected value. This technique is useful for determining the direction of flow in the portal vein

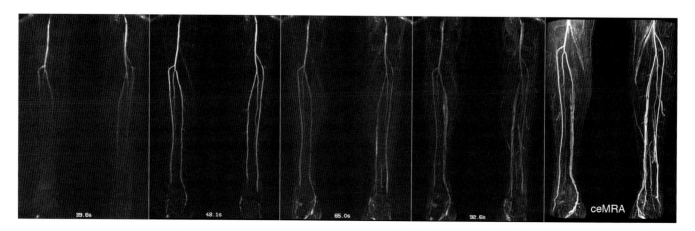

Figure 11.1 *First-pass enhancement of arterial and venous phases.* Time-resolved MRA (trMRA) of the calf showing first-pass enhancement of arterial and venous phases after the administration of 8 mL of gadolinium contrast media (first four images, from left to right). At the time of the second image, there is optimal enhancement of the arteries of the calf. The fourth image shows early venous filling. The last image demonstrates venous contamination of the calf station during multi-station (aortoiliac, thigh, and calf) high-resolution contrast-enhanced MRA (ceMRA). Venous contamination refers to the obscuration of the arterial structures by contrast-enhanced veins and is a consequence of imaging with too much delay after the administration of contrast media. trMRA acquired prior to high-resolution ceMRA allows for discrimination between arteries and veins and provides temporal information about blood flow to the feet.

Box 11.1 ESSENTIALS TO REMEMBER

- 2D-TOF is best used to image vessels that course perpendicular to the slice such as vessels in the extremities. The technique is especially useful for venous mapping in the setting of chronic venous occlusion. However, 2D-OF requires long acquisition times and is susceptible to motion artifact.

- Bright blood imaging without the use of intervenous contrast material is performed with bSSFP.

- Gadolinium-enhanced MR angiography provides high resolution, fast-acquisition vascular imaging and is the sequence of choice for most applications.

- Velocity encoded MR provides assessment of blood flow velocity and direction, which is useful for determining the hemodynamic significance of vascular stenoses and the presence of hepatofugal flow in portal hypertension.

in the setting of portal hypertension or for assessing the vertebral artery in the setting of subclavian artery stenosis; the technique is also good for determining the hemodynamic significance of renal artery stenoses.[1]

THORACIC AORTA AND ABDOMINAL AORTA

The thoracic aorta is the largest artery in the body, receiving the entire systemic cardiac output. It is divided into four sections: aortic root, ascending aorta, transverse aorta, and descending aorta. The aorta is largest at the root, with a mean diameter of 36 mm in adults, and it progressively decreases in size to about 25 mm in the distal thoracic aorta.

The aortic root extends from the annulus of the aortic valve to the sinotubular junction (STJ) and contains three saccular outpouchings, denoted the sinuses of Valsalva. The most anterior of the three is the right sinus of Valsalva, which gives rise to the right coronary artery. The left main coronary artery arises from the left sinus of Valsalva. The third sinus is the posterior, or noncoronary, sinus and is adjacent to the interatrial septum, as noted on imaging parallel to the aortic annulus.

The ascending aorta comprises the tubular portion of the aorta, which extends from the STJ to the innominate, or brachiocephalic, artery. The ascending aorta passes anterior to the left atrium, to the right of the main pulmonary artery, and to the left of the superior vena cava. There are no branches of the ascending aorta and most of this structure is within the pericardial sac.

The transverse aorta, also known as the aortic arch, extends from the brachiocephalic artery to the distal aspect of the left subclavian artery, containing all of the supra-aortic vessels. The normal position of the transverse aorta is to the left of the trachea and esophagus. The normal branching pattern of the supra-aortic vessels is as follows: brachiocephalic artery in the first position, left common carotid in the second position, and left subclavian in the third position (from proximal to distal). The most common variant to this configuration, consisting of a common origin or trunk of the brachiocephalic and left common carotid arteries, occurs in about 15% of the population and has been referred to as a "bovine arch"; this is

a misnomer, however, as ruminant species do not have this configuration. In 5% of the population, the left vertebral arteries arise from the transverse aorta, typically between the left common carotid and left subclavian arteries.

The descending aorta extends from the left subclavian artery to the diaphragm. The aortic isthmus is the portion of the descending aorta between the left subclavian artery and the ligamentum arteriosum. The location of the ligamentum arteriosum can often be identified as the apex of the ductus bump, which is a bulge that is variably present on the lesser curvature of the aorta that should not be confused with an aneurysm. The descending aorta gives rise to visceral (bronchial, esophageal, pericardial, and mediastinal arteries) and parietal (intercostal, subcostal, and superior phrenic arteries) branches. Importantly, the blood supply of the spinal cord arises from the intercostal arteries, and injury and therapeutic intervention to the descending aorta can have catastrophic neurologic impact if this supply is interrupted. The descending aorta is located along the left anterior aspect of the vertebral column, becoming midline in the distal extent.

The aorta passes through the diaphragm at the aortic hiatus, at which point it becomes the abdominal aorta, and extends to the aortic bifurcation. The abdominal aorta gives rise to a number of paired and unpaired visceral and parietal branches, and its diameter decreases from 25 mm proximally to 20 mm distally in the average adult. The visceral branches of the abdominal aorta from proximal to distal include the celiac, superior mesenteric, middle adrenal, renal, gonadal, and inferior mesenteric arteries. The parietal branches are the inferior phrenic, lumbar, and median sacral arteries.

The abdominal aorta bifurcates into paired common iliac arteries at the level of fourth lumbar vertebral body. The common iliac arteries further divide into internal and external branches. Internal branches supply the pelvic organs and musculature, whereas the external iliac branches are conduits that deliver blood to the lower extremities (Figs 11.2 and 11.3)

ANEURYSMAL DISEASE

Aneurysms can be located in any segment of the arterial system but are most common in the aorta, particularly the infrarenal aorta. Aneurysms are generally defined as a segment of vessel

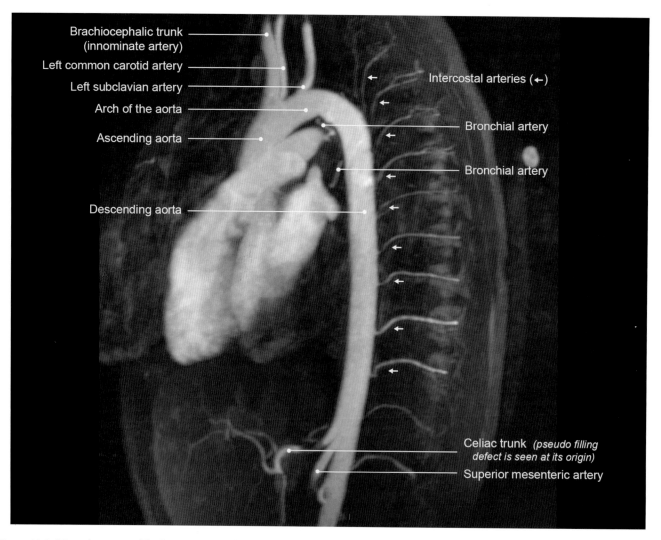

Brachiocephalic trunk
(innominate artery)
Left common carotid artery
Left subclavian artery
Arch of the aorta
Ascending aorta

Descending aorta

Intercostal arteries (←)

Bronchial artery

Bronchial artery

Celiac trunk *(pseudo filling
defect is seen at its origin)*
Superior mesenteric artery

Figure 11.2 *Normal anatomy of the thoracic aorta and branches.* Sagittal sub-volume maximum intensity projection (MIP) image reconstructed from a ceMRA data set acquired in the parasagittal orientation. The pseudo-filling defect in the celiac trunk is due to partial exclusion from the MIP volume. *Small arrows* indicate the intercostal arteries. (This figure was printed in Chapter 2 of Kramer CM, Hundley WG. *Atlas of Cardiovascular Magnetic Resonance Imaging.* Copyright Elsevier, 2010.)

that is 1.5 times larger than the expected diameter of the vessel. The thoracic aorta is considered aneurysmal if the ascending diameter is larger than 4 cm and the descending portion is greater than 3.5 cm. The abdominal aorta is classically considered aneurysmal when the diameter is greater than 3.5 cm. Abdominal aortic aneurysms may extend to included the common iliac arteries, which are considered aneurysmal above 16 mm.

Classification of an aneurysm is based on location and morphology, which suggest the etiology of disease. Location of an aneurysm determines the type of intervention that can be performed and the approach. Thoracic aortic aneurysm locations include sinus of Valsalva, ascending, arch, descending, and a combination thereof. Abdominal aortic aneurysms are classified as suprarenal, juxtarenal, or infrarenal. Thoracoabdominal aneurysms are classified by the Crawford system (Fig. 11.4) into fours classes: (I) complete descending thoracic aneurysm with isolated suprarenal abdominal aneurysm, (II) complete descending thoracic aneurysm extending to the aortic bifurcation, (III) distal descending thoracic aneurysm extending to

the aortic bifurcation, and (IV) abdominal aortic aneurysm from the aortic hiatus to the aortic bifurcation.

Morphology is grouped into saccular, which are eccentric outpouchings from a vessel, and fusiform, which includes centric expansion of the vessel. Alternatively, aneurysm morphology can be grouped into true and false (pseudo-aneurysms). True aneurysms involve dilatation of all three layers of the artery (intima, media, adventitia). Pseudo-aneurysms can represent either a rupture of a vessel that is contained by a hematoma and surrounding connective tissues, or a focal aneurysmal outpouching contained by less than all three layers of the arterial wall. Pseudo-aneurysms can be the result of iatrogenic injury, deceleration injuries, penetrating ulcers, and defects at surgical graft anastomoses. Generally, true aneurysms tend to be fusiform and pseudo-aneurysms tend to be saccular. As it is impossible to resolve the histologic components of the arterial wall involved in an aneurysm, these terms are based on morphology and presumed etiology.

Aneurysm etiologies can be divided into two main groups, congenital and acquired, of which the latter is much

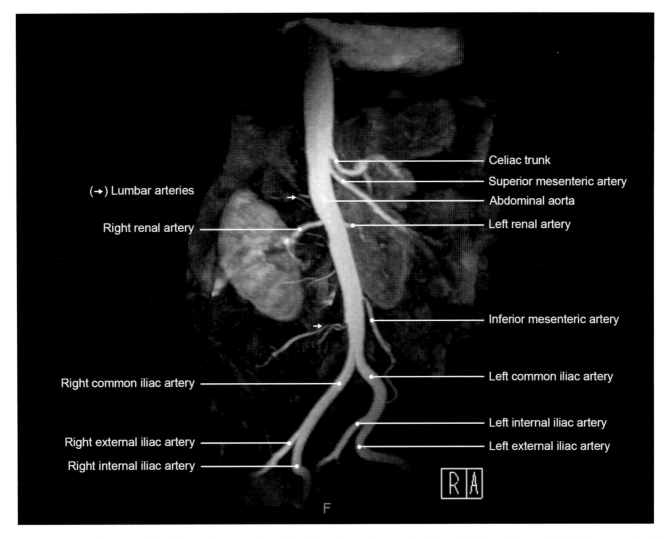

(→) Lumbar arteries

Right renal artery

Right common iliac artery

Right external iliac artery
Right internal iliac artery

Celiac trunk
Superior mesenteric artery
Abdominal aorta
Left renal artery

Inferior mesenteric artery

Left common iliac artery

Left internal iliac artery
Left external iliac artery

Figure 11.3 *Normal anatomy of the abdominal aorta and branches.* Sub-volume right anterior oblique MIP image from a ceMRA data set acquired in the coronal plane. *Small arrows* indicate the lumbar arteries. (This figure was printed in Chapter 2 of Kramer CM, Hundley WG. *Atlas of Cardiovascular Magnetic Resonance Imaging.* Copyright Elsevier, 2010.)

more common. Medial degeneration, a consequence of age-related cyclic repetitive aortic injury and repair, is common to most aortic aneurysms regardless of their cause and location. Atherosclerosis is associated with many aortic aneurysms and may be the inciting cause, as is the case of aneurysms due to penetrating aortic ulcers. Atherosclerosis is less likely to be associated with aneurysms of the ascending aortic compared to elsewhere in the aorta. In Marfan syndromes, genetic abnormalities that affect connective tissue throughout the body result in acceleration of medial degeneration of the aortic root and ascending aorta, leading to bulbous dilatation of the aortic root (annuloaortic ectasia). Aortic aneurysms can also be secondary to infection (mycotic aneurysm), aortoarteritis (Takayasu disease), or an inflammatory aneurysm, which is a rare entity characterized by medial infiltrates and periaortic inflammatory changes. Aortic aneurysm may also be secondary to aortic dissection.[2,3]

The MR imaging protocol used for aneurysms at our institution includes multiplanar bSSFP, ceMRA, and post-contrast 3D gradient-echo with fat-saturation sequences. For patients who cannot receive gadolinium-based contrast agents due to renal insufficiency, multiplanar SSFP is performed in conjunction with TOF of the iliac vessels when appropriate. ECG-gated black blood imaging is added in the thoracic aorta if detailed imaging of the aortic wall is required (e.g., in the determination of coexisting intramural hematoma). In the case of ascending thoracic aortic aneurysms, cine SSFP can be performed at the aortic valve to assess for pathology (Fig. 11.5). ceMRA allows for interrogation of the thoracic and abdominal aorta as well as determination of the patency and location of side branches. Venous-phase ceMRA or subsequent fat-saturated 3D gradient-echo imaging is useful for determining the external diameter of the aneurysmal vessel as well as the amount and location of mural thrombus, both of which are better identified when the adventitia and periaortic tissues become enhanced (Fig. 11.6). These sequences should be reconstructed perpendicular to the vessel axis, which is essential for accurate measurement.[4] bSSFP imaging is quite useful when renal insufficiency precludes use of intravenous contrast media. bSSFP provides good tissue contrast between

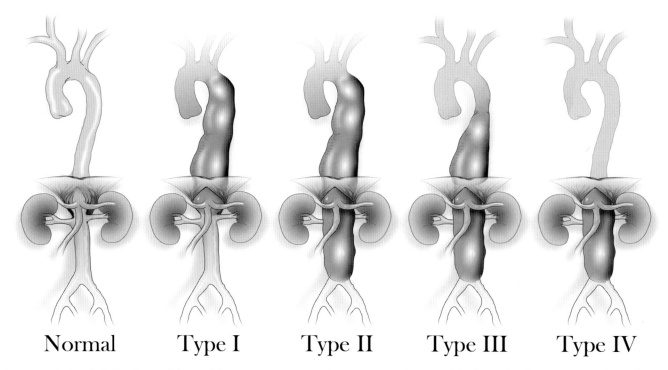

Normal   Type I   Type II   Type III   Type IV

Figure 11.4 *Crawford classification of thoracoabdominal aneurysms. Type I* aneurysms involve most of the descending thoracic aorta, with possible involvement of the ascending aorta (not shown), and extend to the level of the renal arteries. *Type II* aneurysms have a similar extent proximally as type I but also involve the infrarenal aorta. *Type III* aneurysms have less of a proximal extent than type I or II, originating in the mid-thoracic aorta (below the sixth rib), and extend into the infrarenal aorta. *Type IV* aneurysms extend from the aortic hiatus of the diaphragm to the aortic bifurcation. (Artist credit: Philip Cohen)

periaortic tissue, aortic wall, mural thrombus, and lumen. Measurements can be made in the plane of acquisition, but due to the 2D nature of the sequence, MPRs are not very useful. Additionally, bSSFP provides little information regarding luminal narrowing or occlusion of small vessels.[4]

ENDOVASCULAR REPAIR OF AORTIC ANEURYSMS

Over the past decade, endovascular delivery of covered stent-grafts for treatment of aortic aneurysmal disease has become a viable alternative to surgical repair for patients who have suitable anatomy. Thoracic stent-grafts consist of a tubular metallic stent to which a non-porous, biocompatible fabric has been attached, most often along the interior surface. Infrarenal abdominal aortic stent-grafts are modular covered stents, consisting of a main body, which is placed in the aorta and extends into an iliac vessel, and a separately placed contralateral limb, extending from the main body to the contralateral iliac vessel. The goal of stent-grafting is to exclude the aneurysm from blood flow by directing the flow through the stent-graft. Preprocedural assessment of the aortic aneurysm for suitable anatomy is typically performed with CT angiography (CTA) at most centers, but MRA is an important alternative for patients with mild to moderate (glomerular filtration rate [GFR] above 30 mL/min/1.73m2) renal insufficiency. The imaging protocol for aortic stent-graft planning is similar to that for evaluation of aortic aneurysmal disease, consisting of ceMRA with bSSFP and fat-saturated 3D gradient-echo sequences, performed as

needed. The size of the aortic lumen proximal and distal to the aneurysm is measured to determine the appropriate size of the graft. Proximal to the aneurysm, the aorta is assessed for a suitable neck, which is a region of non-aneurysmal aorta at least 1.5 cm long. An adequate neck is needed to ensure a tight seal of the stent-graft to the aortic wall.

Stent-graft placement is performed via a transfemoral approach, and the entire route of access to the aneurysm should therefore also be included in the evaluation. Thus, in the case of a thoracic aneurysm, total coverage of imaging includes the chest, abdomen, and pelvic regions. Venous-phase ceMRA imaging should also be performed to identify potential pitfalls, such as retroaortic renal veins, in case the aneurysm is not suitable for endovascular repair and surgery has to be performed.

Both CT and MR can be used for assessment of stent-graft complications following placement, such as endoleaks and stent failure. An endoleak occurs when the treated aneurysmal sac becomes repressurized due to continued blood flow in the excluded aneurysm sac. There are several types of endoleaks: type 1, leakage around the ends of the graft; type 2, back-flow through side branches of the aorta that are covered by the graft; type 3, structural failure of the graft or leakage between modular components; and type 4, leakage through the fabric of the graft prior to endothelialization. Type 5 endoleak, or endotension, is a controversial entity representing an enlarging aneurysm sac in the absence of a visualized endoleak. Repressurization of the aneurysm sac in the setting of endoleak can lead to progressive growth of the aneurysmal sac and

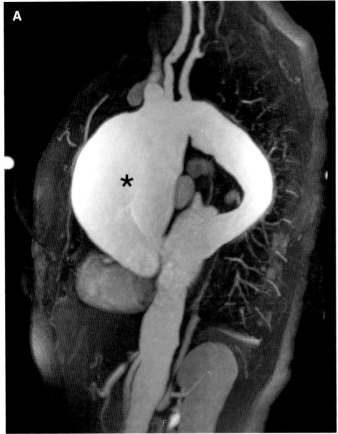

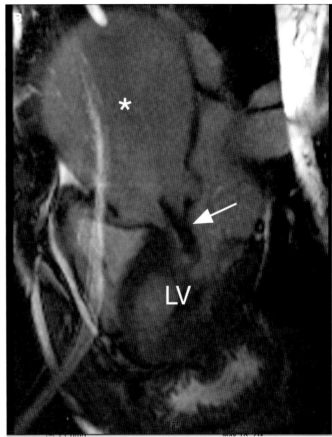

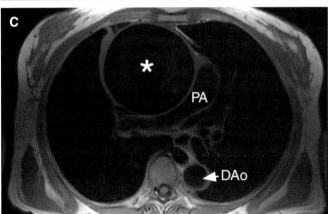

Figure 11.5 *Aneurysm of the ascending thoracic aorta.* A 78-year-old woman presented for evaluation prior to surgery. (**A**) Sagittal sub-volume MIP reconstruction image from an arterial-phase ceMRA shows a large aneurysm (*) of the tubular portion of the ascending thoracic aorta. There is ectasia of the brachiocephalic artery (first branch of aortic arch) and aortic dilatation of the proximal arch, necessitating a complex hemi-arch repair. (**B**) Diastolic image from an ECG-gated SSFP cine image demonstrates a jet (*arrow*) of aortic regurgitation, caused by dilatation of the aortic annulus. *LV*, left ventricle. *, aneurysm of the ascending aorta (**C**) ECG-gated black blood T1-weighted FSE/TSE image shows massive dilatation of the ascending aorta (*), which displaces the main pulmonary artery (*PA*). The wall of the aneurysm is thin and there is no intramural hematoma or aortic dissection. *DAo*, descending aorta.

potentially rupture. Definitive diagnoses of complications, including endoleak, can be made with either MR or CT. MRA surveillance of endograft complications is not practical in case the endografts consist of stainless steel because of the large artifacts produced from susceptibility effects; additionally, there is a theoretical risk of stent migration in these grafts caused by the strong magnetic field. MRA surveillance is therefore currently approved only for nitinol-based grafts. In addition to ceMRA, post-procedural assessment should include unenhanced and contrast-enhanced fat-saturated 3D gradient-echo imaging of the aneurysmal sac. Enhancement in the excluded aneurysm sac represents an endoleak, which is classified by the source of enhancement as above (Fig. 11.7).

ACUTE AORTIC SYNDROME

Compared to uncomplicated aneurysmal disease, which is typically diagnosed in asymptomatic patients, acute aortic disease typically presents with chest and/or back pain in the setting of hypertension. Hemodynamic compromise may also exist at presentation. The three aortic conditions to consider in this setting are intramural hematoma, penetrating athero-sclerotic ulcer, and aortic dissection. Although each of these entities has a different mechanism of origination, several path-ways of progression have been described linking one entity to another. It is not uncommon to observe several coexisting entities in the same patient, making it difficult to identify the inciting cause. *Acute aortic syndrome* is the term used to

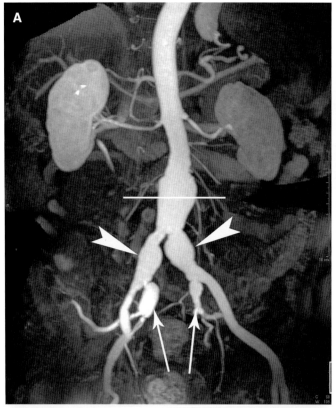

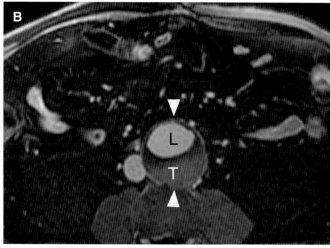

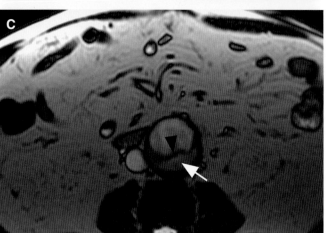

Figure 11.6 *Infrarenal abdominal aortic aneurysm.* A 67-year-old man presented for annual monitoring. (**A**) Sub-volume MIP image of ceMRA acquired in the coronal plane reveals an abdominal aortic aneurysm (at level of *horizontal line*), bilateral common iliac artery aneurysms (*arrowheads*), and bilateral internal iliac artery aneurysm (*arrows*). (**B**) Axial 3D gradient-echo acquisition with fat saturation at the level of the line in image A was performed approximately 5 minutes after the administration of gadolinium contrast agent, delineating the serosal borders of the aneurysm (*arrowhead*). The ceMRA in image A reveals only the lumen (*L*), underestimating the size of the aneurysm when there is significant mural thrombus (*T*). (**C**) Axial SSFP imaging performed prior to contrast agent administration can be used to measure aortic aneurysms when gadolinium is contraindicated. The appearance of the mural thrombus is heterogeneous, with a darker periphery (*arrowhead*) due to hemosiderin or fibrosis, compared to the brighter interior (*arrow*). The similar high intensity of the lumen and central portion of the thrombus can result in the appearance of a dissection flap (*arrowhead*). Hence, additional imaging is sometimes needed to verify the absence of an aortic dissection when contrast media cannot be administered.

denote this heterogeneous group that has similar clinical presentations.

Aortic dissection is the most commonly encountered acute aortic syndrome and also carries the highest mortality rate. A defect in the intima of the aorta allows blood to enter the subintimal space, creating a false lumen that is typically located in the outer third of the media, separated from the true lumen by an "intimal flap." The initial defect, termed the entry site, is caused by abnormal weakness in the vessel wall, most commonly from medial degeneration accelerated by hypertension. The false lumen can propagate either proximally or distally, or in both directions, sometimes involving the entire length of the aorta. Subsequently, connections between the false and true lumen may develop; these are termed re-entry sites or fenestrations. In patients who develop aortic dissection at a young age, there is typically an underlying disorder that weakens the wall, such as Marfan disease, pregnancy, coarctation, bicuspid aortic valve, or cocaine use. The most common place of entry is at the right anterolateral aspect of the ascending aorta, due to the high hydrodynamic stresses in this area. The next most common location is in the descending aorta just distal to the origin of the left subclavian artery. Rarely, an aortic dissection may be isolated to the abdominal aorta. During the development of a dissection, the false lumen tends to spiral around the aorta as it progresses distally, located right anteriorly in the ascending aorta, superiorly and posteriorly in the transverse aorta, and to the left in the descending aorta. The true lumen is typically smaller than the false lumen and

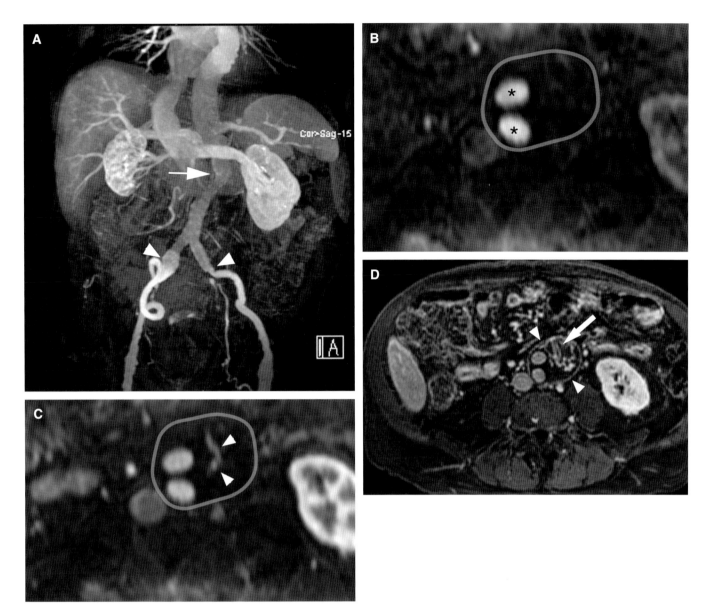

Figure 11.7 *Endograft leak.* An infrarenal abdominal aortic aneurysm was repaired with an endograft in 63-year-old man. (**A**) MIP image of a ceMRA sequence obtained in the coronal plane demonstrates the morphology of an aortic endograft. The proximal landing site of the graft (*arrow*) is in the abdominal aorta, inferior to the renal arteries. The distal landing sites (*arrowheads*) are in the common iliac arteries. The textured appearance of the endograft is caused by the metallic skeleton of the endograft, which reduces the signal from the enhanced blood within the endograft. (**B**) Axial image reconstructed from the arterial-phase ceMRA sequence, demonstrating luminal enhancement of the limbs (*) of the endograft. *Gray outline* represents the border of the aneurysm sac. (**C**) Early-venous-phase reconstructed image reveals an endoleak, as shown by a small focus of enhancement (*arrowheads*) within the aneurysm sac that was not present in the arterial-phase image shown in image B. (**D**) An axial 3D gradient-echo image with fat saturation obtained after the ceMRA shows progressive irregular enhancement (*arrow*) within the aneurysm sac, confirming the presence of an endoleak. The wall of the aneurysm sac shows enhancement on this phase (*arrowheads*).

has high-velocity flow compared to the slow, turbulent flow of the false lumen. The false lumen may enlarge to such an extent that it compromises the flow in the true lumen.

Aortic aneurysms may occur when the weakened exterior wall of the false lumen is exposed to systemic pressures, resulting in dilatation of the aorta and eventual rupture (Fig. 11.8). Aortic dissection may propagate into the branch vessels and occlude them, leading to stroke, renal failure, mesenteric ischemia, or myocardial infarction. If there is retrograde propagation into the aortic root, there can be disruption of the aortic valve, resulting in acute, severe aortic regurgitation and

heart failure. Rupture of ascending aortic dissections into the pericardium can cause cardiac tamponade. Classification of aortic dissections is based on the anatomic location and extension of the intimal flap. By the commonly used Stanford classification, a dissection is type A if it involves the ascending aorta and type B if it spares it. Type A dissections require surgical intervention because of the high risk for extension into the aortic root and for the other catastrophic complications described before. Type B aortic dissections can be treated medically with antihypertensive medication but may require intervention if there is uncontrolled pain, retrograde extension

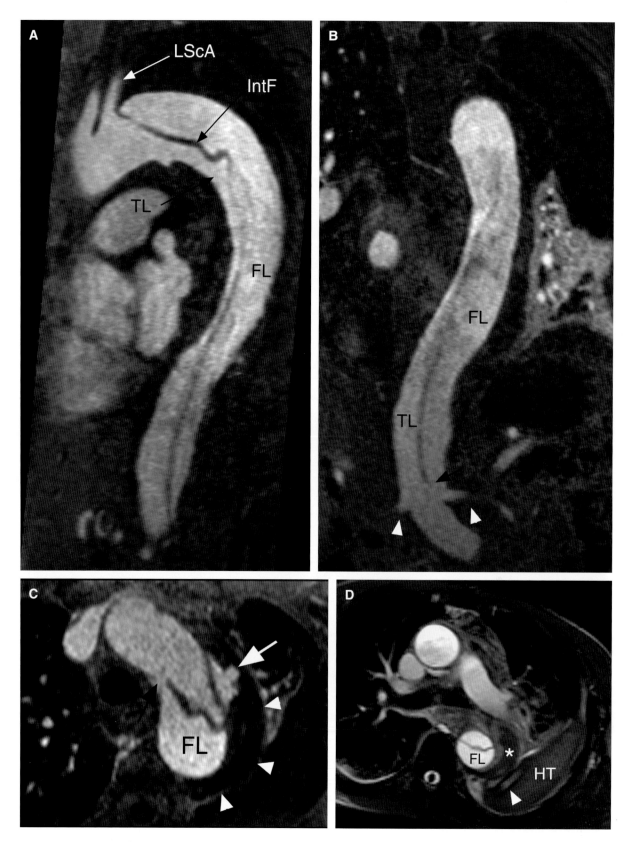

Figure 11.8 *Acute type B aortic dissection.* A 48-year-old man with a history of hypertension initially presented with chest pain and hypotension. Imaging was performed after the patient was stabilized. (**A**) Parasagittal MPR image from ceMRA demonstrates an intimal flap (*IntF*) originating just distal to the left subclavian artery (*LScA*). The false lumen (*FL*) tends to be the larger than the true lumen (*TL*) and in the descending thoracic aorta tends to be located posteriorly. (**B**) Coronal MPR image from ceMRA shows the intimal flap termination (*arrow*) in the abdominal aorta, at the level of the renal arteries (*arrowheads*), due to a re-entry tear. (**C**) The entry tear (*black arrow*) is present in the proximal descending aorta. Due to weakening of the aortic wall from the dissection, there has been a rupture (*white arrow*) of the false lumen (*FL*) into the perivascular space. The perivascular hematoma (*arrowheads*) contains the rupture, in essence forming a large pseudo-aneurysm. (**D**) Axial SSFP image shows an intermediate-signal-intensity fluid collection in the left pleural space representing a hemothorax (*HT*). SSFP is performed without contrast media and is excellent for identifying the intimal flap. The perivascular hematoma (*) and a chest tube (*arrowhead*) are also present in the image.

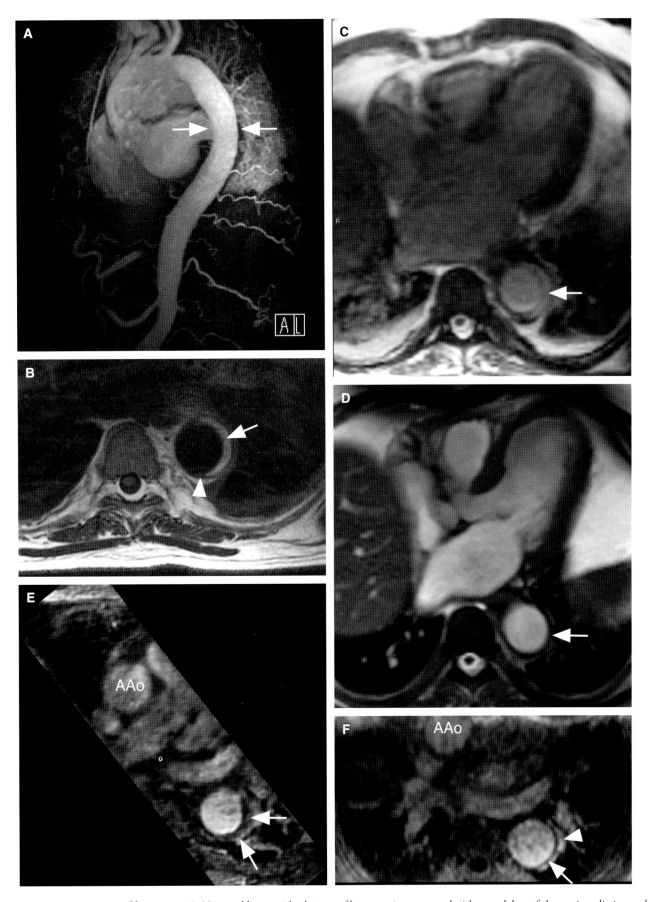

Figure 11.9 *Aortic intramural hematoma.* A 66-year-old man with a history of hypertension presented with several days of chest pain radiating to the back. (**A**) ceMRA image of the thoracic aorta suggests mild luminal narrowing (between *arrows*) in the mid-descending thoracic aorta. (**B**) ECG-gated T1-weighted FSE/TSE axial image of the mid-descending thoracic aorta reveals a relatively high-signal crescentic area within the

(Continued)

Figure 11.9 (*Continued*) aortic wall (*arrow*) compared to the lower-signal, normal-thickness aortic wall (*arrowhead*). (**C**) SSFP gradient-echo image also demonstrates relatively high signal within the aortic wall (arrow), confirming the presence of a subacute intramural hematoma (see text for staging). (**D**) Repeat imaging with SSFP 1 year later shows that there has been reabsorption of the intramural hematoma (arrow). (**E**) Initial venous-phase ceMRA image demonstrates concentric wall thickening (*arrows*) that appears darker in signal intensity than the enhancing lumen; however, differentiating this finding from atheroma on this sequence alone can be difficult. *AAo*, ascending aorta. (**F**) Venous-phase ceMRA image 1 year after initial imaging shows normal-thickness wall (*arrow*). The enhancing atelectatic lung (*arrowhead*) adjacent to the aorta should not be confused with abnormal signal within the aortic wall. *AAo*, ascending aorta.

with transformation to type A, or progressive aneurysmal dilatation. Mortality from aortic dissection is highest during the acute period, which is defined as the first 14 days after initiation of referrable symptoms, with a rate of 1% per hour for the first 24 hours and 75% within the first 2 weeks.[5]

Classically, aortic *intramural hematoma* is defined as rupture of the vasa vasorum in the medial layer resulting in a hematoma of the aortic wall. Unlike an aortic dissection, there is no defect in the intima separating the lumen of the vessel from the hematoma. Arterial hypertension leading to spontaneous rupture of the vasa vasorum is considered the initiating process of intramural hematoma. However, a penetrating aortic ulcer leading to a diseased media as well as blunt chest trauma can result in intramural hematoma. The appearance of intramural hematoma is quite distinct on cross-sectional imaging of the involved aortic segment, appearing as a crescentic thickening of the aortic wall (Fig. 11.9). Clinically, the presentation is common to all acute aortic syndromes, with the primary symptom being tearing chest pain radiating to the back. Prognosis and complications are similar to those associated with aortic dissection, and classification into type A or B using the same system is based on the location and extent of the hematoma. Intramural hematoma is most common within the ascending aorta, with 70% of cases occurring there. In 30% of cases, intramural hematoma will progress to aortic dissection. Intramural hematoma associated with a penetrating aortic ulcer has a less stable course than when no penetrating ulcer is present.

A *penetrating aortic ulcer* is initiated at the site of an atherosclerotic plaque that ruptures and ulcerates, leading to disruption of the internal elastic lamina and blood entering the media. It may result in intramural hematoma or localized intramedial dissection. If the ulceration extends to the adventitia, a focal saccular pseudo-aneurysm extending beyond the normal border of the aortic wall may develop. The adventitia may also rupture, resulting in a hematoma contained by the periaortic tissue or may lead to an uncontained aortic rupture. A unique complication of a penetrating aortic ulcer is the showering of emboli to the distal arterial circulation. Penetrating aortic ulcers are most common in patients who are elderly and hypertensive, with 90% of cases affecting the mid-descending thoracic aorta. Both the depth and maximum diameter are reliable predictors of disease progression.[6]

Imaging of acute aortic syndrome with MR is reserved for patients who are hemodynamically stable. MR is often used as a problem-solving modality when CT results are indeterminate. Several advantages of MR compared to other imaging modalities include the lack of radiation and iodinated contrast material, the ability to image the entire aorta and great vessels,

excellent characterization of the aortic wall, and functional imaging of the aortic valve and intimal flaps. MR is also a choice for patients who have renal insufficiency, with gadolinium contrast agent used only in patients with stage III or above (GFR above 30 mL/min/1.73m^2) renal insufficiency and unenhanced imaging performed in patients with severe renal insufficiency.

In patients with aortic dissection, axial black blood spin-echo sequences reveal the presence of an intimal flap separating the true and false lumens. In the true lumen, the spins in the blood are completely saturated, resulting in signal void. The false lumen shows with higher signal from incomplete saturation of spins due to turbulent, slow-moving blood. Additionally, the false lumen may display webs of crossing tissue, representing remnants of the dissected media. Axial spin-echo and bSSFP images can be used to assess the periaortic tissue for rupture, which can present with a large left pleural effusion, or hemopericardium in the setting of a type A dissection, suggestive of impending rupture into the pericardium. Cine bSSFP imaging is used to differentiate slow flow in the false lumen from a thrombosed false lumen. Additionally, with cine bSSFP the degree of dynamic compression of the true lumen by the intimal flap can be assessed. If a type A dissection is present, cine imaging of the aortic valve can be performed to determine the presence and degree of aortic regurgitation. Aortic regurgitation can be further quantified using velocity-encoded MR. In patients who have adequate renal function, trMRA and ceMRA can be performed to increase the confidence of diagnosis. trMRA demonstrates the temporal sequence of false-lumen perfusion, elucidating the entry tear and providing important information for endovascular treatment of type B dissections. Multi-station, multi-phase ceMRA is performed from the vessels of the neck to the vessels of the femur and provides exquisite detail of the aorta and intimal flap extent. The size of the aorta is important to document, as it is a predictor of future complications. An aortic diameter greater than 40 mm in the proximal descending aorta is predictive of future aneurysmal expansion, as is an initial false-lumen diameter greater than 22 mm. The location of entry and re-entry sites in the aorta should be documented, as well as significant narrowing of the true lumen or obstruction of the branch vessel ostia by the intimal flap, which can result in end-organ ischemia. Malperfusion of organs can also occur when a dissection extends in a branch vessel and the false lumen thromboses, resulting in either high-grade stenosis or occlusion of the involved vessel.

The diagnosis of intramural hematoma relies on the detection of blood within the aortic wall. The process leads to thickening of the aortic wall that is typically eccentric and crescent-shaped but may be concentric. With all modalities, it can be difficult to differentiate aortic wall thickening caused by intramural hematoma from atheroma or mural thrombus. In a comparison of different modalities, MR has the highest accuracy for the identification of intramural hematoma. On ECG-gated black blood spin-echo imaging, which can be T1 or T2 weighted, blood in the wall shows with an abnormal signal different from that of atheroma (Fig. 11.10). During the acute phase (0 to 7 days after onset of symptoms), T1-weighted images demonstrate a crescent-shaped, intermediate intensity within the wall of the aorta. In the subacute phase (more than 8 days), methemoglobin results in high-intensity signal. When the signal from blood in the wall is iso- or hypointense to the unaffected wall, it may be difficult to differentiate intramural hematoma from atheroma on T1-weighted images, requiring the use of T2-weighted images that demonstrate hyperintense signal relative to normal wall. Thus, MR is able to detect recurrent hemorrhage in the aortic wall, a finding that implies instability of a hematoma and the need for intervention.

The imaging diagnosis of penetrating aortic ulcers relies on the visualization of a crater-like ulcer in the aortic wall. Ulceration (and the extensive atheromatous changes that often coexists) is best visualized on ceMRA when images are reconstructed parallel to the long axis of the aorta. Black blood spin-echo imaging is used to detect associated intramural hematoma, indicating extension of the ulcer into the media. ceMRA is also excellent for depicting pseudo-aneurysms that form when there is sufficient compromise of the wall or a contained rupture (Fig. 11.11).

In the setting of suspected acute aortic syndrome, the symptoms can guide the region of coverage for initial imaging: pain in the anterior chest, neck, and jaw suggests ascending aorta involvement, whereas back or abdominal pain suggests descending or abdominal aortic involvement. A comprehensive imaging protocol including ECG-gated black blood spin-echo imaging, bSSFP cine imaging, time-resolved MRA, multiphase high-resolution ceMRA, and gadolinium contrast-enhanced 3D gradient-echo imaging with fat saturation can be tailored as needed for patients with suspected acute aortic syndrome.

LOWER EXTREMITY VASCULATURE

Noninvasive imaging of the lower extremity vasculature is of interest because of the high prevalence of peripheral arterial disease (PAD), particularly in the aging population. PAD, also known as atherosclerotic peripheral arterial occlusive disease, accounts for about 80% of lower extremity arterial disease, with a prevalence of 2.5% in patients older than 50 years of age and about 7% in patients older than 70 years. The symptoms of PAD are secondary to ischemia and subsequent necrosis, and include claudication, rest pain, and tissue loss. Claudication is pain with activity that occurs when the metabolic demand of the muscles exceeds the oxygen-delivering capacity of the arteries. Risk factors for the development of PAD include increasing age, elevated cholesterol, tobacco use, diabetes

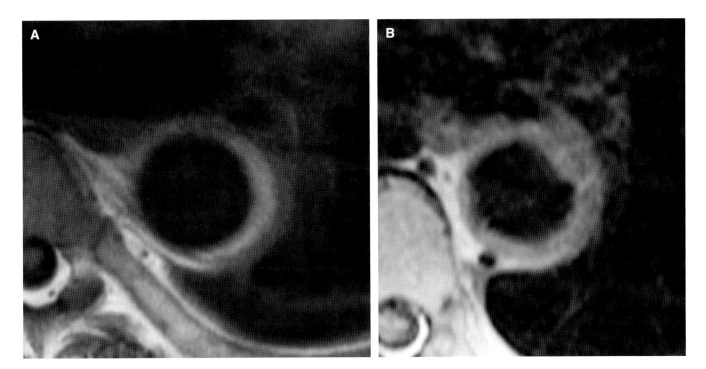

Figure 11.10 *Differentiating intramural hematoma from atheroma.* (**A**) ECG-gated black blood axial T1-weighted FSE/TSE image of an intramural hematoma within the descending aorta. The higher-intensity signal within the wall represents hemorrhage. Note that the hemorrhage has smooth borders as it spreads through the intramedial space. (**B**) ECG-gated black blood axial T1-weighted FSE/TSE image of atheroma within the descending aorta. Note that the signal intensity is intermediate and cannot be separated from the aortic wall. Also note that there is irregularity of the wall. In the setting of intramural hematoma and atheroma at the same level, the high-signal intramural hematoma will have a smooth border, as it is internal to the wall, while the atheroma will be at the luminal border and typically has irregular margins.

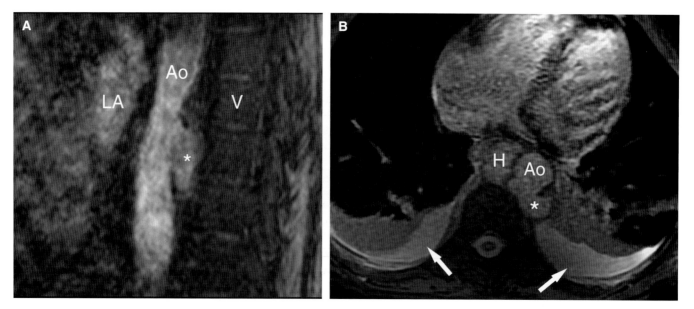

Figure 11.11 *Contained rupture of a penetrating aortic ulcer.* A 68-year-old woman with a history of severe renal insufficiency presented with back pain. Unenhanced CT (not shown) demonstrated an abnormality in the posterior mediastinum requiring further evaluation. (**A**) Sagittal unenhanced ECG-gated and respiratory-gated SSFP MRA image demonstrates an outpouching of the descending aorta (*), representing a pseudo-aneurysm from a penetrating aortic ulcer. *LA,* left atrium; *V,* vertebra; *Ao,* aorta. (**B**) Axial SSFP image with fat saturation (without ECG gating) also demonstrates the pseudo-aneurysm (*) arising from the aorta (*Ao*), as well as the posterior mediastinal hematoma (*H*). On the unenhanced MRA, the hematoma is differentiated from the pseudo-aneurysm by its lack of signal. There are also bilateral pleural effusions (*arrows*) secondary to this acute process.

mellitus, hypertension, and family history. Treatment of PAD involves risk-factor modification and intervention, including both surgical and endovascular therapy. Other causes of chronic arterial occlusion, which account for about 20% of cases, include aneurysmal disease, popliteal entrapment syndrome, cystic adventitial disease, and other vasculitides. Acute thromboembolic events can also present with symptoms of peripheral arterial disease. MRI provides a noninvasive method of interrogating the entire lower extremity vasculature for diagnosis and therapeutic planning without exposing the patient to iodinated contrast agent or ionizing radiation, and the technique does not lead to obscuration of the vessel lumen by calcium, which is a limitation of CT angiography.

The vessels of the lower extremity can be separated into inflow, outflow, and runoff vessels. This classification is impor-

tant because the segments affected directly influence surgical planning. Inflow vessels, also known as aortoiliac vessels, include the abdominal aorta as well as the iliac arterial system. The abdominal aorta bifurcates into the common iliac arteries, which further bifurcate into internal and external arteries. The internal iliac arteries, also known as the hypogastric arteries, have many branches that supply the pelvic organs and musculature. The internal iliac arteries serve as important pathways for collateralization, receiving blood from the inferior mesenteric artery via the rectal arteries when the distal aorta and common iliac arteries are occluded and providing blood to the femoral system via gluteal and femoral circumflex arteries when the external iliac arteries are occluded. The external iliac arteries serve as pelvic conduits that deliver flow to the outflow vessels (Fig. 11.12).

Box 11.2 **ESSENTIALS TO REMEMBER**

- Aneurysms are defined as a segment of an artery that is 1.5 times greater in diameter than the same artery just upstream. Aneurysms of the ascending aorta are defined as larger than 4 cm diameter and of the descending thoracic aorta as larger than 3.5 cm. Differing from the definition, the abdominal aorta is considered aneurysmal when larger than 3.5 cm. An iliac artery aneurysm is present when the vessel is larger than 16 mm diameter.

- Aortic dissection is a potentially life-threatening condition that occurs when a tear in the intima allows blood to dissect the layers of the aortic wall creating a true lumen and a false lumen that may compromise blood flow and occlude branch vessels. MR demonstrates an intimal flap that separates the true and false lumens.

- Penetrating aortic ulcer refers to ulceration of an atherosclerotic plaque that may result in an intramural hematoma, a localized dissection, or a shower of emboli into the distal arterial vessels.

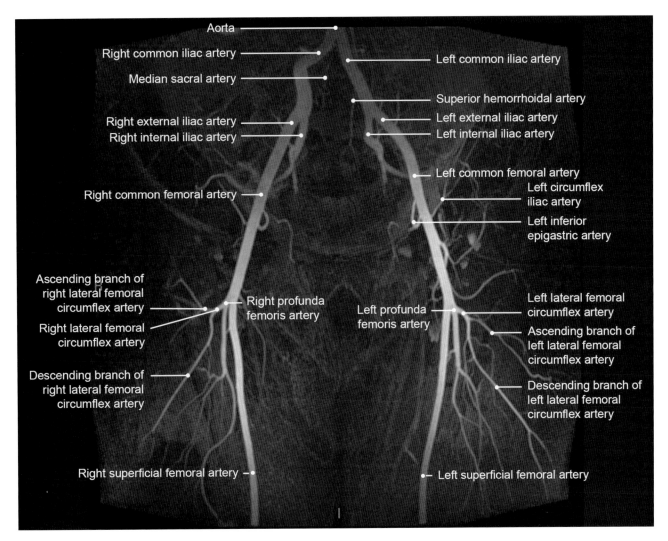

Figure 11.12 *Normal anatomy of the inflow vessels of the lower extremity.* Sub-volume coronal MIP image of the aortoiliac station from a multi-station ceMRA. The inflow territory contains the arteries from the aortic bifurcation to the common femoral arteries. (From Chapter 2 in Kramer CM, Hundley WG. *Atlas of Cardiovascular Magnetic Resonance Imaging.* Copyright Elsevier 2010.)

The femoral arteries and the popliteal artery make up the outflow vessels. The common femoral artery is the continuation of the external iliac artery as it passes deep to the inguinal ligament. The circumflex iliac artery and inferior epigastric are superficial branches of the common femoral artery. These branches become important collateral pathways in the presence of aortoiliac occlusive disease, where the circumflex iliac artery collateralizes with lumbar and intercostal arteries and the inferior epigastric artery collateralizes with the internal mammary arteries. The common femoral artery bifurcates into the superficial femoral artery (SFA) and profunda femoral artery. The profunda femoral artery provides most of the blood to the muscles of the thigh and is a collateral pathway in the setting of SFA occlusion, anastomosing with the geniculate arteries around the knee. The SFA continues inferiorly from its origin, coursing medially to the femur, and passes through the adductor canal (Hunter's canal) to become the popliteal artery at the adductor hiatus. The popliteal artery courses posterior to the knee joint, giving rise to the superior

and inferior geniculate arteries, which anastomose around the knee (Fig. 11.13)

The runoff vessels, also known as the tibioperoneal or crural arteries, arise from the popliteal artery as it passes superficial to the lower border of the popliteus muscle. The runoff vessels and their variant anatomy can be understood by taking a nontraditional approach of considering the peroneal artery as a continuation of the popliteal artery, and the anterior and posterior tibial arteries as branches of the peroneal artery. The approach is useful when the tibial arteries are hypoplastic or absent, in which case the peroneal artery supplies blood to the distal territories.[7] The anterior tibial artery is the first branch, coursing anterolaterally in a horizontal fashion proximally and then descending along the anterior aspect of the interosseous ligament. Distally, the AT follows the anterolateral aspect of the tibia. At the ankle, the AT gives rise to the dorsal pedal artery, which courses over the dorsum of the foot. Beyond the origin of the anterior tibial artery, the peroneal artery continues on for a short segment as the tibioperoneal trunk,

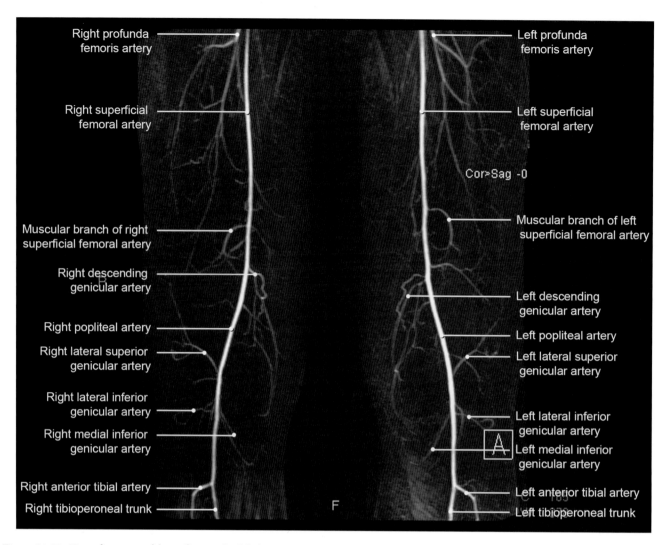

Figure 11.13 *Normal anatomy of the outflow vessels of the lower extremity.* Sub-volume coronal MIP image of the thigh station from a multi-station ceMRA. The outflow territory contains the arteries from the common femoral arteries to the origin of the anterior tibial arteries. (From Chapter 2 in Kramer CM, Hundley WG. *Atlas of Cardiovascular Magnetic Resonance Imaging.* Copyright Elsevier, 2010.)

bifurcating into the posterior tibial artery and the peroneal artery. The posterior tibial artery courses inferomedial from its origin and descends in a slightly posterior fashion relative to the peroneal artery. At ankle, the posterior tibial artery courses posterior to the medial malleolus to become the plantar artery, supplying the plantar aspect of the foot (Fig. 11.14).[8]

ATHEROSCLEROTIC PERIPHERAL ARTERIAL OCCLUSIVE DISEASE

State-of-the-art vascular imaging of the lower extremity vasculature is performed using ceMRA with use of a multi-station acquisition. Two main methods are currently employed: the three-station bolus chase method with a single injection, or a hybrid approach in which the calf station is obtained first, followed by the bolus chase of the aortoiliac and thigh stations, requiring two separate contrast material injections.

In the three-station bolus chase method, scout images of the aortoiliac, thigh, and calf stations are obtained for determination of the MRA coverage. An unenhanced, or mask, acquisition of each station is acquired for background subtraction. Imaging is performed in the coronal plane. Timing is determined either with a test bolus injection or bolus tracking method, as described early. The full data set is acquired with the patient holding his or her breath for acquisition of images at the aortoiliac station, which optimizes the depiction of the proximal aorta and renal arteries, and acquisition of the imaging data at the lower stations is done with the patient breathing freely.

There are many different methods for calculating the amount of contrast material and rate injection to cover the three stations. All injection protocols share the same goal: provide contrast material fast enough to sufficiently enhance the arterial segments at each station but not too fast to cause unwanted venous contamination. One approach is to use a fixed volume for all patients with a fixed injection rate; thus, all patients have the same duration of injection. Another approach is to use a biphasic injection with a higher rate

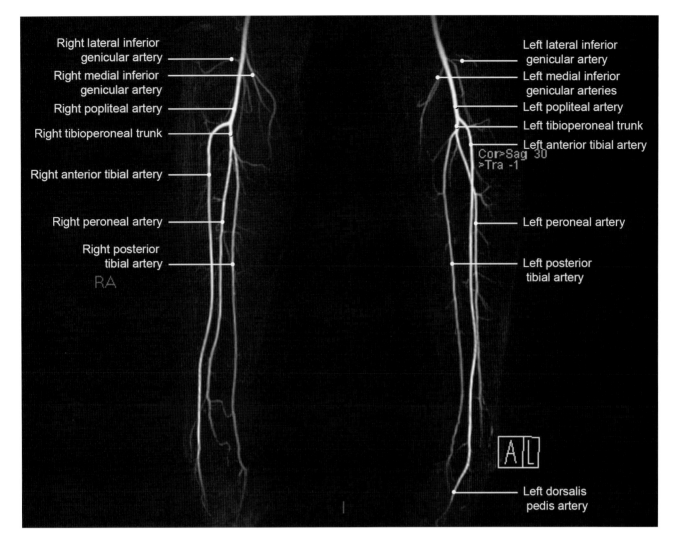

Figure 11.14 *Normal anatomy of the runoff vessels of the lower extremity.* Sub-volume coronal MIP image of the calf station from a multi-station ceMRA. The inflow territory contains the arteries from the aortic bifurcation to the common femoral arteries. (From Chapter 2 in Kramer CM, Hundley WG. *Atlas of Cardiovascular Magnetic Resonance Imaging.* Copyright Elsevier, 2010.)

initially, followed by a slower rate of injection. This tends to lengthen the injection duration, allowing longer arterial enhancement at the distal stations, but may lead to stronger venous contamination. A solution to venous contamination at the calf station is to perform trMRA at the calf station prior to performing the multi-station ceMRA, which requires additional administration of a small amount of contrast medium. trMRA interpretation should be used in conjunction with higher-resolution ceMRA, as trMRA is prone to its own unique artifacts.

In the hybrid approach, venous contamination of the calf station is avoided by imaging this station first with high-resolution ceMRA. As above, a mask is obtained of the calf station to plan the acquisition. Bolus tracking is used for timing to reduce contrast media load. Subsequently, the aortoiliac and thigh stations are imaged with a separate injection. By acquiring a mask after the previous injection, subtracted imaging of the aortoiliac and thigh stations alleviates the problem of venous contamination posed by recirculation of contrast agent from calf imaging. Overall, the hybrid approach uses

more contrast material than the three-station approach but may be more appropriate in patients with chronic critical ischemia than in patients with intermittent claudication.

In patients who are unable to receive contrast media due to the risk of nephrogenic systemic fibrosis, unenhanced MRA methods can be used. 2D TOF is the most widely available of these techniques. The technique suffers from motion artifacts due to long acquisition times, inability to image in-plane flow, and signal loss due to turbulent flow from vessel narrowing, leading to overestimation of stenoses. However, this technique can augment ceMRA and can be quite useful in areas that are difficult to image with ceMRA, such as the foot. Newer techniques, which use a combination of SSFP and ECG gating, can provide imaging that is comparable to ceMRA, but at this time without the robustness that ceMRA offers.

Post-processing the ceMRA data is an essential part of efficient interpretation. The subtracted arterial data sets can be transformed in full-volume MIP that can be presented as a single image or a rotational series of images. These reconstructions allow for an overview of the severity and distribution of disease. However, focused interrogation of lesions should be performed using the unsubtracted source data, as the subtracted data are prone to artifacts that can be caused from misregistration between the mask and the images of the ceMRA acquisition in case the patient moves. Evaluation of source data also allows for identification of surgical clips adjacent to the artery or a stent within the artery that causes loss of signal and can easily be mistaken for stenosis or occlusion on subtracted images (Fig. 11.15).The focused examination of a lesion on source images is performed with subvolume MIP, typically on the order of 10 mm thickness, and MPR viewed at the original slice thickness.[9]

In evaluating the extent of PAD, it is important to note the location, length, and luminal diameter reduction of a stenosis and to describe the pattern of disease, as this is essential to interventional planning and assessing the prognosis for the patient. PAD isolated to the aortoiliac vessels has a better prognosis than disease associated with the outflow and runoff vessels. A cornerstone of vascular therapy is to treat the most proximal disease, as these lesions restrict flow to the greatest extent.

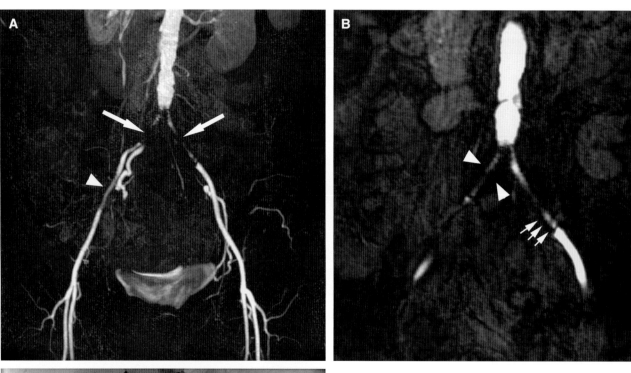

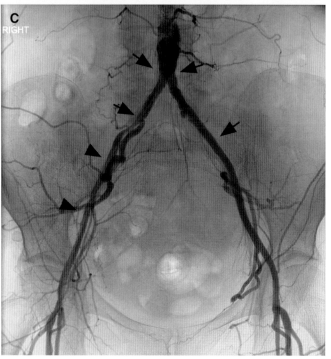

Figure 11.15 *Artifact from stents in the aortoiliac arteries.* (**A**) Sub-volume MIP image created from the background subtracted data set of an arterial-phase ceMRA demonstrates abnormal, decreased signal intensity in the bilateral common iliac arteries (*arrows*), suggesting occlusion; however, there are no identifiable collateral vessels that have developed. There is also segmental loss of signal within the right external iliac artery (*arrowhead*) without narrowing. (**B**) Thin-section coronal unsubstracted source image from ceMRA reveals dark blooming artifact (*arrowheads*) surrounding the right common iliac artery, due to magnetic field distortion from the presence of a metallic stent. Less severe blooming artifact appears as dark dots (*arrows*) from individual metallic components of the stent within the left common iliac artery. Due to the artifact, the lumen of the stent cannot be evaluated. (**C**) Digital subtracted angiogram shows the extent of the bilateral common iliac artery stents (*arrows* denote the ends of the stents) and right external iliac stents (*arrowheads* denote extent) and demonstrates lack of significant narrowing of the stent lumen. Different types of stents produce artifacts to varying degrees. The stent in the right external iliac artery has less metal and a wider-spaced mesh structure compared to common iliac artery stents, resulting in fewer artifacts. In general, stents aligned with long axis parallel to the B_0 magnetic field produce fewer artifacts than stents aligned perpendicular.

Aortoiliac occlusive disease is atherosclerotic occlusive disease that involves the abdominal aorta and the proximal common iliac arteries. The proximal aorta and distal extremities are usually normal with the involvement of the distal iliac and femoral-popliteal arteries being variable but more commonly present. A less common type that involves only the distal aorta and proximal iliac arteries is present in middle-aged female smokers. The sequela of aortoiliac occlusive disease is present in *Leriche syndrome*, which is the clinical presentation of buttock, thigh, and leg claudication, and impotence in the setting of absent femoral pulses. Depending on the extent of occlusion, flow is maintained by collateral pathways including the inferior mesenteric artery to the internal iliac artery via the rectal arteries, internal mammary arteries to the inferior epigastric arteries, and intracostal and lumbar arteries to the superficial circumflex iliac arties. Treatment is typically surgical, with placement of an aortobifemoral bypass graft (Fig. 11.16).

Chronic critical ischemia is characterized by multiple, bilateral stenoses that occur in multiple locations, making treatment difficult. In addition to identifying stenosis or occlusion in inflow and outflow vessels, MRA allows for identification of reconstitution of major runoff vessels, which can be potential targets for bypass grafting. Thus, it is important to identify the largest and least diseased vessel in the calf station that has uninterrupted flow to the foot as the target vessel for bypass grafting (Fig. 11.17). In general, patients with diabetes tend to have distal disease that spares the inflow vessels.

Stenosis grading is typically performed by dividing the diameter of the diseased vessel by that of the normal diameter of a nondiseased portion of the vessel segment and subtracting the result from 1 to calculate a ratio reduction, which can be mutliplied by 100 to get a precentage reduction (e.g., 60% stenosis). In the case of eccentric lesions, the reduction in luminal diameter is best assessed by viewing the lesion in several different longitudinal projections or viewing the cross-sectional extent directly to measure the minimum diameter. A simplified approach to lesion grading is to group the lesions into mild, moderate, severe, and occluded, where mild lesions result in narrowing less than 50%, moderate lesions have narrowing ranging from 50% to 70%, and severe lesions have greater than 70% narrowing. This approach is useful for quick estimation of lesions and, when combined with lesion length and location, it gives a good estimate of the flow limitation caused by a lesion. Historically, ceMRA overestimates stenoses compared to catheter angiography. However, with advances in gradient strength and speed, pulse sequences with very short TR and TE can be achieved, resulting in minimal overestimation.

Surgical bypass grafts require close follow-up for complications, which will be present in as many as 30% of patients within the first 2 years following placement. Early bypass failure is commonly due to intimal hyperplasia within the graft. Alternatively, worsening atherosclerotic disease of vessels either proximal or distal can result in reduced flow through the graft and subsequent thrombosis. The acute complication of graft thrombosis can often be prevented by early intervention on these lesions. Multi-station multiphase ceMRA as described above is used to evaluate lower extremity bypass grafts. Additionally, late-venous-phase 3D gradient-echo imaging with fat saturation is useful for the identification of thrombosed bypass grafts when the surgical anatomy is not previously known. This sequence may also help identify surgical clips as the source of artifact on the ceMRA sequences, visualized as blooming artifact in the region of a metallic clip. Surgical bypass grafts can be grouped into inflow and outflow grafts. Inflow grafts include aortobiiliac, aortobifemoral, and axillobifemoral. Outflow grafts typically arise from the common femoral artery and anastomose distally to the above-knee popliteal artery, running medially in the subcutaneous tissues of the thigh. Outflow grafts may have an infragenicular anastomosis to the popliteal artery or a tibial artery, but these grafts have lower patency rates than their above-knee counterparts.[10]

OTHER CAUSES OF OCCLUSIVE PERIPHERAL DISEASE

Aneurysmal disease in the lower extremity is similar to the disease process in the aorta. The majority of aneurysms are the nonspecific, degenerative type that are often associated with atherosclerotic disease. These aneurysms are most often found in the iliac, femoral, and popliteal arteries. Aneurysms can be a direct result from atherosclerosis, as in the case of penetrating ulcers. Pseudo-aneurysms occurring after surgery or arterial catheterization are common complications. Other causes of aneurysm include connective tissue disease such as Ehlers-Danlos or Marfan syndrome.

The common iliac artery is aneurysmal when the diameter exceeds 16 mm. Iliac artery aneurysms commonly present with abdominal aortic aneurysm or, less likely, can be isolated. Thus, screening of the abdominal aorta for aneurysmal disease should also include the iliac vessels. Detection of femoral and popliteal aneurysms is important as these can lead to complications such as distal emboli and thrombosis. Risk of rupture of aneurysms in the extremities is low. Additionally, all patients with aneurysms of the lower extremity should be screened for an abdominal aortic aneurysm, as there is a 62% and 85% association with popliteal and femoral artery aneurysms, respectively (Fig. 11.18).

Arterial emboli most commonly arise from a cardiac source, either from thrombus in the left ventricle, in the setting of a prior myocardial infarction, or from the left atrium, in the setting of longstanding atrial fibrillation. Alternatively, irregular atheroma in the aorta can be a source for distal emboli, as can penetrating aortic ulcer. Emboli can lodge in any vessel, with small emboli traveling more distal before occluding a vessel. Patients who have developed extensive collaterals from preexisting atherosclerotic disease may be asymptomatic if they have emboli; however, a single embolus can have dramatic effects in patients without collaterals. ceMRA is excellent for detecting emboli, which appear as central signal voids ("filling defects") on images obtained perpendicular to the vessel and show as an inverted meniscus parallel to the long axis of the vessel.

Popliteal entrapment syndrome is caused by a congenital anatomic abnormality that leads to compression of the popliteal artery. Men are typically affected, with most patients presenting before 40 years of age. Classification is based on the anatomic variation compressing the artery (types I through IV), if there is primary venous entrapment (type V), or if the symptoms are based on muscular hypertrophy with normal

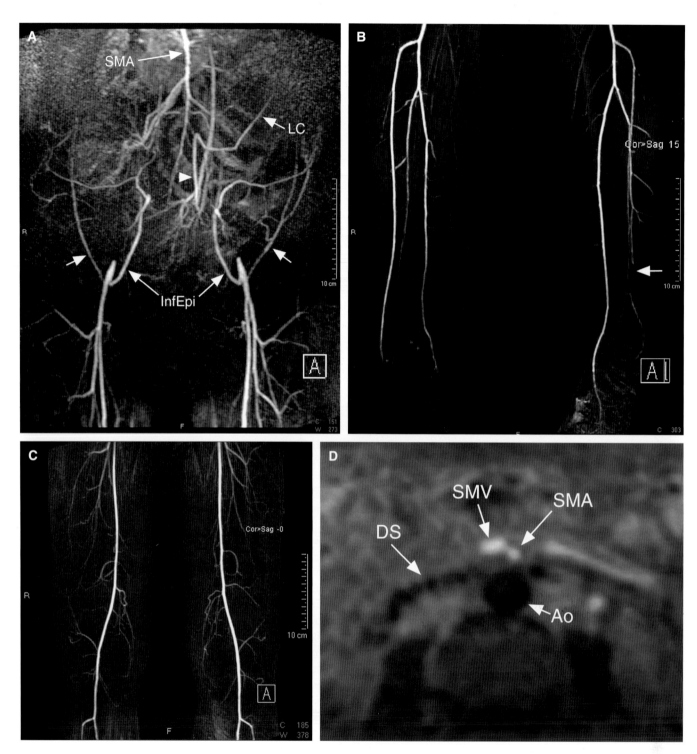

Figure 11.16 *Aortoiliac occlusive disease.* A 45-year-old woman presented with acute renal failure. (**A**) ceMRA image of the abdomen and pelvis displayed as a sub-volume MIP image shows no blood flow within the abdominal aorta or the iliac arteries. Blood flow is reconstituted at the level of the common femoral artery by the iliac circumflex arteries (*unlabeled arrows*) and the inferior epigastric arteries (*InfEpi*). Flow is present in the superior mesenteric artery (*SMA*). The branches of the inferior mesenteric artery provide collateral flow to the pelvis via the left colic artery (*LC*) to the superior rectal artery (*arrowhead*). The inferior mesenteric artery is occluded proximally. No enhancing renal parenchyma is present. (**B**) The outflow vessels (femoral arteries and branches) look relatively normal. (**C**) There is a focal occlusion of the left anterior tibial artery (*arrow*), possibly from prior embolic disease. (**D**) Reconstructed venous-phase ceMRA image in axial orientation at the level of the duodenal sweep (*DS*) shows complete thrombosis of the aorta (*Ao*) with flow in the superior mesenteric artery (*SMA*) and vein (*SMV*).

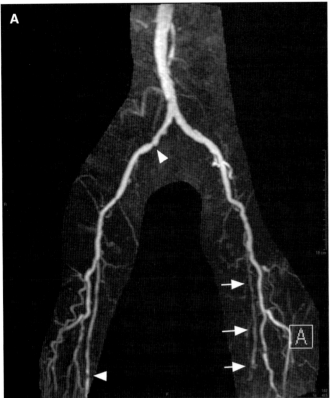

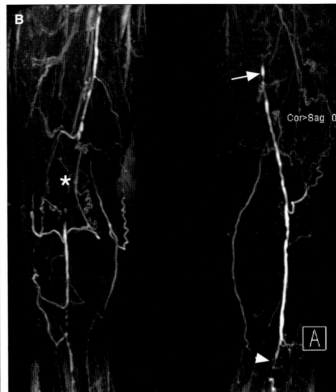

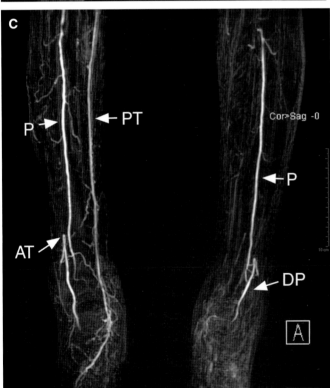

Figure 11.17 *Severe atherosclerotic peripheral arterial occlusive disease.* A diabetic, 89-year-old woman presented with a soft tissue ulcer on her left toe. (**A**) Multi-station ceMRA displayed as MIP images demonstrates significant focal narrowing of the right common iliac artery (*proximal arrowhead*) in the region of the occluded right internal iliac artery and a high-grade stenosis in the right superficial femoral artery (*distal arrowhead*). Both of these could be treated with endovascular therapy. The left inflow arteries are without significant stenosis. There is severe disease of the proximal left superficial femoral artery followed by occlusion (*arrows*). (**B**) Segmental occlusion of the proximal right popliteal artery (*) demonstrates reconstitution of a short segment of the popliteal artery by collaterals of the geniculate artery. The left superficial femoral artery is reconstituted in its midportion (*arrow*) and provides flow to the popliteal artery, which occludes (*arrowhead*) below the knee. (**C**) Collateral vessels reconstitute the right peroneal (*P*) and posterior tibial (*PT*) arteries proximally. The right anterior tibial (*AT*) artery is reconstituted via a collateral of the peroneal artery. The peroneal artery (*P*) is the only identifiable, patent runoff vessel on the left side, reconstituting the dorsalis pedis (*DP*) artery at the foot. A surgical bypass graft from the left common femoral artery to the peroneal artery would be required to treat this patient's left-sided symptoms.

anatomy (type VI, functional entrapment). In a few cases, the disease may be bilateral or have coexisting venous entrapment. The typical clinical presentation is that of a young male athlete presenting with calf claudication. Paresthesia and calf swelling may also be present, but ischemia is rare.

The popliteal artery and vein course normally between the medial and lateral heads of the gastrocnemius and superficial

to the popliteus muscle. During normal embryologic development, the medial head of the gastrocnemius muscle migrates from lateral to medial. Aberration of the migration causes the medial head of the gastrocnemius muscle to compress the popliteal artery. In type I, the popliteal artery is located medial to the medial head of the gastrocnemius. In type II, the medial head of the gastrocnemius is laterally attached. In type III,

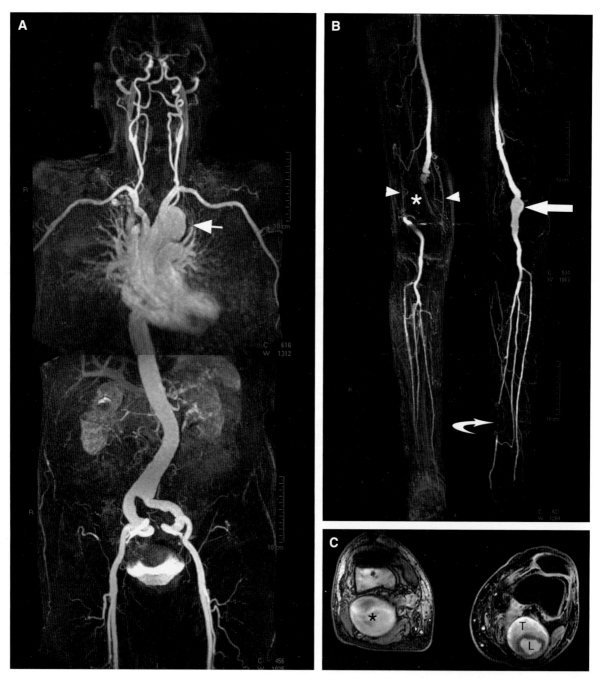

Figure 11.18 *Aneurysm screening.* Screening for aneurysms was performed in a 65-year-old woman with known bilateral popliteal artery aneurysms. Whole-body ceMRA was performed with one contrast material injection for four stations: head, neck and chest; abdomen and pelvis; thigh; and calf. (**A**) MIP image of the superior two stations reveals a thoracic aortic aneurysm (*arrow*) as well as ectasia of the infrarenal abdominal aorta and bilateral common iliac arteries. (**B**) MIP image of the inferior two stations shows segmental occlusion of the right popliteal artery (*) with prominent geniculate collaterals (*arrowheads*). An aneurysm of the left popliteal artery (*straight arrow*) is shown, and there is chronic segmental occlusion of the distal left posterior tibial artery (*curved arrow*) from embolic disease, with reconstitution of the distal vessel via a collateral from the peroneal artery. (**C**) Axial gadolinium-contrast-enhanced 3D gradient-echo image with fat saturation at the level of the popliteal arteries demonstrates a thrombosed right popliteal artery aneurysm (*), accounting for the occluded segment present in image B. The relatively high signal in the aneurysm is due to the T1 shortening caused by the blood products and not due to gadolinium enhancement. The left popliteal artery aneurysm is larger than it appears on ceMRA because the size of the lumen (*L*) contributes only partially to the overall size. A large mural thrombus (*T*), which is the source of the embolic disease in image B, also contributes to the overall size of the aneurysm.

an accessory fibrous slip of the medial head of the gastrocnemius crosses laterally and compresses the popliteal artery. In type IV, the course of the popliteal artery is deep to the popliteus muscle, which compresses the artery. When popliteal entrapment is suspected the imaging protocol needs to include

high-spatial-resolution T1-weighted spin-echo imaging, in addition to ceMRA, to identify the relationship of the popliteal artery to the muscles of the popliteal fossa.[11]

Cystic adventitial disease is a rare chronic occlusive process that affects the popliteal artery in 85% of cases, but it can also affect the external iliac, common femoral, radial, and ulnar arteries. It is characterized by the presence of mucoid cysts in the adventitia of an artery, leading to compression of the lumen. The cysts are associated with arteries near joints and they may be in direct communication with the joint space. The etiology is not completely understood, but possible mechanisms include myxoid degeneration of the adventitia, synovium tracking from the joint into the adventitia, repeated minor trauma, and incorporation of mucoid-producing cells within the adventitia during embryologic development. The typical patient is a 20- to 50-year-old man presenting with symptoms of calf claudication or a soft tissue mass. Symptoms often have an acute onset with physical activity and persist for some time after termination of activity. The disease is most often unilateral and occurs in patients who do not have risk factors for atherosclerotic disease.

Imaging of cystic adventitial disease relies on the detection of stenosis with ceMRA and identification of cysts using T1- and T2-weighted sequences. The cysts may be circumferentially located around the vessel, resulting in a stenosis with a smooth, hourglass appearance of the lumen, or they can be located concentrically, resulting in a smooth eccentric stenosis known as the "scimitar sign." On T1-weighted images, the cysts show variable signal intensity due to variable protein content but are uniformly hyperintense to muscle on T2-weighted images. The natural history of the disease is that it progresses to occlusion of the artery. Treatment requires surgical intervention: either cyst enucleation if there is no arterial occlusion or placement of a bypass graft if the artery has become occluded. If the entire cyst tissue is not removed or if a connection to the joint space is not ligated, there is a high likelihood of recurrence (Fig. 11.19).

MESENTERIC VASCULATURE

The mesenteric vasculature is composed of the arterial supply and venous drainage of the gastrointestinal (GI) viscera. A wide variety of pathologic changes affect these vessels, including trauma, vasculitis, connective tissue disease, aneurysmal disease, and encasement by tumors. However, the most common disease is arterial occlusive disease secondary to atherosclerosis. Arterial and venous occlusive diseases have the potential to result in life-threatening bowel ischemia and infarction. Most patients with mesenteric atherosclerosis remain asymptomatic even where there is severe stenosis or occlusion of a major supplying artery due to the robustness of collateral pathways that form during the slow progression of the disease. MR allows for detailed assessment of both the arterial and venous component of the mesenteric vasculature as well as end-organ status but is typically reserved for patients without life-threatening symptoms.

The blood supply of the GI tract arises from the anterior branches of the abdominal aorta, which include the celiac artery, superior mesenteric artery (SMA), and inferior mesenteric artery. The celiac artery is the most proximal visceral branch of the abdominal aorta and supplies the upper abdominal organs. It arises at the level of the thoracolumbar junction and in 65% of patients gives rise to the left gastric, splenic, and common hepatic arteries. There are many variations to this pattern, and any of the branch vessels may arise directly from the aorta or the SMA. The splenic artery gives rise to the pancreatic arteries that supply the body and tail of the pancreas, the short gastric arteries that supply the stomach, and the left gastroepiploic artery. The proper hepatic artery arises from the common hepatic artery, at the origin of the gastroduodenal artery, and bifurcates into left and right hepatic arteries, a pattern present in 50% of patients. In the other 50%, a replaced or accessory hepatic artery is present, typically arising from the SMA in the case of the right hepatic artery, or from the left gastric artery in the case of the left hepatic artery. The right gastric artery is variable in its origin but most commonly arises from the proper hepatic artery. The gastroduodenal artery arises from the common hepatic artery in 75% of patients and usually has two main branches: the superior pancreaticoduodenal artery and the right gastroepiploic artery.

The SMA supplies most of the small intestine as well as the right and transverse colon. It arises from the anterior aspect of the abdominal aorta, approximately 1 cm below the celiac artery. Rarely, the celiac artery and SMA arise as a single celiomesenteric trunk directly from the aorta. The inferior pancreaticoduodenal artery is typically the first branch of the SMA and originates from a right posterior location from the SMA. In combination with the superior pancreaticoduodenal artery from the gastroduodenal artery, it forms a collateral pathway between the celiac artery and SMA when there is significant proximal disease of either artery. The small bowel is supplied by the jejunal and ileal artery branches that arise from the left side of the SMA and are notable for their interconnected arcades. The SMA gives off three right-sided branches: the middle colic, right colic, and ileocolic arteries. The middle colic artery supplies the hepatic flexure and proximal transverse colon via its right and left branches, respectively. The right and left branches anastomose with the right colic and variably with left colic (branch of the inferior mesenteric artery) artery, respectively. The right colic artery supplies the right colon and anastomoses with the middle colic and ileocolic arteries. The ileocolic artery supplies the terminal ileum and cecum, anastomosing with the right colic and ileal arterial branches (Fig. 11.20).

The inferior mesenteric artery supplies the left colon and sigmoid colon. It arises from the anterior, left aspect of the aorta at approximately the level of the third lumbar vertebral body and is much smaller in diameter than the other two mesenteric arteries. The first branch of the inferior mesenteric artery ascends as the left colic artery, which has an inconsistent anastomosis with the middle colic artery. The sigmoid branch may also arise as the second branch of the inferior mesenteric artery or as a branch of the left colic artery. The terminal branch of the inferior mesenteric artery is the superior rectal artery.

The mesenteric arterial circulation is notable for its robust collateral pathways. The dominant collateral pathway between the celiac artery and the SMA is via the gastroduodenal artery and the pancreaticoduodenal arcades. The marginal artery of Drummond is located along the mesenteric border of the

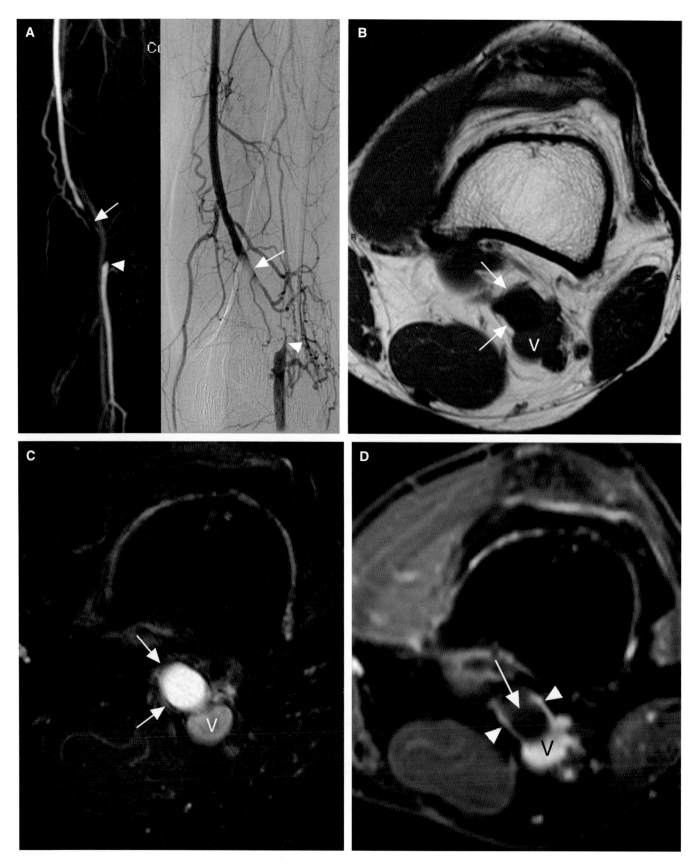

Figure 11.19 *Cystic adventitial disease.* (**A**) ceMRA (*left*) and digital subtraction arteriogram (*right*) images demonstrate an eccentric filling defect and occlusion of the left popliteal artery. The filling defect is outlined by the thin tail of contrast enhancement (*arrow*) proximally ("scimitar sign") and an meniscus distally (*arrowhead*). Venous enhancement is present in the ceMRA as vessels with lower signal intensity. T1-weighted FSE/TSE (**B**) and T2-weighted STIR (**C**) images show mucoid cyst (*arrows*) obstructing the artery, characterized by low signal intensity compared to muscle on T1-weighted images and very bright signal intensity on T2-weighted images. The popliteal vein (*V*) is adjacent to the obstructed artery. (**D**) On late-venous-phase post-contrast-enhanced 3D gradient-echo imaging with fat saturation, there is adventitial enhancement (*arrowheads*) around the cyst (*arrow*), which does not enhance. *V*, popliteal vein.

Box 11.3 ESSENTIALS TO REMEMBER

- MR angiography is increasingly utilized to assess PAD in the extremities. Lesions are classified by location, length, and severity. Compared to catheter angiography ceMRA overestimates the severity of stenoses. Lesions are classified as mild when the vascular narrowing is less than 50%, moderate when narrowing is 50% to 70%, and severe when narrowing exceeds 70%.

- Additional causes of ischemia in the extremities includes emboli, aneurysms, entrapment syndromes, and cystic adventitial disease.

colon and is formed by the distal colonic arcades, allowing blood flow between the right, middle, and left colic arteries. The arc of Riolan is located more centrally within the mesentery and forms an inconsistent connection between the left and middle colic arteries. This collateral pathway is an important connection between the superior and inferior mesenteric artery circulation and becomes hypertrophic when there is significant proximal disease of either vessel (Fig. 11.21). However, when absent, the splenic flexure is a watershed area between the superior and inferior mesenteric artery circulation, which is why it is a frequent site of ischemic colitis. The anastomosis between the superior rectal and middle rectal artery is an important pathway in the setting of aortoiliac disease,

connecting the circulation of the inferior mesenteric and internal iliac arteries.[12]

MESENTERIC ISCHEMIA

Mesenteric ischemia is a disease of the geriatric population and is associated with heart disease and tobacco use. Patients present with abdominal pain, nausea, diarrhea, and abdominal distention. Mesenteric ischemia is grouped into acute and chronic subtypes.

When mesenteric ischemia is suspected, MR imaging with multiphase ceMRA of the aorta and mesenteric vasculature is performed in the coronal plane to include the entire mesenteric

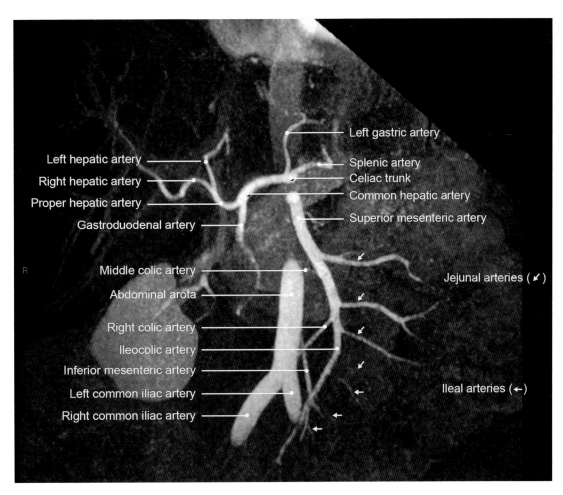

Figure 11.20 *Normal anatomy of the mesenteric arteries.* Sub-volume coronal MIP image of the mesenteric arteries imaged with ceMRA. The three main mesenteric arterial branches arising from the abdominal aorta are the celiac, superior mesenteric, and inferior mesenteric arteries. The entire aorta is not in the imaging volume for simplification. The *tiny arrows* indicate jejunal and ileal artery branches. (From Chapter 2 in Kramer CM, Hundley WG. *Atlas of Cardiovascular Magnetic Resonance Imaging.* Copyright Elsevier, 2010.)

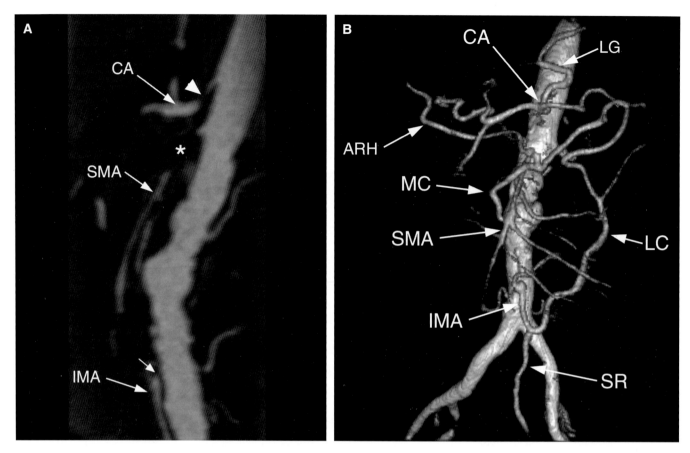

Figure 11.21 *Mesenteric artery collateral pathways.* (**A**) Sagittal MIP image from a ceMRA in a 65-year-old woman with chronic mesenteric ischemia. There is high-grade stenosis (*arrowhead*) at the origin of the celiac artery (*CA*), occlusion (*) of the proximal superior mesenteric artery (*SMA*), and high-grade stenosis (*small arrow*) at the origin of the inferior mesenteric artery (*IMA*). (**B**) 3D volume-rendered ceMRA image shows that most of the blood flow to the mesentery enters via the superior rectal (*SR*) artery, which supplies the inferior mesenteric artery (*IMA*). Flow continues to the superior mesenteric artery (*SMA*) and distributes via the arc of Riolan, which is composed of the left colic (*LC*) artery and the middle colic (*MC*) artery. An accessory right hepatic (*ARH*) artery arises from the SMA, just distal to the proximal occlusion. The celiac artery (*CA*) receives collateral flow from the left gastric (*LG*) artery via an enlarged phrenic artery pathway (not shown).

arterial system as well as the portal-venous system. Post-contrast enhanced T1-weighted gradient-echo imaging with fat saturation is useful for identifying venous clots and vascular wall enhancement in acute occlusions, and assessing perfusion of the gut. Axial T1-weighted gradient-echo and T2-weighted spin-echo imaging with fat saturation are also employed to assess for edema or blood within the intestinal wall and perienteric edema.

Acute mesenteric ischemia (AMI) is a catastrophic event that occurs when there is abrupt interruption of blood flow to the GI tract that cannot be compensated by collateral flow. Other causes include acute failure of cardiac output leading to inadequate perfusion of the tissues and thrombosis of the venous system. The four major causes of AMI are SMA embolus, SMA thrombosis, mesenteric venous thrombosis, and non-occlusive mesenteric vasoconstriction. Aortic or SMA dissections can cause AMI in rare instances. AMI is associated with congestive heart failure, valvular heart disease, cardiac arrhythmias, recent myocardial infarction, and intra-abdominal malignancies. Due to the severe clinical status of patients with AMI, MRA is not typically employed for diagnosis.

Acute SMA embolism accounts for 50% of AMI cases and is typically from a cardiac source but may result from any cause of arterial emboli. Because the SMA is a large vessel with a small angle of origin, it is susceptible to emboli. Emboli typically lodge just beyond the origin of the middle colic artery, may be multiple, and are considered major if they are proximal to the origin of the ileocolic artery. A central signal-void is apparent on cross-sectional MR imaging and a meniscus of the embolus may be seen on long-axis imaging. The vessel is typically enlarged by the embolus and there is perivascular edema. Typically, imaging does not reveal collateral vessels.

Acute SMA thrombosis is secondary to rupture of an atherosclerotic plaque in the proximal aspect of the SMA and accounts for 15% to 25% of AMI cases. The onset is more insidious due to previous development of collateral vessels, and in 50% of patients a history of abdominal angina is present. Occlusion of the SMA occurs within the first 2 cm, distinguishing it from embolic disease. ceMRA can identify the occlusion as well as the collateral vessels.

Mesenteric venous thrombosis affects a younger population than that affected by AMI, with the mean age ranging from 48 to 60 years. Mesenteric venous thrombosis is associated with cirrhosis, neoplasm, trauma, and recent surgery affecting the portomesenteric venous system, with the thrombus occurring at the site of obstruction and propagating distally. In patients with hypercoagulable states, the thrombus starts in the small vessels and propagates centrally. The presentation of mesenteric venous thrombosis ranges from asymptomatic to life-threatening, depending on the degree and location of the thrombosis. Bowel infarction occurs when the thrombosis is widespread and peripheral, resulting in mucosal congestion, hemorrhage, and arterial hypoperfusion. The presence of serosanguineous ascites predicts hemorrhagic infarction of the bowel (Fig. 11.22).

Nonocclusive mesenteric ischemia is a diagnosis of exclusion that occurs in 20% to 30% of AMI cases. It is the result of abnormal vasoconstriction of the mesenteric arteries in response to global hypoperfusion that does not reverse when perfusion is restored. It has a mortality rate as high as 70%. Angiographic findings include narrowing at the origins and irregularities of the SMA branches, and spasm of the arcades. These finding are typically beyond the resolution of ceMRA, and diagnosis of nonocclusive mesenteric ischemia by MRA has yet to been described in humans.

CHRONIC MESENTERIC ISCHEMIA

Despite the widespread prevalence of mesenteric atherosclerosis, chronic mesenteric ischemia (CMI) is rare due to the extensive potential for collateral formation in the mesenteric

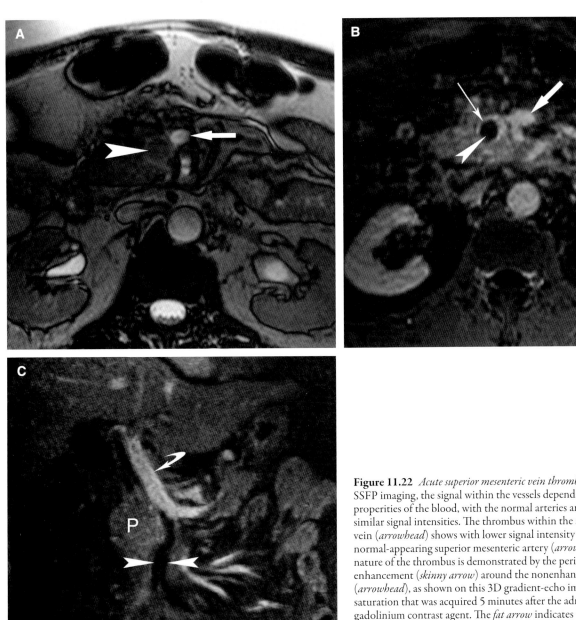

Figure 11.22 *Acute superior mesenteric vein thrombosis.* (**A**) On SSFP imaging, the signal within the vessels depends on the T1 and T2 properities of the blood, with the normal arteries and veins having similar signal intensities. The thrombus within the superior mesenteric vein (*arrowhead*) shows with lower signal intensity than the blood in the normal-appearing superior mesenteric artery (*arrow*). (**B**) The acute nature of the thrombus is demonstrated by the perivascular enhancement (*skinny arrow*) around the nonenhancing thrombus (*arrowhead*), as shown on this 3D gradient-echo image with fat saturation that was acquired 5 minutes after the administration of gadolinium contrast agent. The *fat arrow* indicates the superior mesenteric artery. (**C**) Venous-phase ceMRA image acquired in the coronal plane demonstrates the extent of the thrombus (between *arrowheads*), which is limited to the central superior mesenteric vein and does not extend into the portal vein (*curved arrow*). *P*, head of the pancreas.

vasculature. CMI, also know as abdominal angina, occurs when the delivery of oxygen to the gut is exceeded by the metabolic demand. CMI is most often due to atherosclerotic disease, and thus associated risk factors include increasing age, smoking, hypertension, and hypercholesterolemia. There is a female predominance of symptomatic disease. The classic triad of clinical symptoms is postprandial pain, weight loss, and the avoidance of food due to pain. Notably, patients retain their appetite, differentiating the weight loss from that associated with cancer.

ceMRA is an excellent screening modality for patients who present with symptoms of CMI. It is difficult to gauge the degree of stenosis required to develop intestinal angina, as it depends on the extent of collateralization. In general, symptoms attributable to vascular insufficiency require high-grade stenosis or occlusion of at least two of the three main mesenteric arteries. CMI in the setting of proximal or segmental mesenteric arterial stenosis or occlusion of only one vessel is rare but may occur if there is poor collateral development. Thus, assessment of collaterals is necessary.

ceMRA has excellent performance for detecting stenosis in the celiac artery and SMA; however, due to its small size, assessment of the inferior mesenteric artery for stenosis is less accurate. Furthermore, visualizing the distal and side branches is a diagnostic challenge, so patients suspected of having medium-artery vasculitis should undergo catheter angiography. ceMRA is also employed to monitor mesenteric bypass grafts (Fig. 11.23).

Additional non-atherosclerotic etiologies of CMI include celiac artery compression (median arcuate ligament syndrome), fibromuscular dysplasia, chronic dissection, and vasculitis.

Median arcuate ligament syndrome is caused by extrinsic compression of the origin of the celiac artery or celiac neural plexus by the central tendon of the crura of the diaphragm. The compression is most pronounced during expiration and appears as an abrupt downward deflection of the artery on sagittal images. When severe, the compression may involve the SMA and renal arteries in rare cases. Clinical correlation and assessment of pancreaticoduodenal collateral is important, as this finding can be present in patients without symptoms.

Fibromuscular dysplasia is a rare entity that is most commonly encountered in the renal arteries. It results in areas of stenosis and aneurysmal dilatation of an artery, which can be flow-limiting. Detection of fibromuscular dysplasia by ceMRA is difficult when the disease occurs only as fine webs that limit the flow in the artery. However, fibromuscular dysplasia as a cause of CMI has been described in the literature.

Chronic aortic dissection can result in CMI, either by the intimal flap covering the ostia of the mesenteric vessels or by extending into a vessel and causing flow limitation.

Takayasu arteritis is the most common vasculitis to cause mesenteric ischemia. High-resolution ceMRA is well suited to

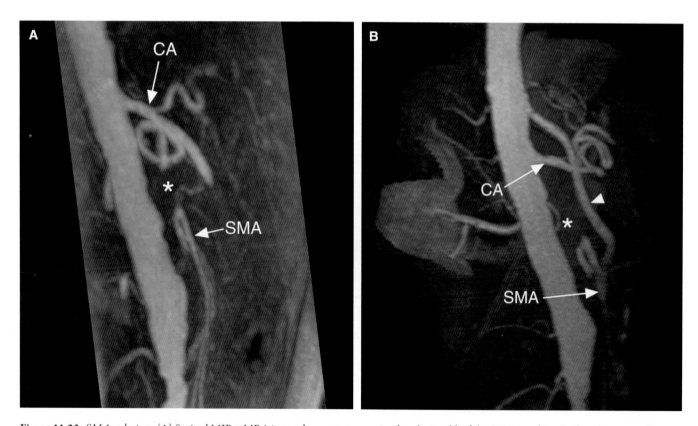

Figure 11.23 *SMA occlusion.* (**A**) Sagittal MIP ceMRA image demonstrates proximal occlusion (*) of the SMA, resulting in chronic mesenteric ischemia. The celiac artery (*CA*) is patent. The inferior mesenteric artery is occluded at the origin and not visualized. (**B**) Oblique reconstructed ceMRA image after a supraceliac SMA bypass graft (*arrowhead*) has been created. The proximal SMA remains occluded (*) and the bypass graft supplies the visceral branches of the SMA.

detect both of these processes. T2-weighted imaging is useful in the case of vasculitis, as it can help differentiate the causes of wall thickening.[13]

VISCERAL ARTERY ANEURYSMS

Visceral artery aneurysms are rare and have a propensity to rupture, making detection and close monitoring essential. Visceral aneurysms are distributed as follows: splenic artery 60%, hepatic arteries 20%, SMA 5.5%, celiac artery 4%, gastric and gastroepiploic arteries 4%, jejunal, ileal, and colic 3%, pancreatic and pancreaticoduodenal arteries 2%, and gastroduodenal 1.5%.

Splenic artery aneurysms are more often found in women (4:1 female to male ratio), with increasing incidence with the number of prior pregnancies. They are located in the distal half of the splenic artery, are usually less then 2 cm, and are typically asymptomatic. Splenic aneurysms are often found during pregnancy when they rupture, resulting in a maternal mortality rate of 70% and a fetal rate of 95%. Splenic artery aneurysms are thought to develop due to degeneration of the media. In pregnancy, this process is accelerated due to the hormonal milieu and increased splenic blood flow. Patients with portal hypertension and splenomegaly have also been found to have a higher incidence of splenic artery aneurysms (Fig. 11.24).

Inflammatory aneurysms of the visceral arteries are almost always associated with pancreatitis, which results in pseudo-aneurysm formation. The splenic, gastroduodenal, and pancreaticoduodenal arteries are most often affected by pancreatitis. Other local inflammatory processes, such as peptic ulcer disease, can rarely result in aneurysm formation.

Post-traumatic aneurysm can occur in the setting of blunt or penetrating trauma. An increasing number of aneurysms are iatrogenic, related to the increased number of interventional diagnostic and therapeutic procedures, particularly in the hepatic circulation.[14]

RENAL VASCULATURE

The kidneys are susceptible to a number of disease states that can be attributed to abnormalities of the vasculature. MRA is most commonly used to assess renal artery stenosis, renal artery aneurysm, renal vein thrombosis, renal vascular malformations, variant arteries that can cause ureteropelvic junction (UPJ) obstruction, and the renal vasculature in potential

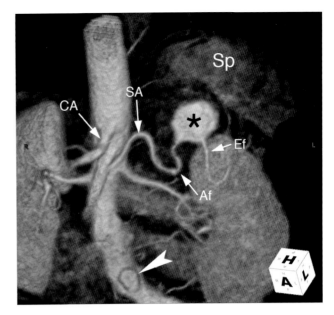

Figure 11.24 *Splenic artery aneurysm.* Volume-rendered ceMRA image in a 58-year-old woman who presented for monitoring of known splenic artery aneurysm. The aneurysm (*) arises directly from the main branch of the splenic artery (*SA*). Thus, most of the blood flow to the spleen passes through the aneurysm. Volume-rendered reconstructions are useful in preprocedural planning for determining the arteries entering and exiting visceral aneurysms. In this case, there is one afferent (*Af*) and one efferent (*Ef*) artery. This configuration is ideal for the placement of a covered stent across the aneurysm for treatment. The proximal connection of the splenic artery with the celiac artery (*CA*) is not included in the imaging volume. A penetrating aortic ulcer is identified (*arrowhead*). *Sp*, spleen.

renal donors. Other pathology may affect the renal vasculature by extrinsic compression or invasion by renal tumors, particularly renal cell carcinoma.

In most people, the renal arteries arise from the abdominal aorta immediately below the SMA, at the level of the L1–L2 vertebral interspace. The origins of the artery are typically at the lateral aspect of the aorta, but it may arise closer to the ventral surface, which occurs more frequently with the right renal artery. Most commonly, the renal artery branches into anterior and posterior divisions at the level of the renal hilum, but in 15% of cases an early bifurcation occurs that has clinical implications for treating ostial and proximal obstructive disease (Fig. 11.25).

Variants to the normal configuration of bilateral single renal arteries occur in 40% of the general population. When multiple,

---

Box 11.4 **ESSENTIALS TO REMEMBER**

- Causes of mesenteric arterial and venous occlusive diseases include atherosclerosis, vasculitis, trauma, connective tissue disease, aneurysms, and encasement by tumor.

- ceMRA is excellent for evaluating patients with suspected mesenteric ischemia. Mesenteric vascular insufficiency typically requires high grade stenosis or occlusion of at least two of the three main mesenteric arteries: the celiac axis, superior mesenteric artery, and inferior mesenteric artery. However, in patients with poor collaterals, stenosis of a single vessel may result in symptoms.

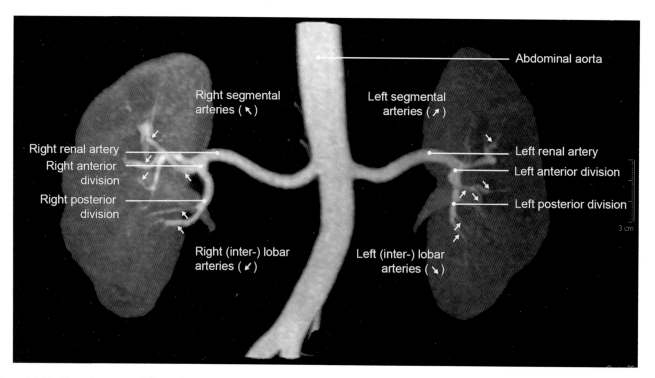

Figure 11.25 *Normal anatomy of the renal arteries.* Sub-volume coronal ceMRA MIP demonstrates the renal arteries and the main branches that can be imaged. *Tiny arrows* indicate the segmental renal arteries. (From Chapter 2 in Kramer CM, Hundley WG. *Atlas of Cardiovascular Magnetic Resonance Imaging.* Copyright Elsevier, 2010.)

renal arteries can arise anywhere from the proximal abdominal aorta to the level of the external iliac arteries, and five or more can be present per side. The identification of small accessory renal arteries can be difficult with MRA due to limitations of spatial resolution; however, imaging should be optimized to identify accessory renal arteries, particularly in potential renal donors.

In a significant portion of UPJ obstructions, the cause can be attributed to a crossing artery (49% of cases in children and 29% of cases in adults). Most commonly, the obstructing artery crosses anterior to the UPJ. Dominant precaval right renal arteries, with a course close to the lower pole of the kidney, are also prone to cause a UPJ obstruction.

The normal renal venous configuration is a single renal vein per side. The left renal vein is longer than the right, due to the location of the inferior vena cava (IVC) being right of the midline. The left renal vein accepts the left gonadal vein before crossing the midline. The right renal vein joins the IVC at the lower aspect of the L1 vertebral body, with the left inserting slightly more superiorly. Most variants of the renal anatomy involve the left renal vein, which has a circumaortic course in 17% of patients or a purely retroaortic course in about 3% of patients. When a retroaortic component is present, it will course inferiorly to meet the IVC, whereas the anterior components always travel horizontally.[15]

RENAL OCCLUSIVE DISEASE

In 90% of cases, renal artery stenosis (RAS) is due to atherosclerotic disease. Risk factors for atherosclerotic RAS are increasing age, hypertension, diabetes mellitus, and coronary artery disease. RAS has a high association with infrarenal abdominal aortic aneurysm and peripheral vascular disease. When untreated, the sequelae of RAS are ischemic nephropathy and end-stage renal disease. RAS accounts for end-stage renal disease in 10% to 30% of all cases.

The evaluation of RAS depends on both morphologic assessment of the obstructing lesion and the physiologic consequences of the lesion. In regards to morphologic assessment, the determination of the degree of stenosis is paramount and high-resolution ceMRA has been shown to be the most accurate sequence for this task. The administration of gadolinium-based contrast agents is not always possible in this population, as the presence of disease may lead to severely diminished renal function and increased risk of nephrogenic systemic fibrosis. Newer bSSFP-based, unenhanced MRA sequences that employ both ECG and respiratory gating show promise for this patient group. These sequences can be augmented with unenhanced flow measurements to add confidence to the diagnosis.

Measurement of the diameter reduction is commonly used for grading of stenosis; however, studies have shown a significant improvement in reproducibility of the measurement as well as accuracy when the area of the reduced lumen is measured. This technique is particularly important to avoid overgrading mild stenosis and to increase accuracy in assessing stenoses with complex cross-sectional morphology. In determining appropriate therapy, the location of the lesion should be separated into ostial lesions that occur within the first centimeter of the vessel and lesions that occur beyond this point. Ostial lesions are primarily stented. In the setting of significant mural thrombus in the abdominal aorta, MR plays an important role in the localization of the stenosis that is caused by atheroma in the renal artery or from narrowing caused by thrombus within the aorta. Given that with catheter angiography only the lumen can be depicted, a stenosis may mistakenly be identified as being within the renal artery when in fact it is in aortic thrombus. This may result in selection of a stent that is too short, leading to inadequate purchase in the renal artery with subsequent migration of the stent. Post-stenotic dilatation greater than 20% of the normal diameter is an additional morphologic finding that suggests a significant stenosis. However, this is more common with moderate- than severe-grade stenoses, where the flow is significantly attenuated.

Flow and perfusion measurement can be performed as part of a comprehensive MR imaging protocol for renovascular disease to assess the hemodynamic effect of stenosis. 3D phase-contrast MRA produces an MRA image where signal intensity correlates with velocity such that flowing blood is bright and stationary tissues are dark. Mild stenoses are typically underestimated due to acceleration of blood that increases brightness at the stenosis. Severe stenosis results in turbulent flow and signal dephasing, producing a black jet at the site of the narrowing and apparent occlusion. Thus, when used in conjunction with ceMRA, 3D phase-contrast MRA provides additional hemodynamic information. 2D phase-contrast imaging was described in the beginning of this chapter, a technique that allows for calculations of flow velocity in a vessel as a function of time. Similar to the approach used in duplex ultrasound, the loss of early peak systolic velocity marks the onset of a hemodynamically significant lesion. In addition to flow measurement, qualitative assessment of renal perfusion is possible with trMRA. In ischemic kidneys, the transit time between cortex and medulla is lengthened compared to that of normal kidneys from about 15 seconds to 40 seconds. Decreased glomerular filtration is evidenced by delayed and

decreased medullary enhancement on trMRA. Arterial spin labeling is an non-contrast enhanced technique that allows for qualitative assessment of renal perfusion based on inflow of magnetically tagged blood to the renal parenchyma: increased signal correlates with increased blood flow.[16]

In addition to focusing on the artery, imaging of the renal parenchyma adds information about the significance of a stenosis. In the normal kidney, the renal cortex is brighter than the medulla on T1-weighted imaging. Loss of differentiation between cortex and medulla on unenhanced imaging is a nonspecific marker of renal dysfunction but is expected in ischemic nephropathy. When this loss of differentiation occurs with contrast-enhanced imaging, it implies decreased blood flow to the cortex. Size discrepancies between the kidneys also are predictive of good therapeutic outcomes. When the kidney ipsilateral to the stenosis is more than 1.5 cm shorter in length than the contralateral kidney, ischemic nephropathy is suggested (Fig. 11.26). However, this finding is less useful in bilateral RAS. An atrophic kidney measuring less than 7.5 cm in length is unlikely to improve after revascularization.

Fibromuscular dysplasia (FMD) is the second most common cause of RAS after atherosclerosis. The classic presentation is a young or middle-aged woman with uncontrollable hypertension. Stenoses tend to occur in the middle or distal aspects of the renal artery, as opposed to the ostial and proximal portion of the vessel in atherosclerotic lesions. FMD has several different phenotypes, characterized by the location of the abnormality within the vessel wall. The most common type is medial fibroplasia, which is composed of alternating webs of stenosis and aneurysmal dilatation, causing a "string of beads" appearance on angiography. As these ridges may be quite thin, detection by ceMRA is limited due to the constraints of spatial resolution. Digital subtraction angiography remains the reference standard for the detection of FMD. The renal arteries are the most common vascular territory

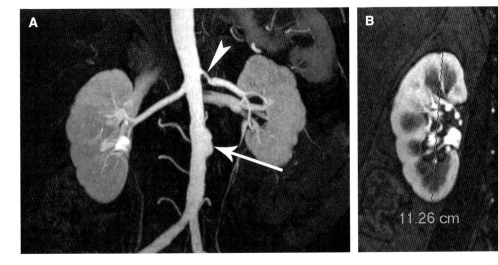

Figure 11.26 *Renal artery stenosis.* A 59-year-old woman presented with poorly controlled hypertension. (**A**) ceMRA optimized for imaging of the renal arteries shows a moderate-grade ostial stenosis of the left renal artery (*arrowhead*). A penetrating ulcer of the abdominal aorta was also discovered (*arrow*). (**B**) Despite the morphologic moderate grade of the stenosis in image A, there is size discrepancy between the left and right kidneys of greater than 1.5 cm. The left kidney ipsilateral to the stenosis is smaller than the normal right kidney, suggesting ongoing ischemic nephropathy of the left kidney.

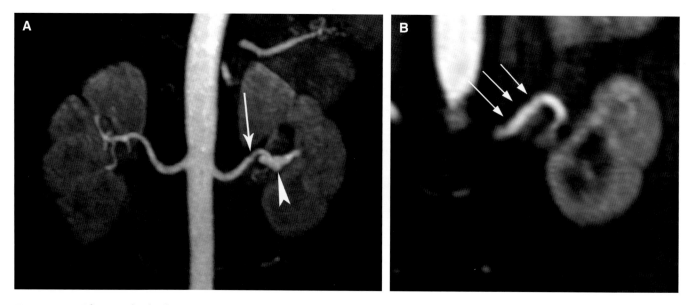

Figure 11.27 *Fibromuscular dysplasia.* A 42-year-old woman presented with new hypertension. (**A**) Sub-volume MIP image from a high-resolution ceMRA of the renal arteries shows irregularity and slight narrowing (*arrow*) of the distal left renal artery. Beyond this, at the bifurcation into anterior and posterior divisions, there is an irregularly shaped aneurysm (*arrowhead*). (**B**) Thin-section MPR image shows the subtle irregularity (*arrows*) of fibromuscular dysplasia.

affected by FMD, followed by the carotid and iliac arteries (Fig.11.27).

As there may be other pathologic processes that present clinically as renovascular disease, a comprehensive imaging protocol should include multiphase (arterial and venous) high-resolution ceMRA, T1- and T2-weighted imaging of the kidneys, and unenhanced and enhanced parenchymal imaging (3D gradient echo with fat saturation). These basic sequences will allow for additional diagnosis of renal infarctions, hemorrhage in the kidney, identification of hydronephrosis, and detection of renal neoplasm and its extent. As above, additional physiologic sequences can provide more information for borderline cases of stenosis or can play a primary role in patients who cannot receive contrast agents due to severely compromised renal function.[17]

RENAL ARTERY ANEURYSMS

Renal artery aneurysms are most often asymptomatic and found incidentally during cross-sectional imaging, averaging about 2 cm in size at identification. There is a 1% prevalence in the general population. Symptoms of these aneurysms are flank pain, hematuria, and hypertension. Aneurysms that are less than 2 cm in size and are asymptomatic do not require intervention but should be followed. Aneurysms found in women of childbearing age should be treated, as there is a risk for rupture during pregnancy due to the elevated blood flow. Symptomatic aneurysms as well as aneurysms that demonstrate continual growth are repaired. Overall, 10% to 20% of renal artery aneurysms rupture, with dire consequences.

Damage to the vessel wall is the underlying cause of renal artery aneurysm formation, most often due to degenerative processes such as atherosclerosis, inflammation such as FMD and polyarteritis nodosa, or trauma. Atherosclerosis leads to

both fusiform and saccular aneurysms that tend to form in the proximal and lobar renal arteries, calcify, and develop mural thrombus. Thrombus within an aneurysm is a source of emboli that lead to clinical symptoms. FMD is the most common cause of renal artery aneurysms, but they are difficult to diagnose when small as they tend to form in the lobar and segmental arteries. Inflammatory diseases such as polyarteritis nodosa lead to microaneurysm within the renal parenchymal and have an increased risk of rupture. Postinfectious (mycotic) aneurysms are also prone to rupture.

Detection of aneurysms is best performed with high-resolution ceMRA, with optimized parameters similar to those used to detect RAS. Newer techniques such as unenhanced respiratory-gated MRA show promise for the detection of aneurysms in the more distal branches, as the resolution is quite high and the signal from the renal parenchyma is suppressed.

RENAL VEIN THROMBOSIS

Renal vein thrombosis (RVT) typically occurs in the setting of a hypercoagulable state. In children, this is commonly due to dehydration or sepsis. In adults, this can be caused by collagen vascular disease, such as systemic lupus erythematosus, or glomerulonephritis. RVT is often present in the setting of renal cell carcinoma that has invaded the renal vein. Other causes include trauma, pancreatitis, extrinsic compression, or extension of left gonadal vein thrombosis.

RVT occurs more frequently in the left renal vein, likely due to its greater length. Thrombus may extend from the renal vein into the right atrium, requiring appropriate coverage when planning imaging. Classic symptoms (flank mass, hematuria, and thrombocytopenia) are often not present, and thus imaging plays an important role in diagnosis.

Box 11.5 ESSENTIALS TO REMEMBER

- MRA for renal artery stenosis is optimally performed with intravenous contrast material. However, a significant number of patients with suspected renal artery stenosis have impaired renal function that may limit the use of intravenous contrast agents. In this setting diagnostic studies may be performed by using bSSSP with respiratory and cardiac gating.

- In addition to MRA assessment of the renal artery additional findings that support a diagnosis of significant renal artery stenosis include size discrepancy, with the affected kidney measuring 1.5 cm or more smaller in length than the unaffected kidney and loss of corticomedullary differentiation on T1-weighted images. Atropic kidneys less than 7.5 cm in length are unlikely to respond to revascularization.

- Most (90%) cases of significant renal artery stenosis are caused by atherosclerotic disease, which nearly always involves the ostia of the renal arteries. Fibromuscular dysplasia is found most commonly in middle aged and young women, affects the mid portion of the renal artery, and has a "string-of-beads" appearance on angiography.

- Renal vein thrombosis occurs in patients with hypercoagulability, dehydration, sepsis, trauma, and invasion of the renal vein by renal carcinoma.

Renal ultrasound is the screening modality of choice in suspected RVT. MRI plays a complementary role when ultrasound is nondiagnostic. MRA reveals a signal void in the renal vein, which typically enlarges the vein in the acute phase and results in venous wall enhancement. The affected kidney swells in the acute phase and can become atrophic and scarred when RVT is chronic. On T1- and T2-weighted imaging, the renal parenchyma shows relatively low signal intensity. Signal loss in the cortex on T2-weighted images is one of the earliest parenchymal signs of abnormality. In the acute phase, congestion can result in hemorrhage that may appear as a dark band in the outer portion of the medulla.

TRANSPLANT IMAGING

MR can be used to evaluate the suitability of donors for organ transplantation as well as follow recipients for complications. The advantages of preoperative assessment of a potential donor with MR include excellent visualization of arterial and venous structures and sensitive assessment for asymptomatic parenchymal disease, all without the need for ionizing radiation. Vascular complications are common to all types of organ transplants and often require immediate diagnosis and assessment to guide appropriate therapy.

RENAL TRANSPLANTATION

Preoperative planning for renal transplantation is performed to assess for any underlying anatomic abnormality or pathologic processes that would put either the donor or the recipient at risk for a poor outcome. Thus, the arterial and venous anatomy, the parenchymal status, and the excretory system must be evaluated.

Standard donor assessments with T1- and T2-weighted imaging combined with unenhanced and enhanced 3D gradient-echo imaging of the parenchyma are used to characterize cysts and masses. ceMRA is performed in the coronal plane from the diaphragm to the external iliac arteries to assess for the location and number of renal arteries. Early branching, defined as branching within 2 cm of the origin, should be noted, as these vessels may not be suitable for anastomosis to the recipient vessels, particularly when on the right. The venous system may have left-sided variation, including circum- and retro-aortic courses, and the presence of enlarged lumbar or gonadal veins is important for surgical planning. Imaging of the collecting system is performed with heavily T2-weighted urography to identify stones or tumors within the ureters as well as duplication of the collecting system and abnormal ureteral insertion on the bladder.

After transplantation, renal ultrasound is the modality of choice for screening for complications. However, MRI is used to confirm an abnormality if there is clinical suspicion and the ultrasound results are discrepant. Common complications of renal transplantation are vascular complications, urinary complications, and rejection. MRI can diagnose all but rejection using a protocol similar to that for assessing the donor transplant.

The vessels of the transplanted kidney are most commonly anastomosed to the external or common iliac vessels, in an end-to-side fashion. Typically, a donor's left kidney is used because it has a long renal vein, but selection depends on the presence of other complicating features such as accessory renal arteries. In most cases, good renal function will permit the use of contrast material, and in these cases standard imaging with ceMRA is performed. However, if the patient's renal function is such that the GFR is less than 30 mL/min/1.73m^2, it is advisable to use unenhanced MRA techniques to assess the vasculature. One advantage of the pelvic location of renal transplants is that respiratory gating for unenhanced bSSFP MRA is not necessary in this location, shortening the time of the acquisition. ECG gating should still be used as required by the sequence.

Stenoses of the renal artery of the transplanted kidney are most commonly located at the anastomotic site and are a consequence of the surgical procedure. Other proximal arterial stenoses may be due to clamp injuries as well as kinking of the artery. In chronic rejection, stenoses tend to occur distally. The significance of a stenosis is primarily determined by its morphology, with physiologic imaging used for borderline cases. Rare complications of renal transplantation include pseudo-aneurysms, renal artery thrombosis, and torsion of the transplant (Fig. 11.28). Venous stenosis is more difficult to assess, as the vein may be significantly compressed yet completely unaffected. When venous obstruction is suspected, evaluation of the kidney may demonstrate enlargement from outflow obstruction. RVT occurs in the setting of acute or chronic rejection, or may be due to kinking of the renal vein in the immediate postoperative period.[18]

Hepatic transplantation is performed for end-stage cirrhosis and for treatment of hepatocellular carcinoma that has limited involvement as defined by the Milan criteria. Liver transplants are either *orthotopic*, in which the entire liver is transplanted, or from a related *living donor*, in which either the right lobe, left lobe, or a portion of the left lobe (segments II and III) is transplanted. In living donor transplantation, the portion of the donor liver is selected that best matches the recipient size. When segments II and III are transplanted, the left hepatic artery, left portal vein, left hepatic vein, and left bile duct are isolated and anastomosed to the recipient's proper hepatic artery, main portal vein, confluence of the left and middle hepatic veins, and jejunum (of a Roux-en-Y loop), respectively. When the right lobe alone is harvested, the right hepatic artery, right portal vein, right hepatic vein, and right bile duct are isolated and anastomosed to the recipient's proper hepatic artery, right portal vein, right hepatic vein, and jejunum of a Roux-en-Y loop. In orthotopic liver harvesting, the arterial supply is dissected proximally to the origin of the celiac artery and the side branches (splenic, left gastric, gastroduodenal, right gastric, cystic arteries) are ligated. The artery is

removed with a patch of aorta (Carrel patch) to be anastomosed to the most appropriate location in the recipient. The donor common bile duct and main portal vein are also isolated and anastomosed to the respective recipient structures. The donor hepatic veins may be directly anastomosed to the recipient IVC, or the portion of the donor IVC that includes the hepatic veins is anastomosed to the IVC of the recipient.

MR is performed for presurgical evaluation of the living donor anatomy (arterial, venous, and biliary system) to reduce surgical risk associated with anatomic variants and to assess the liver volume for appropriate match. The difference in portal vein diameter between the recipient and donor should be 4 mm or less; when there is greater discrepancy a matching conduit may have to be made at the time of surgery. Congenital absence of a right portal vein and trifurcation of the portal vein may prohibit donation. The presence of the right anterior portal vein arising from the left portal vein must be identified preoperatively to prevent inadvertent devascularization of segments IV, V, and VIII. Donor hepatic artery evaluation for significant atherosclerotic disease and the presence of anatomic variants is equally important. Localization of the artery that feeds segment IV is important to prevent devascularization of the medial lobe. Recipient evaluation is performed to assess liver volume, define anatomy (arterial, venous, biliary), to determine the size and patency of the portal and superior mesenteric veins, to identify the location and size of portosystemic varices, and to detect and characterize possible hepatic lesions.

Postoperative evaluation of the transplanted liver is indicated in the setting of suspected vascular complications. The most common arterial complications include hepatic artery narrowing and thromboses, which present with abnormal laboratory findings including elevated liver function tests and abnormal bilirubin levels. Arterial complications typically require ceMRA for diagnosis as the hepatic arteries tend

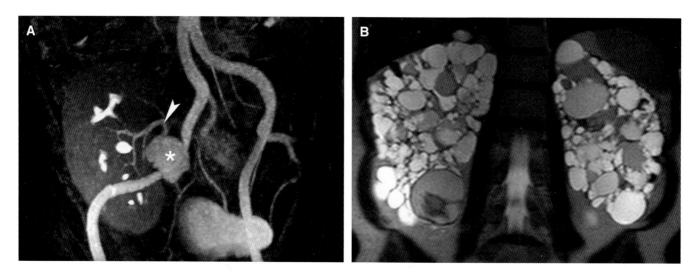

Figure 11.28 *Renal artery pseudo-aneurysm in a renal transplant.* A 54-year-old man presented with neutropenic fever and sepsis 2 months after renal transplantation for polycystic kidney disease. MR was performed to evaluate for abscess in the native kidneys. (**A**) Full-volume MIP image from ceMRA of the pelvis demonstrates a mycotic pseudo-aneurysm (*) at the anastomosis of the right external iliac artery and the renal artery (*arrowhead*) to the transplanted kidney. (**B**) Coronal T2-weighted single-shot FSE/TSE image of this patient's native kidneys demonstrates the multiple cysts with varying intensity that are characteristic of autosomal dominant polycystic kidney disease.

to be small (Fig. 11.29). If diagnosed rapidly, graft salvage is possible; otherwise, biliary necrosis will quickly ensue. Portal venous thrombosis or stenosis is less common than arterial complications and presents with liver dysfunction, ascites, or variceal bleeding. Embolectomy or anticoagulation therapy may be performed depending on the liver status. Often, 2D imaging with bSSFP or TOF MRA is sufficient for diagnosis. In the chronic phase, collateral veins form at the porta hepatis. Narrowing at the hepatic vein anastomosis or hepatic vein thrombosis can complicate transplantation, resulting in an edematous liver and abnormal liver function. Significant hepatic vein stenosis typically occurs with severe narrowing; however, the morphologic appearance of the anastomosis is not a good predictor of the significance of stenosis. In these cases, a monomorphic waveform in the hepatic vein on velocity-encoded imaging is suggestive of a significant stenosis.[19]

PANCREAS TRANSPLANTATION

Pancreas transplantation is most often performed in patients with type 1 diabetes mellitus, often simultaneously with a kidney transplant. Organs are harvested from beating-heart cadaveric donors, who often have multiple organs harvested simultaneously. Pancreatic transplant are typically harvested at the same time a liver is harvested. During harvesting, the common hepatic artery is taken with the liver, and this artery cannot be used to perfuse the pancreatic head via the superior pancreaticoduodenal arteries. The solution to arterial perfusion of the harvested pancreas is to combine the pancreatic perfusion territories of the SMA and the splenic artery into a common arterial circuit. This is performed with the creation of a Y-graft, which is composed of common iliac artery and bifurcation from the cadaveric donor. The donor's external iliac artery is anastomosed to the donor's SMA and the donor's internal iliac artery is anastomosed to the donor's splenic

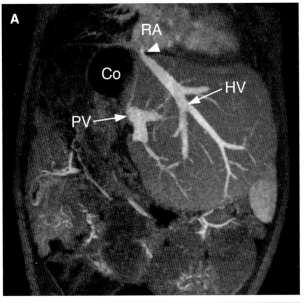

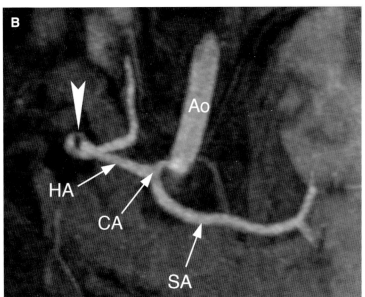

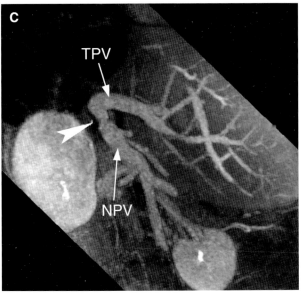

Figure 11.29 *Hepatic arterial stenosis of a liver transplant.* A 9-year-old boy presented 1 month after liver transplantation with elevated serum liver enzymes, causing clinical concern for vascular compromise. (**A**) A left hepatic lobe from an adult donor was transplanted into the left upper quadrant of the abdomen. Venous-phase ceMRA image demonstrates a patent hepatic venous system with mild narrowing (*arrowhead*) of the hepatic vein (*HV*) at the anastomosis with the IVC (not seen on this image), immediately adjacent to the right atrium (*RA*). *PV*, portal vein. *Co*, colon. (**B**) Arterial-phase ceMRA image shows high-grade stenosis (*arrowhead*) at the tortuous anastomosis of the native common hepatic artery (*HA*) with the transplant hepatic artery. *Ao*, aorta; *CA*, celiac artery; *SA*, splenic artery. (**C**) MIP image of venous-phase ceMRA shows the normal appearance of the portal vein anastomosis (*arrowhead*) between the native portal vein (*NPV*) and transplanted portal vein (*TPV*).

artery, with the SMA ligated distal to the inferior pancreaticoduodenal artery and the splenic artery ligated distal to the dorsal pancreatic arteries. The harvested venous system is composed of a portion of the portal vein, the superior mesenteric vein, and the splenic vein. The duodenal sweep is also harvested for exocrine drainage.[20]

The transplanted pancreatic arterial system is most commonly anastomosed to the recipient's common or external iliac artery, but may also be anastomosed to the recipient's infrarenal aorta. The venous drainage of the transplanted pancreas is anastomosed to either the recipient's iliac veins (systemic connection) or superior mesenteric vein (portal connection). The exocrine drainage of the transplanted pancreas is typically anastomosed to the recipient's urinary bladder via an enteric–cystic anastomosis in case a systemic venous connection is made, or is anastomosed to the recipient's gut via an enteric–enteric anastomosis in case a portal venous connection is made.

An arterial stenosis is suspected early after transplantation when the patient develops hyperglycemia. The stenoses occur most commonly at the anastomotic sites, either to the iliac artery or at the site of the Y-graft coupling. Acute rejection consists of an autoimmune arteritis that causes small vessel occlusion and may progress to large artery thrombosis. Chronic rejection is the result of multiple minor bouts of acute rejection, resulting in an atrophic, scarred pancreas. This is apparent as decreased signal intensity on T1- and T2-weighted imaging due to fibrosis; however, enhancement is preserved. Thrombus formation is typical in the ligated arterial stumps (donor SMA and splenic artery) distal to the parenchymal vessels and does not require therapy. Thrombus formation in a venous stump is more likely to propagate and lead to occlusion of draining parenchymal veins, resulting in pancreatic edema, hyperglycemia, and pain. Pancreatitis may occur in the immediate postoperative period due to poor graft-organ quality or may be from acute rejection. A postoperative fluid collection may also develop as a complication, compressing the pancreas or its vascular structures.

Comprehensive pancreas transplant imaging with MR includes T1- and T2-weighted 2D imaging, performed in the axial plane to cover the abdomen and pelvis. Multiphase high-resolution ceMRA is performed to assess the vasculature. 3D gradient-echo imaging with fat saturation, performed after ceMRA, is useful for assessing graft enhancement and detecting thrombus. trMRA can also be used to assess the perfusion characteristics of the graft. In patients with renal failure, unenhanced MRA has been used successfully to identify vascular complications (Fig. 11.30).[21]

DEEP VENOUS THROMBOSIS

In the general population, 5% of people will experience an acute venous thrombosis in their lifetime; the majority of these occur in the deep veins of the lower extremity. Morbidity and mortality rates are high in the setting of thromboembolic disease, as 60% of patients with untreated deep venous thrombosis (DVT) will experience pulmonary emboli. Delay in treatment of DVT also increases the risk of developing post-thrombotic syndrome, which is due to chronic venous insufficiency. Although duplex ultrasonography is the initial imaging modality for suspected DVT of the extremity, MRI plays an important role in the diagnosis of central venous thrombosis within the pelvic veins and the central veins of the chest, as well as for detecting isolated calf vein DVT.

The staging of thrombi has clinical implications for treatment, as the success of thrombolytic therapy increases with earlier intervention. Broadly, staging can be divided into the acute phase, which is the period within the first 2 weeks after developing DVT, and the chronic phase. Acute thrombi on venous-phase ceMRA appear as a signal void within the center of the vein and result in enlargement of the vein. Thrombus is typically occlusive or near occlusive in the acute phase. Due to the inflammatory reaction related to acute thrombosis, there is enhancement of the vessel wall as well as perivascular inflammation, both of which can be appreciated as increased signal on T2-weighted fat-saturated imaging and enhanced T1-weighted fat-saturated imaging. The inflammatory reaction usually resolves over the course of 14 days. As the thrombus evolves, it becomes incorporated into the vessel wall. With progression, the vein becomes fibrotic, decreases in diameter, and becomes less compliant. There may be eventual recanalization of the lumen, which occurs from the center of the vessel to the periphery. The wall of the vein eventually becomes fibrotic, resulting in a small-diameter vein with wall thickening. If the vein remains occluded, the vessel may completely atrophy over time. Eccentric, wall-adherent thrombus within a vein is a finding of chronicity. Additionally, the presence of collateral veins suggests a thrombus is chronic. In longstanding thrombosis of a large vein, the collaterals may become so numerous that it is impossible to identify the primary vein.[22]

LOWER EXTREMITY VENOUS SYSTEM

Ultrasonography remains the primary imaging modality for the initial assessment of DVT of the lower extremity, with high accuracy of detecting the thrombus in the proximal leg. Ultrasound has poor sensitivity for diagnosing isolated calf DVT, which occurs in 10% to 20% of patients with DVT. Furthermore, isolated calf DVT will progress proximally in 20% of patients, placing the patient at risk for pulmonary embolism. MRI is used when ultrasound is not diagnostic or is inconclusive and clinical suspicion for DVT is high. Additionally, MRI is used for determining appropriate intervention based on thrombus age.

The primary sequence used in the diagnosis of DVT is ceMRA. Large-area coverage can be obtained using a multiple-station approach, as was described earlier for the arterial system, in which the aortoiliac, thigh, and calf stations are imaged sequentially. Imaging is performed in the arterial phase as well as two venous phases. Using the arterial images as a mask, the arteries can be subtracted from subsequently acquired venous phases, producing an image similar to a conventional venogram. On ceMRA, the thrombus should appear very dark. Intermediate low signal (showing gray) is not likely

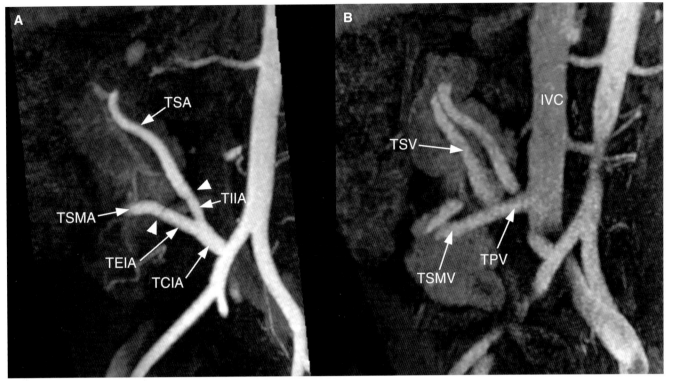

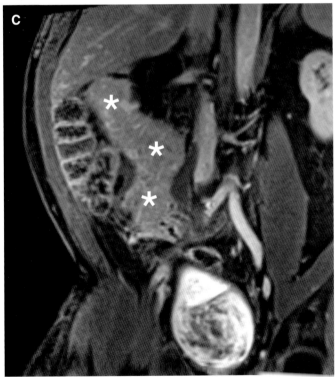

Figure 11.30 *Normal vascular anatomy of a pancreas transplant.*
A 40-year-old patient with type 1 diabetes presented for routine
postoperative assessment of the pancreas transplant. (**A**) Normal
arterial anatomy. The transplanted pancreas arterial Y-graft has been
anastomosed to the right common iliac artery of the recipient. The
arterial Y-graft is composed of the transplanted common iliac artery
(*TCIA*), which is anastomosed to the transplanted superior mesenteric
artery (*TSMA*) via the transplanted external iliac artery (*TEIA*), and
to the transplanted splenic artery (*TSA*) via the transplanted internal
iliac artery (*TIIA*). The normal appearance of the anastomotic sites is
shown at the *arrowheads*. (**B**) Normal venous anatomy. The head of the
transplanted pancreas is drained via the transplanted superior
mesenteric vein (*TSMV*), which drains into the transplanted portal
vein (*TPV*). The tail of the pancreas is drained via the transplanted
splenic vein (*TSV*) and then into the TPV. The TPV is anastomosed
to the recipient inferior vena cava (*IVC*) but can also be connected to
the recipient iliac venous system or portal venous system. (**C**) Coronal
3D gradient-echo image with fat saturation shows normal
enhancement of the transplanted pancreas (*).

to represent a thrombus. Findings should always be confirmed
with a later phase acquisition if possible. Artifacts can occur
that can mistakenly be interpreted as thrombus when there is
incomplete mixing of unenhanced and enhanced blood within
the vessel, leading to foci of decreased signal intensity resembling thrombus, or when there are susceptibility artifacts from
metallic clips in a postoperative patient. 3D gradient-echo

acquisition with fat saturation during the equilibrium phase
of enhancement is a useful complement to ceMRA for venous
imaging, as it provides higher a contrast-to-noise ratio compared to ceMRA, albeit at lower resolution (Fig. 11.31). 2D
TOF imaging is particularly helpful in the setting of chronic
thrombosis with dense collaterals, as the collateral flow is
somewhat suppressed due to their tortuous nature, allowing

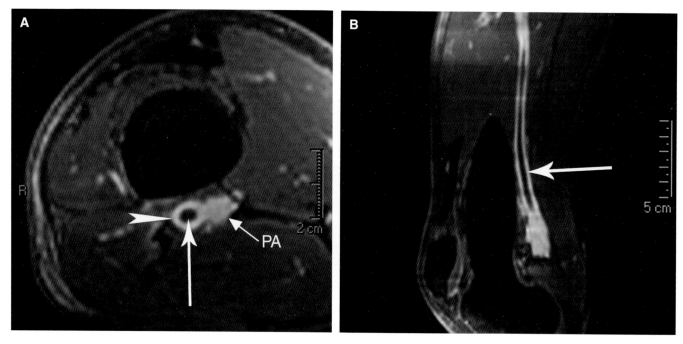

Figure 11.31 *Acute deep venous thrombosis.* A 56-year-old woman with breast cancer presented with leg swelling. (**A**) T1-weighted 3D gradient-echo image with fat saturation shows an occlusive thrombus (*arrow*) within the proximal popliteal vein. Vessel wall enhancement (*arrowhead*) is present during the acute phase. *PA*, popliteal artery. (**B**) Sagittal reconstruction image demonstrates the extent of the thrombus (*arrow*).

for visualization of the primary vein. In addition to imaging the venous system, MR is excellent at identifying external compression as a cause of venous thrombosis.

Severe, extensive thrombosis of the venous system of the lower extremity can result in critical compromise of arterial inflow flow due to backpressure. This process, termed *phlegmasia cerulea dolens*, may progress to frank tissue necrosis. Obstructed venous drainage leads to massive tissue edema and intravascular hypovolemia that can progress to shock and death. Edema, cyanosis, and severe pain are the hallmark clinical findings. Phlegmasia cerulea dolens more commonly affects women, has a left lower extremity predilection (4:1), and most often presents in the fifth and sixth decades. As the presentation may be gradual, it is an important diagnostic consideration in patients with massive thrombus burden and edema, and requires swift intervention to prevent progression.

ILIAC VEINS AND INFERIOR VENA CAVA

Most instances of pelvic vein thrombosis are secondary to extension from the lower extremity. Less than 10% of DVT cases present with isolated pelvic vein thrombosis. The risk of isolated pelvic DVT is increased in the puerperium. More than 90% of cases affect the left iliofemoral system, likely due to compression of the left common iliac vein by the right common iliac artery and the gravid uterus during the final weeks of pregnancy. The risk of pelvic DVT is also increased in the setting of pelvic malignancies. Compared to lower extremity DVT, the risk for pulmonary embolism is greatest in the presence of pelvic DVT. Trauma, surgery, infection, and hypercoagulable states are also risk factors.

Pelvic DVT is suspected in the setting of lower extremity edema in a patient with a known risk factor for thrombosis. MRI is performed when lower extremity ultrasonography reveals monophasic venous waveforms, suggesting an upstream occlusion or stenosis, or when the extent of lower extremity thrombus cannot be visualized by ultrasound. The goal of imaging is to identify the extent of thrombosis, determine its chronicity, and identify anatomic abnormalities that may have led to thrombus formation.

Imaging sequences used for diagnosis of pelvic venous thrombosis are the same as those for the lower extremities. In the setting of a pelvic mass, MRI can differentiate between lower extremity edema caused by extrinsic compression of the iliofemoral vessels and edema resulting from venous thrombosis. MRI can also be used to assess tumor involvement of the pelvic vessels, as this will affect surgical planning if resection is an option. Vascular tumor involvement is best evaluated using T1-weighted spin-echo imaging without fat saturation, and this sequence should be added to protocols intended for such. An intact fat plane between the mass and the vessel suggests against tumor invasion. Enhanced imaging can be used to differentiate between bland thrombus and tumor thrombus, if invasion is suspected.

May-Thurner syndrome, also termed iliac vein compression syndrome, results from compression of the left common iliac vein between the right common iliac artery and the vertebral body. Longstanding pulsatile compression can lead to fibrotic changes in the intima and media, resulting in web-like structures within the lumen. Most commonly, this leads to the development of DVT in the left iliofemoral venous system and left lower extremity veins. Less commonly, patients may present with leg pain and edema from venous hypertension without DVT.

Diagnosis of May-Thurner syndrome requires the identification of left iliofemoral thrombosis in the setting of venous compression. In the absence of thrombosis, venous hypertension is differentiated from asymptomatic vascular compression by the presence of numerous pelvic collateral vessels that shunt blood to the contralateral iliac veins or to the lumbar veins. Therapy includes thrombolysis as well as removing the obstruction, which currently is performed with endovascular stenting (Fig. 11.32).[23]

CENTRAL THORACIC VEINS

Due to the overlying soft tissue, osseous structures, and the air-containing lung, assessment of the central venous structures of

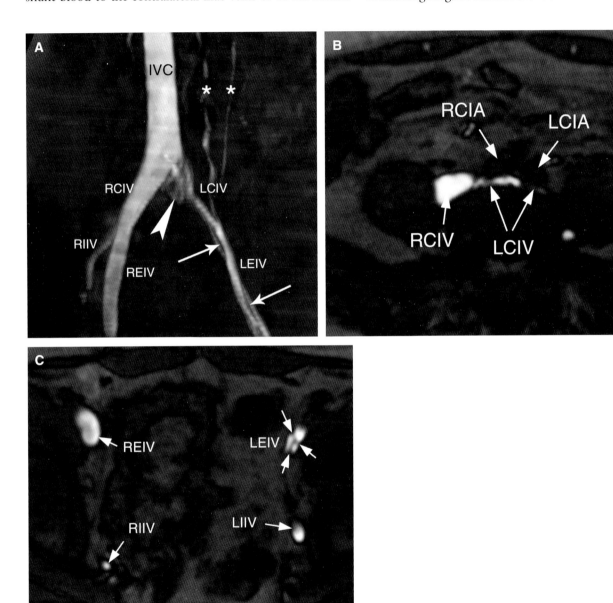

Figure 11.32 *May-Thurner syndrome.* A 51-year-old woman presented with left leg pain and swelling. Duplex ultrasound (not shown) demonstrated monomorphic waveforms in the left common femoral vein without the presence of thrombus. (**A**) MIP image generated from a 2D gradient-echo TOF MRA. The source images were obtained as individual slices in the axial orientation, and flow of the aorta was suppressed by using a spatial presaturation pulse superior to each slice (see Chapter 2 for details of spatial presaturation pulses). The iliac veins (*RCIV, LCIV*) and inferior vena cava (*IVC*) are well shown and there is narrowing of the left common iliac vein (*LCIV*) from chronic compression by the right common iliac artery (not shown on this image). Also seen are web-like structures (*arrowhead*) in the LCIV at the site of compression, synechiae (*arrows*) within the left external iliac vein (*LEIV*), narrowing of the LEIV compared to the right external iliac vein (*REIV*), and left perivertebral lumbar venous collaterals (*) that bypass the obstruction. The right internal iliac vein (*RIIV*) is present, but the left internal iliac vein is chronically occluded in the proximal portion. (**B**) Axial source image from the same 2D TOF sequence reveals compression of the left common iliac vein (*LCIV*) by the right common iliac artery (*RCIA*). The right common iliac vein (RCIV) is normal in caliber. *LCIA*, left common iliac artery. (**C**) On source images obtained inferior to image B, synechiae (*arrows*) are shown in the left external iliac vein (*LEIV*), representing residual fibrous material in the lumen after spontaneous recanalization of prior venous thrombosis. Note that the overall diameter of the LEIV is small compared to that of the right external iliac vein (*REIV*). The left internal iliac vein (*LIIV*) is patent at this level. *RIIV*, right internal iliac vein.

Box 11.6 ESSENTIALS TO REMEMBER

- MRI is well suited for the noninvasive evaluation of the vascular system. High-resolution morphologic imaging, tissue characterization, and hemodynamic assessment are combined in a single examination.

- MRI often complements other modalities when results are inconclusive. In other situations, MRI may be the initial modality of choice, particularly for central venous imaging.

- In patients with mild to moderate renal insufficiency who require imaging of the vessel lumen, MRI provides a high-resolution alternative to CT angiography because it does not require nephrotoxic iodinated contrast material.

- The unique imaging characteristics and the lack of ionizing radiation make MRI an important modality for noninvasive vascular imaging.

the chest with ultrasonography is limited. The proximal axillary and subclavian veins can be evaluated by duplex ultrasound, but the more central structures, including the brachiocephalic veins and superior vena cava, cannot be assessed. MRI provides a noninvasive modality to image the central venous system when DVT is suspected or when preprocedural planning is required for placement of central venous catheters in patients with a known history of DVT.

SVC syndrome is a clinical diagnosis based on the presence of bilateral upper extremity and face swelling, nasal congestion, headaches, and lethargy. It occurs when there is SVC obstruction central to the confluence with the azygos vein. Most commonly it is due to compression of the SVC by a thoracic malignancy, but it can also be the result of fibrosing mediastinitis, aortic aneurysms, or venous occlusion secondary to thrombosis associated with cardiac pacemakers and central venous catheters.

REFERENCES

1. Ersoy H, Zhang H, Prince MR. Peripheral MR angiography. *J Cardiovasc Magn Reson.* 2006;8:517–528.
2. Litmanovich D, Bankier AA, Cantin L, et al. CT and MRI in diseases of the aorta. *AJR Am J Roentgenol.* 2009;193:928–940.
3. Russo V, Renzulli M, Buttazzi K, Fattori R. Acquired diseases of the thoracic aorta: role of MRI and MRA. *Eur Radiol.* 2006;16:852–865.
4. Elefteriades JA, Farkas EA. Thoracic aortic aneurysm: clinically pertinent controversies and uncertainties. *J Am Coll Cardiol.* 2010;55:841–857.
5. Liu Q, Lu JP, Wang F, et al. Three-dimensional contrast-enhanced MR angiography of aortic dissection: a pictorial essay. *Radiographics.* 2007;27:1311–1321.
6. Hayashi H, Matsuoka Y, Sakamoto I, et al. Penetrating atherosclerotic ulcer of the aorta: imaging features and disease concept. *Radiographics.* 2000;20:995–1005.
7. Leiner T, Fleischmann D, Rofsky NM. Lower extremity vasculature. In: Rofsky NM, Rubin GD, eds. *CT and MR Angiography.* Philadelphia: Wolters Kluwer Health/Lippincott Williams & Wilkins, 2009:1316.
8. Snell RS. *Clinical Anatomy by Systems.* Philadelphia: Lippincott Williams & Wilkins, 2007:950.
9. Ersoy H, Rybicki FJ. MR angiography of the lower extremities. *AJR Am J Roentgenol.* 2008;190:1675–1684.
10. Tatli S, Lipton MJ, Davison BD, et al. From the RSNA refresher courses: MR imaging of aortic and peripheral vascular disease. *Radiographics.* 2003;23:S59–78.
11. Holden A, Merrilees S, Mitchell N, Hill A. Magnetic resonance imaging of popliteal artery pathologies. *Eur J Radiol.* 2008;67:159–168.
12. Gore RM, Yaghmai V, Thakrar KH, et al. Imaging in intestinal ischemic disorders. *Radiol Clin North Am.* 2008;46:845–875.
13. Shih MC, Hagspiel KD. CTA and MRA in mesenteric ischemia: part 1, Role in diagnosis and differential diagnosis. *AJR Am J Roentgenol.* 2007;188:452–461.
14. Pasha SF, Gloviczki P, Stanson AW, Kamath PS. Splanchnic artery aneurysms. *Mayo Clin Proc.* 2007;82:472–479.
15. Urban BA, Ratner LE, Fishman EK. Three-dimensional volume-rendered CT angiography of the renal arteries and veins: normal anatomy, variants, and clinical applications. *Radiographics.* 2001;21:373–386.
16. Roditi G, Maki JH, Oliveira G, Michaely HJ. Renovascular imaging in the NSF Era. *J Magn Reson Imaging.* 2009;30:1323–1334.
17. Zhang HL, Sos TA, Winchester PA, et al. Renal artery stenosis: imaging options, pitfalls, and concerns. *Prog Cardiovasc Dis.* 2009;52:209–219.
18. Hohenwalter MD, Skowlund CJ, Erickson SJ, et al. Renal transplant evaluation with MR angiography and MR imaging. *Radiographics.* 2001;21:1505–1517.
19. Saad WE, Lin E, Ormanoski M, et al. Noninvasive imaging of liver transplant complications. *Tech Vasc Interv Radiol.* 2007;10:191–206.
20. Han DJ, Sutherland DE. Pancreas transplantation. *Gut Liver.* 2010;4:450–465.
21. Dobos N, Roberts DA, Insko EK, et al. Contrast-enhanced MR angiography for evaluation of vascular complications of the pancreatic transplant. *Radiographics.* 2005;25:687–695.
22. Haage P, Krings T, Schmitz-Rode T. Nontraumatic vascular emergencies: imaging and intervention in acute venous occlusion. *Eur Radiol.* 2002;12:2627–2643.
23. Gurel K, Gurel S, Karavas E, et al. Direct contrast-enhanced MR venography in the diagnosis of May-Thurner syndrome. *Eur J Radiol* 2010 [E-pub ahead of print].

INDEX